Abbreviations

AD	Alzheimer disease
ADC	apparent diffusion coefficient
ADNI	Alzheimer's Disease Neuroimaging Initiative
AGD	argyrophilic grain disease
ALS	amyotrophic lateral sclerosis
ALS-D	amyotrophic lateral sclerosis with dementia
ALSFRS-R	Amyotrophic Lateral Sclerosis Functional Rating Scale-Revised
AOS	apraxia of speech
bi	behavioural impairment
BIBD	basophilic inclusion body disease
BMAA	β-*N*-methylamino L-alanine
bv	behavioural variant
CBD	corticobasal degeneration
CHMP2B	chromatin modifying protein 2B
ci	cognitive impairment
CMAP	compound motor action potential
CNS	central nervous system
CSF	cerebrospinal fluid
CST	corticospinal tract
DA	axial diffusivity
DAO	D-amino oxidase gene
DLB	dementia with Lewy bodies
DR	radial diffusivity
DTI	diffusion tensor imaging
ELAV	embryonic lethal and abnormal vision (-like proteins)
FA	fractional anisotropy
FBI	Frontal Behavioural Inventory
FLAIR	fluid-attenuated inversion recovery
FLTD	frontotemporal lobar degeneration
fMRI	functional magnetic resonance imaging
FTD	frontotemporal dementia
FUS	fused in sarcoma
GM	grey matter
GRN	progranulin
GWAS	genome-wide association studies
hnRNP	heterogeneous ribonucleoprotein
IBM	inclusion body myopathy
KO	knockout
LMN	lower motor neurone
lv	logopenic variant
MAPT	microtubule-associated protein tau
MD	mean diffusivity
miRNA	microRNA
MND	motor neurone disease
MPS	multiple point stimulation (technique)
MRE	mRNA recognition element
MRI	magnetic resonance imaging
MRS	magnetic resonance spectroscopy
MSTD	multiple system tauopathy with dementia
MT	microtubule
MUNE	motor unit number estimation
NAA	*N*-acetyl aspartate
NCI	neuronal cytoplasmic inclusion
NF	neurofilament (NF_L, NF light chain, NF_M, NF medium chain, NF_H, NF heavy chain)
NFT	neurofibrillary tangles
nfv	non-fluent/agrammatic variant
NIFID	neuronal intermediate filament inclusion disease
NPI	Neuropsychiatric Inventory
PABP	poly(A) binding protein
PDB	Paget's disease of bone
PDC	parkinsonism–dementia complex
PEG	percutaneous endoscopic gastrostomy
PGRN	progranulin
PiD	Pick's disease
PLS	primary lateral sclerosis
PMA	progressive muscular atrophy
PNFA	progressive non fluent aphasia
pRb	retinoblastoma protein
PSP	progressive supranuclear palsy

RBP	RNA binding protein
RNP	ribonucleoprotein
ROI	region of interest
SD	semantic dementia
SNP	single nucleotide polymorphism
SOD	superoxide dismutase
SPECT	single-photon emission computed tomography
STA	spike-triggered averaging
sv	semantic variant
TARDBP	transactive response (TAR) DNA-binding protein of 43 kDa
TBSS	tract-based spatial statistics
TDP-43	transactive response DNA-binding protein of 43 kDa
TG	transgenic
TOD	'tangle-only' dementia
tRNA	transfer RNA
U	ubiquitin
UMN	upper motor neurone
UPS	ubiquitin–proteasome system
UTR	untranslated region
VBM	voxel-based morphometry
VCP	valosin-containing protein
WM	white matter

Chapter 1

Lessons from the study of natural experiments of hyperendemic foci of neurodegeneration

Ralph M. Garruto

One of the most fascinating ways of understanding neurodegenerative disease is through an understanding of what are called natural experimental models (1,2). Natural experiments are represented by anthropological populations that may be culturally, as well as geographically, isolated; they are often small, and represent either closed or semi-closed systems of mating behaviour. They help to address anthropological, biomedical, and evolutionary problems concerning humans that often are difficult to solve because human experimental research design is constrained. Natural experimental models are designed to help lessen the impact of such constraints, in that they take advantage of a population or special circumstance that naturally isolates a particular problem (i.e. a population will be identified as particularly appropriate for addressing an existing scientific problem). Natural experimental models also use populations that have unique attributes or biomedical phenomena that direct inquiry and have relevance locally as well as globally (i.e. a population with unique attributes will identify a new scientific problem). Both cases are opportunistic: in the first case, the problem dictates the population; in the second case, the problem arises from the population.

These natural experiments in small populations usually do not suffer from the confounding factors that exist in more technologically complex societies. Biomedicine has come to recognize the value of such models and populations that provide a natural laboratory for understanding neurodegenerative and other diseases. We believe natural experiments lead us to a quicker understanding not only of the causal and fundamental mechanisms of disease, but ultimately for a more rapid translation of information into clinical practice and prevention (Figure 1.1).

In 1947, D. Carleton Gajdusek, on his way back to the United States from Sir MacFarlane Burnet's laboratory, stopped off in New Guinea. This became an historic visit, with publication of a new focus of neurodegeneration (i.e. kuru among the Fore people of New Guinea), which would lead 20 years later to the awarding of the Nobel Prize for 'discoveries of new mechanisms for the origin and dissemination of infectious diseases' (3), and to a second Nobel Prize some 20 years after Gajdusek to Stanley Pruisner for

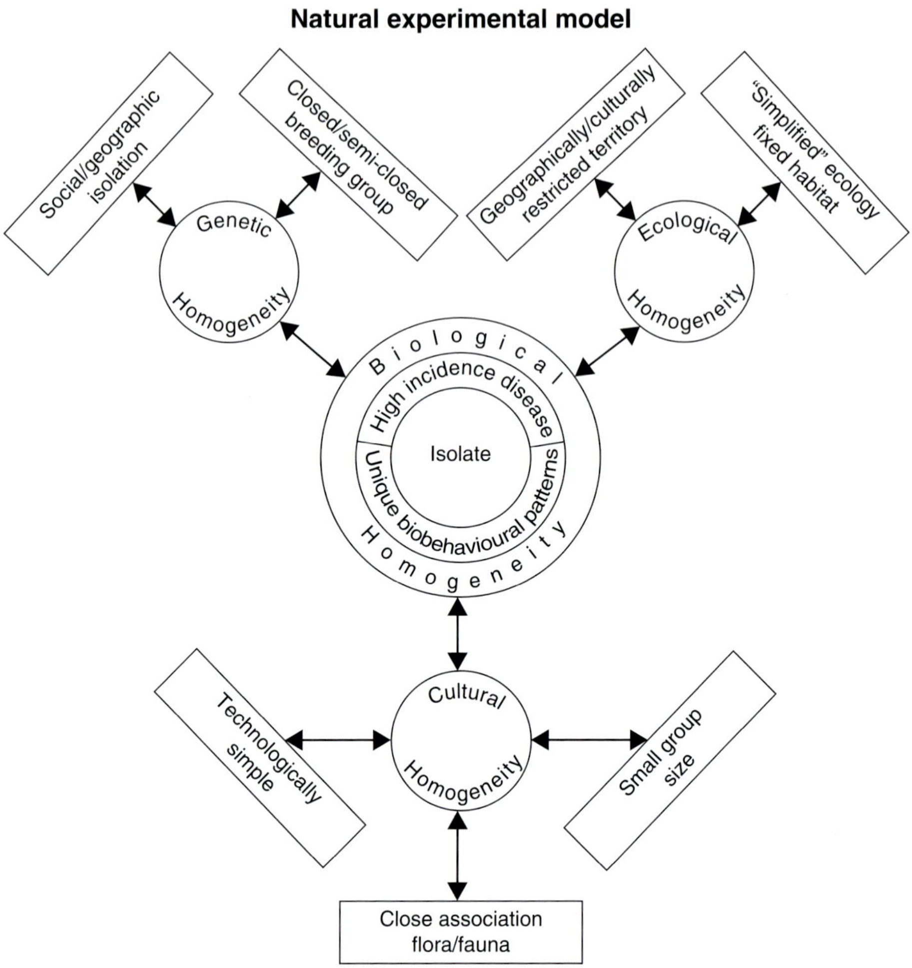

Fig. 1.1 Schematic diagram depicting the characteristics of a natural experimental model using small anthropological populations that provide a natural laboratory for understanding major biomedical phenomena.

characterization of the infectious agent (4). Gajdusek's discovery of this unique focus of neurodegeneration, which changed some of our fundamental thinking in the neurosciences and in biology and medicine, was not the first nor the last discovery of unique foci of hyperendemic neurodegenerative disease in isolated human groups. Subsequent to the discovery of kuru, in the late 1950s and early 1960s in then Dutch New Guinea, Gajdusek described a new focus of motor neurone disease and parkinsonism among a population of about 5000 Auyu and 9000 Jakai speaking people, still headhunters and cannibals at the time, living on a wetland plain in southern West New Guinea (5). In 1974 and in later years he would return to what was known as Irian Jaya or West New Guinea to continue his research, culminating in several important papers on this focus. His discovery would bring another dimension to the already existing knowledge of two other foci of high-incidence amyotrophic lateral sclerosis (ALS) and parkinsonism–dementia complex (PDC) in isolated Pacific populations, one in the Kii Peninsula of Japan (6–8), and the other in the Mariana Islands (9,10) (Figure 1.2).

Only the study of kuru, however, would lead relatively quickly to a significant new discovery and scientific breakthrough. The three high-incidence foci of ALS and PDC, while well poised to lead to new discoveries and major breakthroughs in neurodegenerative disease research, did not readily lead to an understanding of the cause or fundamental mechanisms of neurodegeneration, with diseases that presumably started decades after their initial insults, be they genetic, epigenetic, environmental, or some combination of a gene–environment (GxE) interaction (11).

Discovery of Pacific foci of amyotrophic lateral sclerosis and parkinsonism–dementia complex

One of the most unique and interesting questions in our understanding of the cause of high-incidence neurodegenerative disease is how three foci of ALS and PDC could represent the

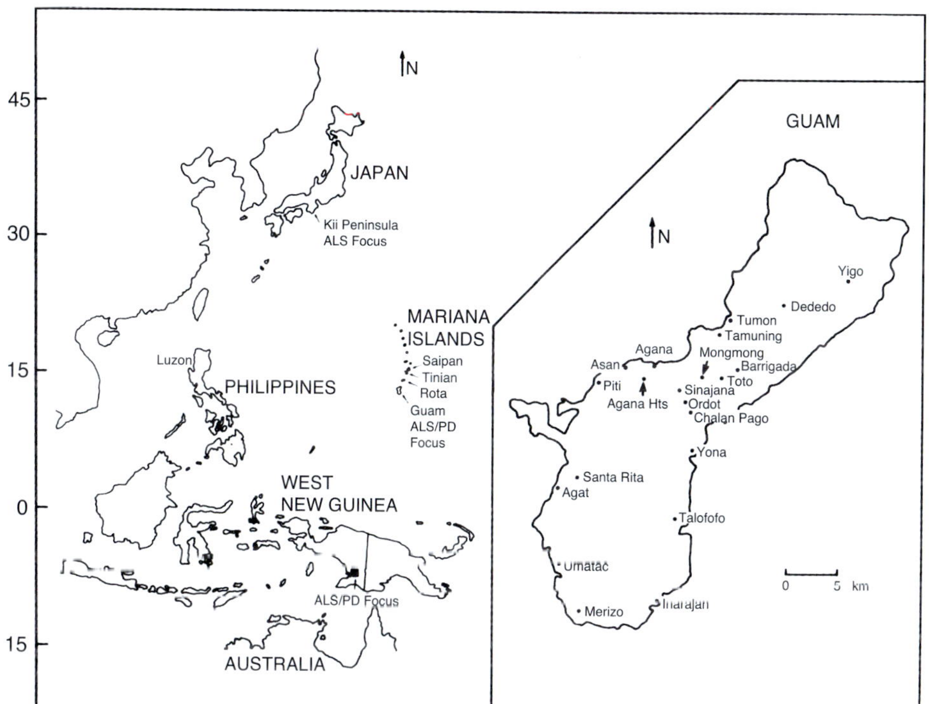

Fig. 1.2 Map of the Western Pacific showing the three high incidence foci of ALS and PDC, all approximately on the same north–south longitude. The insert of the island of Guam shows the traditional villages on Guam, with those in the south having the highest incidence of ALS and PDC.

same neurodegenerative process and likely the same initiating causal factors that arose in three geographically and genetically distinct isolated human groups, all in the Pacific basin, and all approximately on the same north–south longitude (Figure 1.2).

Clinically, ALS in these foci is essentially the same as sporadic ALS described by Charcot more than a century ago (12). It is a disease of the motor neurones and corticospinal tract, characterized by muscle weakness, progressive muscular atrophy, paralysis, and spasticity (13–15). Neuropathologically, Pacific ALS is the same as sporadic ALS, except that neurofibrillary tangles (NFTs) are a hallmark lesion in both brain and spinal cord (Figure 1.3) (8,16). By comparison, parkinsonism in these foci is characterized by slowness of voluntary motor activity, muscular rigidity, and tremor, and most unusually, accompanied by an early-onset progressive dementia (8,16). Neuropathologically, PDC is also associated with severe NFT formation and neuronal loss in a specific distribution within the brain (16). Lewy bodies and senile plaques are rarely observed. ALS and PDC

(a)

(b)

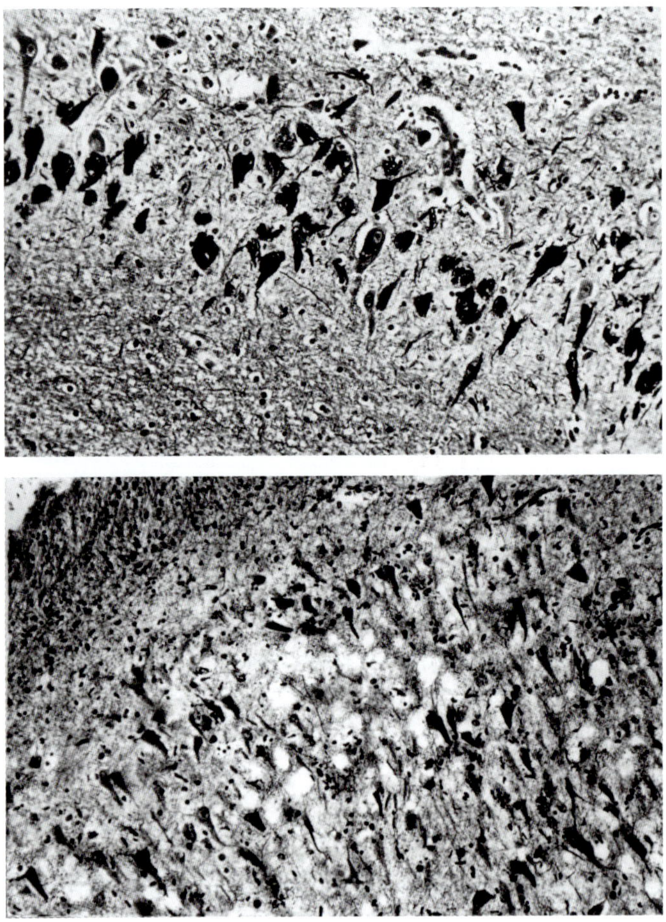

Fig. 1.3 Neurofibrillary tangles in the brain of Guam patients. Silver-stained 6 μm section of the hippocampus of the brain. (a) Guam patient with ALS and (b) Guam patient with PDC.

in these foci are often found in the same families, the same sibship and even the same individual (14,17,18,19), and likely represent different clinical endpoints of the same disease spectrum. Both disorders are late-onset, uniformly fatal, and of unknown aetiology. These hyperendemic foci, all located in the western Pacific, represent natural experimental models of chronic degenerative disease that occur in different cultures, in different ecological zones, and among genetically diverse human groups.

West New Guinea focus

The most isolated and remote of the three foci of ALS and PDC is found among the Auyu and Jakai people living on the southern inland plain of West New Guinea. In 1960, while Gajdusek was searching other regions of New Guinea and Melanesia for kuru-like disease and while he was on the southern coast of West New Guinea, a Dutch medical officer at Kepi brought to his attention several cases of motor neurone disease (5). In this region, about 4000 Auyu and 9000 Jakai-speaking people lived around the lower Digul and Mappi Rivers. The region had been visited by missionaries in 1935, although even in 1960, they were still headhunters and cannibals (5). The ALS/PDC focus in West New Guinea is geographically limited, and neither ALS nor PDC is found in the surrounding larger population residing outside of the focal region.

Originally, Gajdusek reported finding 13 cases of ALS among the Auyu and seven cases among the Jakai, along with at least one patient with PDC. As on Guam, patients with PDC were slower to be recognized. Unlike Guam, where the male/female ratios were 2:1 for ALS and as high as 3:1 for PDC, the sex ratio in the West New Guinea focus was near unity. The mean age at onset of ALS, however, was much younger in the West New Guinea focus than on Guam. Thirty per cent of Auyu and Jakai cases were 30 years of age and younger, with a mean duration of 3.5 years, a duration for ALS that was similar to Guam. After a series of expeditions over the preceding 20 years, Gajdusek summarized a total of 97 cases of ALS and 19 cases of PDC (17). The overall crude average annual incidence rate for ALS alone in this focus was 147 per 100 000 population, more than 100 times higher than rates in the continental United States, and the highest recorded level anywhere in the world (17). In selected villages, the prevalence rate exceeded 1300 per 100 000 population, more than twice that of the village of Umatac, the highest prevalence village on Guam. Gajdusek noted that ALS and PDC had not spread to other villages within the affected area and indeed had dramatically declined in some villages by 1982, and by 1987, ALS had virtually disappeared among the Auyu and Jakai (Gajdusek, personal communication), a fact later confirmed by Peter Spencer and colleagues (20).

Of the three foci, only the West New Guinea focus had no autopsies and thus no neuropathology was available for any cases of ALS or PDC. Thus NFTs, the hallmark lesion found in the brain and spinal cord of ALS and in the brain of patients with PDC from Guam and in the Kii Peninsula of Japan, could not be confirmed in West New Guinea. The reason there was never an autopsy among the Auyu and Jakai was both interesting and unique. Many years ago, Gajdusek stated that the lack of autopsies among the Auyu and Jakai related to his fear that headhunting in the region, which was mostly under control by the 1960s, would again flair up if the sanctioning of the 'taking heads' was resumed (D.C. Gajdusek, personal communication).

Kii Peninsula focus

The first account of the high incidence of ALS in the Kii Peninsula of Honshu Island, Japan, was documented by Miura in 1911 (21). Subsequently, extensive epidemiological surveys disclosed two separate foci of ALS within the Kii Peninsula: the Kozagawa focus (population 6200) in 1966, and the Hohara (Hobara) focus (population 2100) in 1969 (22). The foci are approximately 200 km apart, and both are located in remote, mountainous regions where farming and lumbering are the main occupational activities. The Hohara focus had an incidence rate of 55 per 100 000 compared with 14 per 100 000 for Kozagawa for the 20-year period immediately post-World War II to the mid-1960s. Rates were up to 25–100 times higher than the average annual incidence rate of 0.4 per 100 000 population for the whole of Japan. Subsequent studies showed a decline in the incidence rate in the Kii Peninsula between 1965 and 1989 (23). In the town of Kozagawa itself, the reason for the decline was the dramatic loss in population, some 50% as a result of out migration over the years (24). By 2002, however, the rates had increased and were 53 per 100 000 population with a male/female ratio of 2:1, similar to that found in the 1960s on Guam (23). In the Hohara subfocus in the 1990s the incidence rate for ALS and PDC combined was about 100 per 100 000 population, essentially what it was three decades earlier (22,25). Neuropathologically, patients with ALS and PDC in the Kii Peninsula focus frequently have NFTs and accumulation of neurofilament and other proteins in brain and spinal cord neurones (26), which are hallmark features of patients from the Mariana Island focus.

Mariana Island focus

Of the three known high incidence foci of motor neurone disease and parkinsonism, none has been more closely monitored epidemiologically, clinically, and neuropathologically than that of the Chamorros of the Mariana Islands (27). The striking concentration of ALS on Guam led to the establishment of a field station in 1956 by the National Institute of Neurological Disorders and Stroke. On Guam, ALS is locally referred to as *lytico*, with an original incidence rate in the 1950s of more than 50 times that of the continental United States (10). Subsequent surveys revealed the presence of a second neurological disorder, PDC, locally referred to as *bodig* in the Chamorro language, which also occurred in high incidence (28). Both disorders previously accounted for one in five deaths among Guamanians over 25 years of age. Patients with ALS and PDC both show the hallmark characteristic of NFTs in the brain and spinal cord without associated senile plaques, Lewy bodies, or spongiform change (29).

There is a high incidence rate of the disorders not only among the Chamorros of Guam, but also among the Chamorros of Rota, an island lying 70 km north of Guam. Yet, the Chamorros of Tinian, Saipan, and the more northerly inhabited islands in the Marianas chain do not exhibit high incidence rates of either disease (30). Studies of both Chamorro migrants to the continental United States and long-term Filipino migrants to Guam indicate a 5–10-fold increased risk of developing ALS and PDC, regardless of whether exposure to the Guamanian environment occurred during childhood or adolescence (Chamorro migrants) or during adulthood (Filipino migrants) (30). However, in neither instance have the diseases reached levels observed among Chamorros on Guam. Other ethnic groups, such as the small endogamous Carolinian community and the much larger Caucasian population, consisting predominately of transient American military personnel and their dependants, have not shown any increase in risk of developing disease.

The accumulating epidemiological evidence in each of these three geographically and genetically distinct Pacific foci suggests that environmental factors are involved in the development of these fatal neurological disorders and confirm earlier observations that ALS and PDC are rapidly disappearing from Guam (Figure 1.4) (30,31). The decline in incidence rates on Guam is most dramatic among males and among those from the traditional high-incidence southern villages, so that the male/female ratio for both disorders is now approaching unity (Figure 1.4). Follow-up studies in Hohara indicate a decline in the incidence of ALS from about 52 to 100 000 to 14 per 100 000 population by the 1980s, only to surge again in the 1990s (24,25). However, in the remote West New Guinea focus, the incidence of ALS and PDC has declined and essentially disappeared with increasing Western contact and introduction to new foodstuffs (30,32). Evidence from all three foci suggests a cohort effect and a disease involving exposure to selected environmental factors (9,30,32–34).

Environmental aetiological hypothesis: metals

In 1961, Kimura and colleagues established the high incidence of ALS in the Kii Peninsula of Japan and noted that 20% of the adult population had neurological symptoms (22). It was also observed that ALS occurred in areas where river and drinking water were low in minerals and over the next decade, Yase and colleagues working in both the Kii Peninsula and on Guam began to postulate a possible mechanism for the involvement of manganese and other metals in these disorders (33–36). Additional studies suggested that calcium is linked to the disease process (37) and in all three foci, reports of low environmental levels of calcium and high levels of aluminium began to appear (7,8,17,38–42). Biochemical disturbances in calcium and vitamin D metabolism were also reported in 37% of Guamanian patients with ALS and PDC (43). Animal models were developed based on low-dose chronic exposure through diet or intracisternal inoculations and were largely supportive of the toxicity of aluminium in association with a low calcium diet (9,44–47).

Sophisticated studies by Yase and colleagues in the 1960s (35) had determined by neutron activation analysis, elevated levels of manganese, calcium, and aluminium, in brain and spinal cord tissues in patients with ALS from the Kii Peninsula of Japan. These studies were repeated using other techniques such as neutron activation analysis and X-ray microanalysis (40,48). The chemical imaging of the intraneuronal accumulation of aluminium,

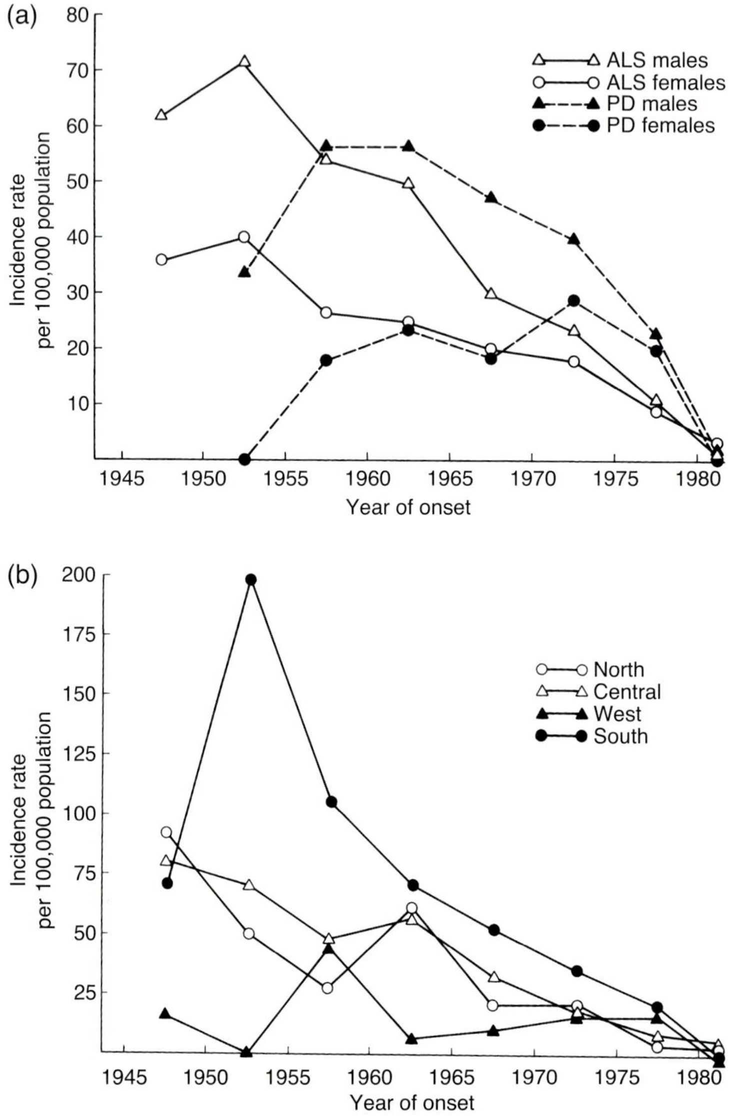

Fig. 1.4 Five-year average annual incidence rates of ALS and PDC on Guam. The increase in incidence depicted between the years 1945 and 1955 represents case finding and ascertainment. The subsequent decrease in incidence from about 1955 onward represents the dramatic decline of the high incidence over approximately 30 years, suggesting a major environmental factor in the disease aetiology. (a) Incidence rates for male and female patients with ALS and PDC island-wide. Note the 2:1 male/female sex ratio for ALS and the almost 3:1 sex ratio for PDC. (b) Incidence by geographic region on Guam. Note the dramatic decrease in the southern region of Guam, which has the most traditional villages on the island, and were the slowest to modernize.

calcium, and silicon in NFT-bearing neurones in brain tissues and spinal cords of Guamanian patients, using X-ray microanalysis and energy and wavelength dispersive spectrometry, secondary ion mass spectrometry, etc., was an important finding (49–56).

It is thought that susceptible individuals in these high-incidence foci, provoked by chronic nutritional deficiencies of calcium and magnesium, leads to enhanced gastrointestinal absorption of aluminium. In addition, the deposition of calcium and aluminium in neurones that disrupt neuronal function induces the accumulation of hyperphosphorylated fibrillary proteins in perikarya and neuronal processes, resulting in cascading neuronal degeneration and cell death (9). More recently, additional support for the role of metals in Guam ALS and PDC comes from studies by Hermosura and colleagues who suggest that mutations in neuronal cell membrane ion channels may lead to metal intoxication and neuronal death (57–59).

Environmental aetiological hypothesis: cycad and β-*N*-methylamino L-alanine

Since the 1960s, like aetiological studies of metals, cycad and its neurotoxic derivatives, in particular β-*N*-methylamino L-alanine (BMAA) have been studied as possible causes of ALS and PDC in the western Pacific. The fruit of *Cycas micronesica* has been used on Guam as an occasional food source for at least 150 years (60). In the 1960s, Whiting (61) and Kurland (62) suggested that an unknown neurotoxin in cycad fruit might be the cause of these neurological disorders. Yet, subsequent research in the 1960s and early 1970s was unable to establish either a chronic toxicity or a causal link with Guam ALS and PDC, and in the Kii Peninsula and West New Guinea foci, the fruit was not eaten. Although Vega and Bell (63) had isolated BMAA from cycad fruit and Polsky and colleagues (64) had shown it to be neurotoxic to chicks, rats, and mice when given acutely and in high concentration, the latter group concluded that it was unlikely to be a major factor in the development of neurological disease in humans. Other toxicological studies using cycad were both positive (65) and negative (16,66–68).

A revival occurred in the 1980s when Spencer and colleagues (69) reported that cynomolgus monkeys (*Macaca fascicularis*) fed huge subconvulsive doses (average 250 mg/kg body weight) of synthetic BMAA daily by gavage developed neurological symptoms and limited pathology, although previous studies demonstrated that washed cycad, as traditionally prepared on Guam, contains only trace amounts of free BMAA (70–74). Furthermore, cycad had traditionally been eaten and used as a poultice in many regions of India, Southeast Asia, and the Pacific basin (75), yet no unusual prevalence of ALS or PDC has ever been described in these regions.

Most recently, a new cycad hypothesis has emerged. Cox and Sacks (76) proposed that biomagnification (bioaccumulation) of BMAA by cycad-eating fruit bats, which were a sought-after delicacy on Guam, could have resulted in ingestion of high levels of cycad toxins, without any consequences to the fruit bat resulting in the development of ALS and PDC decades after exposure during childhood, adolescence, or in adulthood. Subsequent studies by Cox and colleagues found that BMAA occurred at much higher levels in the protein-bound form than as free BMAA, with the implication that protein-bound BMAA would be absorbed through acid hydrolysis in the stomach (77). They also reported that brain tissue from Guamanian patients with ALS and PDC had significant levels of both free and protein-bound BMAA, as did patients with Alzheimer's disease (77,78). Finally, Cox and colleagues reported that diverse taxa of cyanobacteria produce BMAA naturally (79). On Guam, the roots of *C. micronesica*, the fruit from which the flying foxes eat, were infected with cyanobacteria (79). As cyanobacteria appeared to be the culprit, rather than cycad per se, the implication was that it could potentially explain not only ALS and PDC but neurodegenerative diseases such as Alzheimer's disease worldwide (80–82). However, many recent studies are equivocal at this time (83–94).

A half century of genetic studies

In the 1950s, during the early years of the first systematic studies of ALS and PDC on Guam, there was a strong suspicion that these diseases might be of genetic origin. Familial clustering of cases was prevalent on Guam as it was in the Kii Peninsula and in West New Guinea (8,17–19). By the late 1950s, Robert Krooth (with the assistance of James Neel) had developed a prospective registry of patients and their first-degree relatives along with matched controls and their first-degree relatives. This prospective case–control registry involved the long-term follow-up of all first-degree relatives (parents, siblings, and offspring) as well as spouses who acted as non-genetic controls. The registry was closed in 1962 after 5 years, and Chris Plato, a geneticist, was recruited to go to Guam for 2 years to begin the prospective assessment of the registry, and the implementation of a series of genetic studies of ALS and PDC on the island (95–98). His ongoing studies confirmed that parents, siblings, and spouses of patients had a significantly increased risk of developing disease (99), as did offspring once they reached age at risk (96). The increased risk among spouses of patients confirmed a household effect. Forty per cent of probands had at least one affected first-degree relative with many families having more than one affected relative. These long-term studies were combined with analyses of a pedigree for the entire village of Umatac (19), the highest-incidence village on Guam.

Additional genetic studies followed the development of the ALS and PDC case–control relative registry, and included calculation of inbreeding coefficients, segregation analysis, identification of genetic markers, including blood groups, serum proteins, red cell enzymes, HLA antigens, immunoglobulin allotypes, and dermatoglyphics (19,97–102). However, all failed to provide a satisfactory genetic explanation, and the continuing rapid decline of ALS and PDC implicated a major environmental factor (30,31). Studies that were more recent included searching for mutations in the nuclear genome, yet no mutations were found in the superoxide dismutase (*SOD*) gene (103) and mutations discovered in the TAU gene proved only to have a small effect (103,104). Using a larger sample, Sundar and colleagues concluded that genetic changes in the 'TAU region' contributed only a small risk to Guam ALS and PDC, and was unlikely to be the cause (105), and Morris and colleagues in a nuclear genome-wide analysis, could not identify a single gene locus, major or minor, involved in Guam PDC (106).

Efforts to construct a gene–environment interaction model

Using cumulative lifetime risks for developing ALS and PDC in the Chamorro population, Bailey-Wilson and colleagues (107) pursued an updated analysis of the Guam patient–control relative registry discussed above (18,31,96,99). For the first time, it was demonstrated that the best-fit model based on 40 years of empirical data was one involving a GxE interaction. Clearly, neither pure genetic nor pure environmental lines of evidence and inquiry seemed sufficient, obtainable, or convincing enough by themselves and thus active pursuit of a testable GxE interaction model ensued.

A second major step in the search for a GxE interaction came when Hermosura and colleagues discovered a nuclear mutation in the calcium/magnesium membrane ion channel, the transient receptor potential melastatin 7 (*TRPM 7*) gene, in a subset of Guam patients with ALS and PDC (57–59). The channel is a bi-functional protein involved in homeostatic regulation of intracellular calcium and magnesium and trace metal ion concentration. The discovery of the novel mutant channel was shown to have decreased functionality under low cellular levels of magnesium. Effectively, the defective channel could decrease the cellular import of magnesium, causing lipid peroxidation leading to increased oxidative stress and production of reactive oxygen species (57–59,108). Alternatively, low extracellular magnesium may lead to an influx of extracellular calcium into neurones, a prospect supported by studies almost three decades earlier (38,55).

In other studies, the *TRPM 2* calcium ion channel gene was found to be highly expressed in the brain, particularly in neuronal and microglial cells in the hippocampus and in other brain regions (110–112). Subsequently, Hermosura and colleagues discovered, again in a subset of Guam patients, a mutation in the *TRPM 2* gene that produced a heterozygous variant that activates in response to H_2O_2 and adenosine diphosphate ribose, but in the presence of physiological concentrations of extracellular calcium, is quickly inactivated. There is a decreased influx of calcium into the cell in response to H_2O_2, increasing reactive oxygen species and its downstream processing, potentially leading to neuronal death and the ensuing cascade of neuronal loss in neurodegeneration (57).

With an increased emphasis in the neurosciences on mechanisms of cell death and role of the metals and reactive oxygen species in neurodegeneration and their link to mitochondrial dysfunction, we have concentrated our efforts on the mitochondrial genome and search for both somatic and inherited mutations in the further development of a GxE interaction model of Guam ALS and PDC (113). As mitochondria are the main providers of energy for cellular processes through oxidative phosphorylation and the fact that energy requirements vary among and within tissues at different times, mitochondrial transcription and replication must respond to these vulnerable special and temporal demands to provide the enormous energy requirements of cells in the CNS and skeletal muscle. In mitochondria, the light strand promoter (LSP) region (np399–411) is crucial for mitochondrial transcription, replication, and stability of the mitochondrial genome (114) As Coskun *et al.* (115) reported a greater frequency of somatic mutations in the mitochondrial region in Alzheimer brain tissues compared with controls, we sought to determine the presence of LSP mutations in Guam patients and controls. Our finding demonstrated a higher frequency of somatic mutations in the LSP control region in patients, the majority of which were transversions (113). In addition, Guamanian Chamorros, regardless of diagnosis group, had inherited mutations at np73 and np195 in 95% and 56%, respectively, of all individuals sequenced. These are the same mutations that Coskun *et al.* (115) reported as somatic mutations at a greater frequency in brain tissue from patients with Alzheimer disease than in age-matched controls. However, only individuals with an E2 haplogroup inherited both np73 and np195. Thus, we interpreted this to mean that a large majority of the Guam Chamorro population inherits several mutations that may represent a susceptibility or risk for ALS or PDC (113).

Using eight risk factors, including mtDNA somatic LSP mutations and nuclear TRPM7 mutations mentioned above, metals, BMAA, NFTs, family history, village of residence, and age and gender, we developed a first attempt at a GxE interaction model that was overall statistically significant (113), suggesting genetic susceptibility and environmentally induced neurodegeneration. Recently, we also sequenced the entire mitochondrial genome of 21 Guam patients with ALS and PDC and controls. Although we did not find any direct correlation between mitochondrial dysfunction and ALS and PDC using HVS1 to determine haplogroup, we did find that the odds of developing PDC is significantly high if an individual is haplogroup E1, and therefore E1 may be a risk factor (susceptibility allele) in Guam PDC (116). Likewise, we found that the E2 haplogroup may be a protective factor in Guam PDC (116). Thus, we believe that a genetic susceptibility to ALS and PDC may have expanded with the founding population of Guam through genetic drift or as a result of a later population bottleneck in the late eighteenth century. At 90%, the high frequency of haplogroup E (Figure 1.5), a reflection of this expansion, is unmatched anywhere outside of Guam (117,118).

Pacific amyotrophic lateral sclerosis/parkinsonism-dementia and frontotemporal lobar dementia

One of the most important and intriguing aspects of ALS and PDC in these foci, as stated earlier, is the unusual accumulation of fibrillary proteins in a variety of lesions. While proclaimed a tauopathy by some (104,105), the discovery of yet another protein, TDP-43, in ubiquitin-positive, tau-negative inclusion bodies, originally in ALS, but later in frontotemporal lobar dementia (FTLD)-U with motor neurone disease and in FTLD with motor neurone inclusion bodies without clinical disease is most intriguing (119–123). The discovery of TDP-43 pathology in Guam patients with ALS and PDC (124–126) links FTLD-U with the Guam disease and suggests a common pathogenic mechanism of neurodegeneration. TDP-43 is a nuclear protein that appears to repress transcription and enhance exon skipping (alternative splicing) (127,128), but its physiological function is presently unknown (see Buratti, Chapter 24). Recently, TDP-43 has been found to be an mRNA neurofilament light as well as a DNA binding protein and likely contributes to the formation of skeins of neurofilament in the brain and spinal cord of patients with ALS (129). TDP-43 inclusions do not co-localize with tau in Guam ALS and PDC (124–126), and TDP-43-positive inclusions in the brain were not found in Guam controls.

Thus, TDP-43-positive inclusions apparently discriminate patients from controls much better than tau pathology (124). Of note, non-Chamorros with Guam ALS and PDC were TDP-43 positive as well as NFT tau positive (124), a fact that may have aetiological implications. To what extent the expression of, or mutations in, the TDP-43 gene might impact the aetiology of ALS and PDC in these high-incidence foci is as yet unknown. A search for mutations in 11 regions within the *progranulin* gene, four within the *FUS* gene and two within the *TARDBP* gene in Guam patients with ALS/PDC, is currently underway (R.M. Garruto unpublished data).

Population bottlenecks

A most important aspect to understanding ALS and PDC in these foci is to attempt to frame them within a historical context. ALS and PDC on Guam and in the Kii Peninsula of Japan have at least a century-long historical record, and in West New Guinea although the historical perspective is more recent, it still represents some five decades. In order to decipher why there was such an incredibly high incidence of disease in these isolated, genetically and culturally homogeneous groups, each living in a small, circumscribed area, historical information becomes critically important. For example, are there post-contact written records by missionaries, explorers, or indigenous or colonial administrators that shed some light on to the health and disease of these isolated groups? Do particular events in the historical record that could have created a genetic predisposition to ALS and PDC exist? Is the historical record supportive of any current or past aetiological hypotheses? What studies need to be done to provide answers to our remaining questions?

Using Guam as the best studied of the three foci as the example, at the time of the first systematic epidemiological studies in the early 1950s (10,130–132), the disease may already have been in decline (Figure 1.5). Ingestion of cycad likely occurred before 1875 (60) and probably at the time of the Spanish conquest (133), as it was being used by many indigenous populations in Asia and the Pacific basin. Metals in the local environment in all three foci have probably been there in more or less the same concentrations for thousands of years. It would appear that Guam ALS and PDC were not known or recognized before 1875, as there were no indications of their existence in the Spanish record before de la Corte (60). Even then, the record is conflicting: de la Corte mentions 'endemic illnesses which have become hereditary and produce elephantiasis illness, often causing premature aging and short life' (60, p. 101). The question is, therefore, whether the prehistoric high incidence of ALS and PDC could have been missed by the Spanish in 1521 and the succeeding 350 years (Figure 1.6).

One wonders if in the 1783 population bottleneck, which occurred as a result of the Spanish Chamorro War, epidemics, and typhoons (95,134,135), if there occurred an increased frequency of a susceptibility allele(s) for ALS and PDC in the small remaining population of about 1000–1500 Chamorros, from a population at the time of conquest estimated to be 50 000–100 000 (95,134). Figure 1.7 shows the theoretical incidence rate for just such a scenario. Also likely is the probability of developing a susceptibility allele

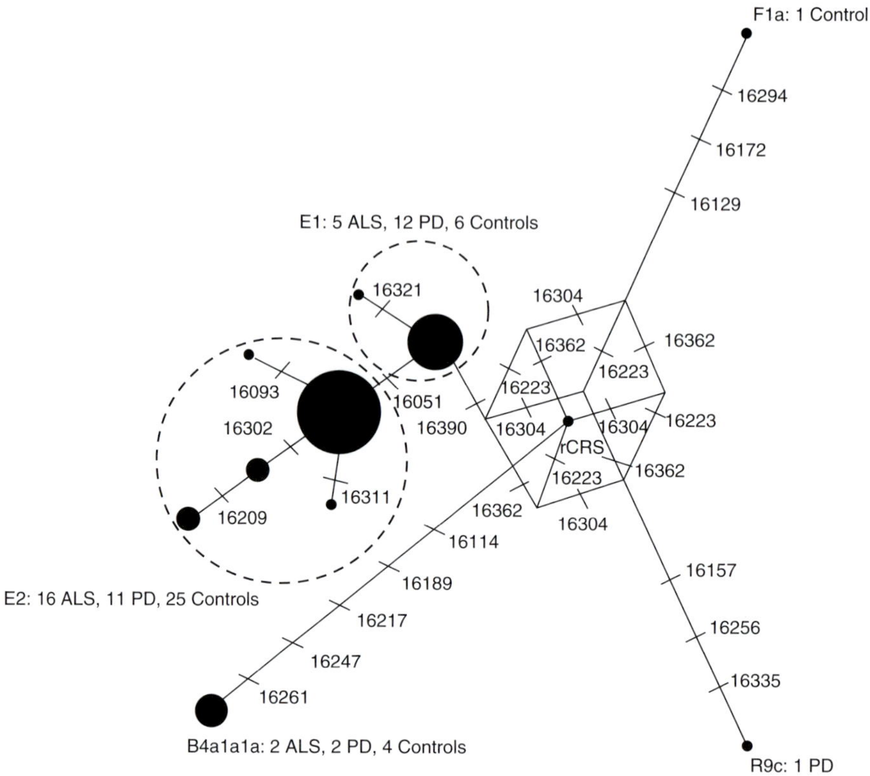

Fig. 1.5 Reduced median network diagram for the hypervariable sequence (HVS1) of the mitochondrial genome. mtDNA HVS1 represent 23 Guam patients with ALS, 26 Guam patients with PDC, and 36 non-neurological Guam controls. Haplogroups B4, E1, and E2 represent Guamanian Chamorros. Haplogroups F1a and R9c represent two Flilipinos on Guam, a non-neurological control and a patient with PDC, respectively.

in the founding population of Guam 3600 years ago. The theoretical incidence curve in Figure 1.8 reflects an envisioned slow increase in the frequency of such an allele in the founding population, which during a second population bottleneck in 1783, may have been nearly lost, or alternately, increased in frequency, resulting in the slow recognition of the disease by the Spanish in 1875 a century later. However, this is simply conjecture, but reflects the importance of thinking about demographic changes and historical events as impacting high-incidence foci of neurodegeneration, be it kuru (arising as a result of a possible case of sporadic Creutzfeldt–Jakob disease in a cannibalistic society that immediately increased the risk) or ALS and PDC on Guam.

Epigenetic influences

C. H. Waddington appears to be the first to use the term 'epigenetics' to describe how genotypes give rise to phenotypes during development and the concept of phenotypic plasticity (136). His classical experiment in 1953 of genetic assimilation was conducted

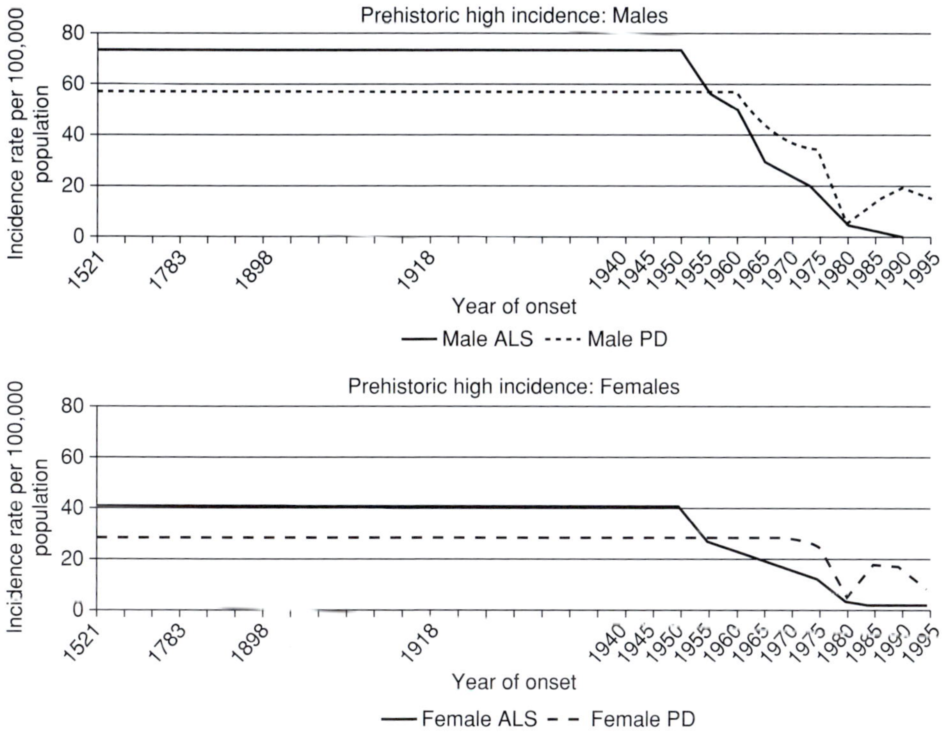

Fig. 1.6 Theoretical incidence curves for male and female patients with ALS and PDC on Guam showing an already high incidence at the time of Spanish conquest in 1521. These curves assume the Spanish did not recognize the disease on Guam over the next 350 years on the island. The curves from 1945 onward represent actual data. With permission from Ralph M. Garruto and Richard Yanagihara (2009), Folia Neuropathol.

with *Drosophila* embryos, which were exposed to the gas ether (137,138). The toxic exposure produced a bithorax phenotype, demonstrating phenotypic plasticity. Eventually 20 generations later, after each generational exposure to ether, mated *Drosophila* produced the bithorax mutant phenotype even when ether was no longer applied, thus, his development of the concept of genetic assimilation and artificial selection.

Today, the concept of epigenetics can have a different meaning, such as changes in gene function that cannot be explained by changes in the DNA sequence (139). In neurobiology, perhaps the best known examples for the molecular basis of heritable epigenetics are methylation of DNA, which plays a key role in memory-associated gene transcription (140,141). A second example is chromatin modification (140–142), which refers to the post translational modification of histone proteins that make up the nucleosomes, which have the DNA double helix coiled around them. Such events may be influenced by teratogins, including metals or organotoxins, and on a broader scale, such things as diet and maternal–fetal interactions. All can influence gene expression and cell differentiation, and result in phenotypic plasticity.

Bird (142) recently offered a unifying definition of epigenetics, 'the structural adaptation of chromosomal regions so as to register, signal, or perpetuate altered activity states',

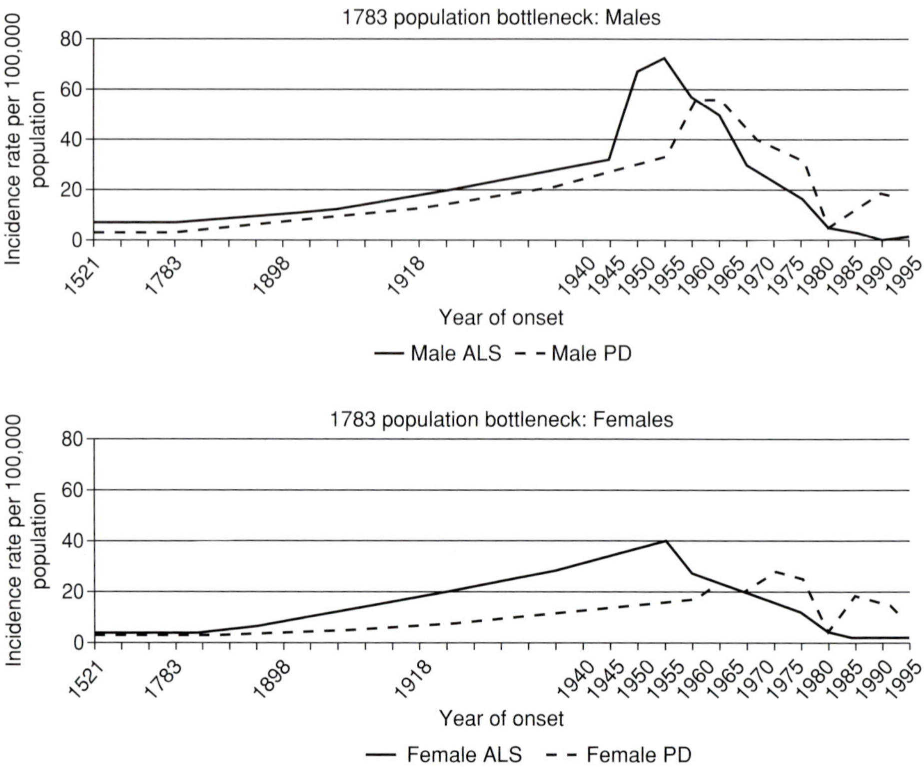

Fig. 1.7 Theoretical incidence curves for male and female patients with ALS and PDC on Guam showing a developing high incidence as a result of a population bottleneck in 1783, which was a function of typhoons, epidemics, and the long and decimating Spanish–Chamorro War. The curves from 1945 onward represent actual data. With permission from Ralph M. Garruto and Richard Yanagihara (2009), Folia Neuropathol.

a definition he feels is inclusive. Irrespective of the definition one is drawn to, it is clear that epigenetics, as a research field, is moving rapidly in the assessment of complex diseases (phenotypes), and in particular those complex phenotypes represented by neurodegenerative disorders.

For ALS, parkinsonism, and FTLD, the future is bright for using epigenetics to help elucidate the cellular and molecular mechanisms of neuronal degeneration. However, for Pacific foci of ALS and PDC, epigenetic prospects have dimmed as the high incidence in these foci has already disappeared, at least on Guam and in West New Guinea. Thus, our attempt to understand the foci of high incidence of ALS and PDC, and the relative contribution of epigenetic marks to the aetiology of ALS and PDC, will likely remain unknown.

Lessons learned

One of the most important aspects in deciphering the cause of Guam ALS and PDC is an appreciation for, and an understanding of, the epidemiology, population biology, and natural

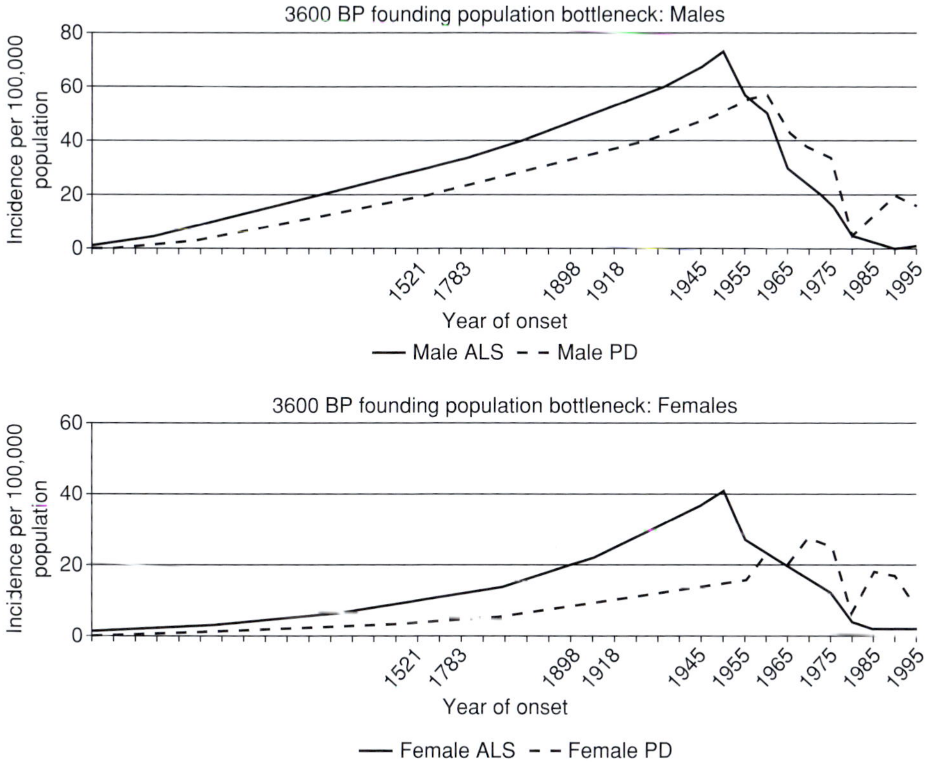

Fig. 1.8 Theoretical incidence curves for male and female patients with ALS and PDC on Guam showing a developing high incidence as a result of a population bottleneck represented by the prehistoric founding population of the island (founder effect). The curves from 1945 onward represent actual data.

history of the disease in the Marianas. How did these diseases arise in the population? When were they first observed clinically? What islands and ethnic groups was the disease confined to? And, how did the high incidence of ALS and PDC disappear in little more than 30 years after the first systematic epidemiological studies in both the Mariana Islands and in West New Guinea? These questions are paramount to understanding what we and others have long sought, the cause and mechanisms of pathogenesis of ALS and PDC in all three Pacific foci. An understanding of the aetiology in one focus will likely translate to all three foci and provide a breakthrough in our understanding ALS and PDC globally.

A haunting question that often plagues those of us who have given our careers to understanding ALS and PDC in these foci is the possibility that we overlooked important information still embedded in research data already collected and/or analysed. These foci are so well studied, particularly in Guam and the Kii Peninsula, that an answer should be apparent from more than a half century of systematic research. The naturalistic model as shown in Figure 1.1 should have yielded an answer, such as kuru, as to the cause(s) and mechanisms of neuronal degeneration. Yet, answers continue to remain elusive.

Critical information that we already know, again using Guam as the primary example, is summarized below:

- ALS and PDC are found in the same families (first-degree relatives and spouses) and sometimes overlap clinically in the same individual.
- NFTs are prominent in the brain (and spinal cord) of patients with ALS, in the brain of patients with PDC, and in nearly 70% of neurologically normal controls. NFTs are likely a neuropathology link to Alzheimer's disease, FTLD, and other neurodegenerative disorders.
- The high incidence of ALS and PDC disappeared from West New Guinea and Guam about 30 years after the first systematic epidemiological studies began.
- A change in the male/female sex ratio in ALS and PDC from 2:1, and even 3:1, to currently 1:1, has occurred during the decline in incidence.
- Neither genetic nor purely environmental models are a best fit aetiologically. Therefore, a GxE interaction model seems most plausible at this time.
- Epigenetic influences such as DNA methylation and chromatin modification could play a major role in Guam ALS and PDC, but to date no epigenetic studies have been conducted.
- As a working hypothesis, it is reasonable to consider ALS and PDC as complex diseases with small genetic effects (inherited or somatic), combined with a major environmental trigger. A major susceptibility allele is also possible, but to date has not yet been found.
- Historical events in these foci are important to document and understand to clarify any impact they may have on the aetiology and mechanisms of pathogenesis.
- And finally, re-evaluation of existing data and/or systematic sifting through already collected data and records may be helpful to make sure important facts have not been overlooked.

Although we know with certainty that there is a sole or at least a major environmental component to ALS and PDC in these foci, we are still not certain what that environmental component may be. We have identified two neurotoxins as potential aetiologies over the past 50 years, but we have fallen short in 'proving' that one or the other is 'the' cause. Causality and causal mechanisms of disease are difficult to demonstrate in biology and medicine; however, it seems reasonable to assume we should be on much more solid scientific ground with respect to either of the proposed candidate neurotoxins. Part of the problem is that the high incidence of these disorders has disappeared, likely the result of changing cultural practices or changes in the level of environmental exposure and, therefore, we may never be able to sort out causality retrospectively. Answers from our long-term genetic studies also have not been forthcoming, despite our long-term prospective case–control relative registry developed in the late 1950s and updated periodically over the past half century (18,96,99). With the lack of a major gene or genetic marker, what is left are small genetic effects for a complex disease. The lantern is clearly dimming on what should have been a solvable naturalistic model, given all the exceptional controls built into the model. The continued search for answers remains frustrating and elusive.

Gajdusek's contributions to the understanding of neurodegenerative diseases through studies of focal disease in isolated human groups is legendary and a landmark in the history of science. We who follow, and who have spent decades in search of answers like our mentor's, are simply running out of time, not only with respect to the disappearance of disease in these foci, but as a result of the limitations of our own mortality. Still, scholars from around the world continue to have a profound interest in these foci, and they pursue ongoing questions of aetiology and mechanisms of pathogenesis, an understanding of which will have consequences for our understanding of neurodegenerative diseases globally.

Acknowledgements

The authors would like to thank the patients, and all those who participated as healthy controls and their families, in each of the three foci of high incidence of ALS and PDC in the Western Pacific. Their long-term participation and cooperation in these studies, along with the assistance of local physicians, administrators, and public health officials, have given all of medicine and neuroscience a much better understanding of the problems of neurodegeneration locally as well as globally. I would also like to acknowledge the contributions of the many scientists, too numerous to mention, who have given a lifetime of effort to advancing our knowledge and understanding of the problems of high-incidence disease in these foci. Finally, I would like to thank Dana Reiff, Chim Chan, and Katie Olszowy for assisting with research and technical aspects and manuscript preparation.

References

1. Garruto RM. (1985). Use of genetic isolates as natural experiments in human biology and medicine. Abstracts of the International Symposium on Genetic Diversity and its Maintenance in Tropical Populations, Proceedings of the Society for the Study of Human Biology. *Ann Hum Biol*, **12**, 560.
2. Garruto RM, Little MA, James GD, Brown DE. (1999). Natural experimental models: the global search for biomedical paradigms among traditional, modernizing and modern populations. *Proc Natl Acad Sci USA*, **96**, 10536–10543.
3. Gajdusek DC. (1977). Unconventional viruses and the origin and disappearance of kuru. In: PA Norstedt and Soner (eds.), *Les Prix Nobel en 1976*, pp. 167–216. Stockholm.
4. Prusiner SB. (2003). Prions. In: Jornvall H (ed.), *Nobel Lectures, Physiology or Medicine 1996–2000*. World Scientific Publishing Co., Singapore.
5. Gajdusek DC. (1963). Motor-neuron disease in natives of New Guinea. *N Engl J Med*, **268**, 474–476.
6. Garruto RM, Yase Y. (1986). Neurodegenerative disorders of the western Pacific: the search for mechanisms of pathogenesis. *Trends Neurosci*, **9** (Suppl 12), 368–374.
7. Shiraki H, Yase Y. (1975). Amyotrophic lateral sclerosis in Japan. In: Vinken PJ, Bruyn GW (eds.), *Handbook Clinical Neurology*, Vol. 22, pp. 353–419. Elsevier Publishing Company, New York.
8. Shiraki H, Yase Y. (1991). Amyotrophic lateral sclerosis and parkinsonism-dementia in the Kii Peninsula: comparison with the same disorders in Guam and with Alzheimer's disease. In: Vinken PJ, Bruyn GW, Klawans HL, de Jong JMBV (eds.), *Handbook of Clinical Neurology*, Vol. 15(59): *Diseases of the Motor System*, pp. 273–300. Elsevier Science Publishing Co., Inc., New York.

9. Garruto RM. (1991). Pacific paradigms of environmentally-induced neurological disorders: clinical, epidemiological and molecular perspectives. *Neurotoxicology*, **12**, 347–378.
10. Kurland LT, Mulder DW. (1954). Epidemiologic investigations of amyotrophic lateral sclerosis. 1. Preliminary report on geographic distributions, with special reference to the Marianas Islands, including clinical and pathological observations. *Neurology*, **4**, 355–378, 438–448.
11. Garruto RM. (2006). A commentary on neuronal degeneration and cell death in Guam ALS and PD: an evolutionary process of understanding. *Curr Alzheimer Res*, **3**, 397–401.
12. Charcot JM, Joffroy A. (1869). Deux cas d'atrophie musculaire progressive avec lésions de la substance grise et des faisceaux antérolateraux de la moëlle épinière. *Arch Physiol*, **3**, 629–744.
13. Chen K-M. (1979). Motor neuron involvement in parkinsonian dementia and its relationship to Guam ALS. In: Japan Medical Research Foundation (ed.), *Amyotrophic Lateral Sclerosis. Proceedings of the International Symposium on Amyotrophic Lateral Sclerosis*, pp. 319–344. University of Tokyo Press, Tokyo.
14. Elizan TS, Hirano A, Abrams BM, Need RL, Van Nuis C, Kurland LT. (1966). Amyotrophic lateral sclerosis and parkinsonism-dementia complex of Guam. *Arch Neurol*, **14**, 356–368.
15. Rodgers-Johnson P, Garruto RM, Yanagihara R, Chen KM, Gajdusek DC, Gibbs CJ Jr. (1986). Amyotrophic lateral sclerosis and parkinsonism-dementia on Guam: a 30-year evaluation of clinical and neuropathologic trends. *Neurology*, **36**, 7–13.
16. Hirano A. (1973). Progress in the pathology of motor neuron diseases. In: Zimmerman HM (ed.), *Progress in Neuropathology*, Vol. II, pp. 181–215. Grune and Stratton, New York.
17. Gajdusek DC, Salazar AM. (1982). Amyotrophic lateral sclerosis and parkinsonian syndromes in high incidence among the Auyu and Jakai people of West New Guinea. *Neurology*, **32**, 107–126.
18. Plato CC, Reed DM, Elizan TS, Kurland LT. (1967). Amyotrophic lateral sclerosis/parkinsonism-dementia complex of Guam. IV. Familial and genetic investigations. *Am J Hum Genet*, **19**, 617–632.
19. Plato CC, Cruz MT, Kurland LT. (1969). Amyotrophic lateral sclerosis/parkinsonism-dementia complex of Guam: further genetic investigations. *Am J Genet*, **21**, 133–141.
20. Spencer PS, Palmer VS, Ludolph AC. (2005). On the decline and etiology of high-incidence motor system disease in West Papua (Southwest New Guinea). *Mov Disord*, **20** (Suppl 12), S119–S126.
21. Miura K. (1911). Amyotrophische lateralclerose unter dem bilde von sog. bulbaparalyse. *Neurol Jpn*, **10**, 366–36.
22. Kimura K, Yase Y, Higashi Y, *et al.* (1961). Epidemiological and geomedical studies on ALS and allied diseases in the Kii Peninsula (Japan). Preliminary Report. *Proc Jpn Acad*, **37**, 417–421.
23. Kihira T, Yoshida S, Hironishi M, Miwa H, Okamato K, Kondo T. (2005). Changes in the incidence of amyotrophic lateral sclerosis in Wakayama, Japan. *Amyo Lat Scler*, **6**, 155–163.
24. Yoshida S, Uebayashi Y, Kihira T, *et al.* (1998). Epidemiology of motor neuron disease in the Kii Peninsula of Japan, 1989–1993: active or disappearing focus? *J Neurol Sci*, **155**, 146–155.
25. Kuzuhara S, Kokubo Y, Narita Y, Ryogen S. (1998). Continuing high incidence rates and frequent familial occurrence of Amyotropic Lateral Sclerosis and Parkinsonism-Dementia complex of the Kii Peninsula of Japan. *American Academy of Neurology 50th Annual Meeting Program*, **50**, A173.
26. Kobubo Y, Shigeki K. (2004). Neurofibrillary tangles in ALS and Parkinsonism-dementia complex focus in Kii, Japan. *Neurology*, **53**, 2399–2401.
27. Garruto RM. (1985). Elemental insults provoking neuronal degeneration: the suspected etiology of high incidence amyotrophic lateral sclerosis and parkinsonism-dementia of Guam. In: Hutton JT, Kenny AD (eds), *Senile Dementia of the Alzheimer Type* (Neurology and Neurobiology Series), **18**, pp. 319–336. Alan R. Liss.
28. Hirano A, Kurland LT, Krooth RS, Lessel S. (1961). Parkinsonism-dementia complex, and endemic disease on the island of Guam. I. Clinical features. *Brain*, **84**, 642–661.
29. Hirano A, Malamud N, Kurland LT. (1961). Parkinsonism-dementia complex, and endemic disease on the island of Guam. II. Pathological features. *Brain*, **84**, 662–279.

30. Garruto RM, Yanagihara R, Gajdusek DC. (1985). Disappearance of high incidence amyotrophic lateral sclerosis and parkinsonism-dementia on Guam. *Neurology*, **35**, 193–198.

31. Plato CC, Garruto RM, Galasko D, *et al.* (2003). Amyotrophic lateral sclerosis and parkinsonism-dementia complex of Guam: changing incidence rates during the past sixty years. *Am J Epidemiol*, **157**, 149–157.

32. Gajdusek DC. (1984). Environmental factors provoking physiological changes which induce motor neurone disease and early neuronal ageing in high incidence foci in the Western Pacific. In: Rose FC (ed.), *Progress in Motor Neuron Disease*, pp. 44–69. Pitman, London.

33. Yase Y. (1972). The pathogenesis of amyotrophic lateral sclerosis. *Lancet*, **ii**, 292–296.

34. Kihara T, Yoshida S, Mitani K, Yasui M, Yase Y. (1993). ALS in the Kii Peninsula of Japan, with special reference to neurofibrillary tangles and aluminum. *Neuropathology*, **13**, 125–136.

35. Yase Y, Kumamoto T, Yoshimasu F, Shinjo Y. (1980). Amyotrophic lateral sclerosis studies using neutron activation analysis. *Neurol India*, **16**, 46–50.

36. Yoshimasu F, Yasui M, Yase Y, *et al.* (1980). Studies on amyotrophic lateral sclerosis by neutron activation analysis. 2. Comparative study of analytical results on Guam PD, Japanese ALS and Alzheimer disease cases. *Psychiat Neurol Jap*, **34**, 75–82.

37. Yanagihara R. (1982). Heavy metals and essential minerals in motor neuron disease. In: Rowland LP (ed.), *Human Motor Neuron Diseases*. Proceedings of the International Conference on Human Motor Neuron Diseases, Scottsdale, Arizona, June 8–11, 1981. *Adv Neurol*, **36**, 233–247.

38. Garruto RM, Fukatsu R, Yanagihara R, Gajdusek DC, Hook G, Fiori CE. (1984). Imaging of calcium and aluminum in neurofibrillary tangle-bearing neurons in parkinsonism-dementia of Guam. *Proc Natl Acad Sci USA*, **81**, 1875–1879.

39. Garruto RM, Yanagihara R, Gajdusek DC, Arion DM. (1984). Concentrations of heavy metals and essential minerals in garden soil and drinking water in the Western Pacific. In: Chen K-M, Yase Y (eds.), *Amyotrophic Lateral Sclerosis in Asia and Oceania*, pp. 265–329. National Taiwan University, Taipei.

40. Iwata S, Sasajima K, Yase Y, Uebayashi Y, Yoshida S. (1976). Studies of amyotrophic lateral sclerosis by neutron activation analysis and X-ray microanalysis. *Ann Rep Res Reactor Inst, Kyoto Univ*, **9**, 44–54.

41. Yanagihara R, Grafton DA, Garruto RM, Gajdusek DC. (1984). Elemental hair analysis in Guamanian Chamorros with amyotrophic lateral sclerosis and parkinsonism-dementia. In: Chen K-M, Yase Y (eds.), *Amyotrophic Lateral Sclerosis in Asia and Oceania*, pp. 331–336. National University of Taiwan, Taipei.

42. Yase Y. (1978). The basic process of amyotrophic lateral sclerosis as reflected in the Kii Peninsula and Guam. In: Hartog Jager WA, Bruyn GW, Heijstee APJ (eds.), *Proceedings of the Eleventh World Congress of Neurology. International Congress Series 434*, pp. 413–427. Excerpta Medica, Amsterdam.

43. Yanagihara R, Garruto RM, Gajdusek DC, *et al.* (1984). Calcium and vitamin D metabolism in Guamanian Chamorros with amyotrophic lateral sclerosis and parkinsonism-dementia. *Ann Neurol*, **15**, 42–48.

44. Strong MJ, Wolff AV, Wakayama I, Garruto RM. (1991). Aluminum-induced chronic myelopathy in rabbits. *Neurotoxicology*, **12**, 9–22.

45. Wisniewski HM, Sturman J, Shenk JW. (1980). Aluminum chloride induced neurofibrillary changes in the developing rabbit: a chronic animal model. *Ann Neurol*, **8**, 479–490.

46. Kihira T, Yoshida S, Komoto J, Wakayama I, Yase Y. (1995). Aluminum-induced model of motor neuron degeneration. Subperineurial injection of aluminum in rabbits. *Neuro Toxicology*, **16**, 413–424.

47. Kihira T, Yoshida S, Yase Y, Ono S, Kondo T. (2002). Chronic low-Ca/Mg high-Al diet induces neuronal loss. *Neuropathology*, **22**, 171–179.

48. Yoshida S. (1977). X-ray microanalytic studies on amytrophic lateral sclerosis. I. Metal distribution compared with neuropathological findings in cervical spinal cord. *Rinsho Shinkeigaku*, **17**, 299–309.

49. Ikuta F, Makifuchi T. (1977). Distribution of aluminum in the spinal motor neurons of ALS, examined by wavelength-dispersive X-ray microanalysis. *Annual Report of the Research Committee of Motor Neuron Disease*, pp. 66–69. The Ministry of Health and Welfare of Japan, Tokyo.

50. Perl DP, Gajdusek DC, Garruto RM, Yanagihara RT, Gibbs CJ Jr. (1982). Intraneuronal aluminum accumulation in amyotrophic lateral sclerosis and parkinsonism-dementia of Guam. *Science*, **217**, 1053–1055.

51. Garruto RM, Swyt C, Fiori CE, Yanagihara R, Gajdusek DC. (1985). Intraneuronal deposition of calcium and aluminum in amyotrophic lateral sclerosis of Guam. *Lancet*, **ii**, 1353.

52. Garruto RM, Swyt C, Yanagihara R, Fiori CE, Gajdusek DC. (1986). Intraneuronal co-localization of silicon with calcium and aluminum in amyotrophic lateral sclerosis and parkinsonism with dementia of Guam. *N Engl J Med*, **315**, 711–712.

53. Linton RW, Bryan SR, Griffis DP, Shelburne JD, Fiori CE, Garruto RM. (1987). Digital imaging studies of aluminum and calcium in neurofibrillary tangle-bearing neurons using secondary ion mass spectrometry. *Trace Elem Med*, **4**, 99–104.

54. Perl DP, Good PF. (1990). Microprobe studies of aluminum accumulation in association with human central nervous system disease. *Environ Geochem Health*, **12**, 97–101.

55. Yase Y. (1980). The role of aluminum in CNS degeneration with interaction of calcium. *Neurotoxicology*, **1**, 101–109.

56. Yoshida S, Kihira T, Mitani K, *et al.* (1990). Intraneuronal localization of aluminum: possible interaction with nucleic acids and pathogenic role in amyotrophic lateral sclerosis. In: Rose FC, Norris FH (eds.), *Amyotrophic Lateral Sclerosis—New Advances in Toxicology and Epidemiology*, pp. 211–223. Smith-Gordon, London.

57. Hermosura MC, Ciu AM, Go RCV, *et al.* (2008). Altered functional properties of a TRPM2 variant in Guamanian ALS and PD. *Proc Natl Sci USA*, **105**, 18029–18034.

58. Hermosura M, Garruto RM. (2007). TRPM7 and TRPM2—candidate susceptibility genes for western Pacific ALS and PD? *Biochim Biophys Acta*, **1772**, 822–835.

59. Hermosura MC, Nayakanti H, Dorovkov MV, *et al.* (2005). A TRPM7 variant shows altered sensitivity to magnesium that may contribute to the pathogenesis of the Guamanian neurodegenerative disorders. *Proc Natl Acad Sci USA*, **102**, 11510–11515.

60. Rogers RF. (1996). *Destiny's Landfall: A History of Guam*. University of Hawai'i Press, Honolulu.

61. Whiting MG. (1964). Food practices in ALS foci in Japan, the Marianas and New Guinea. *Fed Proc*, **23**, 1343–1345.

62. Kurland LT. (1964). Introductory remarks. Proceedings of the Third Conference on Toxicity of Cycads. *Fed Proc*, **23**, 1337–1339.

63. Vega A, Bell EA. (1967). Alpha-amino-beta-methylaminopropionic acid: a new amino acid from seeds of Cycas circinalis. *Phytochemistry*, **6**, 759–762.

64. Polsky RI, Nunn PB, Bell EA. (1972). Distribution and toxicity of α-amino-β-methylaminopropionic acid. *Fed Proc*, **31**, 1473–1475.

65. Dastur DK, Palekar RS. (1974). The experimental pathology of cycad toxicity with special reference to oncogenic effects. *Indian J Cancer*, **11**, 33–49.

66. Garruto RM, Shankar SK, Yanagihara R, Salazar AM, Amyx HL, Gajdusek DC. (1989). Low calcium, high aluminum diet-induced motor neuron pathology in cynomolgus monkeys. *Acta Neuropathol*, **78**, 210–219.

67. Sieber SM, Correa P, Dalgard DW, McIntire KR, Adamson RH. (1980). Carcinogenicity and hepatoxicity of cycasin and its algycone methylazoxymethanol acetate in nonhuman primates. *J Natl Cancer Inst*, **65**, 177–189.

68. Yang MG, Mickelsen O, Campbell ME, Laqueur GL, Keresztesy JC. (1966). Cycad flour used by Guamanians: effects produced in rats by long-term feeding. *J Nutr*, **90**, 153–156.

69. Spencer PS, Nunn PB, Hugon J, *et al.* (1987). Guam amyotrophic lateral sclerosis-parkinsonism-dementia linked to a plant excitant neurotoxin. *Science*, **237**, 517–522.
70. Garruto RM, Yanagihara R, Gajdusek DC. (1988). Cycads and amyotrophic lateral sclerosis/parkinsonism dementia. *Lancet*, **ii**, 1079.
71. Duncan MW, Kopin IJ, Garruto RM, Lavine L, Markey SP. (1988). 2-amino-3 (methylamino)-propionic acid in cycad-derived foods is an unlikely cause of amyotrophic lateral sclerosis/parkinsonism. *Lancet*, **ii**, 631–632.
72. Duncan MW, Marini AM, Kopin IJ, Markey SP. (1989). BMAA and ALS-PD: A causal link? *International ALS◆MND Update*, 2Q89, 31.
73. Borenstein AR, Mortimer JA, Schofield E, *et al.* (2007). Cycad exposure and risk of dementia, MCI, and PDC in the Chamorro population of Guam. *Neurology*, **68**, 1764–1771.
74. Gajdusek DC. (1990). Cycad toxicity not the cause of high-incidence amyotrophic lateral sclerosis-parkinsonism-dementia on Guam, Kii Peninsula of Japan, or in West New Guinea. In: Hudson AH (ed.), *Amyotrophic Lateral Sclerosis: Concepts in Pathogenesis and Etiology*, pp. 317–325. University of Toronto Press, Toronto.
75. Burkill IH. (1935). *A Dictionary of the Economic Products of the Malay Peninsula*, Vol. 1 (A–H), pp. 729–731. Ministry of Agriculture and Co-operatives, Malaysia, Kuala Lumpur.
76. Cox PA, Sacks OW. (2002). Cycad neurotoxins, consumption of flying foxes, and ALS-PDC disease in Guam. *Neurology*, **58**, 956–959.
77. Murch SJ, Cox PA, Banack SA, Steele JC, Sacks OW. (2004). Occurrence of β-N-methylamino-L-alanine (BMAA) in ALS/PDC patients from Guam. *Acta Neurol Scand*, **110**, 267–269.
78. Pablo J, Banack SA, Cox SA, *et al.* (2009). Cyanobacterial neurotoxin BMAA in ALS and Alzheimer's disease. *Acta Neurol Scand*, **120**, 216–225.
79. Cox PA, Banack SA, Murch SJ, *et al.* (2005). Diverse taxa of cyanobacteria produce β-N-methylamino-L-alanine, a neurotoxic amino acid. *Proc Natl Acad Sci USA* **102**, 5074–5078.
80. Metcalf JS, Banack SA, Lindsay J, Morrison LF, Cox PA, Codd GA. (2008). Co-occurrence of β-N-methylamino-L-alanine, a neurotoxic amino acid with other cyanobacterial toxins in British waterbodies, 1990–2004. *Environ Microbiol*, **10**, 702–708.
81. Murch SJ, Cox PA, Banack SA. (2004). A mechanism for slow release of biomagnified cyanobacterial neurotoxins and neurodegenerative disease in Guam. *Proc Natl Acad Sci USA*, **101**, 12228–12231.
82. Cox PA, Bradley WG (eds.) (2009). Amyotrophic lateral sclerosis: beyond Guam, Cyanobacteria, BMAA, and sporadic amyotrophic lateral sclerosis. *Amyotrophic Lateral Sclerosis (Supplement)*, **10**, 1–126.
83. Rosén J, Hellenäs KE. (2008). Determination of neurotoxins BMAA (β-N-methylamino-L-alanine) in cycad seed and cyanobacteria by LC-MS/MS (liquid chromatography tandem mass spectrometry). *Analyst*, **133**, 1785–1789
84. Buenz EJ, Howe CL. (2007). Beta-methylamino-alanine (BMAA) injuries hippocampal neurons in vivo. *Neurotoxicology*, **28**, 702–704.
85. Lobner D, Piana PMT, Salous AK, Peoples RW. (2007). β-N-methylamino-L-alanine enhances neurotoxicity through multiple mechanisms. *Neurobiol Dis*, **25**, 360–366.
86. Rao SD, Banack SA, Cox PA, Weiss JH. (2006). BMAA selectively injures motor neurons via AMPA/kainate receptor activation. *Exp Neurol*, **201**, 244–252.
87. Ly PTT, Singh S, Shaw CA. (2007). Novel environmental toxins: steryl glycosides as a potential etiological factor for age-related neurodegenerative diseases. *J Neurosci Res*, **85**, 231–237.
88. Karamyan VT, Speth RC. (2008). Animal models of BMAA neurotoxity: a critical review. *Life Sci*, **82**, 233–246.

89. Papapetropoulos S. (2007). Is there a role for naturally occurring cyanobacterial toxins in neurodegeneration? The beta-N-methylamino-L-alanine (BMAA) paradigm. *Neurochem Int*, **50**, 998–1003.
90. Ince PG, Codd GA. (2005). Return of the cycad hypothesis—does the amyotrophic lateral sclerosis/parkinsonism dementia complex (ALS/PDC) of Guam have new implications for global health? *Neuropathol Appl Neurobiol*, **31**, 345–353.
91. Steele JC, McGeer PL. (2008). The ALS/PDC syndrome of Guam and the cycad hypothesis. *Neurology*, **70**, 1984–1990.
92. Cruz-Aguado R, Winkler D, Shaw CA. (2006). Lack of behavioral and neuropathological effects of dietary β-methylamino-L-alanine (BMAA) in mice. *Pharmacol Biochem Behav*, **84**, 294–299.
93. Santiago M, Matarredona ER, Machado A, Cano J. (2006). Acute perfusion of BMAA in the rat's striatum by in vivo microdialysis. *Toxicol Lett*, **167**, 34–39.
94. Montine TJ, Li K, Perl DP, Galasko D. (2005). Lack of β-N-methylamino-L-alanine in brain from controls, AD, or Chamorros with PDC. *Neurology*, **65**, 768–769.
95. Plato CC, Cruz M. (1967). Blood group and haptoglobin frequencies of the Chamorros of Guam. *Am J Hum Genet*, **19**, 722–731.
96. Plato CC, Galasko D, Garruto RM, *et al.* (2002). ALS and PDC of Guam: forty-year follow-up. *Neurology*, **58**, 765–773.
97. Blake NM, Kirk RL, Wilson SR, *et al.* (1983). Search for a red cell enzyme or serum protein marker in amyotrophic lateral sclerosis and parkinsonism-dementia of Guam. *Am J Med Genet*, **14**, 299–305.
98. Garruto RM, Plato CC, Myrianthopoulos NC, Schanfield MS, Gajdusek DC. (1983). Blood groups, immunoglobulin allotypes and dermatoglyphic features of patients with amyotrophic lateral sclerosis and parkinsonism-dementia of Guam. *Am J Med Genet*, **14**, 289–298.
99. Plato CC, Garruto RM, Fox KM, Gajdusek DC. (1986). Amyotrophic lateral sclerosis and parkinsonism-dementia on Guam: a 25-year retrospective case-control study. *Am J Epidemiol*, **124**, 643–656.
100. Sieh W, Choi Y, Chapman NH, *et al.* (2009). Identification of novel susceptibility loci for Guam Neurodegenerative disease: challenges of genome scans in genetic isolates. *Hum Mol Genet*, **18**(19), 3725–3738.
101. Hoffman PM, Robbins DS, Gibbs CJ Jr, Gajdusek DC, Garruto RM, Terasaki PI. (1977). Histocompatability antigens in amyotrophic lateral sclerosis and parkinsonism-dementia on Guam. *Lancet*, **ii**, 717.
102. Reed DM, Torres JM, Brody JA. (1975). Amyotrophic lateral sclerosis and parkinsonism-dementia on Guam, 1945–1972. II. Familial and genetic studies. *Am J Epidemiol*, **101**, 302–310.
103. Figlewicz DA, Garruto RM, Krizus A, Yanagihara R, Rouleau GA. (1994). The Cu/Zn superoxide dismutase gene in ALS and parkinsonism-dementia of Guam. *Neuroreport*, **5**, 557–560.
104. Poorkaj P, Tsuang D, Wijsman E, *et al.* (2001). TAU as a susceptibility gene for amyotrophic lateral sclerosis-parkinsonism dementia complex of Guam. *Arch Neurol*, **58**, 1871–1878.
105. Sundar PD, Yu CE, Sieh W, *et al.* (2007). Two sites in the MAPT region confer genetic risk for Guam ALS/PDC and dementia. *Hum Mol Genet*, **16**, 295–306.
106. Morris HR, Steele JC, Crook R, *et al.* (2004). Genome-wide analysis of the parkinsonism-dementia complex of Guam. *Arch Neurol*, **61**, 1889–1897.
107. Bailey-Wilson JE, Plato CC, Elston RC, Garruto RM. (1993). Potential role of an additive genetic component in the cause of amyotrophic lateral sclerosis and parkinsonism-dementia in the western Pacific. *Am J Med Genet*, **45**, 68–76.
108. Chinopoulos C, Adam-Vizi V. (2006). Calcium, mitochondria and oxidative stress in neuronal pathology. Novel aspects of an enduring theme. *FEBS J*, **273**, 433–450.

109. Kraft R, Grimm C, Grosse K, *et al.* (2004). Hydrogen peroxide and ADP-ribose induced TRPM2-mediated calcium influx and cation currents in microglia. *Am J Physiol*, **286**, C129-C137.

110. Kaneko S, Kawakami S, Hara Y, *et al.* (2006). A critical role of TRPM2 in neuronal cell death by hydrogen peroxide. *J Pharmacol Sci*, **101**, 67–76.

111. Perraud AL, Fleig A, Dunn CA, *et al.* (2001). ADP-ribose gating of the calcium-permeable LTRPC2 channel revealed by Nudix motif homology. *Nature*, **411**, 595–599.

112. Sano Y, Inamura K, Miyake A, *et al.* (2001). Immunocyte Ca^{2+} influx system mediated by LTRPC2. *Science*, **293**, 1327–1330.

113. Lynch D, Wanglund C, Spathis R, *et al.* (2007). The contribution of mitochondrial dysfunction to a gene-environment model of Guamanian ALS and PD. *Mitochondrion*, **8**, 109–116.

114. Gaspari M, Larson NG, Gustafsoon CM. (2004). The transcription machinery in mammalian mitochondria. *Biochim Biophys Acta*, **1659**, 148–152.

115. Coskun PE, Beal M, Wallace DC. (2004). Alzheimer's brains harbor somatic mtDNA control-region mutations that suppress mitochondrial transcription and replication. *Proc Natl Acad Sci USA*, **101**, 10726–10731.

116. Reiff DM, Spathis S, Chan CW, *et al.* (2011). The role of inherited and somatic mitochondrial DNA mutations in Guam ALS and PD. *Neurological Sciences*, **32**, 883–892.

117. Friedlander JS, Friedlander FR, Hodgson JA, *et al.* (2007). Melanesian mtDNA complexity. *PLoS ONE*, **2**, e248.

118. Hill C, Soares P, Mormina M, *et al.* (2007). A mitochondrial stratigraphy for Island Southeast Asia. *Am J Hum Gene*, **80**, 29–43.

119. Bergmann M, Kuchelmeister K, Schmid KW, Kretzschmar HA, Schröder R. (1996). Different variants of frontotemporal dementia: a neuropathological and immunohistochemical study. *Acta Neuropathol (Berl)*, **92**, 170–179.

120. Iseki E, Li F, Odawara T, Hino H, *et al.* (1998). Ubiquitin-immunohistochemical investigation of atypical Pick's disease without Pick bodies. *J Neurol Sci*, **159**, 194–201.

121. Jackson M, Lennox G, Lowe J. (1996). Motor neuron disease-inclusion dementia. *Neurodegeneration*, **5**, 339–350.

122. Okamoto K, Murukami N, Kusada H, *et al.* (1992). Ubiquitin-positive intraneuronal inclusions in the extramotor cortices of presenile dementia patients with motor neuron disease. *J Neurol*, **239**, 426–430.

123. Wightman G, Anderson VER, Martin AJ, *et al.* (1992). Hippocampal and neocortical ubiquitin-immunoreactive inclusions in amyotrophic lateral sclerosis with dementia. *Neurosci Lett*, **139**, 269–274.

124. Geser F, Winton MJ, Kwong LK, *et al.* (2008). Pathological TDP-43 in parkinsonism-dementia complex and amytrophic lateral sclerosis of Guam. *Acta Neuropathol*, **115**, 133–145.

125. Hasegawa M, Arai T, Akiyama H, *et al.* (2007). TDP-43 is deposited in the Guam parkinsonism-dementia complex brains. *Brain*, **130**, 1386–1394.

126. Miklossy J, Steele JC, Yu S, *et al.* (2008). Enduring involvement of tau, β-amyloid, α synuclein, ubiquitin and TDP-43 pathology in the amyotrophic lateral sclerosis/parkinsonism-dementia complex of Guam (ALS/PDC). *Acta Neuropathol*, **116**, 625–637.

127. Ayala Y, Pantano S, D'Ambrogio A, *et al.* (2005). Human, drosophila, and C. elegans TDP43: nucleic acid binding properties and splicing regulatory function. *J Mol Biol*, **348**, 575–588.

128. Buratti E, Brindisi A, Giombi M, Tisminetzky S, Ayala YM, Baralle FE. (2005). TDP-43 binds heterogeneous nuclear ribonucleoprotein A/B through its C terminal tail. *J Biol Chem*, **280**, 37572–3758.

129. Strong MJ, Volkening K, Hammond R, *et al.* (2007). TDP43 is a human low molecular weight neurofilament (*h*NFL) mRNA-binding protein. *Mol Cell Neurosci*, **35**, 320–327.

130. Arnold A, Edgren DC, Palladino VS. (1953). Amyotrophic lateral sclerosis: Fifty cases observed on Guam. *J Nerv Ment Dis*, **177**, 135–139.
131. Tillema S, Wijnberg CJ. (1953). 'Endemic' amyotrophic lateral sclerosis on Guam; epidemiological data. A preliminary report. *Doc Med Geogr Trop*, **5**, 366–370.
132. Zimmerman HM (June 1, 1945). Monthly report to medical officer in command, U.S. Naval Medical Research Unit Number 2.
133. Safford WE. (1905). *The Useful Plants of the Island of Guam*. Smithsonian Institution, Government Printing Office, Washington DC.
134. Carano P, Sanchez P. (1964). *A Complete History of Guam*, Charles Tuttle Company, Rutland, Vermont.
135. Yanagihara RT, Garruto RM, Gajdusek DC. (1983). Epidemiological surveillance of amyotrophic lateral sclerosis and parkinsonism-dementia in the Commonwealth of the Northern Mariana Islands. *Ann Neurol*, **13**, 79–86.
136. Waddington CH. (1942). The epigenotype. *Endeavour*, **1**, 18–20.
137. Waddington CH. (1953). Genetic assimilation of an acquired character. *Evolution*, **7**, 118–126.
138. Waddington CH. (1956). Genetic assimilation of the bithorax phenotype. *Evolution*, **10**, 1–13.
139. Russo VEA, Martienssen RA, Riggs AD (eds.). (1996). *Epigenetic Mechanisms of Gene Regulation.* Cold Spring Harbor Laboratory Press, Woodbury.
140. Feinberg AP. (2008). Epigenetics at the center of modern medicine. *J Am Med Assoc*, **299**, 1345–1350.
141. Penner MR, Roth TL, Barnes CA, Sweat JD. (2010). An epigenetic hypothesis of aging-related cognitive dysfunction. *Frontiers Aging Neurosci*, **2**, 1–11.
142. Bird A. (2007). Perceptions of epigenetics. *Nature*, **447**, 396–398.

Chapter 2

The motor neurone diseases

Jeffrey Rosenfeld

Motor neurone disease (MND) refers to a spectrum of disorders resulting from degeneration of the upper (UMN) and/or lower motor neurone (LMN) population. Currently, the diagnostic distinctions within this spectrum of MND are dependent upon clinical and electrophysiological evidence of UMN versus LMN involvement as well as the distribution of clinical signs along the neuraxis (Table 2.1). The contrast between bulbar and limb predominance, UMN versus LMN predominance, rapid versus slow progression and the extent of cognitive involvement can be striking. Recently, an increasing number of genetic abnormalities have been identified, which further define specific inherited variants of MND and serve as a diagnostic standard in those specific clinical settings (1,2). In addition, historically there have been geographical regions identified worldwide where the incidence rates of MND subtypes are disproportionately high, implicating a distinct potential aetiology in those patients (3–7).

The clinical variability underlying the MND disorders has been a challenge in identifying therapeutic strategies in heterogeneous treatment groups. Distinct aetiologies have been proposed, including genetic, biochemical, metabolic, cytoskeletal, and inflammatory mechanisms (8,9). These may serve as either a primary or secondary processes underlying the disparate clinical presentations.

The term amyotrophic lateral sclerosis (ALS) and MND are often used synonymously. However, MND is more accurately thought of as a category of disease presentations encompassing a great variety of clinical phenotypes. In the UK and in some European countries, the term MND is synonymous with ALS. In the United States and Canada, however, MND refers to a more general spectrum of disorders involving degeneration of motor neurones. ALS, by contrast, is limited to those clinical syndromes where *both* UMN and LMN clinical pathology exists along the neuraxis, often affecting bulbar and limb regions. Historically, there have been four categories of ALS clinical variants recognized despite the solitary ALS nomenclature.

1. The classical sporadic variant as originally described by Charcot (10).
2. A familial form of ALS defined by an increasing number of mutations affecting several genes (1,2) (see Tables 2.2, 2.3).
3. A geographical variant of ALS restricted to an area in the western Pacific implicating an environmental aetiology (3,11,12).

Table 2.1 The diversity of motor neurone disease

Disorder	Pathology	Clinical signs/symptoms	Genetics	Disease course
Amyotrophic lateral sclerosis	UMN and LMN	Varies widely: weakness, atrophy, spasticity, dysarthria, dyspnoea, dysphagia	By definition, sporadic	Varies widely often dependent upon the degree of supportive care
Primary lateral sclerosis	UMN	Spasticity and rigidity	Familial patterns identified, no specific genes implicated yet	Often prolonged, >10 years
Progressive muscular atrophy	LMN	Weakness and atrophy	Familial forms referred to as spinal muscular atrophy	Varies widely, some rapidly progressive forms have been described
Bulbar ALS	UMN and/or LMN (usually both)	Predominant dysarthria, dysphagia, dyspnoea, sialorrhoea AND weakness, atrophy, spasticity	Some forms of bALS are familial see Table 2.3	Usually more aggressive, disease course depends heavily upon the degree of supportive interventions
Progressive bulbar palsy	UMN > LMN	Dysarthria, dysphagia, dyspnoea, sialorrhoea	Sporadic	Similar to bALS
Familial myotrophic lateral sclerosis	UMN and/or LMN (usually both)	Varies widely: weakness, atrophy, spasticity, dysarthria, dyspnoea, dysphagia	>50 mutations implicated on 12 genes	Varies widely by phenotype

LMN, lower motor neurone; UMN, upper motor neurone.

4. Anatomical variants of ALS where clinical pathology is restricted to either bulbar *or* limb involvement (predominantly). Patients affected solely with bulbar pathology are also often referred as having progressive bulbar palsy (also known as progressive bulbar atrophy), whereas patients affected with bulbar predominant symptoms are referred to as bulbar ALS (13–16).

Furthermore, our traditional view of ALS as a disorder restricted to the motor system has been greatly modified by recognition of comorbid syndromes of frontotemporal dysfunction in up to 30–50% of patients (17,18). As discussed elsewhere in this text, patients with ALS are now identified as having primarily cognitive or behavioural pathology versus primary motor symptoms and more subtle cognitive involvement. ALS is therefore best viewed a multisystem disorder in which the motor system is affected early and the patient's symptoms are progressive (19). Multisystem involvement is supported by the range of concurrent cognitive, behavioural, or dysexecutive symptoms. In a subgroup, a more florid dementia consistent with a frontotemporal dementia will be evident (see subsequent chapters).

The heterogeneity of clinical presentation in patients diagnosed with 'ALS' has presented a great challenge to the discovery of underlying mechanisms; it remains unclear if

Table 2.2 Genetic heterogeneity of familial amyotrophic lateral sclerosis (ALS). All mutations are transmitted via autosomal dominant inheritance except ALS2 and ALS5, which are autosomal recessive. Multiple unique mutations exist in many of loci listed below (2)

Onset	Name	Linkage	Gene	Protein
Adult	ALS1	21q22.1	*SOD1*	Cu/Zn SOD
Juvenile	ALS2	2q33–35	*ALS2*	Alsin
Adult	ALS3	18q21	Unknown	
Juvenile	ALS4	9q34	*SETX*	Senataxin
Juvenile	ALS5	15q15–q22	Unknown	
Adult	ALS6	16q12	Unknown	
Adult	ALS7	20p	Unknown	
Adult	ALS8	20q13.33	*VAPB*	VAMP
Adult	ALS9	14q11	*ANG*	Angiogenin
Adult	ALS10	1q36	*TARDBP*	TDP-43
Adult	ALS/FTD	9q21–22	Unknown	
Juvenile	ALS/FTD2	9p13.2–21.3	Unknown	
Juvenile		7q34–q36	Unknown	

this clinical spectrum reflects disparate aetiologies with distinct pathogenesis or multiple presentations of a single pathogenic mechanism.

Historical understanding of motor neurone disease/ amyotrophic lateral sclerosis

Duchenne and Aran first described a LMN disorder, which we accept today as progressive muscular atrophy (PMA) (20–22). Recognition of a MND affecting speech and swallowing was next characterized 10 years later by Duchenne as progressive bulbar palsy. In 1874, Charcot and Cuveilheir described a syndrome of corticospinal tract pathology and anterior horn cell degeneration. The concept of generalized motor neurone involvement was thus introduced as ALS (10). Shortly after this report, a syndrome of isolated UMN pathology was introduced as primary lateral sclerosis (PLS) (Erb), not associated with atrophy or weakness (23).

Currently, there remains significant controversy whether ALS, progressive bulbar palsy, bulbar ALS, PLS, and PMA are all variations along a continuum of a single disease entity. This controversy has been further strained by the increasing recognition of cognitive involvement in some affected patients.

In 1994, the World Federation of Neurology drafted formal guidelines in an attempt to standardize diagnostic criteria primarily for research purposes (24). These criteria were subsequently modified in response to desire from the research community to include patients at earlier stages of disease progression as well as recognition of the great variety of disease phenotypes that were being excluded using the original criteria (25). These diagnostic criteria have been further refined to define a patient population based primarily on their electrophysiological abnormalities (26,27).

World Federation Diagnostic Criteria (24)

These criteria remain the most widely accepted for diagnostic and research purposes. Upper *and* lower motor signs found in the bulbar region *and* at least two regions along the neuraxis (cervical, thoracic, lumbosacral) are required for **definite ALS**. Alternatively, UMN *and* LMN signs can be present in three regions, sparing bulbar areas at the time of diagnosis. **Probable ALS** requires UMN *and* LMN signs in at least two spinal regions. At least one UMN sign should be present rostral to at least one LMN sign. For patients with minimal signs and symptoms, **probable laboratory supported ALS** can include patients with UMN and LMN signs in only one region; however, electrophysiological evidence of denervation in at least two regions where other aetiologies have been excluded. Patients with **possible ALS** have UMN *and* LMN findings in only one region or UMN findings in at least two regions or LMN signs rostral to UMN signs.

Clinical features

Weakness and atrophy are the most common clinical symptoms triggering medical attention in the early stages of MND/ALS. Although the signs, symptoms, and distribution vary widely, the diagnostic hallmark of UMN and LMN signs are required for confirmation in all forms of ALS. Bulbar presentation of impaired speech, swallowing, and/or breathing is less common but still requires the clinical signs of UMN and LMN pathology.

Fasciculations (muscle twitching) are a common source of patient concern for the possibility of an underlying motor neurone disease. In the absence of weakness and atrophy, fasciculations are typically benign and even in the presence of concurrent weakness are neither specific nor sensitive enough to be used in routine practice for definitive diagnosis (28).

Clinical detection of LMN disease includes muscle weakness, atrophy, and loss of deep tendon reflexes. These findings should always be associated with abnormal electromyography. The presence of spontaneous activity (acutely, fibrillations, and positive sharp waves) and/or reduced recruitment and motor unit remodelling are the electrical correlates of denervation due to motor neurone loss. An electromyogram reported to be normal in a muscle weakened by lower MND is not physiological. Conversely, electromyography can often be abnormal before the onset of muscle weakness in lower motor involvement. This might ultimately be the earliest preclinical disease marker (27). The most convincing LMN sign suggestive of MND includes atrophy of the tongue muscle, a muscle not commonly affected in other conditions (Figure 2.1).

UMN signs largely result from the loss of descending corticospinal tract pathways. The disinhibition of the LMN, resulting from the absence of these upper motor pathways, causes both rigidity and spasticity. Poor control from the central nervous system due to UMN loss, can result in discoordination, brisk reflexes, and the presence of pathological reflexes not usually present (i.e. jaw jerk, palmomental response, persistent glabellar

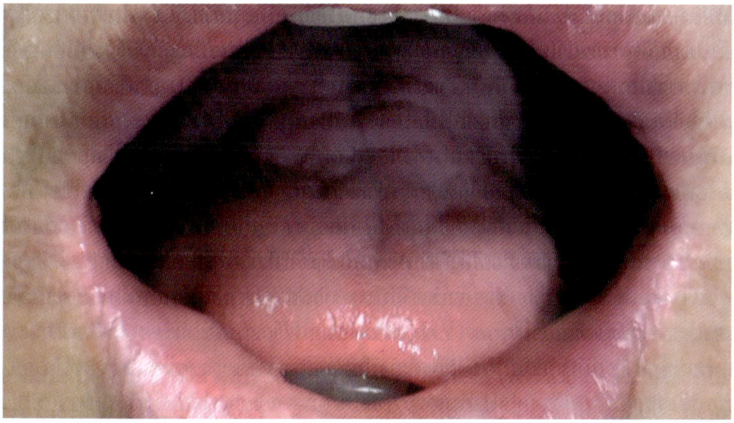

Fig. 2.1 Atrophy and weakness of the tongue muscle, frequently a confirming sign of motor neurone disease.

response, finger flexion (Tromner) and Hoffman's reflex). Emotional lability, also known as pseudobulbar affect, is another consequence of central disinhibition (29).

Clinical variability

As noted earlier, the diagnostic criteria summarized above only allow for the description of the motor manifestations of ALS. They do not address the considerable clinical heterogeneity with which ALS can present, including wide variability with respect to the affected areas, rates of disease progression, associated non-motor manifestations, and the nature of the patient disability, as well as the impact on quality or duration of life. These observations have resulted in the now commonly held belief that ALS is a syndrome rather than a specific disease. Furthermore, the clinical variability coupled with the disparate proposed mechanisms of motor neurone death has led to the suggestion that various subgroups of patients affected with 'ALS' may be due to different aetiologies.

This heterogeneity in disease presentation can present both a challenge and an opportunity. If, for example, certain therapeutic agents work in one 'type' of ALS but not another, then the failure of the current diagnostic criteria to discriminate between the two would confound efforts in drug discovery, particularly if the natural history of the two variants differed significantly. Alternatively, recognition of individual disease presentations, in conjunction with available biomarkers, drugs, and therapies may allow for more rapid progress in our understanding of underlying disease mechanism(s) that may apply.

Variations in classical amyotrophic lateral sclerosis/motor neurone disease

As described by Charcot the diagnostic criteria of UMN and LMN involvement includes both significant regional involvement on the neuraxis (bulbar, limb, extra motor) and anatomical involvement (extent of UMN versus LMN). Recently, there has been more acceptance of distinct groups where upper versus lower motor pathology is predominant and persists through the course of the disease (30–34). UMN predominant ALS (UMN/ALS) is generally accepted as having a more benign course and prognosis (35). Diagnostic classification schemes for UMN/ALS distinguish clinically pure upper motor pathology (PLS) from mixed UMN and LMN pathology (36,37). Several reports suggest that survival is negatively impacted by the degree to which LMN pathology evolves in the patient with UMN/ALS. PLS is accepted as generally having the most prolonged and benign course whereas UMN/ALS followed by generalized ALS are more aggressive forms of MND (16,38–40). Axial or bulbar involvement is a significant factor confounding estimates of disease course and mortality even in PLS and UMN/ALS. Patients with prominent bulbar presentations of either condition may progress more like what is expected in generalized ALS (16).

Lower motor syndromes also tend to be heterogeneous with respect to disease progression and mortality. Pure LMN disease (PMA) can be quite benign, particularly when the disease is limited to few extremities, sparing bulbar function. By contrast, some patients with PMA experience a very virulent course with rapid progression of both bulbar and extremity involvement despite aggressive supportive care (15,30,31,41). There are, as yet, no clinical markers that will crisply differentiate between those with a more benign versus aggressive course of PMA. Specific phenotypes of LMN disease (PMA variants) have been identified affecting primarily the upper extremities (23,42,43) or the lower extremities (23,44). These conditions can be fairly indolent for years, limited to the initially affected extremities. A subset of these patients will progress to generalized MND.

LMN disease affecting only one extremity is referred to as monomelic amyotrophy. This was originally described in Japanese children or young adults as weakness of the distal upper extremity and has been referred to as either 'Hirayama's syndrome' or the 'Sobue variant' (45–47). A variant affecting older individuals is often referred to as the 'flail arm variant'. This rare condition is usually limited to cervical myotomes (75%) with weakness affecting mostly hand and forearm muscles. Men are preferentially affected (by almost ninefold). Typically, the condition progresses very slowly and is always limited to LMN pathology in the absence of UMN signs. Sensory symptoms of hypesthesia to pin and touch in the affected limb have been described in approximately 20% of patients. A subset of these patients (≤50%) will progress to involve the contralateral limb. Magnetic resonance imaging studies may reveal cervical spinal cord atrophy due to laxity of the dura, stretched across the cord during neck flexion (48). Detection of this magnetic resonance imaging finding may require imaging of the neck in full flexion.

Variations in genetically defined amyotrophic lateral sclerosis/ motor neurone disease

The majority of patients presenting with ALS have a sporadic onset. Approximately 5–10% of patients, however, have a familial (usually autosomal dominant) pattern of inheritance. Mutations affecting the *SOD1* gene were originally described in 1993 in families affected by ALS (49). Since then many additional genes, proteins, and phenotypic presentations have been identified but mutations in the *SOD1* gene still account for the majority (20%) of all the familial presentations. Over 120 different mutations have

Table 2.3 Phenotypic variability of *SOD* mutations in familial amyotrophic lateral sclerosis

Phenotype	*SOD1* mutation
LMN predominant	A4V, L84V, D101N
UMN predominant	D90A
Slow progression	G37 R (18 years), G41D (11 years), G93C, L144S, L144F
Fast progression	A4T (1.5 years), N86S (homozygous 5 months), L 106V (1.2 years), V148G (2 years)
Late onset	G85R, H46R
Early onset	G37R, L38V
Female predominant	G41D
Bulbar onset	V148I
Low penetrance	D90A, I113T
Posterior column involvement	E100G

LMN, lower motor neurone; SOD, superoxide dismutase; UMN, upper motor neurone

been identified in the *SOD1* gene (see http://alsod.iop.kcl.ac.uk for an up to date summary of *SOD1* mutations associated with both familial and sporadic (less than 7% of cases)), many of which are associated with specific disease phenotypes that correlate with the rate of disease progression. While it is generally accepted that the toxicity of the mutated SOD1 protein is a primary pathogenic mechanism in the disease, there is less agreement with respect to the mechanism by which this toxicity occurs. In reality, it is most likely that the toxicity of mutated SOD1 is multifactorial and includes perturbations in DNA and RNA metabolism, mitochondrial function, axonal transport, and immunologically mediated pathways (2,50).

Recently, mutations in the *TARDBP* gene have been shown to affect RNA processing in both familial and some sporadic forms of ALS (see Buratti (Chapter 24) and Volkening and Strong (Chapter 22) for a detailed discussion). The transactive response DNA-binding protein of 43 kDa (TDP-43) has been implicated as impairing transcriptional regulation, binding both RNA and DNA. Abnormalities in TDP-43 protein have also generated significant interest in the overlap between frontotemporal dementia and ALS.

To date, at least 10 different genes affecting at least 15 different loci have been implicated as a primary disease pathogenesis (see Table 2.2). These implicated genes have been associated with approximately 25 different phenotypic presentations, supporting the contention that there is more than one primary pathological mechanism responsible for disease presentation. However, there are no phenotypic characteristics that distinguish between patients with familial and sporadic ALS. Indeed, there are likely to be greater numbers of patients with sporadic ALS identified to have an underlying genetic basis than is classically believed. Such a concept is supported by twin studies of affected patients resulting in heritability estimates ranging from 0.38 to 0.85, higher than originally suspected (51). Although not the specific focus of this chapter, it is also important to recognize that genome-wide association studies identified an abundance of candidate genes and proteins appropriate for subsequent study (51,52) (see also Traynor, Chapter 20).

Variations in geographically defined amyotrophic lateral sclerosis/motor neurone disease

The incidence of ALS on the Pacific island of Guam has been documented to be at least 50 times greater than the incidence found in the United States (53) (see also Garruto, Chapter 1). The clinical characteristics of patients with ALS offer interesting clues and speculation on the potential overlap of the clinically distinct neurological conditions in this endemic area. Post-mortem analyses of this patient population reveal the formation of extensive neurofibrillary tangles (54,55). Several of these cytoskeletal abnormalities are identical to those found in Alzheimer's disease leading to speculation of common mechanisms of cell death in these two otherwise distinct conditions (56). The incidence of parkinsonism was also higher among the Chamorro people of Guam and the surrounding islands compared with incidence rates reported elsewhere (55). Similar pathological changes with neurofibrillary tangles and accumulations of abnormal protein have been reported in these patients further contributing to the speculation of common mechanisms leading to cell death in these distinct neurological conditions. Understanding the overlap in post-mortem findings from patients with ALS, Parkinson's disease, and Alzheimer's disease is also confounded by the recognition that patients in this region commonly share multiple characteristics of Parkinson's disease, ALS as well as dementia (ALS/parkinsonism–dementia complex), a phenomenon originally thought to be largely limited to the Chamorros in this area of the Pacific.

Such endemic clusters of ALS have been provocative areas of investigation as they offer the potential to elucidate important clues to disease aetiology. Although these high incidence rates suggest an underlying genetic predisposition, to date only linkage to the mammalian transient receptor potential melastatin 2 (*TRPM2* and *TRPM7* genes) has proven to be robust (57). The place-specific incidence rates suggested a significant environmental trigger for this variant of ALS. A popular concept has been that this environmental factor was the consumption of a traditional Chamorro diet, in which cycad was a major component (58). The presence of the neurotoxin β-methyl-amino-L-alanine (BMAA) in unprocessed cycad, as well as its ability to function as a potent glutamate antagonist on motor neurones, led to its implication as a causative agent in this susceptible population (59,60). In support of this, high concentrations of BMAA (mean 627 μg/g) were observed in the superior frontal gyrus of six patients with ALS/parkinsonism–dementia complex in contrast to the mean levels (82 μg/g) observed in asymptomatic Chamorro controls (59). BMAA was not observed in 13 non-neurological disease controls obtained from outside Guam.

The Pacific islands around Guam are not the only region where a common overlap between ALS, Parkinson's disease, and Alzheimer's disease exists. The Kii Peninsula of Japan is home to another endemic area of patients with symptoms of Parkinson's disease, ALS, and cognitive impairment. Initial symptoms include a parkinsonian gait or hypobulia/amnesia, akinesia, rigidity, tremor, and eventually akinetic mutism. Several years after onset, most of the patients develop features of ALS, including muscle atrophy, bulbar palsy, and UMN signs. Neurofibrillary tangles and abnormal accumulations of tau protein are found in these patients, similar to that found in patients with Alzheimer's disease. Multiple hypotheses have been offered to link risk factors among the Chammoros and patients in this region. However, a causative toxic or environmental agent has not been definitively identified and this still remains an active area of investigation.

In summary, since the early clinical descriptions, much has been added to our understanding of ALS as a complex clinical and pathological condition. The phenotypic heterogeneity of both sporadic and familial forms of ALS is vast. It is generally accepted that ALS is a multisystem disorder variably affecting components of the motor system and often behaviour and cognition. The presentation and distribution of affected areas and disease course are quite variable. Currently, significant supportive and adjunctive therapies exist, which significantly impact the quality and duration of a patient's life. These successful therapeutic measures further contribute a source of variability confounding the study of potential therapies.

Advances in our understanding of the pathophysiology of ALS have also rapidly grown. Similar to the clinical heterogeneity, the mechanism(s) leading to motor neurone cell death are diverse and exist in parallel. It remains unresolved whether different pathological mechanisms predominate in different clinical variations of the disease. The requirement for multidrug, 'cocktail' therapy is likely an inevitable consequence of our current understanding. Future clinical trials may require stratification to address the clinical diversity and impact on disease-modifying therapies; both of which confound efforts to identify a new pharmacological agent to treat the syndrome of ALS.

References

1. Orrell RW, Figlewicz DA. (2001). Clinical implications of the genetics of ALS and other motor neuron diseases. *Neurology*, **57**, 9–17.
2. Beleza-Meireles A, Al-Chalabi A. (2009). Genetic studies of amyotrophic lateral sclerosis: controversies and perspectives. *Amyotroph Lateral Scler*, **10**, 1–14.
3. Tillema S, Wijnberg CJ. (1953). 'Epidemic' amyotrophic lateral sclerosis on Guam: epidemiologic data. *Doc Med Geog Trop*, **5**, 366–370.
4. Horner RD, Grambow SC, Coffman CJ, *et al.* (2008). Amyotrophic lateral sclerosis among 1991 Gulf War veterans: evidence for a time-limited outbreak. *Neuroepidemiology*, **31**, 28–32.
5. Uccelli R, Binazzi A, Altavista P, *et al.* (2007). Geographic distribution of amyotrophic lateral sclerosis through motor neuron disease mortality data. *Eur J Epidemiol*, **22**, 781–790.
6. Cox PA, Richer R, Metcalf JS, *et al.* (2009). Cyanobacteria and BMAA exposure from desert dust: a possible link to sporadic ALS among Gulf War veterans. *Amyotroph Lateral Scler*, **10**(Suppl. 2), 109–117
7. Bharucha NE, Schoenberg BS, Raven RH, *et al.* (1983). Geographic distribution of motor neuron disease and correlation with possible etiologic factors. *Neurology*, **33**, 911–915.
8. Strong MJ, Rosenfeld J. (2003). Amyotrophic lateral sclerosis: a review of current concepts. *Amyotroph Lateral Scler Other Motor Neuron Disord*, **4**, 136–143.
9. Strong MJ. (2010). The evidence for altered RNA metabolism in amyotrophic lateral sclerosis (ALS). *J Neurol Sci*, **288**, 1–12.

10. Charcot JM, Joffroy A, (1869). Deux cas d'atrophie musculaire progressive avec lésions de la substance grise et des faisceaux antérolatéraux de la moelle épinière. *Arch Physiol Norm Pathol*, **2**, 354–744.
11. Garruto RM. (1991). Pacific paradigms of environmentally-induced neurological disorders: clinical, epidemiological and molecular perspectives. *NeuroToxicology*, **12**, 347–378.
12. Zhang ZX, Anderson DW, Mantel N, *et al.* (1996). Motor neuron disease on Guam: geographic and familial occurrence, 1956–85. *Acta Neurol Scand*, **94**, 51–59.
13. Van den Berg-Vos RM, Van den Berg LH, Visser J, *et al.* (2003). The spectrum of lower motor neuron syndromes. *J Neurol*, **250**, 1279–1292.
14. Lambrechts D, Robberecht W, Carmeliet P. (2007). Heterogeneity in motoneuron disease. *Trends Neurosci*, **30**, 536–544.
15. Rowland LP. (2010). Progressive muscular atrophy and other lower motor neuron syndromes of adults. *Muscle Nerve*, **41**, 161–165.
16. Soraru G, Ermani M, Logroscino G, *et al.* (2010). Natural history of upper motor neuron-dominant ALS. *Amyotroph Lateral Scler*, **11**, 424–429.
17. Strong MJ, Grace GM, Freedman M, *et al.* (2009). Consensus criteria for the diagnosis of frontotemporal cognitive and behavioural syndromes in amyotrophic lateral sclerosis. *Amyotroph Lateral Scler*, **10**, 131–146.
18. Strong MJ. (2008). The syndromes of frontotemporal dysfunction in amyotrophic lateral sclerosis. *Amyotroph Lateral Scler*, **9**, 323–338.
19. Strong MJ. (2001). The evidence for ALS as a multisystems disorder of limited phenotypic expression. *Can J Neurol Sci*, **28**, 283–298.
20. Duchenne (De Boulogne). (1860). Paralysie musculaire progressive de la langue, du voile du palais et des levres; affection non encore decrite comme espece morbide distincte. *Arch Gen Med*, **16**, 283–296.
21. Aran FA. (1850). Recherches sur une maladie non encore décrite du systéme musculaire (atrophie musculaire progressive). *Arch Gén de Méd*, **24**, 5–35.
22. Aran FA. (1850). Recherches sur une maladie non encore décrite du systéme musculaire (atrophie musculaire progressive)(2e article—suite et fin). *Arch Gén de Méd*, **24**, 172–214.
23. Swash M, Desai J. (2000). Motor neuron disease: classification and nomenclature. *Amyotroph Lateral Scler Other Motor Neuron Disord*, **1**, 105–112.
24. World Federation of Neurology Research Group on Neuromuscular Disease. (1994). El Escorial World Federation of Neurology criteria for the diagnosis of amyotrophic lateral sclerosis. *J Neurol Sci*, **124**(Suppl.), 96–107.
25. Brooks BR, Miller RG, Swash M, *et al.* (2000). El Escorial revisited: revised criteria for the diagnosis of amyotrophic lateral sclerosis. *Amyotroph Lateral Scler Other Motor Neuron Disord*, **1**, 293–299.
26. Carvalho MD, Swash M. (2009). Awaji diagnostic algorithm increases sensitivity of El Escorial criteria for ALS diagnosis. *Amyotroph Lateral Scler*, **10**, 53–57.
27. Douglass CP, Kandler RH, Shaw PJ, *et al.* (2010). An evaluation of neurophysiological criteria used in the diagnosis of motor neuron disease. *J Neurol Neurosurg Psychiatry*, **81**, 646–649.
28. Rosenfeld J. (2000). Fasciculations without fibrillations: the dilemma of early diagnosis. *Amyotroph Lateral Scler Other Motor Neuron Disord*, S53–S56.
29. Brooks BR, Thisted RA, Appel SH, *et al.* (2004). Treatment of pseudobulbar affect in ALS with dextromethorphan/quinidine: a randomized trial. *Neurology*, **63**, 1364–1370.
30. Visser J, de Jong JMBV, de Visser M. (2008). The history of progressive muscular atrophy: syndrome or disease? *Neurology*, **70**, 723–727.
31. Maragakis NJ. (2010). Motor neuron disease: progressive muscular atrophy in the ALS spectrum. *Nat Rev Neurol*, **6**, 187–188.

32. Yoshida M. (2004). Amyotrophic lateral sclerosis with dementia: the clinicopathological spectrum. *Neuropathology*, **24**, 87–102.
33. Jackson CE, Rosenfeld J. (2001). Motor neuron disease. *Phys Med Rehabil Clin N Am*, **12**, 335–33x.
34. Ludolph AC, Knirsch U. (1999). Problems and pitfalls in the diagnosis of ALS. *J Neurol Sci*, **165** (Suppl 1), S14–S20.
35. Traynor BJ, Codd MB, Corr B, *et al.* (2000). Clinical features of amyotrophic lateral sclerosis according to the El Escorial and Airlie House diagnostic criteria. *Arch Neurol*, **57**, 1171–1176.
36. Mortara P, Chio A, Rosso MG, *et al.* (1984). Motor neuron disease in the province of Turin, Italy, 1966–1980. Survival analysis in an unselected population. *J Neurol Sci*, **66**, 165–173.
37. Mortara P, Bardelli D, Leone M, *et al.* (1981). Prognosis and clinical varieties of ALS disease. *Ital J Neurol Sci*, **2**, 237–242.
38. Kuipers-Upmeijer J, de Jager AEJ, Hew JM, *et al.* (2001). Primary lateral sclerosis: clinical, neurophysiological, and magnetic resonance findings. *J Neurol Neurosurg Psychiatry*, **71**, 615–620.
39. Le Forestier N, Maisonobe T, Piquard A, *et al.* (2001). Does primary lateral sclerosis exist? A study of 20 patients and a review of the literature. *Brain*, **124**, 1989–1999.
40. Cedarbaum JM, Stambler N, Malta E, *et al.* (1999). The ALSFRS-R: a revised ALS functional rating scale that incorporates assessments of respiratory function. BDNF ALS Study Group (Phase III). *J Neurol Sci*, **169**, 13–21.
41. Van den Berg-Vos RM, Visser J, Kalmijn S, *et al.* (2009). A long-term prospective study of the natural course of sporadic adult-onset lower motor neuron syndromes. *Arch Neurol*, **66**, 751–757.
42. Katz JS, Wolfe GI, Andersson PB, *et al.* (1999). Brachial amyotrophic diplegia: a slowly progressive motor neuron disorder. *Neurology*, **53**, 1071–1076.
43. Hu MTM, Ellis CM, Al-Chalabi A, *et al.* (1998). Flail arm syndrome: a distinctive variant of amyotrophic lateral sclerosis. *J Neurol Neurosurg Psychiatry*, **65**, 950–951.
44. Rosenfeld J, Chang S, Jackson C, *et al.* (2002). Lower extremity amyotrophic diplegia (LAD): A new clinical entity in the spectrum of motor neuron disease. *Neurology*, **58**, A412.
45. Hirayama K, Tomonaga M, Kitano K, *et al.* (1987). Focal cervical poliopathy causing juvenile muscular atrophy of distal upper extremity: a pathological study. *J Neurol Neurosurg Psychiatry*, **50**, 285–290.
46. Hirayama, K. (1991). Non-progressive juvenile spinal muscular atrophy of the distal upper limb (Hirayama's disease). In: de Jong JMBV (ed.), *Handbook of Clinical Neurology*, Vol. **15**(59), pp. 107–120. Elsevier Science Publishers BV, Amsterdam.
47. Sobue I, Saito N, Iida M, *et al.* (1978). Juvenile type of distal and segmental muscular atrophy of upper extremities. *Ann Neurol*, **3**, 429–432.
48. Hirayama K, Tokumaru Y. (2000). Cervical dural sac and spinal cord in juvenile muscular atrophy of distal upper extremity. *Neurology*, **54**, 1922–1926.
49. Siddique T, Figlewicz DA, Pericak-Vance MA *et al.* (1991). Linkage of a gene causing familial amyotrophic lateral sclerosis to chromosome 21 and evidence of genetic-locus heterogeneity. *N Engl J Med*, **324**, 1381–1384.
50. Andersen PM, Morita M, Brown RH, Jr. (2000). Genetics of amyotrophic lateral sclerosis: an overview. In: Brown RH, Jr, Meininger V, Swash M (eds.), *Amyotrophic Lateral Sclerosis*, pp. 223–250. Martin Dunitz Ltd, London.
51. Graham AJ, Macdonald AM, Hawkes CH. (1997). British motor neuron disease twin study. *J Neurol Neurosurg Psychiatry*, **62**, 562–569.
52. Al-Chalabi A, Fang F, Hanby MF, *et al.* (2010). An estimate of amyotrophic lateral sclerosis heritability using twin data. *J Neurol Neurosurg Psychiatry*, **81**, 1324–1326.
53. Kurland LT, Mulder DW. (1954). Epidemiological investigations of amyotrophic lateral sclerosis. 1. Preliminary report on geographic distribution, with special reference to the Mariana Islands, including clinical and pathological observations. *Neurology*, **4**, 355–378, 438–448.

54. Rodgers-Johnson P, Garruto RM, Yanigahara R *et al.* (1986). Amyotrophic lateral sclerosis and parkinsonism-dementia on Guam: a 30-year evaluation of clinical and neuropathological trends. *Neurology*, **36**, 7–13.
55. Garruto RM. (1989). Amyotrophic lateral sclerosis and Parkinsonism-dementia of Guam: clinical, epidemiological and genetic patterns. *Am J Hum Biol*, **1**, 367–382.
56. Guiroy DC, Miyazaki M, Multhaup G, *et al.* (1987). Amyloid of neurofibrillary tangles of Guamanian parkisonism-dementia and Alzheimer disease share identical amino acid sequence. *Proc Natl Acad Sci USA*, **84**, 2073–2077.
57. Hermosura MC, Garruto RM. (2007). TRPM7 and TRPM2—candidate susceptibility genes for western Pacific ALS and PD? *Biochim Biophys Acta*, **1772**, 822–835.
58. Garruto RM, Yanagihara R. (2009). Contributions of isolated Pacific populations to understanding neurodegenerative diseases. *Folia Neuropathol*, **47**, 149–170.
59. Murch SJ, Cox PA, Banack SA, *et al.* (2004). Occurrence of beta-methylamino-l-alanine (BMAA) in ALS/PDC patients from Guam. *Acta Neurol Scand*, **110**, 267–269.
60. Banack SA, Murch SJ. (2009). Multiple neurotoxic items in the Chamorro diet link BMAA with ALS/PDC. *Amyotroph Lateral Scler*, **10** (Suppl 2), 34–40.

Chapter 3

Amyotrophic lateral sclerosis–parkinsonism–dementia complex in the Kii Peninsula of Japan (Muro disease): a review on recent research and new concept

Shigeki Kuzuhara and Yasumasa Kokubo

More than a century ago, Kin-no-suke Miura, Professor of Internal Medicine of the University of Tokyo discovered a high prevalence of amyotrophic lateral sclerosis (ALS) in the Muro district, the mountainous areas of the southern Kii Peninsula (including the southern parts of the Mie and Wakayama prefectures) (Figure 3.1) (1). In the early 1960s, Kimura, Yase and their colleagues performed a door-to-door survey on patients with ALS in the whole of the Muro district, and discovered two foci of extremely high ALS incidence (i.e. Hohara in the Mie prefecture and Kozagawa in the Wakayama prefecture; see Figure 3.1) (2–4). ALS in these foci showed clinical signs and symptoms produced by selective anatomical involvement of the upper and lower motor neurones in the same manner as Charcot had described in sporadic ALS (5), unique neuropathological features were characterized by the presence of many neurofibrillary tangles (NFTs) throughout the central nervous system (4,6) as in ALS of the Chamorro people in Guam, another high-incidence ALS focus (7,8). In the 1960s, Gajdusek discovered a new ALS focus among the Auyu and Jakai people of southeastern West New Guinea (9). Foci of high-incidence ALS in the Kii Peninsula was thus segregated from classical ALS and classified as 'Kii ALS' or 'Muro disease', a member of the hyperendemic western Pacific ALS family (10).

In Guam, another peculiar neurodegenerative disease or 'parkinsonism–dementia complex' (PDC) was discovered (11,12). PDC was characterized clinically by a combination of progressive dementia and atypical progressive parkinsonism poorly responsive to drugs, and neuropathologically by frontotemporal brain atrophy with presence of many NFTs in the whole central nervous system. Mixed ALS and PDC in which both features were clinically and neuropathologically overlapped were also identified, and ALS and PDC in these high-incidence foci were thus regarded as a spectrum of one disease entity or ALS/PDC (13). Extensive studies failed to solve the cause and pathogenesis of

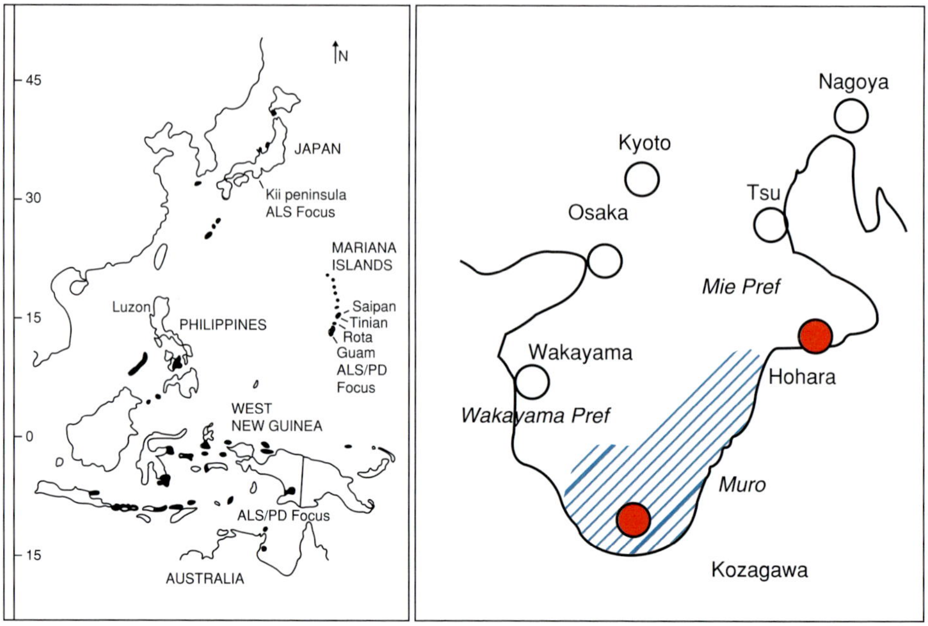

Fig. 3.1 Western Pacific ALS/PDC foci (left) and enlargement of the Kii Peninsula. The shaded areas are the Muro district. Kozagawa and Hohara were the high-incidence ALS foci during 1950–90. (The left map is a modification of the original map in figure 1 of Garruto *et al.* (14).)

high-incidence ALS/PDC. Meanwhile, high-incidence rates of ALS markedly declined in the 1960s and 1970s, and spontaneously disappeared by the early 1980s in Guam (14). A similar decline of high-incidence rates of ALS during the 1980s was also reported in foci of the Kii Peninsula (15) and West New Guinea (16).

In early 1990s, Kuzuhara paid attention to the reoccurrence of ALS among residents in the Hohara focus. After several years' investigations, we confirmed not only the high-incidence rates of ALS but also the coexistence of a high incidence of progressive parkinsonism and dementia associated with many NFTs in the central nervous system neuropathologically, reminiscent of PDC of Chamorro in Guam (11,12,17,18). The focus of this chapter is to review findings of recent research with respect to the Kii ALS/PDC from the Hohara focus, particularly regarding clinical features, neuroimaging studies, immunohistochemical findings of the brain and spinal cord, genetic studies, and recent epidemiological trends. We will also discuss new disease concepts derived from these findings.

Clinical features of Kii amyotrophic lateral sclerosis/parkinsonism–dementia complex

At onset, patients developed signs and symptoms of motor neurone disease (MND), parkinsonism, or dementia. Of the 26 new cases of ALS/PDC neurologically confirmed during 1996 and 1999 in Hohara, four patients developed MND signs consistent with ALS, while 22 patients developed parkinsonism and dementia almost simultaneously (Figure 3.2) (19). Patients with MND who did not demonstrate features of parkinsonism

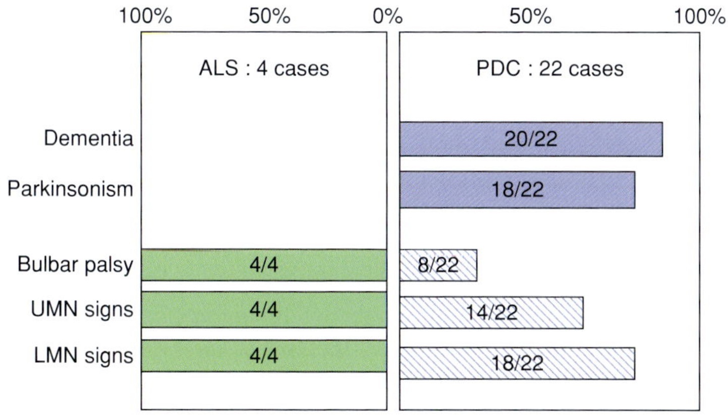

Fig. 3.2 Clinical manifestations of 26 cases of ALS and PDC examined during 1996 and 1999. All four patients with ALS manifested the signs and symptoms of selective motor neurone involvement, while patients with PDC presented with motor neurone disease symptoms several years after the establishment of parkinsonism and dementia (19).

or dementia during their disease progression were classified into 'pure ALS'. Patients with PDC at onset who developed signs of MND during their disease course were classified into 'PDC/ALS'. Rarely, patients who simultaneously developed signs of MND and dementia at onset were classified into the 'ALS–dementia complex (ALSDC)'. Similar clinical overlap of ALS and PDC was described in patients with Guam ALS/PDC in the 1980s (20).

Patients with pure ALS presented with the same clinical signs and symptoms caused by the selective involvement of the upper and lower motor neurones as described by Charcot in sporadic ALS (5). Three main clinical subtypes of ALS were observed: classic ALS, progressive bulbar palsy, and progressive muscular atrophy. Patients with ALS died due to either respiratory paralysis or complications of bulbar palsy. Parkinsonism presented with bradykinesia, rigidity, and postural instability in all cases, and tremor of resting or postural type in some. Parkinsonian motor symptoms responded poorly to levodopa and other antiparkinsonian drugs. Dementia was characterized by deficits of such fundamental frontal functions as basic attention, motivation/initiation, and information processing speed, which were consistent with those of frontal–subcortical dementia (21). Forgetfulness, difficulty in memory retrieval, and slowing in cognition, mental processing, and speech were present, although mild. Patients with PDC fell into akinetic mutism at the late stage. Any patients with PDC and other dementia–ALS/parkinsonism complex (PDC/ALS and ALSDC) did not manifest severe amnesia, aphasia, apraxia, agnosia, disorientation in time and place, and behavioural psychological syndromes frequently seen in Alzheimer's disease, severe personality changes, abnormal behaviours and speech disturbances suggestive of frontotemporal dementia, or severe psychosis and hallucination implying dementia with Lewy bodies.

In summary, Kii ALS/PDC presented clinically with three core features: ALS/MND, frontal–subcortical dementia, and progressive atypical parkinsonism unresponsive to levodopa and other antiparkinsonian drugs. These features occurred individually or in combination, and pure ALS, PDC, and other dementia–ALS/parkinsonism complex were differentiated on the basis of clinical features at the onset and subsequent overlapping symptoms.

Neuroimaging

Either computed tomography or magnetic resonance imaging were applied for anatomical studies and single photon emission computed tomography (SPECT) with a tracer technetium (^{99m}Tc) ethylcysteinate dimer for cerebral blood flow (22). Patients with pure Kii ALS did not show obvious brain atrophy on computed tomography and magnetic resonance imaging (Figure 3.3a), but demonstrated reductions in cerebral blood flow on SPECT (Figure 3.3b). In contrast, patients with PDC and PDC/ALS developed rapidly progressing symmetrical brain atrophy on computed tomography and magnetic resonance imaging, most prominently at the pole of the frontal and temporal lobes with marked dilatation of the lateral ventricles and inferior horns (Figure 3.3c). This was associated with a marked

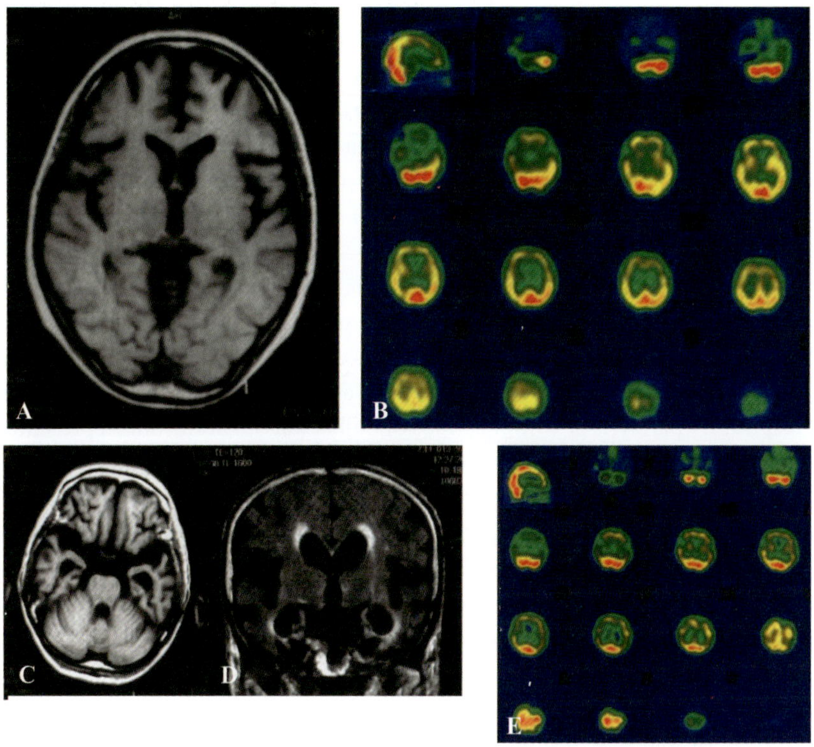

Fig. 3.3 Neuroimaging of Kii ALS and PDC. Kii ALS cases show no or mild atrophy of the frontal and temporal lobes on magnetic resonance imaging (a) with obvious decrease in cerebral blood flow of the frontal and temporal lobes on SPECT with a tracer technetium (^{99m}Tc) ethyl cysteinate dimer (b), while Kii PDC cases show marked atrophy of the frontal and temporal lobes with ventricular dilatation on magnetic resonance imaging (c) with marked loss in cerebral blood flow of the frontal and temporal lobes on SPECT (d). Note that the atrophy and decrease in cerebral blood flow are symmetrical.

reduction in cerebral blood flow on (^{99m}Tc) ethylcysteinate SPECT (Figure 3.3d). In the neuroimaging study, findings of the frontal and temporal lobes, exact symmetry in atrophy, and hypometabolism were characteristic of Kii ALS/PDC, in contrast to the marked asymmetry in the frontotemporal dementias, including behavioural variant, semantic dementia, and progressive non-fluent dementia (23).

Neuropathological findings

Typical ALS pathology combined with neurofibrillary degeneration of mild to moderate degrees in the neurones of the brainstem and cortex of the temporal and frontal lobes was reported in pure Kii ALS cases from the Kozagawa focus (4,10,24). We reported similar findings in pure ALS cases from the Hohara focus and the first neuropathological findings of Kii PDC in 2001 (17). More than 12 autopsy cases have been studied to date (18).

Motor neurone degeneration and neurofibrillary degeneration

The neuropathological findings of 12 autopsy cases of ALS/PDC from seven different families (families A–G) in the Hohara focus are shown in Table 3.1. Macroscopically, the brains of pure ALS and ALSDC cases showed mild atrophy, while brains of PDC and PDC/ALS cases showed marked atrophy of the frontal and temporal lobes (Figure 3.4a).

Table 3.1 Neuropathological findings of 12 ALS/PDC cases

Case number according to their families (A–G)	Clinical diagnosis	Brain weight	Motor neurone disease pathology			NFT			SP	LB
		(g)	UMN	LMN	Bunina body	Mesial temporal	Brainstem	Spinal cord		
A-1	ALS	1190	1+	3+	–	1+	1+	–	–	–
B-1	ALS	1275	1+	3+	1+	3+	3+	–	–	–
C-1	ALS	1140	1+	2+		1+	1+	–	–	–
D-1	ALS	1190	3+	3+	2+	1+	2+	–	–	2+
E-1	ALSDC	ND		NA	NA	3+	2+	NA	2+	2+
B-2	ALSDC	1210	1+	3+ (XII)	NA	3+	2+	NA	–	2+
E-2	ALSDC	1320	1+	NA	NA	2+	2+	NA	–	1+
E-3	ALSDC	1300	–	2+	2+	3+	3+	1+	–	–
A-2	PDC	935	1+	2+		3+	2+	1+	–	–
F-1	PDC	1085	1+	2+		3+	3+	1+	–	–
E-4	PDC/ALS	960	3+	2+	1+	3+	3+	1+	–	–
G-1	PDC/ALS	875	3+	1+	1+	3+	3+	–	–	–

ALS, amyotrophic lateral sclerosis; ALSDC, ALS-dementia complex; LB, Lewy body; LMN, lower motor neurone; NA, not available; ND, not described; NFT, neurofibrillary tangle; PDC, parkinsonism–dementia complex; PDC/ALS, PDC overlapping ALS; SP, senile plaque; UMN, upper motor neurone; 1+, mild; 2+, moderate; 3+, marked.

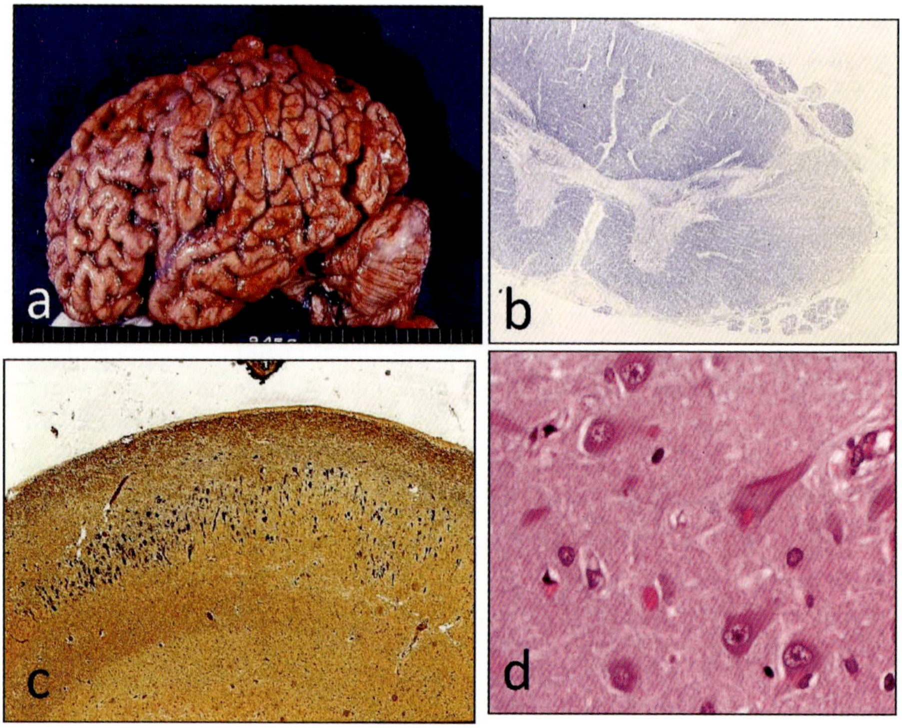

Fig. 3.4 Neuropathological findings of Kii PDC. (a) Fresh unfixed brain shows marked atrophy of the frontal and temporal lobes, particularly in the poles. (b) The spinal cord shows degeneration of the lateral tracts and loss of anterior horn cells (Klüver–Barrera stain). (c) Many NFTs in the hippocampus demonstrated with Bielschowsky stain. (d) Basophilic NFTs and Hirano bodies in the hippocampus (haematoxylin–eosin stain). Reprinted from Shigeki Kuzuhara et al., *Annals of Neurology*, Wiley 2001.

Spinal cords and anterior spinal roots were thin in ALS, ALSDC, and PDC/ALS cases. Pure Kii ALS cases showed classical pathology of sporadic ALS, including pallor of the corticospinal tracts (Figure 3.4b), degeneration and loss of anterior horn cells, and Bunina bodies in the anterior horn cells. Similar degeneration of the upper and lower motor neurones was present in the PDC cases without obvious clinical signs of MND.

Neurofibrillary degeneration associated with no or few senile plaques was observed throughout the cerebral cortex, brainstem, and spinal cord. This was most prominent in cases of PDC, PDC/ALS, and ALSDC, and mildly to moderately evident in pure ALS cases. They were most numerous in the brainstem, hippocampus, parahippocampal gyrus, and cortex of the temporal and frontal lobes (Figure 3.4c). NFTs in pure ALS cases were quantitatively less in number than in PDC and other dementia–ALS/parkinsonism complex, but qualitatively the same in the distribution pattern (25). A similar overlap of the neuropathological findings of ALS and PDC, namely coexistence of selective motor system degeneration and widespread neurofibrillary degeneration, has also been reported in ALS/PDC of Guam (20). As observed with either silver staining or immunohistochemistry (amyloid β-protein), senile plaques were absent or very few in number. Haematoxylin and eosin preparations of the hippocampus revealed numerous basophilic and eosinophilic NFTs, granulovacuolar degeneration and Hirano bodies (Figure 3.4d). Lewy body pathology was present in approximately one-third of cases examined on preparations with haematoxylin and eosin stain or α-synuclein immunohistochemistry (Table 3.1).

Transactive response DNA-binding protein of 43 kDa deposition

In 2006, Neumann and colleagues (26) and Arai and colleagues (27) reported independently from each other that the transactive response DNA-binding protein of 43 kDa (TDP-43) was the primary component of the ubiquitinated inclusions and skein-like inclusion of frontotemporal lobar degeneration and ALS. Subsequently, TDP-43 deposition in brains of Guam PDC cases was reported (28). We subsequently demonstrated the deposition of TDP-43 in brains of both ALS and PDC cases of Kii ALS/PDC on Western blotting and immunohistochemistry (29). Using a polyclonal antibody against TDP-43 (ProteinTech Group, Chicago, IL, USA), we observed neuronal cytoplasmic inclusions within neurones of the dentate gyrus of the hippocampus (Figure 3.5a), and skein-like inclusions (Figure 3.5b), granular inclusions (Figure 3.5b), and round bodies (Figure 3.5c) in anterior horn cells. We also observed neuritic inclusions and glial inclusions in the spinal cord. Intranuclear type inclusions were not detected.

In summary, selective degeneration of the upper and lower motor neurones consistent with ALS, widely distributed NFTs throughout the central nervous system, and TDP-43-immunoreactive inclusions in the neurones of the brain and spinal cord were the core neuropathological changes common to all clinical phenotypes of ALS/PDC. However, the severity of each individual pathological change varied among the different clinical phenotypes.

Pathogenesis

Environmental factors

Yase reported low calcium and magnesium and high aluminium and manganese in water taken from wells, rivers, and soil in the high-incidence ALS foci in the Kii Peninsula and Guam (30). On the basis of these observations, he proposed the 'metal-induced calcified neurone degeneration hypothesis' that chronic hypocalcaemia and hypomagnesaemia, which had been produced by long-term intake of excess aluminium and too low calcium levels in drinking water and food might have caused secondary hyperparathyroidism and induced motor neurone degeneration. Experimental studies in rodents and primates, which had been fed with diet and water containing low calcium and/or high aluminium, succeeded in producing widespread neuronal degeneration of the central nervous system, but failed to produce selective motor neurone degeneration of ALS and NFTs (31). In the 1990s, Iwami and colleagues re-examined the levels of minerals in the drinking water and food in Hohara and neighbouring control areas, and compared the data with the incidence rates of ALS (32). They found excess manganese intake from food coupled with low

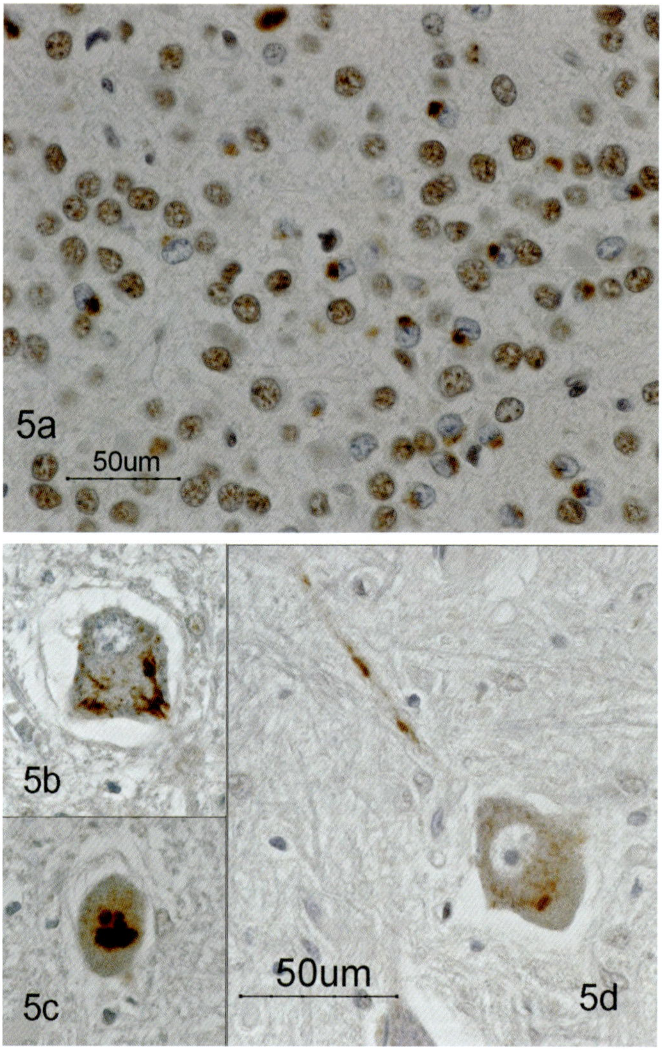

Fig. 3.5 Transactive response DNA-binding protein 43 (TDP-43) immunohistochemistry. A polyclonal antibody against TDP-43 (ProteinTech Group, Chicago, IL, USA) immunolabels many cytoplasmic inclusions in neurones of the dentate gyrus of the hippocampus, with the nuclei of the nerve cells containing inclusions unlabelled (a). TDP-43 immunoreactive skein-like inclusions (b), round inclusions (c), and granular inclusions (d) were observed in the anterior horn cells of the spinal cord.

magnesium in drinking water, and concluded that these findings could account for the high incidence rates of ALS in this focus. We examined serum contents of minerals such as calcium, phosphate, magnesium, and aluminium together with serum levels of alkaline phosphatase and parathyroid hormone in residents in Hohara and neighbouring control areas. We observed that all mineral levels as well as alkaline phosphatase and parathyroid hormone levels were within normal limits, with no significant differences between Hohara and control regions (unpublished data). These findings suggested that the *in vivo* metabolism of calcium and other minerals could be modulated normally even if the levels of minerals and metals in the drinking water and food were far higher or lower than average. Of note, Ahlskog and colleagues reported normal levels of calcium, aluminium, potassium, and parathyroid hormone in the serum of patients with ALS/PDC in Guam (33).

In the Guam focus of ALS and ALS/PDC, toxins derived from cycad, including β-*N*-methylamino l-alanine, were suspected to have caused neurodegeneration and produced ALS/PDC (34,35) (see also Garruto, Chapter 1). Subsequent research failed to convincingly establish a causal link with cycad consumption and ALS/PDC. However, in recent years, Cox and colleagues have proposed a new cycad hypothesis in which β-*N*-methylamino l-alanine was originally biosynthesized by cyanobacteria in cycad roots and then biomagnified in the body of cycad-eating fruit bats (36,37). They postulated that Chamorro people had ingested high levels of toxins by eating the bats, and developed ALS/PDC decades later. Disappearance of fruit bat populations by overhunting resulted in cessation of eating bats and led to the decline of ALS/PDC decades later. Borenstein and colleagues subsequently reported that eating cycad in young adulthood was a risk factor for dementia, mild cognitive impairment, and PDC on Guam, but that there were no associations with the outcomes for consumption of fruit bats or exposure to cycad used as a tropical medicine (38). In the 1980s, cycad had been suspected as the culprit of Kii ALS, but people in Japan, including the Kii Peninsula, had never consumed cycad as daily food although a small amount of cycad flour might have been taken by a few people as an ingredient of herb medicine (39,40). Our survey on medical history revealed that none of the patients with ALS/PDC in the Hohara focus had taken cycad or bats before onset of the disease. While exposure to cycad may be in part related to the pathogenesis of ALS/PDC in Guam, there is thus no evidence that it played a pathogenic role in the Kii Peninsula.

Genetic studies

In the Hohara focus, approximately 70% of patients with ALS/PDC had a positive family history of ALS/PDC in the 1960s and approximately 80% in the 1990s (unpublished data). In some families, the disease occurred vertically in several generations or horizontally in siblings, suggestive of either an autosomal-dominant or autosomal-recessive transmission. Consanguineous marriage was frequent in the 1960s in Hohara (4). We confirmed more than 10 patients who had developed ALS/PDC many years (24–51 years) after they had left the village, and most of them had affected relative(s) of the first or second degree (unpublished data). A high frequency of positive family history in the residents in the high-incidence ALS focus and development of ALS/PDC after long latent periods from migration from the focus suggested genetic abnormalities in the pathogenesis of Kii ALS/PDC.

Gene abnormalities, which had been previously established as the cause or risk of familial or sporadic ALS, dementia, familial Parkinson's disease, and parkinsonism were analysed, but all of them were negative (Table 3.2) (17,41). Gene analyses were performed on

Table 3.2 Causative and risk gene analysis

Neurodegenerative disease	Causal and risk genes
Alzheimer's disease	ApoE-ε4
Familial ALS/motor neurone disease	SOD1, TDP-43, FUS
Spinal muscular atrophy	SMN
Frontotemporal dementia/lobar degeneration	MAPT (exons and introns), PPGN, TDP-43, GSK3
Familial parkinsonism/Parkinson's disease	SNCA, LRRK2 (dardarin), PRKN, DJ-1, PINK1, ATP13A2, MAPT
Progressive supranuclear palsy	MAPT intron polymorphism in dinucleotide repeats
Guam ALS/PDC	TRPM7

ApoE-ε4, apolipoprotein E4 gene; ATP13A2, ATPase type 13A2 gene; DJ-1, oncogene and causative gene of PARK7; FUS/TLS, fused in sarcoma/translated in liposarcoma; GSK3B, glycogen synthase kinase-3β gene; LRRK2 (dardarin), leucine-rich repeat kinase 2 gene; MAPT, tau gene; PGRN, progranulin gene; PINK1, PTEN-induced putative kinase 1 gene; PRKN, parkin gene; SMN, survival motor neurone gene; SNCA, α-synuclein gene; SOD1, Cu/Zn superoxidase dismutase-1 gene; TDP-43, transactive response (TAR) DNA-binding protein of 43 kDa gene; TRPM7, transient receptor potential melastatin 7 gene; UCH-L1, ubiquitin carboxy-terminal hydrolase L1.

apolipoprotein E4 genotype (apoe-ε4) phenotype as well as for mutations in the amyloid precursor protein gene, Cu/Zn superoxidase dismutase-1, *TDP-43* gene, survival motor neurone gene, progranulin, microtubule-associated protein *tau*, glycogen synthase kinase-3β, α-synuclein, leucine-rich repeat kinase 2 (dardarin), parkin, DJ-1, PTEN-induced putative kinase 1, and ATPase type 13a2. All were negative.

Hermosura *et al.* have recently discovered a nuclear mutation in the calcium/magnesium membrane ion channel transient receptor potential melastatin 7 (*TRPM7*) gene in a subset of patients with Guam ALS/PDC (42). They speculated that the defective channel might have caused abnormal metabolism of these metals and induced neuronal degeneration resulting in ALS/PDC in Guam, as the channel is a bifunctional protein involved in homeostatic regulation of intracellular calcium and magnesium and trace metal concentration. In patients with Kii ALS/PDC, however, no mutation was found in the *TRPM7* gene (43). Further studies to identify the susceptible loci or genes of Kii ALS/PDC are ongoing.

Epidemiology

Kimura, Yase and their colleagues started a continuous epidemiological survey and enrolment of patients with ALS in Hohara and Kozagawa in the 1960s, including a retrospective survey of the 1940s (2,3). The diagnoses were confirmed based on neurological examination and information from patients' families, medical records, and charts from hospitals, clinics, and nursing homes. The survey was discontinued in the late 1980s when no new cases had been identified over the course of several years (15). In the early 1990s, however, we restarted the survey after having observed new patients with ALS from Hohara, and included other neurodegenerative disorders (17).

Changing patterns and incidence rates of the Kii amyotrophic lateral sclerosis/parkinsonism–dementia complex in Hohara (1950–2004)

Eighty-four patients were enrolled in the survey between 1950 and 2004 (Table 3.3). This included 40 cases of pure ALS, 14 ALSDC, 22 PDC, and eight PDC/ALS (44). The 5-year-average annual incidence rates per 100 000 population age-adjusted to the Japanese population in 1985 were calculated for pure ALS cases versus PDC and other dementia–ALS/parkinsonism complex (Figure 3.6). The annual incidence rate of pure ALS per 100 000 sharply declined from 107 in the 1950s to 20 in the 1980s, while that of PDC and other dementia–ALS/parkinsonism complex sharply arose from 20 before 1980 to 60 after 1980, mainly due to increase of PDC and PDC/ALS.

The cause(s) of the marked declines of pure ALS and increases of PDC and other dementia–ALS/parkinsonism complex remains unsolved. Using the urinary 8-hydroxydeoxyguanosine (8-OHDG)/creatinine ratio as a marker of oxidative stress, we examined 11 patients with Kii ALS/PDC and eight normal controls and observed an elevation of the mean level of urinary 8-OHDG/creatinine ratio of patients with Kii ALS/PDC in comparison with that of control subjects (45). This suggests that oxidative stress might be related to pathogenesis of Kii ALS/PDC and that changes of environmental factors related to oxidative stress may have influenced the change in phenotypic patterns of Kii ALS/PDC.

For the 50 years after World War II, both the natural and socio-cultural environments and lifestyle of residents in Hohara dramatically westernized, as in other areas in Japan. Drinking water from the well was changed to tap water supplied from the reservoir or

Table 3.3 Number of new cases of ALS, PSC, PDC/ALS, and ALSDC, during each 5 year period

Years	Population of the beginning year	Pure ALS	PDC and other ALS/PDC			
				PDC	PDC/ALS	ALSDC
1950–54	2681	9	1	0	0	1
1955–59	2163	4	2	1	0	1
1960–64	2185	6	0	0	0	0
1965–69	2125	3	2	0	1	1
1970–74	2160	3	2	0	1	1
1975–79	1816	4	0	0	0	0
1980–84	1745	2	2	0	0	2
1985–89	1684	1	2	0	0	2
1990–94	1642	4	10	7	2	1
1995–99	1543	3	15	11	1	3
2000–04	1441	1	8	3	3	2
		40	44	22	8	14

ALS, amyotrophic lateral sclerosis; ALSDC, ALS–dementia complex; PDC, parkinsonism–dementia complex; PDC/ALS, PDC overlapping ALS.

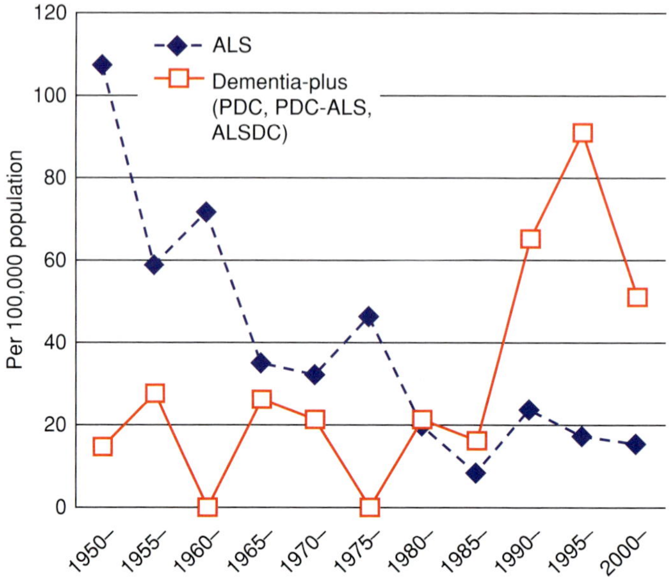

Fig. 3.6 Five-year average incidence rates of Kii ALS/PDC (age-adjusted to the Japanese population in 1985). The incidence of pure ALS sharply declined during 1950 and 1980, while the incidence of PDC and other dementia–ALS/parkinsonism complex jumped up in 1990s.

mineral water bought in supermarkets and food was changed from traditional Japanese style to Western style. Another dramatic change was an increase in the elderly population, as the average life expectancy of Japanese people rose from 58.0 years in men and 61.5 years in women in 1950, to 77.7 years in men and 84.6 in women in 2000 (46). We have postulated that a combination of changes in diet, water source, and lifestyle and rapid progression of ageing of population in these 50 years may have modulated the pathogenesis of Kii ALS/PDC and resulted in the decrease in pure ALS and increase in PDC and other dementia–ALS/parkinsonism complex affecting the elderly.

Comparison with the epidemiological trends of amyotrophic lateral sclerosis/parkinsonism–dementia complex in Guam

In Guam, the occurrence of ALS rapidly declined after World War II, and high incidence of ALS disappeared by the early 1980s (14) (see also Garruto, Chapter 1). Incidence rates of PDC also declined but still remain common (47). Similarly, in the Kii ALS/PDC focus, the incidence rates of pure ALS rapidly declined for these 50 years, while PDC and other dementia–ALS/parkinsonism complex rates sharply increased after 1980 (Figure 3.5). Recent epidemiological studies in Guam ALS/PDC have, however, indicated high prevalence rates of late-onset dementia or 'Mariana dementia' among elderly Chamorro people (48). While the clinical features of the Mariana dementia resemble those of Alzheimer's disease, it is not yet known whether the neuropathological characteristics are those of Alzheimer's disease or those of the ALS/PDC spectrum. A similar survey on dementia-only cases in late life has not been done in the Kii Peninsula ALS foci.

ALS/PDC in the Kii Peninsula and ALS/PDC in Guam seem quite akin to each other clinically and neuropathologically, but quite different from each other not only in their racial and ethnic backgrounds but also in environmental factors such as food, drinking water, culture, lifestyle, and others. It is also very intriguing that there are similar changes in the incidence rates and clinical phenotypes in both Guam and the Kii Peninsula, although the causes remain unknown for either. As discussed by Garruto and Yanagihara, the western Pacific hyperendemic foci of ALS/PDC, represent natural experimental models of chronic neurodegenerative disease that occur in different cultures, different ecological zones, and among genetically diverse human groups (49). In these hyperendemic areas, some hitherto unknown environmental factor(s) may exist that interact with susceptible gene(s) of the indigenous people, giving rise to both a tauopathy and a TDP-43 proteinopathy in the central nervous system, which clinically manifests ALS, parkinsonism, and dementia (Figure 3.7).

In summary, we have reviewed recent findings of current concepts in Kii ALS/PDC. This complex is composed of three core features (i.e. ALS, dementia, and parkinsonism). The clinical features of ALS were identical to those of classical sporadic ALS while the dementia was characterized by deficits of frontal functions that differed from both Alzheimer's disease and the frontotemporal dementias. Rigid akinetic parkinsonism unresponsive to levodopa was present in many, while parkinsonism tremor in a few. Regardless of clinical phenotype, all patients showed both ALS pathology and NFT pathology of varying degrees. TDP-43 immunohistochemistry revealed positive cytoplasmic inclusions in neurones of the dentate nucleus of the hippocampus, and skein-like inclusions and other inclusions in the spinal anterior horn cells in all clinical phenotypes. Lewy bodies were seen in approximately one-third of autopsy cases. Senile plaques were absent or few. Although the genetic basis of this disorder remains unknown, epidemiological studies suggest that environmental

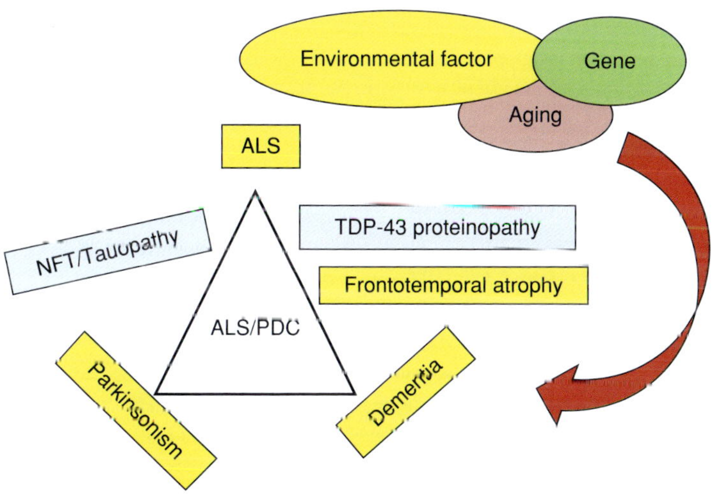

Fig. 3.7 A scheme of the gene–environmental interaction hypothesis in the hyperendemic ALS/PDC foci in the western Pacific isolated islands.

factors interacting with susceptible gene(s), combined with ageing of the population, have contributed to a change in phenotypic patterns of Kii ALS/PDC. Further studies are necessary to clarify the pathogenesis and cause of this hyperendemic neurodegenerative disease.

Acknowledgements

We are grateful to our patients and their family members for their assistance and collaboration. We thank Professor Yase and his collaborators, and all our collaborators including researchers, physicians, residents, medical school students, nurses, medical and laboratory technicians and assistants. These works were supported by Grants-in-Aid from the Research Committee of CNS Degenerative Diseases, the Ministry of Health, Labour and Welfare of Japan, and Grants-in-Aid for Scientific Research (Kakenhi), Japan Society for the Promotion of Science (JSPS), and the Ministry of Education, Culture, Sports, Science and Technology (MEXT) of Japan.

References

1. Miura K. (1911). Amyotrophische Lateralsklerose unter dem Bilde von sog. Bulbaerparalyse. *Neurol Centralblatt Neurol Psychiatr Psychol Wiss*, **10**, 366–369.
2. Kimura K, Yase Y, Higashi Y, *et al.* (1963). Epidemiological and geomedical studies on amyotrophic lateral sclerosis. *Dis Nerv Syst* **24**, 155–159.
3. Kimura K, Yase Y, Higashi Y, *et al.* (1961). Epidemiological and geomedical studies on ALS and allied diseases in Kii peninsula (Japan). Preliminary report. *Proc Jpn Acad*, **37**, 417–420.
4. Shiraki HK, Yase Y. (1975). Amyotrophic lateral sclerosis in Japan. In: Vinken PJ, Bruyn GW (eds.), *Handbook of Clinical Neurology*, pp. 353–419. Elsevier Publishing, New York.
5. Charcot JM, Joffroy A, (1869). Deux cas d'atrophie musculaire progressive avec lésions de la substance grise et des faisceaux antérolatéraux de la moelle épinière. *Arch Physiol Norm Pathol*, **2**, 354–744.
6. Yase Y, Matsumoto N, Azuma K, *et al.* (1972). Amyotrophic lateral sclerosis. Association with schizophrenic symptoms and showing Alzheimer's tangles. *Arch Neurol*, **27**, 118–128.
7. Kurland LT, Mulder DW. (1954). Epidemiological investigations of amyotrophic lateral sclerosis. 1. Preliminary report on geographic distribution, with special reference to the Mariana Islands, including clinical and pathological observations. *Neurology*, **4**, 355–378, 438–448.
8. Malamud N, Hirano A, Kurland LT. (1961). Pathoanatomic changes in amyotrophic lateral sclerosis on Guam. *Arch Neurol*, **5**, 401–415.
9. Gajdusek DC. (1963). Motor-neuron disease in natives of New Guinea. *N Engl J Med*, **268**, 474–476.
10. Yase Y, Yoshida S, Kihira T, *et al.* (2001). Kii ALS dementia. *Neuropathology*, **21**, 105–109.
11. Hirano A, Kurland LT, Krooth RS, *et al.* (1961). Parkinsonism-dementia complex, an endemic disease on the island of Guam. I. Clinical features. *Brain*, **84**, 642–661.
12. Hirano A, Malamud N, Kurland LT. (1961). Parkinsonism-dementia complex, an endemic disease on the island of Guam. II. Pathological features. *Brain*, **84**, 662–679.
13. Hirano A, Malamud N, Elizan TS, *et al.* (1966). Amyotrophic lateral sclerosis and Parkinsonism-dementia complex on Guam. Further pathologic studies. *Arch Neurol*, **15**, 35–51.
14. Garruto RM, Yanagihara R, Gajdusek DC. (1985). Disappearance of high-incidence amyotrophic lateral sclerosis and parkinsonism-dementia on Guam. *Neurology*, **35**, 193–198.
15. Yoshida S. (1991). [Environmental factors in western Pacific foci of ALS and a possible pathogenetic role of aluminum (Al) in motor neuron degeneration]. *Rinsho Shinkeigaku*, **31**, 1310–1312.

16. Spencer PS, Palmer VS, Ludolph AC. (2005). On the decline and etiology of high-incidence motor system disease in West Papua (southwest New Guinea). *Mov Disord,* **20** (Suppl 12), S119–S126.
17. Kuzuhara S, Kokubo Y, Sasaki R, *et al.* (2001). Familial amyotrophic lateral sclerosis and Parkinsonism-dementia complex of the Kii Peninsula of Japan: clinical and neuropathological study and tau analysis. *Ann Neurol,* **49**, 501–511.
18. Kuzuhara S, Kokubo Y. (2005). Atypical parkinsonism of Japan: amyotrophic lateral sclerosis-parkinsonism-dementia complex of the Kii Peninsula of Japan (Muro Disease): an update. *Mov Disord,* **S12**, S108–S113.
19. Kokubo Y, Kuzuhara S. (2001). [Neurological and neuropathological studies of amyotrophic lateral sclerosis/parkinsonism-dementia complex in the Kii Peninsula of Japan]. *Rinsho Shinkeigaku,* **41**, 769–774.
20. Rodgers-Johnson P, Garruto RM, Yanigahara R, *et al.* (1986). Amyotrophic lateral sclerosis and parkinsonism-dementia on Guam: a 30-year evaluation of clinical and neuropathological trends. *Neurology,* **36**, 7–13.
21. Mendez MF, Cummings JL. (2003). Diagnosis of dementia. In: Mendez MF, Cummings JL (eds.), *Dementia. A Clinical Approach*, pp. 41–45. Butterworth Heinemann, Philadelphia.
22. Kokubo Y, Kuzuhara S. (2003). Neuroradiological study of patients with amyotrophic lateral sclerosis and parkinsonism-dementia complex on the Kii peninsula of Japan. *Arch Neurol,* **60**, 1257–1261.
23. Nesator PJ. (2007). Neuroimaging and other investigative findings. In: Hodges JR (ed.), *Frontotemporal Dementia*, pp. 134–160. Cambridge University Press, Cambridge
24. Wakayama I, Kihira Y, Yoshida S, *et al.* (1993). Rare neuropil threads in amyotrophic lateral sclerosis and parkinsonism-dementia on Guam and in the Kii Peninsula of Japan. *Dementia,* **4**, 75–80.
25. Mimuro M, Kokubo Y, Kuzuhara S. (2007). Similar topographical distribution of neurofibrillary tangles in amyotrophic lateral sclerosis and parkinsonism-dementia complex in people living in the Kii peninsula of Japan suggests a single tauopathy. *Acta Neuropathol,* **113**, 653–658.
26. Neumann M, Sampathu DM, Kwong LK, *et al.* (2006). Ubiquitinated TDP-43 in frontotemporal lobar degeneration and amyotrophic lateral sclerosis. *Science,* **314**, 130–133.
27. Arai T, Hasegawa M, Akiyama H, *et al.* (2006). TDP-43 is a component of ubiquitin-positive tau-negative inclusions in frontotemporal lobar degeneration and amyotrophic lateral sclerosis. *Biochem Biophys Res Commun,* **351**, 602–611.
28. Hasegawa M, Arai T, Akiyama H, *et al.* (2007). TDP-43 is deposited in the Guam parkinsonism-dementia complex brains. *Brain,* **130**, 1386–1394.
29. Kuzuhara S. (2007). Revisit to Kii ALS—the innovated concept of ALS-Parkinsonism-dementia complex, clinicopathological features, epidemiology and etiology. *Brain Nerve,* **59**, 1065–1074.
30. Yase Y. (1972). The pathogenesis of amyotrophic lateral sclerosis. *Lancet,* **ii**, 292–296.
31. Strong MJ, Garruto RM. (1997). Motor neuron disease. In: Yasui M, Strong MJ, Ota K, Verity MA (eds.), *Mineral and Metal Neurotoxicity*, pp. 107–112. CRC Press, Boca Raton.
32. Iwami O, Watanabe T, Moon CS, *et al.* (1994). Motor neuron disease on the Kii Peninsula of Japan: excess manganese intake from food coupled with low magnesium in drinking water as a risk factor. *Sci Total Environ,* **149**, 121–135.
33. Ahlskog JE, Waring SC, Kurland LT, *et al.* (1995). Guamanian neurodegenerative disease: investigation of the calcium metabolism/heavy metal hypothesis. *Neurology,* **45**, 1340–1344.
34. Kurland LT. (1972). An appraisal of the neurotoxicity of cycad and the etiology of amyotrophic lateral sclerosis on Guam. *Fed Proc,* **31**, 1540–1542.
35. Spencer PS, Nunn PB, Hugon J, *et al.* (1987). Guam amyotrophic lateral sclerosis-parkinsonism-dementia linked to a plant excitant neurotoxin. *Science,* **237**, 517–522.

36. Cox PA, Sacks OW. (2002). Cycad neurotoxins, consumption of flying foxes, and ALS-PDC disease in Guam. *Neurology*, **58**, 956–959.
37. Cox PA, Banack SA, Murch SJ. (2003). Biomagnification of cyanobacterial neurotoxins and neurodegenerative disease among the Chamorro people of Guam. *Proc Natl Acad Sci USA*, **100**, 13380–13383.
38. Borenstein AR, Mortimer JA, Schofield E, *et al.* (2007). Cycad exposure and risk of dementia, MCI, and PDC in the Chamorro population of Guam. *Neurology*, **68**, 1764–1771.
39. Spencer PS, Ohta M, Palmer VS. (1987). Cycad use and motor neuron disease in Kii Peninsula of Japan. *Lancet*, **ii**, 1462–1463.
40. Iwami O, Niki Y, Watanabe T, *et al.* (1993). Motor neuron disease on the Kii Peninsula of Japan: cycad exposure. *Neuroepidemiology*, **12**, 307–312.
41. Tomiyama H, Kokubo Y, Sasaki R, *et al.* (2008). Mutattion analysis in amyotrophic lateral sclerosis/parkinsonism-dementia complex of the Kii peninsula, Japan. *Mov Disord* **23**, 2344–2348.
42. Hermosura MC, Nayakanti H, Dorovkov MV, *et al.* (2005). A TRPM7 variant shows altered sensitivity to magnesium that may contribute to the pathogenesis of two Guamanian neurodegenerative disorders. *Proc Natl Acad Sci USA*. **102**, 11510–11515.
43. Hara K, Kokubo Y, Ishiura H, *et al.* (2010). TRPM7 is not associated with amyotrophic lateral sclerosis-parkinsonism dementia complex in the Kii peninsula of Japan. *Am J Med Genet B Neuropsychiatr Genet,* **153B**, 310–313.
44. Kuzuhara S. (2009). Amyotrophic lateral sclerosis-parkinsonism-dementia complex of the Kii peninsula, Guam and New Guinea. *Jpn J Neuropsychol,* **25**, 182–191.
45. Morimoto S, Kuzuhara S, Kokubo Y. (2009). Increased oxidative stress in patients with amyotrophic lateral sclerosis/Parkinsonism-dementia complex in the Kii peninsula, Japan. *Mov Disord,* **24**, 123–126.
46. Annual Health, Labour and Welfare Report 2008–2009 of the Department of Health, Labor and Welfare of Japan. http://www.mhlw.go.jp/english/index.html. 2010.
47. Plato CC, Garruto RM, Galasko D, *et al.* (2003). Amyotrophic lateral sclerosis and parkinsonism-dementia complex of Guam: changing incidence rates during the past 60 years. *Am J Epidemiol,* **157**, 149–157.
48. Galasko D, Salmon DP, Craig UK, *et al.* (2002). Clinical features and changing patterns of neurodegenerative disorders on Guam, 1997–2000. *Neurology*, **58**, 90–97.
49. Garruto RM, Yanagihara R. (2009). Contributions of isolated Pacific populations to understanding neurodegenerative diseases. *Folia Neuropathol,* **47**, 149–170.

Chapter 4

The frontotemporal dementias: an overview

Alexandre Henri-Bhargava and Morris Freedman

More than a century ago, Arnold Pick described cases of dementia (1) associated with circumscribed or focal brain atrophy that presented with progressive aphasia (2) or changes in behaviour (3). Since then, a group of related disorders in which there is degeneration of the frontal and temporal lobes has been studied anew and named 'frontotemporal lobar degeneration' (FTLD) (4). Once thought to be rare, FTLD is now recognized as a common cause of dementia, especially in individuals presenting under the age of 70 (5–8). There has recently been an explosion in new observations and research regarding these conditions. Although much has been learned about the phenomenology and biology of syndromes associated with FTLD, the different clinical and pathological phenotypes of these related disorders continue to be defined (3–12). There is considerable overlap between phenotypes with ill-defined boundaries that may change over time. In addition, clinical and pathological categorizations do not necessarily correspond to each other in a convenient one-to-one manner (13,14).

The ongoing development of nosology for the FTLD syndromes has resulted in a confusing array of terminology (15). The eponymous term 'Pick's disease' has become restricted to the specific pathological subtype of FTLD with focal cortical atrophy, and tau-positive Pick bodies and ballooned cells on histology (16). 'Pick complex' has been proposed as an eponym for the general class of diseases (17) but this term has not been universally adopted. The label 'frontotemporal dementia' (FTD) is particularly problematic as its meaning changes depending upon the classification system: it has been used to describe the overarching disorder as a whole (18,19) while at other times 'FTD' is used in a more restricted manner to describe only the frontal/behavioural presentation of this illness. Some experts favour using the term FTLD to describe the group of pathological diagnoses, and using the term FTD to describe the group of clinical syndromes (20). In this chapter, we use the term FTLD to refer to the overarching group of pathological disorders that can result in a variety of clinical syndromes; we use the more specific term 'behavioural variant frontotemporal dementia' (bvFTD) to refer to the behavioural phenotype of this disease, while avoiding the use of the term FTD altogether.

Diagnostic criteria (4,18,21) for syndromes produced by FTLD allow for diagnosis based solely upon clinical presentation. Neuroimaging and other tests provide supporting information but the clinical features remain paramount for diagnosis. The 1998 international consensus criteria proposed by Neary and colleagues contain well-defined, detailed descriptions of the principal syndromes produced by FTLD, which are suitable for clinical application and for selection of participants for research (4,22). FTLD results in three clinical syndromes that present with either (a) behavioural manifestations (bvFTD), (b) impairment of speech with intact comprehension (progressive non-fluent aphasia (PNFA)), or (c) loss of word meaning and/or object identity (semantic dementia (SD)). Other names for SD include 'progressive fluent aphasia'. It has been argued that such terms define distinct clinical entities (23), but we shall use SD to refer to the syndrome as a whole without making such distinctions. PNFA and SD were initially captured under the umbrella term 'primary progressive aphasia' by Mesulam (24). Although many continue to use the term primary progressive aphasia (25), we shall not employ this label and simply refer to PNFA and SD as separate, distinct clinical syndromes.

The clinical criteria for the syndromes associated with FTLD have been found to be 90–99% specific in predicting, ante mortem, a pathological diagnosis of FTLD (26,27). Sensitivity has been reported to be as high as 85% (27), but this may be variable. In one study, sensitivity of the diagnostic criteria was only 56%, and only 33 of 45 patients with a putative diagnosis of bvFTD followed for at least 3 years fulfilled all five core diagnostic criteria for this condition (28). It has been suggested that the predictive value of the criteria could be significantly enhanced by more stringently incorporating structural and functional neuroimaging criteria (29). Although widespread neurodegeneration involving the frontal and temporal lobes is seen at late stages of FTLD, at onset the neurodegenerative disease is often quite localized (30,31). The initial clinical manifestations depend upon the location of the focal neurodegenerative process, and thus, correlating these clinical manifestations with focal atrophy or dysfunction on neuroimaging can lead to a more precise diagnosis.

Behavioural variant frontotemporal dementia

The Neary criteria for bvFTD are listed in Table 4.1. Five core features are required for diagnosis. The first criterion is insidious symptom onset and gradual progression over at least 6 months. This is a criterion for all three forms of FTLD, and serves to exclude static focal lesions that can mimic FTLD symptoms (32) and rapidly progressive syndromes such as vasculitis or prion disease.

The second core criterion is early decline in social interpersonal conduct. The patient with bvFTD will begin to neglect rules of etiquette and make lapses of social decorum. The word 'decline' implies that this represents a real and significant change from the patient's premorbid personality. These changes can be subtle at the beginning. It is not unusual for a patient to be initially misdiagnosed with a psychiatric condition. Interestingly, affected persons often possess intact knowledge about proper social conduct but are unable to judge and reflect upon their own behaviour to act in accordance with this knowledge. Examples of disordered social behaviour range from loss of manners and intrusions into personal space, to verbal, physical, or sexual disinhibition. These behaviours resemble those seen in patients with focal injury to the orbitofrontal cortex (33),

Table 4.1 Diagnostic criteria for bvFTD (reprinted with permission from Neary *et al.* (4))

Character change and disordered social conduct are the dominant features initially and throughout the disease course. Instrumental functions of perception, spatial skills, praxis, and memory are intact or relatively well preserved.

I. Core diagnostic features
- A. Insidious onset and gradual progression
- B. Early decline in social interpersonal conduct
- C. Early impairment in regulation of personal conduct
- D. Early emotional blunting
- E. Early loss of insight

II. Supportive diagnostic features
- A. Behavioural disorder
  1. Decline in personal hygiene and grooming
  2. Mental rigidity and inflexibility
  3. Distractibility and impersistance
  4. Hyperorality and dietary changes
  5. Perseveration and stereotyped behaviour
- B. Speech and language
  1. Altered speech output
     a. Aspontaneity and economy of speech
     b. Press of speech
  2. Stereotypy of speech
  3. Echolalia
  4. Perseveration
  5. Mutism
- C. Physical signs
  1. Primitive reflexes
  2. Incontinence
  3. Akinesia, rigidity, and tremor
  4. Low and labile blood pressure
- D. Investigations
  1. Neuropsychology: significant impairment on frontal lobe tests in absence of severe amnesia, aphasia, or perceptual disorder
  2. EEG: normal conventional EEG despite clinically evidence dementia
  3. Brain imaging (structural and/or functional): predominant frontal and/or anterior temporal abnormality

and are due to dysfunction in that part of the frontal lobe, which undergoes focal degeneration early in the course of the disease (34–36). The symptoms can be quite dramatic and include mania-like symptoms with ideas of grandiosity (37,38) (see Box 4.1), and acquired sociopathy (39). One patient with bvFTD came to medical attention after spending his entire retirement savings on prostitutes. Although he was a previously gentle, regular churchgoer, he had developed a controlling personality towards his wife and kept her virtually imprisoned in one room of their house.

Box 4.1 Behavioural variant frontotemporal dementia: case example

A 62-year-old man with 17 years of formal education, including an MBA had been a manager at a medium-sized company but his partners asked him to leave due to increasingly erratic decisions over the preceding 5 years. His wife was also concerned because of new reckless spending. He stopped filing income taxes 4 years earlier and spent half of his life savings on trivial things such as a $9000 gift for a casual friend. He borrowed a large sum of money from his sister, placing her in financial peril. He acknowledged the situation, but was not bothered by it and laughed when it was mentioned to him. His wife remarked, 'It's as if he has no remorse. He understands what he should feel intellectually but does not seem to feel it. He has no feelings of regret or shame.' The patient knew he had 'Pick's disease' but could not understand that this could affect his ability to return to work. In fact, he talked about planning a multimillion dollar business acquisition. Despite his plans, he spent his days watching TV with very little initiative to do anything else. He developed a craving for sweets, particularly candy bars, and gained over 20 kg. He would call friends and relatives in the middle of the night. He continued to spend time at his former tennis club where he would make inappropriate jokes about other people and intrusions into the personal space of strangers. He talked incessantly to the guests.

Four years later he was living in a long-term care facility. He had developed urinary incontinence and anosmia. He refused to shower and slept with his clothes on. On several occasions when he wanted to leave his locked facility, he pulled the fire alarm to get the doors to open. As he liked to eat breakfast early, before the usual time, he would go into other residents' rooms and wheel them into the dining room in various stages of undress. He would compulsively clap his hands and count numbers out loud. He developed a mildly shuffling gait that was exacerbated by neuroleptic medications.

On initial presentation, standard neuropsychological assessment did not reveal widespread deficits. However, he had difficulty performing the object alternation task, a measure that is sensitive to orbitofrontal function (50). He was also impaired on the Wisconsin Card Sorting Test. He had no insight into his poor performance, which he estimated as superior. MRI showed atrophy accentuated in the frontal regions, worse on the right than the left.

The third core criterion is early impairment in regulation of personal conduct. This is somewhat of a misnomer as it refers more specifically to a quantitative alteration in psychomotor behaviour. It can manifest as either decreased psychomotor behaviour (e.g. passivity and inertia) or as increased psychomotor behaviour (e.g. pacing, wandering, and excessive laughing).

The fourth core criterion for bvFTD is early emotional blunting. This includes blunting of the patient's own affect as well as a loss of emotional responses to others; the latter manifests as indifference, loss of emotional warmth, and lack of empathy and sympathy. Empathy is the awareness of others' feelings whereas sympathy is the ability to share those feelings. Many bvFTD patients are described as being emotionally very cold and this causes great strain on relationships with family and friends.

The final core criterion is early loss of insight. In the Neary criteria, this is defined as 'lack of awareness of mental symptoms . . . or unconcern about the consequences of mental failure' (4). This criterion captures two related, but distinct concepts that must be carefully evaluated: anosognosia (where patients are unaware that they are ill), and anosodiaphoria (where patients are aware but are unconcerned that they are ill) (40). For example, a patient may state that he has FTD and acknowledge that persons with dementia should not operate a motor vehicle but the same patient may still insist on driving his own automobile. It has been suggested that anosodiaphoria represents prefrontal dysfunction, whereas anosognosia also depends upon parietal dysfunction (41). Patients with bvFTD may have either anosognosia, or anosodiaphoria, or both. It has been proposed that for Alzheimer's disease, the development of anosognosia marks the transition from a predementia state to dementia (42). In bvFTD, however, Evers and colleagues demonstrated preserved insight in three of eight patients whose clinical and neuroimaging features were otherwise characteristic of typical bvFTD (43). These patients viewed their symptoms as a problem and tried to compensate for them. It was suggested that loss of insight may not occur as early in some patients who otherwise meet the criteria for bvFTD, especially in patients with high premorbid cognitive function.

The supportive diagnostic criteria for bvFTD include other features that may be frequently seen in bvFTD. Abnormal behaviours include decline in personal hygiene and grooming (Diogenes' syndrome) (38) and perseverative and stereotyped behaviour. Examples of perseverative behaviour include repeatedly turning on all the lights in the house; one bvFTD patient spent entire days repeatedly writing hundreds of letters that were totally devoid of content to a small group of friends. Simpler motor or vocal stereotypies such as finger tapping, body rocking, or throat clearing are also frequently seen (44). A related behaviour is mental rigidity and inflexibility. A patient may develop new routines and refuse to break from them. One patient with bvFTD was content to sit peacefully in his room all day repeatedly reading the same book. When asked to leave his room to attend a new activity or test, he became very agitated and anxious, and shouted that he was busy and did not want to leave his room. Environmentally dependent behaviours such as distractibility and impersistence are also frequently seen, as is utilization behaviour, the tendency to use all objects available within one's personal space. One patient's wife could no longer bring him to the grocery store because he would try to fill their cart with everything within reach. Hyperorality and dietary changes are typical and can include cravings for new or unusual foods, often especially sweets, or a compulsion to eat anything in sight. Significant weight gain may accompany this.

Symptoms related to language include aspontaneity and economy of speech, stereotypy of speech, perseverative speech, and mutism. Echolalia refers to the automatic repetition of vocalizations made by another person. This may be another example of environmentally-dependent behaviour (45), or it may represent a purposeful mode of discourse adopted by patients who are responding to being spoken to as a child, a manner they were not previously accustomed to (46). Press of speech can also be seen. Patients can be so incessantly talkative that caregivers can no longer live with them. As the disease progresses, physical signs develop. Urinary incontinence reflects degeneration of anterior cingulate and insular regions that contribute to the conscious regulation of micturition (47). The appearance of primitive reflexes reflects degeneration of the prefrontal cortex. Extrapyramidal symptoms of akinesia and rigidity develop as neurodegeneration spreads to involve the basal ganglia (48). Although tremor is listed in the diagnostic criteria as an extrapyramidal sign supportive of bvFTD, this sign was rarely seen in the only study to systematically evaluate extrapyramidal signs in bvFTD (49).

Semantic dementia

This term is used to describe a syndrome that is primarily a semantic disorder, referring to impaired understanding of word meaning and/or object identity. Like other syndromes associated with FTLD, onset is insidious, followed by gradual progression. The core criteria distinguish between two overlapping presentations of SD: one is a language disorder characterized by fluent but empty spontaneous speech, loss of word meaning manifest by impaired naming, and semantic paraphasias. The other is a perceptual disorder characterized by impaired recognition of familiar faces (prosopagnosia) and/or impaired recognition of object identity (associative agnosia). The perceptual disorder affects multiple modalities (51), with the 'prosopagnosia' affecting recognition of people from their faces, voices, and even from a name or description, although in some patients it has been demonstrated to be modality-specific (e.g. only face recognition is impaired) (52). This variation may depend upon the extent to which the right, left, or both temporal lobes are affected by disease (53,54). In both the language and the perceptual disorder, there is loss of higher-order (i.e. semantic) concept representation; but primary auditory, verbal, and visual perceptual processing are preserved. To account for this, the core criteria indicate that perceptual matching and drawing reproduction, single-word repetition, and the ability to read and write orthographically regular words should be preserved.

The supportive diagnostic features in the Neary criteria describe additional language features that may be present in SD. Concurrent with the behavioural loss of inhibition there can be press of speech. Patients with SD also present with anomia, which is difficulty in finding words. They complain of loss of knowledge of the meaning of the words; despite the word-finding difficulties, the phonology and grammar of speech are preserved. This is

Table 4.2 Diagnostic criteria for SD (reprinted with permission from Neary *et al.* (4), with numbering format corrected)

Semantic disorder (impaired understanding of word meaning and/or object identity) is the dominant feature initially and throughout the disease course. Other aspects of cognition, including autobiographic memory, are intact or relatively well preserved.

I. Core diagnostic features
- A. Insidious onset and gradual progression
- B. Language disorder characterized by:
  1. Progressive, fluent, empty spontaneous speech
  2. Loss of word meaning, manifest by impaired naming
  3. Semantic paraphasias *and/or*
- C. Perceptual disorder characterized by
  1. Prosopagnosia: impaired recognition of identity of familiar faces *and/or*
  2. Associative agnosia: impaired recognition of object identity
- D. Preserved perceptual matching and drawing reproduction
- E. Preserved single-word repetition
- F. Preserved ability to read aloud and write to dictation orthographically regular words

II. Supportive diagnostic features
- A. Speech and language
  1. Press of speech
  2. Idiosyncratic word usage
  3. Absence of phonemic paraphasias
  4. Surface dyslexia and dysgraphia
  5. Preserved calculation
- B. Behaviour
  1. Loss of sympathy and empathy
  2. Narrowed preoccupations
  3. Parsimony
- C. Physical signs
  1. Absent of late primitive reflexes
  2. Akinesia, rigidity, tremor
- D. Investigations
  1. Neuropsychology
     - a. Profound semantic loss, manifest in failure of word comprehension and naming and/or face and object recognition
     - b. Preserved phonology and syntax, and elementary perceptual processing, spatial skills, and day-to-day memorizing
  2. EEG: normal
  3. Brain imaging (structural and/or functional): predominant anterior temporal abnormality (symmetric or asymmetric)

distinct from the anomia seen in patients with PNFA, who report that they know the word but are unable to say it. In SD, there is an absence of phonemic paraphasias, which are sound substitutions (e.g. 'clable' instead of 'table'). Phonemic paraphasias are more characteristically seen in PNFA. Patients with SD, on the other hand, are more likely to display semantic paraphasias, which are word selection errors where a word is substituted by a different sounding word that belongs to the same general class (e.g. 'dog' instead of 'horse' or 'daughter' instead of 'wife'). As memory for whole classes of words are lost, there is increasingly idiosyncratic word usage. Specific words (e.g. 'cat') are often replaced with more general words (e.g. 'animal,' and eventually 'thing'). One patient with SD substituted the term 'little thing' for almost every noun in a sentence. Another used the word 'mother' to refer to any person. Circumlocutions are very common: a 'fork' may be described as 'the thing you eat with.' Because the mechanics of language are preserved, there is often surface dyslexia and dysgraphia. This means that orthographically regular words, such as 'street' or 'mango' can be read or written by sounding them out, whereas irregular words such as 'yacht' or 'syncope' would be written as 'yot' or read as 'sin-copeh.' As would be expected with a primarily temporal lobe disorder, calculation is preserved.

A second set of supportive features in the diagnostic criteria for SD centres on behavioural features seen in the syndrome. Loss of sympathy and empathy is similar to the diagnostic criterion for bvFTD, but these symptoms may be qualitatively different. Whereas recognition of emotion may be more impaired in bvFTD (55), leading to a more profound loss of empathy, loss of sympathy may be more profound in SD. Patients with both bvFTD and SD are impaired in the cognitive aspects of empathy, for example, the ability to accurately understand another person's perspective, but patients with SD are also impaired in the emotional aspects of empathy: even if they are able to understand accurately the emotional state and perspective of the other person, they are less able to mount an appropriate emotional response of their own (56). Patients with SD score higher on clinical scales of 'cold-heartedness' than do patients with bvFTD (57).

Parsimony refers to a broad range of different 'parsimonious behaviours', including preoccupations with financial matters, thriftiness, and hoarding. One patient with SD bought over 17 used stereo systems because 'they were such a great deal'. He completely filled his house with plastic flowers as a cheaper alternative to taking care of real flowers. The same patient also demonstrated narrowed preoccupations in that he became obsessed with scouting thrift shops in lieu of carrying out his usual household chores.

Other behavioural features not included in current diagnostic criteria are often observed in SD. Hyperorality and impaired regulation of personal conduct may be as common in SD as in bvFTD (58). There are qualitative differences between the two syndromes. Whereas indiscriminate eating and gluttony are more typical of bvFTD, food fads may be more common in SD (59). Compulsive and repetitive behaviour patterns such as clock-watching and preoccupation with time, fixation upon and adherence to routines, and verbal stereotypies may be more common in SD than in bvFTD. For example, a patient with SD was admitted to a behavioural neurology ward. He had previously been told that he should take his medication 'about 20 minutes before meals'. He became fixated on requesting his lunch medication at exactly 11:40 and became very anxious if he did not receive it at that time. Any attempt to introduce a new schedule was met with resistance. He would also appear at the nursing station several times throughout the morning to inquire about the time and remind the nurses that his medications should be administered at 11:40. The complete range of behavioural symptoms in SD continues to be described. It is likely that future diagnostic criteria will encompass a wider array of such features and perhaps accord them more importance. The ubiquitous presence of such non-language symptoms supports the proposition that SD is a distinct syndrome that should be considered more than a primary progressive aphasia (60).

Physical signs are often absent early in SD. However, as the neurodegenerative process progresses and begins to involve basal ganglia structures, extrapyramidal symptoms of akinesia, rigidity, and tremor may develop. However, early development of these features is not characteristic of SD and should prompt consideration of alternative diagnoses. The diagnostic criteria list the absence of late primitive reflexes as a supportive feature of SD; however, this has not been systematically studied. Given a certain prevalence of primitive reflexes in the general population and in all neurodegenerative diseases, in general (61), absence or presence of primitive reflexes should not be considered too strongly when making a diagnosis of an FTLD syndrome.

Patients diagnosed with SD are more likely to have focal left-sided than right-sided temporal atrophy (62). Given the historical description of the syndrome as a primary progressive aphasia and the ongoing importance of language symptoms in the diagnostic criteria, this should not be surprising given that language functions usually localize to the left hemisphere. However, patients may also present with symptoms attributed to right-sided temporal lobe dysfunction, including progressive prosopagnosia, topographagnosia, and more pronounced or earlier behavioural disturbances (63,64). For this reason, some have proposed replacing the term 'SD' with 'temporal variant FTD', specifying both a left- and a right-predominant form (65). There may be unique behavioural characteristics to right temporal lobe atrophy that include somatic complaints, hyper-religiosity, visual hallucinations, and cross-modal sensory experiences (e.g. seeing the whole world as coloured red, except when moving) (66). Many patients with SD with initial left-sided temporal symptoms eventually show features of right temporal lobe atrophy as the disease progresses, and vice versa (67).

Progressive non-fluent aphasia

The Neary criteria for PNFA (4), reproduced in Table 4.3, list two core features necessary for the diagnosis of this syndrome. In addition to insidious onset with gradual progression, there must be non-fluent spontaneous speech with agrammatism, phonemic paraphasias, or anomia. Non-fluent speech refers to effortful, hesitant production and a markedly reduced speaking rate. On average, patients with PNFA use two-thirds less words per sentence and their sentences are one-third shorter than healthy persons (68). Agrammatism refers to a reduction, omission, or inappropriate use of grammatical parts

Box 4.2 Semantic dementia: case example

A 62-year-old man was initially treated for possible depression when he developed problems at work. He had developed difficulties with his memory, forgetting the names of people and of common objects. He maintained vivid memories of his personal history, including time spent travelling in South America. He became increasingly ruminative, anxious, and obsessive, extremely concerned about the financial future of his children, and obsessed with saving money. He did very little to help at home. His wife said that 'he putters around the garden and pool at home, but does little otherwise.'

During cognitive testing, the patient displayed rapid, pressured speech and anxiety regarding test instructions. He had obvious word-finding difficulty and semantic paraphasias. Even high-frequency words such as 'watch' or 'shave' were forgotten. When asked about his mood, he replied 'what is mood?' When asked to name items found in a supermarket, he did not know what a supermarket was. When shown a partial picture of an elephant, he called it 'the lovely animal with the long . . . you know they used them for work . . . you know they would carry the white stuff that people drink.' When asked how a dog and lion are similar, he replied, 'the lion is bigger . . . with lions you can tell the men and women apart.' He spelled 'who' as 'hu', 'ghost' as 'gost', and 'biscuit' as 'biscet'. On the other hand, he had no difficulty reading and writing orthographically regular words. He was able to copy and recall a complex abstract figure (the Rey-Osterrieth Complex Figure) without difficulty. Brain SPECT scan showed decreased perfusion to the left hemisphere, especially the anterior temporal lobe.

Three years after his initial assessment, he had developed an obsession with eating ketchup, loss of initiative, repetitive behaviours such as checking the weather every half-hour, and decreased hygiene. He answered many questions by saying 'I'm sorry . . . something is wrong with my brain.' He could not point to a door or ceiling and apologized for not being able to do so. When asked to write the word 'house,' he did not know what a house was. With letter-by-letter dictation, he was able to write 'hose' because he no longer knew what a 'u' was. When asked to read what he had written out loud, he said 'hoseh'. He did not know what a 'hose' was. He did not know how to mime using a comb when asked to do so, but could mimic the gesture perfectly when shown. His general neurological exam revealed mild cogwheeling.

of speech such as articles, auxiliary verbs, and prepositions. Sentence structure regresses, becoming grammatically simpler and containing a greater proportion of nouns. Sentences become progressively more laconic and telegraphic speech develops. Anomia refers to difficulty finding words: In PNFA, the patient retains knowledge about the word but cannot bring the word itself to mind, whereas in SD, the patient loses knowledge about what the word represents. The distinctive characteristic about the anomia in PNFA is long pauses between words (more than 8 seconds). In SD, there are semantic paraphasias (word substitutions), but speech is fluent without long pauses (68).

Table 4.3 Diagnostic criteria for PNFA (reprinted with permission from Neary *et al.* (4))

Disorder of expressive language is the dominant feature initially and throughout the disease course. Other aspects of cognition are intact or relatively well preserved.

I. Core diagnostic features
  A. Insidious onset and gradual progression
  B. Non-fluent spontaneous speech with at least one of the following: agrammatism, phonemic paraphasias, anomia

II. Supportive diagnostic features
  A. Speech and language
    1. Stuttering or oral apraxia
    2. Impaired repetition
    3. Alexia, agraphia
    4. Early preservation of word meaning
    5. Late mutism
  B. Behaviour
    1. Early preservation of social skills
    2. Late behavioural changes similar to FTD
  C. Physical signs: late contralateral primitive reflexes, akinesia, rigidity, and tremor
  D. Investigations
    1. Neuropsychology: non-fluent aphasia in the absence of severe amnesia or perceptuospatial disorder
    2. EEG: normal or minor asymmetric slowing
    3. Brain imaging (structural and/or functional): asymmetric abnormality predominantly affecting dominant (usually left) hemisphere

Brain imaging (structural and/or functional): asymmetric abnormality predominantly affecting dominant (usually left) hemisphere.

Supportive diagnostic features help add specificity to the diagnosis of PNFA. Additional language symptoms that may be present in PNFA include stuttering. Oral apraxia is often described and usually refers to apraxia of speech, a motor speech disorder characterized by incoordination of fine movements necessary for articulation (69). Studies have shown that in early PNFA, phonemic (language sound) errors are more common than phonetic (language pronunciation) errors. This suggests that the apparent apraxia of speech may result from an early deficit in language processing rather than solely from a problem with motor co-ordination (70). Early perceptual processing of complex non-verbal sounds is also disturbed in PNFA (71), giving further credence to this notion. Taken together, these deficits may also explain impairments in prosody (patterns of stress, rhythm, and intonation) that are also seen in PNFA, which can lead to patients adopting a 'foreign accent' (72). Orofacial apraxia is an inability to co-ordinate craniofacial muscles (independently of the muscles of articulation) and may frequently occur in PNFA (73). Indeed, limb apraxia, although not mentioned in the diagnostic criteria, may also occur in a substantial minority of patients with PNFA (73).

Box 4.3 Progressive non-fluent aphasia: case example

A 64-year-old man sought consultation in a cognitive disorders clinic due to increasing difficulty pronouncing words that had developed over several months. On initial exam, he had normal cognition outside of language functions. Speech was fairly fluent but he had decreased phrase length and had phonemic paraphasias.

He took early retirement from his job as an accountant because he was embarrassed to speak in front of his clients. One year later, speech was no longer fluent and had become telegraphic. Two years later he preferred to write instead of speak, but even his writing was not perfect. He developed difficulty reading. He had difficulty repeating single words and complained of severe word-finding problems: 'I can't picture the words in my head'. Despite this, when a word was named for him, he could give an adequate description of what it referred to. Brain SPECT scan showed decreased perfusion to the left frontal lobe.

Four years after diagnosis, despite a Mini-Mental Status Examination score of 28/30, he was mute. He began to use a specialized 'Lightwriter' to communicate. Eight years after diagnosis he developed asymmetric apraxia, rigidity, and akinesia. He experienced frequent falls. He had difficulties in reasoning and problem-solving despite preserved memory.

Alexia and agraphia also develop in PNFA, though not necessarily at the same rate as the speech disorder (74) (see Box 4.3). An interesting observation is that patients with PNFA and their first-degree relatives have a greater premorbid prevalence of learning disabilities, including developmental dyslexia (75). Impaired repetition is seen in PNFA whereas repetition tends to be spared in SD. In PNFA, there is early preservation of word meaning; however, comprehension of syntactically complex sentences is impaired, for example, 'the car that the truck hit was green: which vehicle was hit?' (76). Recent studies have stressed the importance of altered grammatical competence as the hallmark language feature of PNFA, over and above loss of fluency (68,77,78). PNFA may therefore be considered a disorder of language processing (grammar and syntax, verbs more impaired than nouns) whereas SD is a disorder of language content (semantics, nouns more impaired than verbs) (79). As PNFA progresses, there is a gradual reduction of all parts of speech leading to late mutism with a total cessation of language. Despite the emergence of mutism, other cognitive functions may be only mildly or moderately impaired.

The second group of supportive diagnostic features highlights the fact that early in the disease, behavioural problems are mild or often subclinical and there is early preservation of social skills. Compared with patients with bvFTD, who are usually brought to medical attention by others due to concerns over changing behaviours, in PNFA decorum and insight are initially preserved and many patients present to their physicians due to their own concerns over troubles expressing themselves. Given the progressive nature of the disease, late behavioural changes similar to bvFTD may occur as the neurodegenerative process becomes more widespread.

The third group of supportive diagnostic features involves physical signs. Extrapyramidal features develop in PNFA similarly to bvFTD. This may reflect the shared pathology and clinical overlap between the syndromes of bvFTD, PNFA, progressive supranuclear palsy (PSP), and corticobasal syndrome (CBS) (see below). Diagnostic criteria also mention the appearance of late contralateral primitive reflexes (cortical release signs). Although this clinical observation has been made, the prevalence of such signs in PNFA has not yet been systematically studied.

Neuropsychological and speech-language pathology assessments in the diagnosis of frontotemporal lobar degeneration

Neuropsychological assessment can confirm the absence of a severe amnesia or visuospatial perception disorder that would be more typical of Alzheimer's disease. Specific impairments on neuropsychological testing can also help to corroborate the clinical diagnosis of a specific syndrome associated with FTLD. For example, in bvFTD, there may be significant impairment on frontal lobe tests in the absence of aphasia or perceptuospatial disorder. Early in bvFTD, the neurodegenerative process affects anterior insular, orbitofrontal, and other paralimbic prefrontal cortical areas before affecting other areas of the frontal lobes (80). Many neuropsychological 'frontal lobe tests' are insensitive to damage in these areas of the prefrontal cortex and are more sensitive to dorsolateral frontal functions. Thus, early on in the disease, patients with bvFTD may show very few deficits on standard clinical neuropsychological assessments (81,82), although test batteries are being developed that show more sensitivity for the deficits typically present in early bvFTD (83,84).

Assessment by a speech-language pathologist with expertise in dementia can contribute additional information, for example, in helping to distinguish between PNFA and SD. In PNFA, a combination of neuropsychological and speech-language assessments can demonstrate the characteristic non-fluent aphasia without impairment of elementary spatial skills or short-term episodic memory (85). In SD, such assessments should reveal profound visual and/or verbal semantic loss with preserved phonology and syntax (thus excluding PNFA). Elementary perceptual processing skills should be preserved, confirming true semantic loss (i.e. an associative agnosia instead of an apperceptive agnosia).

Diagnostic tests to support diagnosis in frontotemporal lobar degeneration

Diagnostic tests are particularly useful to rule out other diseases in the differential diagnosis of FTLD. Electroencephalography is normal in bvFTD and SD, and is usually normal in PNFA although the diagnostic criteria allow for minor asymmetric slowing. The excess slow activity that may be seen in other dementias such as Alzheimer's disease, vascular dementia, or Lewy body dementia is not usually present in FTLD (86).

Brain imaging in FTLD usually shows structural (atrophy) and/or functional abnormalities involving the distinct brain regions responsible for the primary initial symptoms. In bvFTD, the abnormality involves predominantly frontal and/or temporal lobes. This can be subtle, particularly early on in the disease, and requires interpretation by a skilled radiologist alerted to the possible diagnosis of bvFTD. Even then, cases exist where atrophy is so subtle as to be subjective, even in patients with marked behavioural symptoms (87). In SD, characteristic findings include symmetric or asymmetric anterior temporal abnormalities. In contrast to bvFTD, these changes may be more dramatic and severe by the time the patient comes to medical attention. The degree of temporal atrophy tends to correlate with the degree of semantic impairment (62). In SD, there is almost always accompanying frontal atrophy, particularly as the disease advances (87), although this is not mentioned in the diagnostic criteria. In PNFA, there is usually an asymmetric abnormality predominantly affecting the dominant hemisphere, particularly in regions encompassing the brain's language network, such as the inferior and middle frontal gyri, and anterior insula (88,89).

Logopenic progressive aphasia

A syndrome presenting with word-finding difficulties, as well as impairments in repetition and comprehension of syntax, has been recently described and named logopenic progressive aphasia (90). It is thought that the underlying pathology in logopenic progressive aphasia is more often Alzheimer's disease (91,92) (whereas this is only the case in the minority of PNFA and SD cases), although there clearly are cases reported with FTLD pathology (25), including one in a patient with a known progranulin mutation (93). Diagnostic criteria are being proposed (94), but there are no published consensus guidelines for the diagnosis of this syndrome, whose complete characterization is still in its infancy.

Frontotemporal lobar degeneration associated with extrapyramidal disease

The association and overlap of FTLD with extrapyramidal syndromes, particularly CBS and PSP, is increasingly being recognized and studied (95–97). PSP was originally described in 1964 as a heterogeneous neurodegeneration with symptoms of axial rigidity, supranuclear palsy, dysarthria, and dementia (98), although subsequent observations focused particularly on the motor aspects of this disorder. Corticobasal degeneration (CBD), initially called 'corticodentatonigral degeneration with neuronal achromasia', was described 3 years later in three patients with initially unilateral, progressive bradykinesia and awkward limb movements (99). The original patients described did not develop noticeable cognitive deficits until later in their illness, and consequently this disorder was primarily considered a movement disorder until the wider spectrum of presentations, commonly including early dementia, was recognized (100). PSP and CBD, in their canonical forms, were described in association with specific histologic findings. However, as more cases have been identified and studied, it has become clear that some clinical cases of PSP and CBD do not have typical pathology at autopsy. To highlight this fact, the clinical syndrome originally associated with CBD pathology is now often referred to as CBS. Many clinical cases of PSP and CBS have pathological features of FTLD. It appears that the common pathological denominator between many, but not all, CBD/FTLD and PSP/FTLD overlap cases is tau-positive pathology, in contrast to the tau-negative pathology that appears to be a common pathological denominator in FTLD cases that overlap with amyotrophic lateral sclerosis (ALS).

In addition to the pathological overlap between PSP, CBS, and FTLD, there is significant clinical overlap between syndromes. This is particularly true of bvFTD and PNFA; both PNFA and bvFTD may be associated with features of PSP or CBS as the disease progresses, or vice versa (101–106). The dementia in PSP was first described as a prototypical 'subcortical dementia' (107); cortical features were only appreciated later. Neuropsychological features common to bvFTD, PSP, and CBS include impairments in verbal fluency, set shifting, attention, abstraction, inhibition, and planning. Furthermore, 'subcortical frontal deficits' described in PSP, such as lack of initiation and slowed processing speed, are also seen in syndromes produced by FTLD despite often not being the prominent feature. Finally, many language features associated with PNFA are often present early in both PSP and CBS. In one case series, nine of 13 patients initially presenting with PNFA had a final diagnosis of PSP or CBS (108). On the other hand, SD-like features rarely overlap with PSP or CBS.

Frontotemporal lobar degeneration associated with amyotrophic lateral sclerosis

The relationship between FTLD and ALS, which forms the subject of this book, is being increasingly recognized. Although the canonical description of ALS is of a disease affecting exclusively motor neurones, it is now known that up to one-half of patients with ALS will have some cognitive dysfunction (109). The consensus guidelines for diagnosing the overlapping FTLD/ALS syndrome propose a multi-axis diagnostic schema (110). Axis II focuses on characterizing the cognitive and behavioural dysfunction present. A minor proportion of patients with ALS will also meet full criteria for one of the FTLD syndromes. These patients are termed to have 'ALS/FTD', which is further divided into ALS/bvFTD, ALS/PNFA, or ALS/SD. (For clarification, it should be emphasized that the term 'ALS/FTD' refers to any of the FTLD syndromes with concomitant ALS, not just the behavioural variant; 'bvFTD/ALS' is used for the latter.) Many of these patients will present with behavioural/cognitive dysfunction before developing signs of motor neurone disease (111). Invariably they will have a shorter lifespan than patients with FTLD alone (112).

Most patients with an FTLD/ALS overlap syndrome will not fulfil criteria for a diagnosis of ALS/FTD. At one end of the spectrum, patients with FTLD may have subclinical motor neurone disease. The term 'FTLD/MND-like' refers to a neuropathological diagnosis where the pathological criteria for FTLD are fulfilled and there is pathological evidence of motor neurone degeneration that is insufficient for an additional diagnosis of ALS. On the other end of the spectrum are patients with ALS and cognitive and/or behavioural manifestations that do not fulfil criteria for a diagnosis of FTLD. Patients who meet at least two non-overlapping supportive diagnostic features from either the Neary and/or Hodge's criteria are considered to have 'ALS with behavioural impairment' (ALSbi). Patients who suffer from cognitive impairment without dementia, particularly in the executive function domain (defined as less than 5th percentile performance on two or more standardized tests of executive function) are termed 'ALS with cognitive impairment' (ALSci). ALSbi and ALSci are more common than ALS/FTD.

There are ways in which the behavioural and cognitive symptoms in ALS appear to differ from those in isolated FTLD (113). Several small studies suggest that psychotic symptoms, especially delusions, may occur earlier, more frequently, and more prominently (111). Apathy is also frequently seen, particularly in patients with ALSbi (114); it may be more frequent in patients with bulbar-onset ALS. In terms of cognitive dysfunction, there is evidence that executive dysfunction is prevalent in up to one-half of patients with ALS (115). Carefully conducted studies that have controlled for dysarthria and motor weakness have shown that phonemic verbal fluency, an indicator of executive function, is often impaired in ALS (116). Episodic memory and short-term memory deficits are also frequently seen, although these are not typically impaired to the extent that they are in amnestic disorders such as Alzheimer's disease (109). Impairment may reflect deficiencies in frontal-lobe-specific memory processes (117).

The ramifications of behavioural and cognitive symptoms in ALS are significant (118,119). Impaired social functioning can lead to interpersonal conflicts that impact on the caregiver relationship when the patient is physically impaired and requires assistance. Reduced insight can impact on issues related to ALS symptoms. It can lead to decreased adherence to medical prescriptions and difficulty with treatment decisions such as the use of feeding tubes and mechanical ventilation. Executive dysfunction can impair the patient's ability to use communication assistance devices. The future of ALS therapies may also rely on brain–computer interfaces to operate artificial limbs and other assistance devices (120), the operation of which would be considerably hampered in a patient with executive dysfunction.

Summary and conclusions

FTLD describes a group of pathologically heterogeneous, yet related neurodegenerative diseases with focal onset primarily in the frontal and/or temporal lobes. There are three well-defined clinical syndromes associated with FTLD: bvFTD, SD, and PNFA. All have insidious onset and gradual progression. The core features of bvFTD include derangements of social and emotional functioning, lack of insight and impaired psychomotor activity. The characteristic feature of SD is progressive loss of semantic knowledge, in the verbal (recognition of word meaning) and visual (recognition of faces, recognition of object meaning) domains (121). Behavioural abnormalities are also often pronounced in SD. The specific symptoms of SD may depend upon whether the left or right temporal lobe is more affected at initial presentation, and to highlight this some prefer to use the terms left and right temporal variant FTD instead of SD. The hallmark of PNFA is progressively worsening non-fluent, agrammatical speech.

Another syndrome potentially associated with FTLD is logopenic progressive aphasia, although the underlying pathology of this syndrome is often AD. FTLD syndromes may overlap with PSP, CBS, or both. There is also an ALS overlap syndrome that includes ALSbi, ALSci, and ALS/FTD. Features specific to the ALS overlap syndrome include more frequent and earlier occurring executive dysfunction, as well as a greater prevalence of early psychotic symptoms, particular delusions.

Concepts regarding FTLD syndromes are undergoing rapid revision, as experience with these diseases has increased exponentially since the mid-1990s. Diagnosis remains heavily dependent upon accurate clinical description, based upon a careful case history, with assistance from physical exam and neuroimaging results, as well as neuropsychological and speech-language pathology assessments. These syndromes are becoming increasingly recognized, and refinements in clinical diagnostic criteria are currently underway (20).

Acknowledgements

Dr Freedman is supported in part by the Saul A. Silverman Family Foundation Toronto, Canada, as part of a Canada International Scientific Exchange Program Project.

References

1. Kertesz A. (2004). Frontotemporal dementia/pick's disease. *Arch Neurol,* **61**(6), 969–971.
2. Pick A (1892). Über die Beziehungen der senilen Hirnatrophie zur Aphasie. *Prag Med Wochenschr,* **17**, 165–167.
3. Pick A. (1904). Über primäre progressive Demenz bei Erwachsenen. *Prag Med Wochenschr,* **29**, 417–420.
4. Neary D, Snowden JS, Gustafson L, *et al.* (1998). Frontotemporal lobar degeneration: a consensus on clinical diagnostic criteria. *Neurology,* **51**(6), 1546–1554.
5. Ratnavalli E, Brayne C, Dawson K, Hodges JR. (2002). The prevalence of frontotemporal dementia. *Neurology,* **58**(11), 1615–21.
6. Ikeda M, Ishikawa T, Tanabe H. (2004). Epidemiology of frontotemporal lobar degeneration. *Dement Geriatr Cogn Disord,* **17**(4), 265–268.
7. Borroni B, Alberici A, Grassi M, *et al.* (2010). Is frontotemporal lobar degeneration a rare disorder? Evidence from a preliminary study in Brescia county, Italy. *J Alzheimers Dis,* **19**(1), 111–116.
8. Feldman H, Levy AR, Hsiung GY, *et al.* (2003). A Canadian cohort study of cognitive impairment and related dementias (ACCORD): study methods and baseline results. *Neuroepidemiology,* **22**(5), 265–274.
9. Pickering-Brown SM. (2010). Review: Recent progress in frontotemporal lobar degeneration. *Neuropathol Appl Neurobiol,* **36**, 4–16
10. Mackenzie I, Neumann M, Bigio E, *et al.* (2010). Nomenclature and nosology for neuropathologic subtypes of frontotemporal lobar degeneration: an update. *Acta Neuropathol,* **119**, 1–4.
11. Kaye ED, Petrovic-Poljak A, Verhoeff NP, Freedman M. (2010). Frontotemporal dementia and pharmacotherapy. *J Neuropsychiatry Clin Neurosci,* **22**, 19–29.

12. Bozoki AC, Farooq MU. (2009). Frontotemporal lobar degeneration insights from neuropsychology and neuroimaging. *Int Rev Neurobiol*, **84**, 185–213.
13. Kertesz A, McMonagle P, Blair M, Davidson W, Munoz DG. (2005). The evolution and pathology of frontotemporal dementia. *Brain*, **128**(9), 1996–2005.
14. Kertesz A. (2009). Clinical features and diagnosis of frontotemporal dementia. *Front Neurol Neurosci*, **24**, 140–148.
15. Kertesz A, Munoz DG, Hillis A. (2003). Preferred terminology. *Ann Neurol*, **54**(Suppl. 5), S3–6.
16. Zhukareva V, Mann D, Pickering-Brown S, *et al.* (2002). Sporadic Pick's disease: a tauopathy characterized by a spectrum of pathological tau isoforms in gray and white matter. *Ann Neurol*, **51**(6), 730–739.
17. Kertesz A, Hudson L, Mackenzie I, Munoz DG. (1994). The pathology and nosology of primary progressive aphasia. *Neurology*, **44**(11), 2065–2072.
18. McKhann GM, Albert MS, Grossman M, Miller B, Dickson D, Trojanowski JQ. (2001). Clinical and pathological diagnosis of frontotemporal dementia: report of the work group on frontotemporal dementia and pick's disease. *Arch Neurol*, **58**(11), 1803–1809.
19. Hodges JR, Miller B. (2001). The classification, genetics and neuropathology of frontotemporal dementia. Introduction to the special topic papers: Part I. *Neurocase*, **7**, 31–35.
20. Rascovsky K, Hodges JR, Kipps CM, *et al.* (2007). Diagnostic criteria for the behavioral variant of frontotemporal dementia (bvFTD): current limitations and future directions. *Alzheimer Dis Assoc Disord*, **21**(4), S14–18.
21. The Lund and Manchester Groups. (1994). Clinical and neuropathological criteria for frontotemporal dementia. *J Neurol Neurosurg Psychiatry*, **57**(4), 416–418.
22. Freedman M. (2006). Clinical phenomeneology and treatment of frontotemporal dementia, in Strong MJ (ed.). *Dementia and Motor Neuron Disease*, pp. 23–29. Informa Healthcare, Abingdon.
23. Adlam AL, Patterson K, Rogers TT, *et al.* (2006). Semantic dementia and fluent primary progressive aphasia: two sides of the same coin? *Brain*, **129**(11), 3066–3080.
24. Mesulam MM. Primary progressive aphasia: a 25-year retrospective. *Alzheimer Dis Assoc Disord*, **21**(4), S8–S11.
25. Grossman M. (2010). Primary progressive aphasia: clinicopathological correlations. *Nat Rev Neurol*, **6**(2), 88–97.
26. Pijnenburg YA, Mulder JL, van Swieten JC, *et al.* (2008). Diagnostic accuracy of consensus diagnostic criteria for frontotemporal dementia in a memory clinic population. *Dement Geriatr Cogn Disord*, **25**(2), 157–164.
27. Knopman DS, Boeve BF, Parisi JE, *et al.* (2005). Antemortem diagnosis of frontotemporal lobar degeneration. *Ann Neurol*, **57**(4), 480–488.
28. Piguet O, Hornberger M, Shelley BP, Kipps CM, Hodges JR. (2009). Sensitivity of current criteria for the diagnosis of behavioral variant frontotemporal dementia. *Neurology*, **72**(8), 732–737.
29. Mendez MF, Shapira JS, McMurtray A, Licht E, Miller BL. (2007). Accuracy of the clinical evaluation for frontotemporal dementia. *Arch Neurol*, **64**(6), 830–835.
30. Rosen HJ, Gorno-Tempini ML, Goldman WP, *et al.* (2002). Patterns of brain atrophy in frontotemporal dementia and semantic dementia. *Neurology*, **58**(2), 198–208.
31. Short RA, Broderick DF, Patton A, Arvanitakis Z, Graff-Radford NR. (2005). Different patterns of magnetic resonance imaging atrophy for frontotemporal lobar degeneration syndromes. *Arch Neurol*, **62**(7), 1106–1110.
32. Hornberger M, Piguet O, Kipps C, Hodges JR. (2008). Executive function in progressive and nonprogressive behavioral variant frontotemporal dementia. *Neurology*, **71**(19), 1481–1488.

33. Namiki C, Yamada M, Yoshida H, Hanakawa T, Fukuyama H, Murai T. (2008). Small orbitofrontal traumatic lesions detected by high resolution MRI in a patient with major behavioural changes. *Neurocase*, **14**(6), 474–479.
34. Broe M, Hodges JR, Schofield E, Shepherd CE, Kril JJ, Halliday GM. (2003). Staging disease severity in pathologically confirmed cases of frontotemporal dementia. *Neurology*, **60**(6), 1005–1011.
35. Viskontas IV, Possin KL, Miller BL. (2007). Symptoms of frontotemporal dementia provide insights into orbitofrontal cortex function and social behavior. *Ann N Y Acad Sci*, **1121**, 528–545.
36. Kril JJ, Halliday GM. (2004). Clinicopathological staging of frontotemporal dementia severity: correlation with regional atrophy. *Dement Geriatr Cogn Disord*, **17**(4), 311–315.
37. Woolley JD, Wilson MR, Hung E, Gorno-Tempini ML, Miller BL, Shim J. (2007). Frontotemporal dementia and mania. *Am J Psychiatry*, **164**(12), 1811–1816.
38. Gálvez-Andres A, Blasco-Fontecilla H, González-Parra S, Molina JD, Padín JM, Rodriguez RH. (2007). Secondary bipolar disorder and Diogenes syndrome in frontotemporal dementia: behavioral improvement with quetiapine and sodium valproate. *J Clin Psychopharmacol*, **27**(6), 722–723.
39. Mendez MF, Chen AK, Shapira JS, Miller BL. (2005). Acquired sociopathy and frontotemporal dementia. *Dement Geriatr Cogn Disord*, **20**(2–3), 99–104.
40. Banks SJ, Weintraub S. (2009). Generalized and symptom-specific insight in behavioral variant frontotemporal dementia and primary progressive aphasia. *J Neuropsychiatry Clin Neurosci*, **21**(3), 299–306.
41. Mangone CA, Hier DB, Gorelick PB, *et al.* (1991). Impaired insight in Alzheimer's disease. *J Geriatr Psychiatry Neurol*, **4**(4), 189–193.
42. Barrett AM, Eslinger PJ, Ballentine NH, Heilman KM. (2005). Unawareness of cognitive deficit (cognitive anosognosia) in probable AD and control subjects. *Neurology*, **64**(4), 693–699.
43. Evers K, Kilander L, Lindau M. (2007). Insight in frontotemporal dementia: conceptual analysis and empirical evaluation of the consensus criterion 'loss of insight' in frontotemporal dementia. *Brain Cogn*, **63**(1), 13–23.
44. Mateen FJ, Josephs KA. (2009). The clinical spectrum of stereotypies in frontotemporal lobar degeneration. *Mov Disord*, **24**(8), 1237–40.
45. Bathgate D, Snowden JS, Varma A, Blackshaw A, Neary D. (2001). Behaviour in frontotemporal dementia, Alzheimer's disease and vascular dementia. *Acta Neurol Scand*, **103**(6), 367–378.
46. Mikesell L. (2010). Repetitional responses in frontotemporal dementia discourse: asserting agency or demonstrating confusion? *Discourse Stud*, **12**(4), 465–500.
47. Fowler CJ, Griffiths D, de Groat WC. (2008). The neural control of micturition. *Nat Rev Neurosci*, **9**(6), 453–466.
48. Brun A, Passant U. (1996). Frontal lobe degeneration of non-Alzheimer type. Structural characteristics, diagnostic criteria and relation to other frontotemporal dementias. *Acta Neurol Scand*, **168**(Suppl), 28–30.
49. Diehl-Schmid J, Schülte-Overberg J, Hartmann J, Förstl H, Kurz A, Häussermann P. (2007). Extrapyramidal signs, primitive reflexes and incontinence in fronto-temporal dementia. *Eur J Neurol*, **14**(8), 860–864.
50. Freedman M, Black S, Ebert P, Binns M. (1998). Orbitofrontal function, object alternation and perseveration. *Cereb Cortex*, **8**, 18–27.
51. Hailstone JC, Crutch SJ, Vestergaard MD, Patterson RD, Warren JD. (2010). Progressive associative phonagnosia: a neuropsychological analysis. *Neuropsychologia*, **48**(4), 1104–1114.
52. Gainotti G, Ferraccioli M, Marra C. (2010). The relation between person identity nodes, familiarity judgment and biographical information. Evidence from two patients with right and left anterior temporal atrophy. *Brain Res*, **1307**, 103–114.

53. Gainotti G. (2007). Different patterns of famous people recognition disorders in patients with right and left anterior temporal lesions: a systematic review. *Neuropsychologia*, **45**(8), 1591–1607.
54. Snowden JS, Thompson JC, Neary D. (2004). Knowledge of famous faces and names in semantic dementia. *Brain*, **127**(4), 860–872.
55. Rosen HJ, Pace-Savitsky K, Perry RJ, Kramer JH, Miller BL, Levenson RW. (2004). Recognition of emotion in the frontal and temporal variants of frontotemporal dementia. *Dement Geriatr Cogn Disord*, **17**(4), 277–281.
56. Rankin KP, Kramer JH, Miller BL. (2005). Patterns of cognitive and emotional empathy in frontotemporal lobar degeneration. *Cogn Behav Neurol*, **18**, 28–36.
57. Rankin KP, Kramer JH, Mychack P, Miller BL. (2003). Double dissociation of social functioning in frontotemporal dementia. *Neurology*, **60**(2), 266–271.
58. Rosen HJ, Allison SC, Ogar JM, *et al.* (2006). Behavioral features in semantic dementia vs other forms of progressive aphasias. *Neurology*, **67**(10), 1752–1756.
59. Snowden JS, Bathgate D, Varma A, Blackshaw A, Gibbons ZC, Neary D. (2001). Distinct behavioural profiles in frontotemporal dementia and semantic dementia. *J Neurol Neurosurg Psychiatry*, **70**(3), 323–332.
60. Rankin KP, Santos-Modesitt W, Kramer JH, Pavlic D, Beckman V, Miller BL. (2008). Spontaneous social behaviors discriminate behavioral dementias from psychiatric disorders and other dementias. *J Clin Psychiatry*, **69**, 60–73.
61. Walterfang M, Velakoulis D. (2005). Cortical release signs in psychiatry. *Aust NZ J Psychiatry*, **39**(5), 317–327.
62. Hodges JR, Davies RR, Patterson K. (2009). Semantic dementia. In: Miller BL, Boeve BF (eds.), *The Behavioral Neurology of Dementia*, pp. 264–278. Cambridge University Press, Cambridge.
63. Josephs KA, Whitwell JL, Knopman DS, *et al.* (2009). Two distinct subtypes of right temporal variant frontotemporal dementia. *Neurology*, **73**(18), 1443–1450.
64. Thompson SA, Patterson K, Hodges JR. (2003). Left/right asymmetry of atrophy in semantic dementia: behavioral-cognitive implications. *Neurology*, **61**(9), 1196–1203.
65. Viskontas IV, Miller BL. (2009). Frontotemporal dementia. In: Miller BL, Boeve BF (eds.). *The Behavioral Neurology of Dementia*, pp. 45–55. Cambridge University Press, Cambridge.
66. Chan D, Anderson V, Pijnenburg Y, *et al.* (2009). The clinical profile of right temporal lobe atrophy. *Brain*, **132**(5), 1287–1298.
67. Seeley WW, Bauer AM, Miller BL, *et al.* (2005). The natural history of temporal variant frontotemporal dementia. *Neurology*, **64**(8), 1384–1390.
68. Ash S, Moore P, Vesely L, *et al.* (2009). Non-fluent speech in frontotemporal lobar degeneration. *J Neurolinguistics*, **22**(4), 370–383.
69. Ogar J, Slama H, Dronkers N, Amici S, Gorno-Tempini ML. (2005). Apraxia of speech: an overview. *Neurocase*, **11**(6), 427–432.
70. Ash S, McMillan C, Gunawardena D, *et al.* (2010). Speech errors in progressive non-fluent aphasia. *Brain Lang*, **113**, 13–20.
71. Goll JC, Crutch SJ, Loo JH, *et al.* (2010). Non-verbal sound processing in the primary progressive aphasias. *Brain*, **133**, 272–285.
72. Luzzi S, Viticchi G, Piccirilli M, *et al.* (2008). Foreign accent syndrome as the initial sign of primary progressive aphasia. *J Neurol Neurosurg Psychiatry*, **79**, 79–81.
73. Rohrer JD, Rossor MN, Warren JD. (2010). Apraxia in progressive nonfluent aphasia. *J Neurol*, **257**(4), 569–574.
74. Fukui T, Lee E. (2008). Progressive agraphia can be a harbinger of degenerative dementia. *Brain Lang*, **104**(3), 201–210.

75. Rogalski E, Johnson N, Weintraub S, Mesulam MM. (2008). Increased frequency of learning disability in patients with primary progressive aphasia and their first-degree relatives. *Arch Neurol*, **65**(2), 244–248.
76. Grossman M, Moore P. (2005). A longitudinal study of sentence comprehension difficulty in primary progressive aphasia. *J Neurol Neurosurg Psychiatry*, **76**(5), 644–649.
77. Mesulam MM, Wieneke C, Rogalski E, Cobia D, Thompson C, Weintraub S. (2009). Quantitative template for subtyping primary progressive aphasia. *Arch Neurol*, **66**(12), 1545–1551.
78. Peelle JE, Troiani V, Gee J, *et al.* (2008). Sentence comprehension and voxel-based morphometry in progressive nonfluent aphasia, semantic dementia, and nonaphasic frontotemporal dementia. *J Neurolinguistics*, **21**(5), 418–432.
79. Hillis AE, Oh S, Ken L. (2004). Deterioration of naming nouns versus verbs in primary progressive aphasia. *Ann Neurol*, **55**(2), 268–275.
80. Seeley WW, Crawford R, Rascovsky K, *et al.* (2008). Frontal paralimbic network atrophy in very mild behavioral variant frontotemporal dementia. *Arch Neurol*, **65**(2), 249–255.
81. Gregory CA, Serra-Mestres J, Hodges JR. (1999). Early diagnosis of the frontal variant of frontotemporal dementia: how sensitive are standard neuroimaging and neuropsychologic tests? *Neuropsychiatry Neuropsychol Behav Neurol*, **12**(2), 128–135.
82. Rahman S, Robbins TW, Sahakian BJ. (1999). Comparative cognitive neuropsychological studies of frontal lobe function: implications for therapeutic strategies in frontal variant frontotemporal dementia. *Dement Geriatr Cogn Disord*, **10**(Suppl 1), 15–28.
83. Torralva T, Roca M, Gleichgerrcht E, Bekinschtein T, Manes F. (2009). A neuropsychological battery to detect specific executive and social cognitive impairments in early frontotemporal dementia. *Brain*, **132**(5), 1299–1309.
84. Manes F, Torralva T, Roca M, Gleichgerrcht E, Bekinschtein T, Hodges J. (2010). Frontotemporal dementia presenting as pathological gambling. *Nat Rev Neurol*, **6**(6), 347–352.
85. Patterson K, Graham NL, Ralph MA, Hodges JR. (2006). Progressive non-fluent aphasia is not a progressive form of non-fluent (post-stroke) aphasia. *Aphasiology*, **20**(9), 1018–1034.
86. Liedorp M, van der Flier WM, Hoogervorst EL, Scheltens P, Stam CJ. (2009). Associations between patterns of EEG abnormalities and diagnosis in a large memory clinic cohort. *Dement Geriatr Cogn Disord*, **27**, 18–23.
87. Nestor PJ. (2007). Neuroimaging and other investigative findings. In Hodges JR (ed.), *Frontotemporal Dementia Syndromes*, pp. 134–160. Cambridge University Press, Cambridge.
88. Nestor PJ, Graham NL, Fryer TD, Williams GB, Patterson K, Hodges JR. (2003). Progressive non-fluent aphasia is associated with hypometabolism centred on the left anterior insula. *Brain*, **126**(11), 2406–2418.
89. Rohrer JD, Warren JD, Modat M, *et al.* (2009). Patterns of cortical thinning in the language variants of frontotemporal lobar degeneration. *Neurology*, **72**(18), 1562–1569.
90. Gorno-Tempini ML, Dronkers NF, Rankin KP, *et al.* Cognition and anatomy in three variants of primary progressive aphasia. *Ann Neurol*, **55**(3), 335–346.
91. Gorno Tempini ML, Brambati SM, Ginex V, *et al.* (2008). The logopenic/phonological variant of primary progressive aphasia. *Neurology*, **71**(16), 1227–1234.
92. Rohrer JD, Rossor MN, Warren JD. (2010). Alzheimer's pathology in primary progressive aphasia. *Neurobiol Aging*, 2010 Jun 24 [Epub ahead of print].
93. Rohrer JD, Crutch SJ, Warrington EK, Warren JD. (2010). Progranulin-associated primary progressive aphasia: a distinct phenotype? *Neuropsychologia*, **48**, 288–297.
94. Bonner MF, Ash S, Grossman M. (2010). The new classification of primary progressive aphasia into semantic, logopenic, or nonfluent/agrammatic variants. *Curr Neurol Neurosci Rep*, 2010 Sep 1 [Epub ahead of print].

95. Kertesz A, Munoz D. (2004). Relationship between frontotemporal dementia and corticobasal degeneration/progressive supranuclear palsy. *Dement Geriatr Cogn Disord*, **17**(4), 282–286.

96. Boeve BF, Lang AE, Litvan I. (2003). Corticobasal degeneration and its relationship to progressive supranuclear palsy and frontotemporal dementia. *Ann Neurol*, **54**(Suppl 5), S15–S19.

97. Sha S, Hou C, Viskontas IV, Miller BL. (2006). Are frontotemporal lobar degeneration, progressive supranuclear palsy and corticobasal degeneration distinct diseases? *Nat Clin Pract Neurol*, **2**(12), 658–665.

98. Steele JC, Richardson JC, Olszewski J. (1964). Progressive supranuclear palsy. A heterogeneous degeneration involving the brain stem, basal ganglia and cerebellum with vertical gaze and pseudobulbar palsy, nuchal dystonia and dementia. *Arch Neurol*, **10**, 333–359.

99. Rebeiz JJ, Kolodny EH, Richardson EP. (1968). Corticodentatonigral degeneration with neuronal achromasia. *Arch Neurol*, **18**, 20–33.

100. Grimes DA, Lang AE, Bergeron CB. (1999). Dementia as the most common presentation of cortical-basal ganglionic degeneration. *Neurology*, **53**(9), 1969–1974.

101. Sanchez-Valle R, Forman MS, Miller BL, Gorno-Tempini ML. (2006). From progressive nonfluent aphasia to corticobasal syndrome: a case report of corticobasal degeneration. *Neurocase*, **12**(6), 355–359.

102. Kertesz A, Martinez-Lage P, Davidson W, Munoz DG. (2000). The corticobasal degeneration syndrome overlaps progressive aphasia and frontotemporal dementia. *Neurology*, **55**(9), 1368–1375.

103. Sakurai Y, Hashida H, Uesugi H, *et al.* (1996). A clinical profile of corticobasal degeneration presenting as primary progressive aphasia. *Eur Neurol*, **36**(3), 134–137.

104. Ioannides P, Karacostas D, Hatzipantazi M, Ioannis M. (2005). Primary progressive aphasia as the initial manifestation of corticobasal degeneration. A 'three in one' syndrome? *Funct Neurol*, **20**(3), 135–137.

105. Moreno F, Indakoetxea B, Barandiaran M, *et al.* (2009). 'Frontotemporoparietal' dementia: clinical phenotype associated with the c.709–1G>A PGRN mutation. *Neurology*, **73**(17), 1367–1374.

106. Mathuranath PS, Xuereb JH, Bak T, Hodges JR. (2000). Corticobasal ganglionic degeneration and/or frontotemporal dementia? A report of two overlap cases and review of literature. *J Neurol Neurosurg Psychiatry*, **68**(3), 304–312.

107. Albert ML, Feldman RG, Willis AL. (1974). The 'subcortical dementia' of progressive supranuclear palsy. *J Neurol Neurosurg Psychiatry*, **37**(2), 121–130.

108. Josephs KA, Petersen RC, Knopman DS, *et al.* (2006). Clinicopathologic analysis of frontotemporal and corticobasal degenerations and PSP. *Neurology*, **66**, 41–48.

109. Ringholz GM, Appel SH, Bradshaw M, Cooke NA, Mosnik DM, Schulz PE. (2005). Prevalence and patterns of cognitive impairment in sporadic ALS. *Neurology*, **65**(4), 586–590.

110. Strong MJ, Grace GM, Freedman M, *et al.* (2009). Consensus criteria for the diagnosis of frontotemporal cognitive and behavioural syndromes in amyotrophic lateral sclerosis. *Amyotroph Lateral Scler*, **10**(3), 131–146.

111. Lillo P, Garcin B, Hornberger M, Bak TH, Hodges JR. (2010). Neurobehavioral features in frontotemporal dementia with amyotrophic lateral sclerosis. *Arch Neurol*, **67**(7), 826–830.

112. Josephs KA, Parisi JE, Knopman DS, Boeve BF, Petersen RC, Dickson DW. (2006). Clinically undetected motor neuron disease in pathologically proven frontotemporal lobar degeneration with motor neuron disease. *Arch Neurol*, **63**(4), 506–512.

113. Phukan J, Pender NP, Hardiman O. (2007). Cognitive impairment in amyotrophic lateral sclerosis. *Lancet Neurol*, **6**(11), 994–1003.

114. Grossman AB, Woolley-Levine S, Bradley WG, Miller RG. (2007). Detecting neurobehavioral changes in amyotrophic lateral sclerosis. *Amyotroph Lateral Scler*, **8**, 56–61.

115. Gordon PH, Goetz RR, Rabkin JG, *et al.* (2010). A prospective cohort study of neuropsychological test performance in ALS. *Amyotrophic Lateral Scler,* **11**(3), 312–320.
116. Abrahams S, Leigh PN, Harvey A, Vythelingum GN, Grise D, Goldstein LH. (2000). Verbal fluency and executive dysfunction in amyotrophic lateral sclerosis (ALS). *Neuropsychologia*, **38**(6), 734–747.
117. Strong MJ. (2008). The syndromes of frontotemporal dysfunction in amyotrophic lateral sclerosis. *Amyotroph Lateral Scler*, **9**(6), 323–338.
118. Lomen-Hoerth C. (2004). Characterization of amyotrophic lateral sclerosis and frontotemporal dementia. *Dement Geriatr Cogn Disord*, **17**(4), 337–341.
119. Merrilees J, Klapper J, Murphy J, Lomen-Hoerth C, Miller BL. (2010). Cognitive and behavioral challenges in caring for patients with frontotemporal dementia and amyotrophic lateral sclerosis. *Amyotroph Lateral Scler*, **11**(3), 298–302.
120. Nijboer F, Sellers EW, Mellinger J, Jordan *et al.* (2008). A P300-based brain-computer interface for people with amyotrophic lateral sclerosis. *Clin Neurophysiol,* **119**(8), 1909–1916.
121. Neary D, Snowden J, Mann D. (2005). Frontotemporal dementia. *Lancet Neurol*, **4**(11), 771–780.

Chapter 5

Language profiles in amyotrophic lateral sclerosis

J.B. Orange and A.E. Hillis

Amyotrophic lateral sclerosis (ALS) is a neurodegenerative disorder linked to cell death of lower motor neurones of the brainstem and spinal cord, and of upper motor neurones of the cerebral cortex. It is the third most common adult-onset neurodegenerative disease (1). ALS was considered to be restricted largely to motor neurones while cognition was thought to be intact. More recently, however, ALS has been recognized as a multisystem disorder (2). Cognitive impairment (CI) (35–55%) but not dementia has been demonstrated in a substantial proportion of individuals with ALS who also show deficits on tests of executive function (3). Typical CIs include disruptions to attention systems and processes, to executive functions, to multiple memory systems, and to visuospatial skills. In particular, studies revealed deficits in verbal and nonverbal fluency tasks (4,5), working memory (6), cognitive flexibility (7), and sustained attention (8). Deficits also are found in recognition memory for words and faces, visual perception, reasoning, word generation, word fluency (7,9), and executive functions such as planning, organizing, and self-monitoring (10). Greater detail of the cognitive profiles of persons with ALS is found in associated chapters in this volume.

The language and behavioural disorders associated with ALS discussed in this chapter will be presented as a spectrum of overlapping clinical syndromes, under the umbrella term 'frontotemporal disease'. Although the former umbrella term was frontotemporal lobar degeneration (11), this term is now used predominantly to refer to histopathologically confirmed pathology. That is, FTLD is the neuropathological correlate of the majority of individuals with frontotemporal dementia (FTD). The specific association between ALS and frontal lobe impairment has been postulated with symptoms, including emotional changes, memory, language, and general intellectual problems, prominent bulbar features, and bilateral frontal and/or temporal lobar atrophy (10,12–14).

The clinical syndromes of FTD will be referred to in this chapter as behavioural variant frontotemporal dementia (bvFTD), and three variants of primary progressive aphasia (PPA). The focus of the language components in ALS in this chapter will, of course, be on PPA, because the chapter is about language and communication behaviours in ALS. However, the language of individuals with bvFTD is not unaffected, so it will be covered briefly as well. We will first describe the language profiles of the variants of PPA, recognizing that they all overlap, both clinically and pathologically. Individuals with ALS can display symptoms and signs of each of the PPA variants over time. Any of the variants can be and are associated with ALS, although the bvFTD and non-fluent/agrammatic variant of PPA (nfvPPA) are the most commonly associated with clinical ALS, perhaps because they are localized to the frontal lobes (predominantly the left posterior fronto-insular regions in nfvPPA), near the motor strip. The key question of whether individuals with ALS develop neuropsychological evidence of FTD before or after progression of the disease is still unclear. ALS with frontotemporal dementia (ALS/FTD) is estimated to occur in 3% of sporadic cases and 15% of the familial type (15,16). The 5–15% of individuals with ALS and dementia generally evolve to the ALS/bvFTD (17). The nfvPPA is sometimes the primary clinical diagnoses in individuals who eventually develop ALS/FTD (18).

Primary progressive aphasia

PPA was first described by Mesulam (19) as a progressive deterioration in language for at least 2 years before the decline in other cognitive functions (other than perhaps praxis). This requirement remains a core element of the diagnosis. Since Mesulam's original description, there have been several attempts to define subtypes. One of the original distinctions was between 'fluent' versus 'non-fluent' PPA. However, fluency parameters are often difficult to define, to quantify consistently and very difficult to agree upon across examiners. Individuals may be fluent in some tasks and dysfluent in other contexts, or fluent on some measures and not others. Fluency often is measured by rate of speech, number, length and location of pauses in the spoken stream, grammatically, articulation accuracy, prosody, etc. Depending on the weight assigned to each dimension of fluency by the examiner, the rating of fluency can be very different over time and across evaluators. Therefore, over the course of several years, gradual consensus developed among investigators of PPA based on a series of video conferences that culminated in guidelines for distinguishing three variants of PPA, which were not based entirely on fluency versus non-fluency dichotomies (20). The three subtypes that were characterized and agreed upon were nfvPPA, semantic variant PPA (svPPA), and logopenic variant (lvPPA), as described below.

Non-fluent/agrammatic primary progressive aphasia

The nfvPPA, formerly known as progressive non-fluent aphasia, is characterized by at least one of two core features: (a) a motor speech disorder best characterized as apraxia of speech (AOS) in all spoken output (effortful, halting, and inaccurate in: repetition, reading aloud, and spontaneous speech), with greater difficulty producing polysyllabic than monosyllabic words, and numerous and varied off-target attempts at producing particular speech sounds, not attributable to muscle weakness, disrupted reflexes, auditory comprehension or cognitive problems, reduced rate or range of movement of the lips, tongue, palate, vocal folds, or respiratory muscles, or (b) agrammatic sentence production, even with anagrams (not attributable to reduced working memory), including simplified language production. Typically, individuals with nfvPPA also have more difficulty naming verbs (actions) than nouns (persons, places and objects). Their spoken output is often telegraphic, and frequently limited to single nouns. They typically speak very little, and may write better than they speak, although writing is typically agrammatic as well. They may, however, be able to write simple sentences long after they no longer produce any sentences verbally.

It can be difficult to assess the presence or influence of AOS in individuals with ALS, particularly those with emerging bulbar symptoms, because they also exhibit a mixed flaccid–spastic dysarthria (even anarthria) that can mask an AOS. It is very useful clinically to assess oral reading of sentences, particularly sentences of varying phonological and morphosyntactic complexity. Patients with ALS who exhibit the mixed-dysarthria only (i.e. without AOS) will have consistent imprecise consonants (i.e. same slurred speech sounds), slowed but prosodically even speaking rate, monopitch, hypernasality, and a harsh voice (21). It usually is possible to understand some or much of what they are saying because the correct sounds in the words are present, although distorted. An examiner generally understands what words individuals with ALS are attempting to say unless the individuals have progressed to a more advanced stage. The overlay of an AOS in persons with ALS typically yields inconsistent speech errors described as 'errors of complication', such as sounds being deleted, added, substituted, an obvious halting, disrupted prosody (i.e. flow), and oral groping or posturing to articulate sounds, all of which are not typical in the mixed-dysarthria profile in ALS.

Most clinicians posit that nfvPPA is the most common variant of PPA associated with ALS. This variant of PPA is, however, more commonly associated with tau pathology than ubiquitin pathology at autopsy (22,23), which is surprising, given that ubiquitin is the pathology classically associated with ALS. A few studies have found corticobasal degeneration to be particularly common in nfvPPA. Voxel-based morphometry studies show that areas of greatest atrophy in nfvPPA are in the left posterior frontal cortex and insula (24). Positron emission tomography studies confirm hypometabolism in these areas (25).

Semantic variant primary progressive aphasia

Individuals with svPPA (formerly known as semantic dementia) must possess the two core features of impaired single-word comprehension and poor confrontation naming of pictures or objects, particularly those of low frequency of occurrence or of low familiarity (e.g. 'emu') (20). A striking feature is that they frequently ask the meaning of words. They will often say something of the sort, 'Peach? What does peach mean? I have heard that word. What is it? Is it something to eat? I think I might like it, but maybe not. Maybe you would.' Their speech is effortless, and their spoken and written language is replete with verbs and functors, but with little meaningful content (i.e. semantically empty). There is a strong effect of familiarity in both comprehension and naming tasks, such that they comprehend highly familiar words ('comb', 'fork', 'car', 'eat', 'shop') far better than less familiar words (e.g. depending on their culture, perhaps 'cactus' or 'pretzel'). Later in its course, many individuals with svPPA develop difficulty understanding the meaning of objects themselves, particularly unfamiliar objects. They might use objects inappropriately, such as using a corkscrew to eat a salad. Speech articulation and prosody are fluid and effortless. Grammatical aspects of spoken and written language are generally spared. They often produce verbs more accurately than nouns (26,18). The noun/verb ratio in their spontaneous spoken language is even higher than normal controls.

The reading comprehension and writing of individuals with svPPA often deteriorates early in the disease, but often has a particular quality known as 'surface dyslexia' and 'surface dysgraphia'. In these cases, the person cannot read or spell irregular words (e.g. 'yacht', 'business', 'phone'), but can read and spell them plausibly, using 'phonics' or orthography–phonology mapping. Thus, scissors might be spelled 'sizzers' and read aloud as 'skissors'.

The most common pathology in svPPA is ubiquitin, frequently TDP-43 (transactive response DNA-binding protein of 43 kDa) (22,23,27), which is the same pathology reported in ALS. Nevertheless, clinical ALS associated with svPPA is relatively rare. The uncommon association may be due to the fact that svALS is associated with atrophy in the left greater than right anterior and lateral inferior temporal cortex (24,25), relatively far from the motor cortex. Individuals with svPPA nearly always (or always) have some right-sided atrophy as well as left, which may be necessary for the deficit in object meaning. Individuals with right greater than left anterior and inferior temporal atrophy have predominant proposognosia and object agnosia more than aphasia.

An illustrative case of a patient with svPPA and ALS is provided in Box 5.1.

Logopenic progressive aphasia

This form of PPA will be mentioned only briefly for completeness to contrast it with nfvPPA and svPPA, as it is not typically associated with ALS. lvPPA is characterized by disproportionately impaired phrase and sentence repetition, and phonological errors, (much like the vascular syndrome of conduction aphasia) and single-word retrieval and confrontation naming problems. Both lvPPA and conduction aphasia are associated with impaired phonological working memory and damage or atrophy in the inferior parietal lobule (supramarginal gyrus and angular gyrus), and/or superior temporal cortex. Motor speech, grammatical sentence production (at least if given anagrams, or sentences to read, thus removing the working memory component), and word comprehension are spared. At autopsy, lvPPA is typically associated with Alzheimer's disease pathology, and most individuals have positive amyloid imaging with positron emission tomography (25).

Behavioural variant frontotemporal dementia

A recent working group put together a new set of criteria for diagnosing bvFTD, which includes several levels of certainty, based on clinical evidence (possible), clinical + imaging

Box 5.1 Illustrative case of amyotrophic lateral sclerosis with semantic variant primary progressive aphasia

Mr V is a 60-year-old man who developed fasciculations and word-finding problems while working in a high-level position. He was highly motivated and exercised avidly to maintain strength. He participated in language therapy to maintain language skills. He continued working despite some clear deficits for another year. His spelling and reading were understandable, but he had trouble understanding irregular words. He became somewhat disinhibited and inappropriate, obsessive-compulsive about exercise, and frustrated about his language deficits. He was particularly disinhibited when he drank, so it was necessary to stop him from drinking. Eventually he was convinced to stop working and driving. He became mildly weak with hyper-reflexia and bilateral Babinksi signs, but no bulbar signs. He continued to have diffuse fasciculations throughout the limbs. His comprehension deteriorated. He developed fluent, meaningless spoken language. He developed difficulty using objects appropriately except for familiar ones. For example, he used a can-opener to spread peanut butter. In short, over time he developed clear signs and symptoms of semantic variant primary progressive aphasia and amyotrophic lateral sclerosis, with some features of behavioural variant frontotemporal dementia as well.

evidence (probable), or pathological/genetic evidence (definite) of the disease (28). With the focus of this chapter on language in ALS, we will discuss only the clinical evidence relative to bvFTD, stressing cognitive–communication issues. The clinical syndrome of bvFTD is essentially a progressive deterioration in comportment. Individuals with bvFTD can become progressively apathetic or disinhibited, but the change is always very striking. Likewise, their spoken language can become either minimal (aphemic) or copious (logorrheic). The apathetic person often has a paucity of spoken language, rarely initiating conversation; and what is said may be mostly perseverative. The disinhibited individual may be digressive and tangential, never coming to the point of what he or she is trying to say. Neither of the individuals who are apathetic or disinhibited are very functional in terms of communication. Both subtypes have difficulty understanding abstract language such as metaphor, and both have trouble understanding facial expressions and prosody of spoken language (although the latter has not been as carefully studied to date). Therefore, there are breakdowns in communication both in terms of expression and comprehension.

Family members and clinicians often report obvious disturbances in the pragmatics (i.e. appropriate use and understanding of language based on social contexts and forces) of those with bvFTD. In these instances, the language of and communication by individuals with bvFTD is inherently inappropriate to the social context(s). That is, individuals with bvPPA may use words, phases or sentences that are unacceptable to the circumstances (i.e. viewed as disinhibited), may not use or understand the subtleties of figurative or sarcastic forms of language, or may digress, shift or reintroduce the topics of conversation (i.e. tangential or off-topic). It is these elements of pragmatics that frequently are perplexing to family, friends, and co-workers, often leading them to refer the individual for assessment.

Specific studies of language in individuals with amyotrophic lateral sclerosis

Speech problems are a prominent feature of individuals with ALS. The mixed flaccid–spastic dysarthria associated with ALS, as noted previously, resulting from involvement of multiple motor systems includes the predominant speech features of imprecise consonants, hypernasality, harsh voice quality, slow speaking rate, monopitch, and short phrases (21). The progression of mixed dysarthria leading to anarthria contributes to their overall communication problems.

Language processing in individuals with ALS without CI or FTD has not been studied in depth but rather as one part of general cognitive testing (29). Recent studies that considered the language performance of individuals with ALS have shown subtle but consistent deficits (3,29). The most commonly reported language deficit in individuals with ALS without CI or FTD is word retrieval problems (3,5,7,9,30,31). Other language deficits include reduced single-word vocabulary comprehension (7), moderately impaired auditory comprehension (31), and verbal and semantic paraphasias on confrontation and generative noun naming (7,30). Cooper *et al.* (30) found a subgroup of ALS participants who made significantly more semantic errors than controls on a generative verbal fluency naming task (i.e. semantic categories). Cobble (29) found auditory comprehension problems of linguistically complex stimuli, spelling errors, and word finding difficulties in individuals with ALS but no CIs or FTD.

Discourse analysis of spoken and written outputs of individuals with ALS using samples from a topic-directed interview and the 'Cookie theft' picture description task from the Boston Diagnostic Aphasia Examination (32) at baseline and then again at 6 months revealed that individuals with ALS produced significantly fewer self-corrected utterances compared with controls (7). Bak and Hodges (33) showed that individuals with ALS without CI or FTD exhibit significant verb naming deficits. Narasimha (34) showed, using discourse tasks, that individuals with ALS without CI or FTD produced more obligatory 1 and 2 place arguments (simplified verb structures) versus controls who produced more obligatory 3 place, optional 2 place and optional 3 place arguments (i.e. more complex verb structures). In addition, Narasimha's ALS participants produced significantly more verbs in the topic-directed interview versus the picture description task. Moreover, the ALS participants produced more parenthetical remarks versus controls on both picture description and topic-directed interview tasks. Parenthetical remarks generally are considered non-propositional language structures adding limited semantic content to the primary information being conveyed. Increased use of parenthetical remarks suggests possible lexical access and linguistic difficulties. The high use of parenthetical remarks also can indicate underlying word finding and semantic memory difficulties, which get masked through the use of the parenthetical remarks. Despite these collective findings, it remains uncertain whether language deficits are a common but under-recognized feature of individuals with ALS without CI or FTD (35). Further study of the language in individuals with ALS but without CI or FTD is warranted.

Individuals with ALS and dementia (typically with FTD), as noted above, exhibit obvious impairments in language functions (36). The most frequently noted language problem in individuals with ALS/FTD is reduced verbal output, often leading to complete mutism (12,15). Other language disturbances include word retrieval deficits on confrontation naming, category naming, and letter fluency problems, impaired comprehension for both complex sentences and single-word semantic processing tasks, and reading and writing difficulties (5,29,36–39). Doran *et al.* (39) found that individuals with ALS/FTD showed significant auditory comprehension problems.

Anomia, impaired language comprehension, semantic paraphasias, and spelling errors also have been reported in individuals with ALS/FTD (5,12,33,35,40–43). On tests of verbal repetition, individuals with ALS/FTD ranged from normal, mildly impaired to echolalic (12,40). Although naming and comprehension are impaired for both verbs and nouns, a consistently larger impairment was noticed in verbs on both naming and comprehension tasks (15,18,35). Neuroimaging studies have confirmed the involvement of language areas such as Broadman areas 44 and 45 in individuals with ALS/FTD (35). Bak and Hodges (35) found that language deficits can be an early and a prominent feature of individuals with ALS/FTD. They also stated that language deficits could be unrelated to a dementia and that the language impairment could be more pronounced than what is expected on cognitive tests. Clearly, further study is warranted.

Assessment of language

An important goal of language and cognitive–communication assessments in the ALS clinic is to characterize carefully the deficits such that clinicians can distinguish among the PPA variants. Moreover, a second goal is to determine the relative contributions among speech, language, and cognitive–communication deficits per se to the overall communication profile. Therefore, specific tools and tasks are needed to distinguish the variants, as described above, as well as those that provide useful guides for language and communication therapies, including counselling regarding work decisions, level of supervision required, and capacity assessments, among others. A minimum set of tasks and tests is listed in Table 5.1.

Tests of word comprehension

Word comprehension subtests of standardized language batteries typically involve pointing to named pictures (forced choice, word/picture matching tests), such as in the Western Aphasia Battery–Enhanced (44), Boston Diagnostic Aphasia Battery (3rd edition) (32), among other comprehensive tests of language. However, simple word/picture verification tasks (e.g. presenting a picture of a dog, and asking, ‘Is this a cat?’) are even more sensitive to word comprehension deficits (45). Nevertheless, most word/picture or word/object comprehension tests are adequate. Even providing an array of not-too familiar objects (e.g. stethoscope, hammer, cotton, gauze, plastic glove, tongue blade) and asking the person to

Table 5.1 Essential tasks for assessment of speech, language, and cognitive-communication in amyotrophic lateral sclerosis

Motor speech assessment—rate of speech, intelligibility scores, sound error profiles
Single word comprehension
Semantic associations (e.g. picture-word matching; word associations—see Pyramids and Palm Trees Test, among others)
Spoken and written sentence production (including anagrams)
Sentence reading aloud and comprehension, and sentence repetition
Naming actions (regular versus irregular verbs in present and then past tense, for example walk-walked versus dive-dove/sleep-slept versus go-went) and objects
Reading aloud and spoken and written spelling of irregular (e.g. shove, touch) and regular words (lend, pair, fresh)
Spoken and/or written language samples using picture description or topic directed interview (Tell me about your current/former jobs, family, where you were born and raised, what you do on a typical day)
Discourse and conversation analysis measures include the following: Mean length of utterance, verb: noun ratios, number and proportion of pronouns, number and proportion of verb argument types, spelling and grammar errors, number and proportions of self-corrections per utterance, wording finding error patterns (paraphasias), number of propositions, number and proportion of on- and off-topic utterances

pick up each named item provides a reasonable assessment of single word comprehension. Individuals with svPPA will be impaired on this test, whereas individuals with the other variants of PPA will perform normally, at least until very late in the course.

Test of semantic association

It is important for the family to understand that their relative with svPPA may have trouble understanding the meaning of objects as well as words. Therefore, a test of non-verbal semantic association is helpful, at least in svPPA. These tests may be less important to give individuals with other forms of PPA. There are published tests, such as the Pyramids and Palm Trees Test (46), which requires the person to select one of two pictures that is most clearly associated with a third picture. For example, the person must decide if a palm tree or a fir tree is more associated with a pyramid. Other tests of semantic association require the person to decide which of two picture pairs are more closely related. Some tests use action pictures (i.e. verbs) (e.g. the Kissing and Dancing Test by Thomas Bak, unpublished).

Tests of sentence production

To distinguish nfvPPA from lvPPA it is often important to detect agrammatism, present in nfvPPA, because both sound relatively hesitant and 'non-fluent'. Both variants produce sentence fragments and exhibit long pauses. It is useful to obtain a spoken, and where possible written, language sample based on a picture description task, much like what is done in the Western Aphasia Battery-Revised and the Boston Diagnostic Aphasia Examination-III.

In addition to this elicited language sample, provide written words that comprise a sentence but which are presented in scrambled order (i.e. disrupted syntax) and ask individuals to reorder the words into a grammatically and syntactically correct sentence. It is important to encourage them to produce some 'non-canonical' or passive sentences, such as 'The man was kicked by the girl'. Avoid unfamiliar vocabulary, which would conflate grammatical and semantic difficulties.

Many individuals with nfvPPA with impairments in grammatical sentence production also will be impaired in reading aloud and repeating sentences. Individuals with lvPPA, on the other hand, should be relatively unimpaired in the anagram task and reading aloud, but very impaired in repeating the same sentences. Sentences that can be used for reading aloud and for repeating are provided in Table 5.2. These sentences permit evaluation of the effects of sentence length versus grammatical and syntactic complexity. Similar sentences can be used in the anagram task.

Naming actions and objects

Impairment in naming is ubiquitous in PPA and apparent in many with ALS. However, stimuli that elicit naming errors are different across variants of PPA and in ALS, and the types of errors vary across variants to some extent (47). Individuals with nfvPPA make more errors on objects, whereas individuals with svPPA make more errors on actions (18,26). Individuals with ALS/FTD who also have motor speech impairments showed the same pattern of performance as those with nfvPPA with more impaired naming of actions than objects; however, persons with ALS/FTD who had fluent aphasia consistent with svPPA showed the opposite pattern (48). Action naming can be tested with the Kissing and Dancing Test (Thomas Bak, unpublished) or the Action Naming Test (49) wherein individuals with ALS might have more trouble with actions than objects. Recent work by Narasimha (34) showed that performance on the Action Naming Test was poorer when individuals with ALS were asked to produce the verbs in past tense form, particularly for irregular verbs ('dig' versus 'dug', 'win' versus 'won'). Individuals with ALS are impaired particularly on letter and semantic category fluency tasks (3,5,7,9,30,31,50). Action fluency (naming as many actions as possible in 1 minute) can be particularly sensitive (51). Circumlocutions are the most common error type among those with svPPA and lvPPA, but semantic coordinate errors (e.g. snail named as fish) are common across all variants of PPA (47) with semantic paraphasia predominant in selected subgroups of those with ALS (30). Therefore, it is important to assess naming both of actions and objects, as well as letter and semantic category and action fluency. Again, a sensitive test should include

Table 5.2 Sentence for oral reading and repetition

The cat ate the caterpillar.
Justin is taller than Henry.
A teacher bought three pairs of gloves.
We walked to the lake and then to the store.
The rabbit was given to the child by a fireman.

items that are not highly familiar. Ideally, actions and objects should be matched for word frequency, familiarity, and word length. Most published naming tests include only objects. The Boston Diagnostic Aphasia Examination-III has some pictures actions in the Word Discrimination test, but they are all of high familiarity.

Reading and writing

There is little published systematic research on the reading comprehension and written expressive skills of individuals with ALS with or without CI or FTD, other than clinical observations regarding written spelling errors. No patterns in spelling errors have been observed in the few samples from participants in the Strong, ALS Clinic, London, Canada other than a small number of instances of problems with irregularly spelled words. As noted previously, the most commonly described reading pattern in PPA is surface dyslexia, with 'regularization' of irregular words (and the mirror deficit in spelling, known as surface dysgraphia). Ichikawa *et al.* (52) reported that individuals with bulbar-onset ALS showed dysgraphia, particularly omission and substitution of kana, associated with hypoperfusion of the frontotemporal cortex, that could not be attributed to aphasia or dementia. This same group reported that dysgraphia in persons with ALS–dementia was associated with anosognosia for writing errors in a retrospective review of a separate group (53).

Other patterns of breakdown in spelling associated with svPPA, lvPPA, and nfvPPA are described (54). These patterns of spelling impairment are similar to those reported, as a result of focal brain damage. In addition, they can be ascribed to loss of one or more of the cognitive processes underlying spelling, such as the graphemic buffer (i.e. a working memory system for holding the series of abstract letter identities while each is written or spelled aloud). This latter pattern is reported in association with nfvPPA. Instead of producing phonologically plausible errors in spelling (e.g. 'leopard' spelled 'lepperd'), individuals insert, delete, transpose, or substitute one or more letters resulting in phonologically implausible errors (e.g. 'leopard' spelled 'leotad').

To evaluate reading and spelling, it is important to obtain spontaneous and elicited writing samples, such as written description of a complex picture (such as the 'Cookie theft' picture from the Boston Diagnostic Aphasia Examination-III) or responses to the questions of a topic-directed interview, as described previously. In accordance with the task protocol, instruct individuals to write complete, grammatical sentences about what is happening in the picture, rather than merely to list items in the picture. For elicited tasks, instruct individuals to spell a list of regular and irregular verbs and nouns to dictation (see Table 5.3 for examples). Pseudowords (e.g. glamp) also can be given to get an idea of phoneme-grapheme (i.e. sound to letter) mapping abilities.

Motor speech assessment

Individuals with ALS display a mixed flaccid–spastic dysarthria, with its speech parameters as described previously. Traditional oral peripheral mechanism assessments (i.e. oral anatomy and physiological evaluation) and speech motor control assessments (single and multiple sound productions and repetitions, single and multiple syllable word repetitions, etc.) should be completed as part of a comprehensive routine evaluation. The topic of AOS remains controversial, as it is not universally recognized as a distinct entity. Nevertheless, we will assume that it is a deficit in motor planning and programming of speech articulation. AOS is characterized by effortful and inaccurate repetition, disrupted oral reading, and halting spontaneous speech. Individuals with AOS exhibit greater difficulty producing polysyllabic than monosyllabic words, particularly for individual and sound blends and clusters, particularly in the initial position of syllables. Individuals with AOS make numerous and varied off-target attempts at producing particular speech sounds, which are not attributable to weakness, reduced rate or range of movement of the lips, tongue, palate, vocal folds, or respiratory muscles (i.e. not attributable to dysarthria), disrupted reflexes, auditory comprehension problems or CIs. AOS often can be detected by asking individuals to produce polysyllabic words (e.g. refrigerator) three to five times or words of increasingly length such as 'jab', 'jabber', and 'jabberwocky' or 'zip', zipper', 'zippering'). Individuals with AOS produce errors of complication (i.e. additions, substitutions, transpositions) as the length of words increase and make different errors across repetitions of the same word or words of increasing length. In contrast, individuals with ALS who show only mixed dysarthria will say the polysyllabic words and those of increasing length nearly the same imprecise way each time.

Language and communication treatments in amyotrophic lateral sclerosis

Medications have uncertain benefit for reducing the rate of decline in ALS. Cholinesterase inhibitors have not been helpful in reducing the rate of decline in cognition in any form

Table 5.3 Regular and irregular words matched for frequency, length, and word class

Irregularly spelled words	Regularly spelled words
earth	book
ghost	road
sword	leaf
tongue	cane
heir	deer
limb	door
word	ball
choir	rope
laugh	speak
sigh	kick
gauge	shave
seize	shoot
sieve	hang
knock	pray
sew	cut

of frontotemporal disease, and so there is no reason to believe they would be helpful in ALS, given its histopathology and neuropathophysiology. Memantine has been used in open-label trials, but not for language function in ALS to our knowledge. On the other hand, language and communication therapy can be helpful not only in maintaining communicative success in ALS and PPA, but also for temporarily improving language function at least on trained sets of items that might be important for the individual (e.g. numbers written on cheques, names of family members, or favourite places or foods) and for caregivers with concerns for functional communication (e.g. use of telephone, work-related communication, etc.).

The authors of one published study of PPA treatment reported success in naming, which showed at least temporary improvement to trained items and (in the case of a person with lvPPA, but not in a case of svPPA) generalization to untrained items (55). This study used a cueing hierarchy approach to treating naming that incorporated teaching participants to use a communication notebook. That is, when each participant was unable to name an item independently, the participant was encouraged to find it in a word communication notebook (organized by theme), and then to read it aloud. This self-cueing strategy provided a functional means of communication that carried over to everyday life. Many persons with mild PPA can carry a word communication notebook (i.e. a form of augmentative communication) containing the names of family members, important people (e.g. beauticians, bankers, lawyers, doctors, etc.), favourite places to go, topics of conversation, and so on. Those who commonly use electronic devices (computer-assisted speech systems, cell phones, tablets and I-pads) can use these more technical versions to produce relatively clear electronic speech from text voices if their dysarthria reduces significantly the intelligibility of their speech. Augmentative and alternate communication devices are used commonly among those with moderate- to advanced-staged ALS with compromised speech intelligibility as result of their mixed dysarthria. An overarching concern with complex augmentative and alternative communication devices among those of ALS and suspected FTD is the cognitive and linguistics loads, in concert with the limb motor movement demands. Some simple communication programs for the I-phone can be learned by individuals with ALS, ALS/PPA, or ALS/FTD. More complex augmentative communication devices (text to speech devices) used by individuals with pure ALS are usually abandoned toward the advanced stage because they require too high level language and/or cognitive skills. This is particularly the case for those with ALS/PPA or ALS/FTD. However, referral to a speech–language pathologist either for direct speech, language and cognitive–communication therapies or for appropriate communication devices is very important for individuals with ALS and all variants of ALS/PPA and ALS/FTD to enhance communication in all its forms, to retain social connectedness, and to optimize health-related quality of life.

As with all aspects of disease progression, speech, language, and communication therapy for individuals with ALS, ALS/PPA, or ALS/FTD must be discontinued when no progress is documented. It is crucial for the medical and healthcare professionals to support those with ALS and their family to understand that the goals of therapy are to find ways to maintain or to optimize speech, language, and cognitive-communicative functions, sometimes within the contexts of a coexisting CI or a FTD. Moreover, clinicians also must implement and train strategies that can be continued by family or other caregivers without the clinician being present to maximize communication. It often is appropriate for speech and language therapies to be brief in duration, but to resume in 6 months to optimize communication at the new (lower) baseline. Medical and other healthcare professionals can access, where available, university-based speech–language pathology graduate programme clinics where new graduate students provide therapy each semester. Websites of the National Aphasia Association (www.aphasia.org), the American-Speech-Language-Hearing Association (www.asha.org), the Canadian Association of Speech-Language Pathologists and Audiologists (www.caslpa.ca), and state or provincial professional associations often contain information on and links to speech–language pathologists who provide therapy for patients with ALS, PPA, or FTD in the United States or Canada.

Concluding remarks

Although language disorders may not be the most common or noticeable impairments in individuals with ALS/FTD, they can be the most bothersome and disabling problems to the person and to her/his family, who sometimes relies on failing written language skills to communicate in the face of profound anarthria. Although challenging to assess and to treat, it is critical to do so. We have made every attempt to provide practical recommendations, stimuli, and resources for this purpose, more than details of all of the research in this domain.

References

1. Brockington A, Ince P, Shaw PJ. (2006). The clinical and pathological spectrum of ALS. In: Strong MJ (ed.), *Dementia and Motor Neuron Disease*, pp. 31–57. Informa UK Ltd.
2. Strong MJ. (1999). Simplifying the approach: What can we do? *Neurology,* **53**, S31–S34.
3. Abrahams S, Leigh PN, Goldstein LH. (2005). Cognitive change in ALS: a prospective study. *Neurology,* **64**, 1222–1226.
4. Ludolph AC, Langen KJ, Regard M, *et al.* (1992). Frontal lobe function in amyotrophic lateral sclerosis: A neuropsychologic and positron emission tomography study. *Acta Neurol Scand,* **85**, 81–89.
5. Rakowicz WP, Hodges JR. (1998). Dementia and aphasia in motor neuron disease: an under recognized association? *J Neurol Neurosurg Psychiatry,* **65**, 881–889.
6. Portet F, Cadilhac C, Touchon J, Camu W. (2001). Cognitive impairment in motor neuron disease with bulbar onset. *ALS Other Motor Neuron Disord,* **2**, 23–29.
7. Strong MJ, Grace GM, Orange JB, Leeper HA, Menon RS, Aere C. (1999). A prospective study of cognitive impairment in ALS. *Neurology,* **53**, 1665–1670.
8. Abe K, Fujimura H, Toyooka K, Sakoda S, Yorifuji S, Yanagihara T. (1997). Cognitive function in Amyotrophic Lateral Sclerosis. *J Neurol Sci,* **148**, 95–100.
9. Abrahams S, Leigh PN, Harvey A, Vythelingum GN, Grise D, Goldstein LH. (2000). Verbal fluency and executive dysfunction in amyotrophic lateral sclerosis (ALS). *Neuropsychologia,* **38**, 734–747.
10. Talbot PR, Goulding PJ, Lloyd JJ, Snowden JS, Neary D, Testa HJ. (1995). Inter-relation between 'classic' motor neuron disease and frontotemporal dementia: neuropsychological and single photon emission computed tomography study. *J Neurol Neurosurg Psychiatry,* **58**, 541–547.

11. Neary D, Snowden JS, Gustafson L, *et al.* (1998). Frontotemporal lobar degeneration: a consensus on clinical diagnostic criteria. *Neurology*, **51**(6), 1546–1554.
12. Neary D, Snowden JS, Mann DMA, Northen B, Goulding PJ, Macdermott N. (1990). Frontal lobe dementia and motor neuron disease. *J Neurol Neurosurg Psychiatry*, **53**, 23–32.
13. Abrahams S, Goldstein LH, Kew JJ, *et al.* (1996). Frontal lobe dysfunction in amyotrophic lateral sclerosis: a PET study. *Brain*, **119**, 2105–2120.
14. Massman PJ, Sims J, Cooke N, Haverkamp LJ, Appel V. (1996). Prevalence and correlates of neuropsychological deficits in amyotrophic lateral sclerosis. *J Neurol Neurosurg Psychiatry*, **61**, 450–455.
15. Bak TH, Hodges JR. (2001). Motor neuron disease, dementia and aphasia: coincidence, co-occurrence or continuum? *Neurology*, **248**, 260–270.
16. Lomen-Hoerth C, Murphy J, Langmore S, Kramer JH, Olney RK, Miller B. (2003). Are amyotrophic lateral sclerosis patients cognitively normal? *Neurology*, **60**, 1094–1097.
17. Strong MJ. (2008). The syndromes of frontotemporal dysfunction in amyotrophic lateral sclerosis. *Amyotroph Lateral Scler*, **9**, 323–338.
18. Hillis AE, Oh S, Ken L. (2004). Deterioration of naming nouns versus verbs in primary progressive aphasia. *Ann Neurol*, **55**(2), 268–275.
19. Mesulam MM. (1982). Slowly progressive aphasia without generalized dementia. *Ann Neurol*, **11**(6), 592–598.
20. Gorno-Tempini ML, Hillis AE, Weintraub S, *et al.* (2011) International guidelines for the diagnosis of primary progressive aphasia and its variants. *Neurology*, **76**, 1006–1014.
21. Darley FL, Aronson AE, Brown JR. (1975). *Motor Speech Disorders*. WB Saunders Company, West Washington Square, Philadelphia.
22. Davies RR, Hodges JR, Kril JJ, Patterson K, Halliday GM, Xuereb JH. (2005). The pathological basis of semantic dementia. *Brain*, **128**(Pt 9), 1984–1995.
23. Kertesz A, McMonagle P, Blair M, Davidson W, Munoz DG. (2005). The evolution and pathology of frontotemporal dementia. *Brain*, **128**(Pt 9), 1996–2005.
24. Gorno-Tempini ML, Dronkers NF, Rankin KP, *et al.* (2004). Cognition and anatomy in three variants of primary progressive aphasia. *Ann Neurol*, **55**(3), 335–346.
25. Rabinovici GD, Jagust WJ, Furst AJ, *et al.* (2008). Abeta amyloid and glucose metabolism in three variants of primary progressive aphasia. *Ann Neurol*, **64**(4), 388–401.
26. Hillis AE, Tuffiash E, Caramazza A. (2002). Modality-specific deterioration in naming verbs in nonfluent primary progressive aphasia. *J Cogn Neurosci*, **14**(7), 1099–1108.
27. Grossman M, Wood EM, Moore P, *et al.* (2007). TDP-43 pathologic lesions and clinical phenotype in frontotemporal lobar degeneration with ubiquitin-positive inclusions. *Arch Neurol*, **64**(10), 1449–1454.
28. Rascovsky K, Hodges JR, Kipps CM, *et al.* (2007). Diagnostic criteria for behavioral variant of frontotemporal dementia (bvFTD): Current Limitations and Future Directions. *Alzheimer Dis Assoc Disord*, **21**(4), S14–S18.
29. Cobble M. (1998). Language impairment in motor neurone disease. *J Neurol Sci*, **160**, S47–S52.
30. Cooper E, Orange JB, Strong MJ, *et al.* (2008). Generative naming in amyotrophic lateral sclerosis. Poster presented at the Annual Convention of the American Speech-Language-Hearing Association, Chicago, IL. *The Asha Leader*, **13**(11), 130
31. Mantovan MC, Baggio L, Barba GD, *et al.* (2003). Memory deficits and retrieval processes in ALS. *Eur J Neurol*, **10**, 221–227.
32. Goodglas H, Kaplan E, Baressi B. (2001). *Boston Diagnostic Aphasia Examination*, 3rd edn. Lippincott, Williams, Wilkins, Baltimore, MD.
33. Bak T, Hodges JR. (1997). Noun-verb dissociation in three patients with motor neuron disease and Aphasia. *Brain Language*, **60**, 38–41.

34. Narasimha AM. (2009). *Verb Use in ALS*. Unpublished master's thesis, University of western Ontario, Ontario, Canada.
35. Bak TH, Hodges JR. (2004). The effects of motor neuron disease on language: Further evidence. *Brain Language,* **89**, 354–361.
36. Haley M, Raymer AM. (2000). Speech, language and cognitive impairments in ALS. *Neurophysiol Neurogenic Speech Lang Disord,* **4**, 2–5.
37. Caselli RJ, Windebank AJ, Petersen RC, *et al.* (1993). Rapidly progressive aphasic dementia and motor neuron disease. *Ann Neurol,* **33**(2), 200–207.
38. Cooper E. (2008). *Generative Naming in ALS: a longitudinal study*. Unpublished Master's Thesis. University of Western Ontario, London Canada.
39. Doran M, Xuereb J, Hodges JR. (1995). Rapidly progressive aphasia with bulbar motor neurone disease: a clinical trial and neuropsychological study. *Behav Neurol,* **8**, 169–180.
40. Cavelleri F, DeRenzi E. (1994). Amyotrophic lateral sclerosis with dementia. *Acta Neurol Scand,* **89**, 391–394.
41. Deymeer F, Smith TW, DeGirolami U, Drachman DA. (1989). Thalamic dementia and motor neuron disease. *Neurology,* **38**, 58–61.
42. Ferrer I, Roig C, Espino A, Piero G, Guiu M. (1991). Dementia of the frontal lobe type and motor neuron disease: a Golgi study of the frontal cortex. *J Neurol Neurosurg Psychiatry,* **54**, 932–934.
43. Gentileschi V, Sperber S, Spinnler H. (1999). Progressive defective recognition of familiar people. *Neurocase,* **5**, 407–423.
44. Kertesz A. (2006). *The Western Aphasia Battery–Enhanced*. Grune Stratton, New York.
45. Breese EL, Hillis AE. (2004). Auditory comprehension: is multiple choice really good enough? *Brain Language*, **89**, 3–8.
46. Howard D, Patterson K. (1992). *The Pyramids and Palm Trees Test*. Thames Valley Test Company, Bury St Edmunds.
47. Budd M, Kortte K, Cloutman L, *et al.* (2010). The nature of naming errors in primary progressive aphasia versus acute post-stroke aphasia. *Neuropsychology*, **24**(5), 581–589.
48. Hillis AE, Heidler-Gary J, Newhart M, Chang S, Ken L, Bak T. (2006). Naming and comprehension in primary progressive aphasia: the influence of grammatical word class. *Aphasiology*, **20**, 246–256.
49. Obler L, Albert M. (1986). *Action Naming Test*. Aphasia Research Center, Boston, MA.
50. Heidler-Gary J, Hillis AE. (2007). Distinctions between the dementia in amyotrophic lateral sclerosis with frontotemporal dementia and the dementia of Alzheimer's disease. *Amyotroph Lateral Scler*, **8**(5), 276–282.
51. Davis C, Heidler-Gary J, Gottesman R, *et al.* (2010). Action versus animal naming fluency in subcortical dementia, frontal dementias, and Alzheimer's disease. *Neurocase*, **16**, 259–266.
52. Ichikawa H, Takahashi N, Hieda S, Ohno H, Kawamura M. (2008). Agraphia in bulbar-onset amyotrophic lateral sclerosis: not merely a consequence of dementia or aphasia. *Behav Neurol*, **20**(3), 91–99.
53. Ichikawa H, Koyama S, Ohno H, Ishihara K, Nagumo K, Kawamura M. (2008). Writing errors and anosognosia in amyotrophic lateral sclerosis with dementia. *Behav Neurol*, **19**(3), 107–16.
54. Sepelyak K, Crinion J, Molitoris JJ, *et al. Patterns of Breakdown in Spelling in Primary Progressive Aphasia*. Cortex, in press.
55. Newhart M, Davis C, Kannan V, Heidler-Gary J, Cloutman L, Hillis AE. (2009). Therapy for naming deficits in two variants of primary progressive aphasia. *Aphasiology*, **23**, 823–834.

Chapter 6

Language impairment in amyotrophic lateral sclerosis from an historical review: kana and kanji versus alphabetical languages

Hiroo Ichikawa, Sotaro Hieda, Hideki Ohno, Kenji Ishihara, and Mitsuru Kawamura

Amyotrophic lateral sclerosis (ALS) has traditionally been thought to affect the upper and lower motor neurones and sparing behaviour, language, and other cognitive domains. However, psychiatric symptoms were identified in the early 1900s (1,2) and Japanese cases of ALS with dementia (ALS-D) were reported by Yuasa (3,4) and Mitsuyama and colleagues (5–7) in the 1960s to 1980s. However, the absence of similar findings worldwide led to an assumption that this condition was a disorder characteristic of Japanese subjects. Thereafter, similar cases were reported, mostly in Japan, and the condition was identified as ALS of the Yuasa–Mitsuyama type (8–11).

In the 1990s, the concept of frontotemporal lobar degeneration (FTLD) was proposed (12–15) and the association of motor neurone diseases (MND) and cognitive impairment came to international attention. More recently, immunohistochemical advances have revealed that FTLD with tau-negative and ubiquitin-positive inclusions (FTLD-U) is linked to ALS and/or MND (ALS/MND) (16–18). The discovery of transactivation response DNA-binding protein with a molecular weight of 43 kDa (TDP-43) has shown that ALS/MND is a multisystem disorder identifiable with most FTLD-U (19–23) (see Highley and Ince, Chapter 19 and Cairns, Chapter 19). Moreover, in addition to identification of mutations in fused sarcoma in familial ALS (24,25), fused sarcoma pathology has recently been found in atypical FTLD-U (26). These discoveries indicate that ALS/MND and FTLD share the same pathology and molecular basis, but have different clinical phenotypes (23,27). Thus, selective ALS motor system involvement was shown to be incorrect for over 100 years after the initial description of ALS by Charcot and Joffroy.

What does this mean for language function as one aspect of cognitive function? Patients with ALS often have accompanying dysarthria due to bulbar or pseudo-bulbar palsy in association with involvement of upper or lower motor neurones, and bulbar symptoms are often an initial symptom. Therefore, language impairment may have been overlooked in ALS. However, historical accounts suggest language impairment in patients with ALS (28) and we believe that evaluation of writing is the key to detect language problems in ALS (9,10).

Descriptions of writing errors in amyotrophic lateral sclerosis

The first historical account of aphasia in Japan is a report of patients with ALS by Watanabe (Figure 6.1) in 1893, as discussed by Kawamura (28). The title of this article was interpreted in English as 'a patient with medullary bulbar palsy and progressive muscular atrophy accompanied by cortical motor aphasia'. This report has largely passed unnoticed, but appears to be the first description of language problems in ALS. It was published about 20 years after the first account of ALS by Charcot and Joffroy, and about 70 years before the description of ALS-D (also called Yuasa–Mitsuyama type) in Japan. Watanabe described the language impairment as incomplete motor aphasia, but spontaneous speech was already lost and aphasia was identified by writing errors with paragraphia. The evidence is incomplete, but it is clear that writing errors disclose language problems of an aphasic nature. We think that the descriptions given by Watanabe are of great importance for discussing language problems, including writing errors, in ALS, and that the aphasia–ALS link has been overlooked.

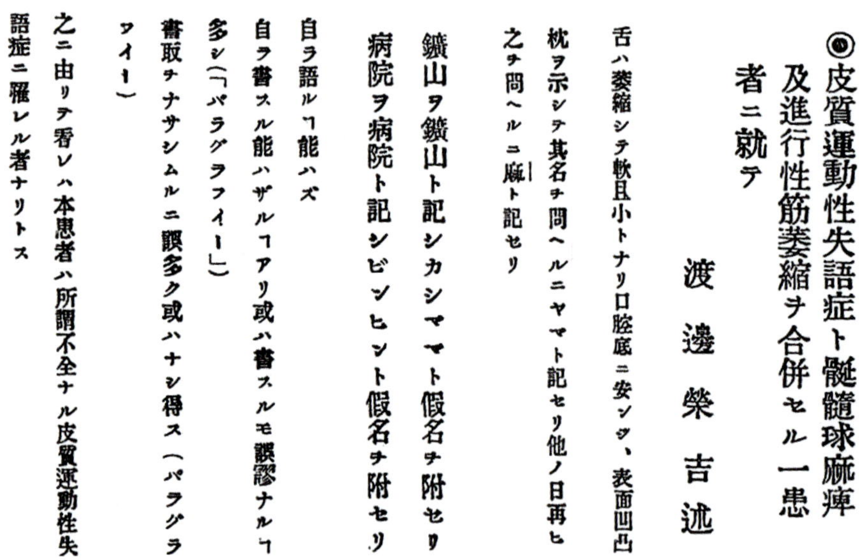
◉皮質運動性失語症ト延髓球麻痺及進行性筋萎縮ヲ合併セル一患者ニ就テ

渡邊榮吉述

舌ハ萎縮シテ軟且小トナリ口腔底ニ安ンジ、表面凹凸
枕ヲ示シテ其名ヲ問ヘルニヤマト記セリ他ノ日再ヒ
之ヲ問ヘルニ麻ート記セリ
鑛山ヲ鑛山ト記シカシママト假名ヲ附セリ
病院ヲ病院ト記シビンヒント假名ヲ附セリ
自ラ語ルヿ能ハズ
自ラ書スル能ハザルヿアリ或ハ書スルモ誤謬ナルヿ
多シ(「パラグラフイー」)
書取ヲナサシムルニ誤多ク或ハナシ得ズ(パラグラ
フイー)
之ニ由リテ看レハ本患者ハ所謂不全ナル皮質運動性失
語症ニ罹レル者ナリトス

Fig. 6.1 Watanabe's 1893 article and its interpretation in English. The title is (translated) 'A patient with medullary bulbar palsy and progressive muscular atrophy accompanied by cortical motor aphasia'. A description of the tongue as atrophied, softened and uneven is given. Incorrect writing without actual meaning was evident in kana letters rather than complex kanji letters: 'ヤマト' in kana, pronounced 'yamato', for '枕', pronounced 'makura', meaning 'pillow' in English; 'カシママ', pronounced 'kashimama', for '鉱山' pronounced 'kouzan', meaning 'mine'; 'ビンヒン', pronounced 'binhin', for '病院', pronounced 'byouin', meaning 'hospital'. Reprinted with permission from the *Journal of Okayama Medical Association* **5**: 138–144, Watanabe, 1893

The Japanese system of writing consists of two types of letters: kana (phonograms) and kanji (ideograms). A kana letter represents a spoken syllable, with a strict one-to-one correspondence of sound-to-script. Kana words consist of one or more kana and always have only one phonetic pronunciation. Therefore, kana words correspond to complete regular words in alphabetical languages (29–32). On the other hand, a kanji letter, which is not used in spoken language, conveys a particular meaning but has different pronunciations. Kanji words consist of one or more kanji and usually have one pronunciation attached to the meaning. Therefore, Kanji words are comparable with irregular words in alphabetical languages (29–32). Generally, a Japanese sentence is written by mixing kana and kanji: kanji letters are usually used for writing most nouns and verb roots, adverbs and adjectives; and kana letters are mainly used to write inflectional endings, conjunctions, and postpositions (prepositions) that integrate syntax. In Japanese literature, dissociated impairment between kana and kanji letters has been frequently described, mostly in patients with cerebrovascular diseases. Double dissociation between kana and kanji has also been documented in localized frontal lobe infarctions (32). Interestingly, although the patient reported by Watanabe made errors in both kana and kanji, dissociated errors between kana and kanji letters were also mentioned (28). For example, when intending to write '盃', pronounced 'sakazuki' and meaning a saké cup, the patient wrote '盃' in kanji, but wrote 'ヨウリ' in kana, pronounced 'youri' and without a meaning. When intending ' 病院', pronounced 'byouin' and meaning a hospital, the patient correctly wrote '病院' in kanji, but incorrectly wrote 'ビンヒン' in kana, pronounced 'binhin' and without a meaning. Overall, the patient made writing errors more frequently in kana than in kanji, suggesting dissociated impairment.

Outside Japan, writing errors in ALS were first documented by Ferguson and Boller in 1977 in a report of two cases of bulbar-onset ALS presenting with syntactic errors and spelling errors without aphasia (33). One of the patients was diagnosed neuropathologically with ALS. Speech was almost abolished in these patients and detailed neuropsychological evaluations were not performed. The features of the writing errors were described as 'pure agraphia' (33). However, subsequent descriptions of language problems or writing errors in ALS did not appear until the 1980s and 1990s (34,35). A breakthrough in language problems in ALS/MND was provided by Caselli and colleagues in 1993 through documentation of seven cases with development of progressive aphasic dementia and MND (36). In this report, the authors stated that 'the aphasic nature of their disturbance only became evident when written language abilities were assessed' (36). This report and subsequent development of the concept of FTLD (12–15) has drawn attention to language problems in ALS/MND.

Accumulation of language problems, including writing errors, in patients with ALS/MND, including primary lateral sclerosis has emerged from many reports (37–57). Thus, although early economy of speech and mutism is considered an important sign in ALS-D (7,8), we believe that language problems of an aphasic nature exist behind such conditions. In support of this, we have found frequent writing errors in ALS-D cases, most of which were bulbar-onset and showed loss of speech in association with severe dysarthria (9).

Language impairment in frontotemporal lobar degeneration subtypes

FTLD is a clinicopathological entity that predominantly involves the frontotemporal lobes and is now the third most common cause of cortical dementia, following Alzheimer's disease and dementia with Lewy bodies (13). ALS and FTLD have been shown to share the same pathological and molecular bases (19–23,26). FTLD consists of three phenotypic neurobehavioural syndromes: frontotemporal dementia (FTD), progressive non-fluent aphasia (PNFA), and semantic dementia (SD) (13). Among the phenotypic subtypes, FTD is divided into frontal lobar degeneration, Pick type, and MND type (15). The typical full-blown dementia observed in ALS is usually FTD, and FTD of the MND type is now generally considered to correspond to ALS-D in Japan. However, cases of ALS with PNFA (36–46) or SD (47,55) have been reported and development of MND supports a diagnosis of both FTD and PNFA in the clinical diagnostic criteria for FTLD (15). These criteria are consistent with recent pathological evidence, which show that many patients with PNFA and SD have tau-negative and ubiquitin-positive inclusions and TDP-43 pathology (20,58–60). Thus, the MND type applies not only to FTD but also to PNFA and SD (Figure 6.2). The recent monograph by Snowden and colleagues (15) describes spelling errors, omissions, and grammatical errors in PNFA and surface dysgraphia in SD, but the nature of writing in FTD is not indicated, except for a description of language problems, including economy of speech leading to mutism; concrete, echolalic, and stereotypic speech; and semantic paraphasia in naming.

PNFA is a disorder of expressive language, characterized by effortful speech production, phonologic, and grammatical errors, and word retrieval difficulties, while understanding of word meaning is relatively well preserved (13). In PNFA, brain atrophy is asymmetric, involving chiefly the left frontotemporal lobes (13). Caselli and colleagues reported patients with rapidly progressive aphasic dementia and MND and described impaired fluency with effortful, halting, paraphasic, and oligosyllabic speech, resembling the characteristic features of PNFA (36). In SD, atrophy is typically bilateral and is most marked in the anterior temporal neocortex, with inferior and middle temporal gyri being

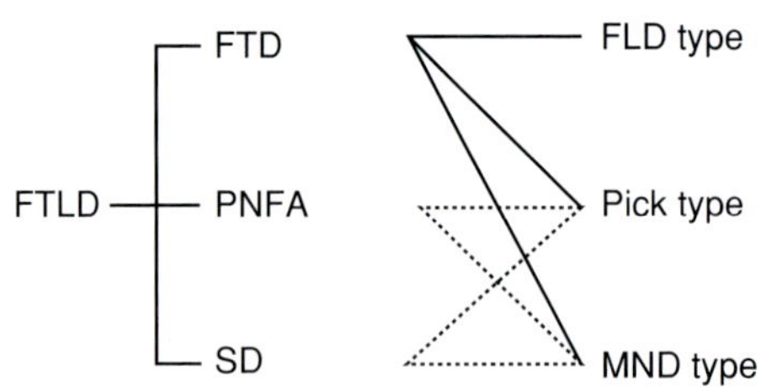

Fig. 6.2 Subtypes of FTLD (15). The MND type was indicated only for FTD by Snowden *et al.* (solid lines), but we believe this subtype is applicable for both PNFA and SD (dotted lines). FLD, frontal lobe degeneration; FTD, frontotemporal dementia; FTLD, frontotemporal lobar degeneration; MND, motor neuron disease; PNFA, progressive non-fluent aphasia; SD, semantic dementia. With permission from Snowden, J.S., Neary, D. & Mann, D.M.A. (1996) Fronto-temporal lobar degeneration: fronto-temporal dementia. Progressive aphasia, semantic dementia. Clinical Neurology and Neurosurgery Monographs. NY: Churchill Livingstone.

predominantly affected (12). Although a combination of SD and clinically manifested ALS is rare (20,58–60), cases of ALS with features of SD have been reported (47,55). Iroi and colleagues described a patient with a history of being 'unable to read Kanji letters in newspapers and reading with effort using a dictionary' and neurological findings were alexia of kanji characters and semantic aphasia (47). A pathological examination was not performed, but left-sided dominant bilateral temporal lobes were predominantly affected on single-photon emission tomography (SPECT) images (47).

As shown above, the clinical nature of aphasia, including PNFA or SD in ALS/MND has been occasionally documented, with most cases appearing to be PNFA (36–46). In most cases, aphasia preceded or was simultaneous with ALS symptoms, and cases in which ALS symptoms preceded aphasia became evident only through writing (36–46). Because motor symptoms progress rapidly in ALS, the patients may not survive until aphasic symptoms develop or aphasia may be masked by severe dysarthria and use of artificial ventilation. It is of interest that most reported cases with aphasia or writing errors were of bulbar-onset ALS. Although the reason for this is unclear, we have found a high prevalence of writing errors in bulbar-onset ALS and speculated that this is due to the proximity of Broca's area with the orolingual motor cortex connecting to bulbar areas (9,10). This may also explain why PNFA is the major type of aphasia in ALS. Notably, Bak and colleagues reported three cases of bulbar-onset MND that showed PNFA with selective impairment of verb production and comprehension relative to noun comprehension, and selective involvement of Broca's area (Broadmann 44 and 45) neuropathologically (42). Interestingly, Hillis and colleagues compared impairment of naming verbs and nouns in patients with fluent primary progressive aphasia (PPA) probably corresponding to SD and non-fluent PPA probably corresponding to PNFA. They found that patients with non-fluent PPA and ALS-FTD were significantly more impaired in verb naming than noun naming, and that non-fluent PPA showed the opposite pattern (46) (see also Orange and Hillis, Chapter 5).

In addition to the aphasia findings described above, word retrieval impairment has also been documented in classical ALS, and recent studies using functional magnetic resonance imaging and ^{11}C-flumazenil positron emission tomography have shown that poor performance on confrontation naming correlates with localized dysfunction in the prefrontal region, including the middle or inferior frontal gyrus extending to Broca's area (61,62). These results indicate that language dysfunction is present even in classical ALS, and suggest that this condition occurs due to selective involvement of extra-motor regions, rather than wider brain dysfunction (61,62).

Insights into language impairment through writing

As emphasized above, patients with ALS often have accompanying dysarthria due to bulbar or pseudo-bulbar palsy, and evaluation of language function is not easy. Therefore, evaluation of writing is necessary to understand language problems in ALS. Writing errors reflect underlying aphasic characteristics, including PNFA or SD, which are obscured if dysarthria is mild enough to evaluate oral language. In other words, hidden aphasic problems can be detected via writing errors. A summary of reported writing errors in ALS/MND, including primary lateral sclerosis, and descriptions of paragraphia

Table 6.1 Reported writing errors in motor neurone disease

Authors	Year	Cases	Features of writing errors
Watanabe (28)	(1893)	1	Paragraphia
Ferguson and Boller (33)	(1977)	2	Grammatical error, spelling error
Ferror *et al.* (35)	(1991)	1	Spelling error
Caselli *et al.* (36)	(1993)	7	Semantic paraphasia, syntatic violation
Strong *et al.* (40)	(1999)	4	Paraphasia in written language
Bak *et al.* (42)	(2001)	6	Paraphasia, grammatical error
Iroi *et al.* (47)	(2002)	1	Impaired writing of kanji, paragraphia
Hyodo *et al.* (43)	(2002)	1	Paraphasia, grammatical error
Zago *et al.* (49)	(2003)	6	Dysgraphia
Kanzaki *et al.* (48)	(2004)	1	Omission of kana, paragraphia
Lucchelli and Papagno (50)	(2005)	1	Deletion, substitution, transposition, insertion
Piquard *et al.* (52)	(2006)	20	Grammatical error, spelling error
Ichikawa *et al.* (9)	(2008)	6	Paraphasia, omission, grammatical error
Ichikawa *et al.* (10)	(2008)	15	Paraphasia, omission, grammatical error
Zago *et al.* (54)	(2008)	16	Spelling error
Ichikawa *et al.* (56)	(2008)	2	Isolated agraphia
Satoh *et al.* (57)	(2009)	3	Isolated agraphia

(dysgraphia), spelling errors, grammatical errors, and omission of letters are given in Table 6.1 (9,10,28,33,35,36,40,42,43,48–50,52,54,56,57). For example, in 1977 Ferguson and Boller (33) described syntactic errors (e.g. 'I wish for my correction instead me walk for seep pills') and spelling errors (e.g. 'graps' for 'grasp'). In 1993, Caselli and colleagues reported patients with MND and progressive aphasia resembling PNFA and described paraphasic spelling (e.g. 'stritch' for the name of a pen) (36). In 2004, Kanzaki and colleagues described a Japanese patient with ALS who presented with omission of kana letters while his general orientation, intelligence and comprehension were preserved (48).

We recently reported a high prevalence of writing errors in Japanese patients with bulbar-onset ALS, with 15 of 19 patients showing these errors (10). Omission of kana was the most frequent error, and paragraphia (substitution of letters) and syntactic errors were also common (10). In addition, we observed dissociated impairment between kana and kanji, with kana errors being more frequent in some patients and kanji errors more common in others. Representative samples of writing that exhibit fairly well preserved complex kanji but frequent errors in simple kana, including omission, paragraphia, and syntactic mistakes, are shown in Figure 6.3. Samples from another patient who showed almost exclusive impairment in writing kana are shown in Figure 6.4. This patient understood the meaning of kanji and words, suggesting that the condition was not alexia of kanji or semantic aphasia as presented by Iroi and colleagues (47). Interestingly, the writing errors resembled those reported by Watanabe (28). SPECT images of the patient referred to in Figure 6.4 revealed reduced uptake in left-sided dominant bilateral frontotemporal

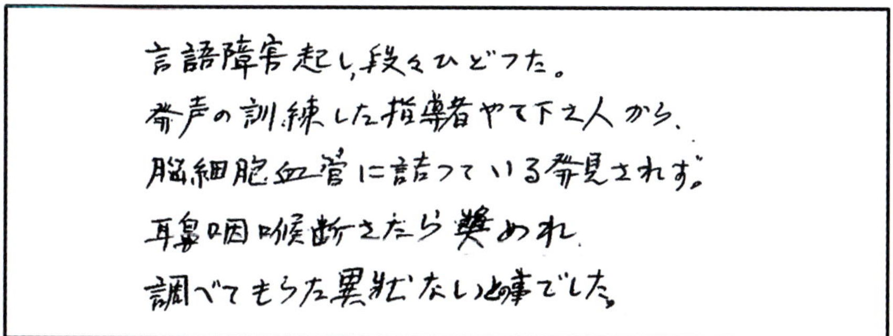

言語障害起 し, 段々 ひどつた(ひどくなった)

発声 の 訓練 した 指導者 やて(やって) 下 さ(さった) 人 から

脳細胞血管 に 詰 まっている(いるのは) 発見 されず

耳鼻咽喉科 (で) 診断 さたら(されたらと) 奨 められ

調 べて もらた(もらったら) 異状 ないとの 事 でした

Fig. 6.3 Writing sample of a 67-year-old man with bulbar-onset ALS. A sample of letters written by the patient is shown above and a typed version with corrections is shown below. Shadowed characters are kanji and errors are corrected in parentheses in the typed version. The patient initially developed bulbar symptoms and brought a record of his medical history. He was polite, intellectual, and aware of his illness without behavioural changes, although already aphonic. Many writing errors were observed in simple kana, including omission, paragraphia, and syntactic errors, whereas complex kanji was written correctly.

lobes (Figure 6.5), which differed from the SPECT images reported by Iroi *et al.* (47). The patients referred to in Figures 6.3 and 6.4 both developed apathetic features without disinhibited behaviour, whereas another patient showed almost exclusive impairment in writing kanji (Figure 6.6) and exhibited disinhibited behaviour.

Based on these findings, we conducted a study in which we counted erroneous characters in samples obtained in 14 patients with ALS and calculated the error rates of kana and kanji characters separately. The results indicated dissociated impairment of kana and kanji in these patients (Figure 6.7). This may reflect involvement of areas of the brain such as the frontal lobe or temporal lobe, and an underlying aphasic condition, including PNFA or SD. In addition, these dissociated patterns of writing errors in Japanese (i.e. kana versus kanji) may partly correspond to observations in English represented as verb versus noun dissociation (42,46).

The inability to write under articulatory suppression has been described in a progressive dysgraphic patient, with the argument that the patient could not write because the task precludes the rehearsal of phonological representation of words (51). However, we believe that writing errors are not derived from vocal rehearsal inability, as we experienced isolated

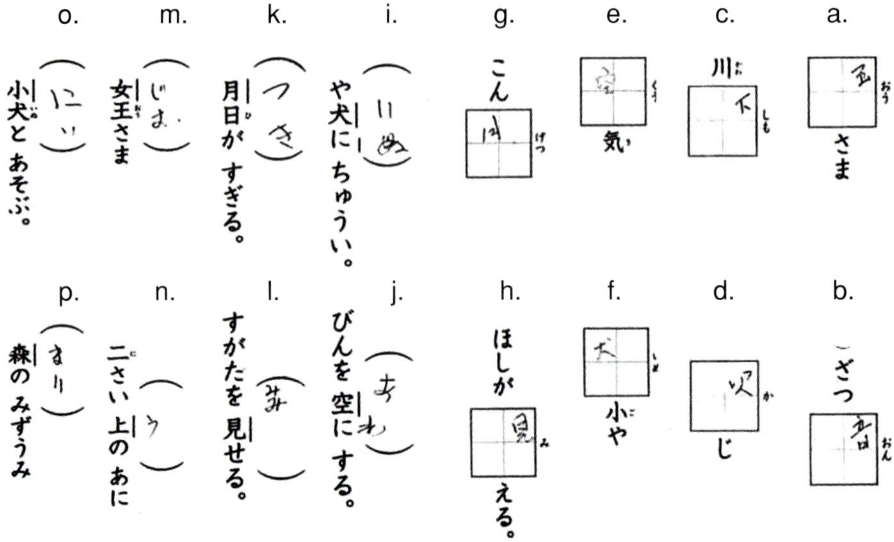

Fig. 6.4 Dictation in a 68-year-old man with bulbar-onset ALS. The patient initially developed bulbar symptoms. He was polite, intellectual, and aware of his illness without behavioural changes, but he was already aphonic. In a dictation drill for elementary school children, all kanji letters were written correctly (a–h), but many writing errors were present in kana (i–p): 'あわ', pronounced 'awa', instead of 'から', pronounced 'kara', meaning empty (j); 'みみ', pronounced 'mimi', instead of 'み', pronounced 'mi', meaning 'look' (l); 'じお', pronounced 'jio', instead of 'じょう', pronounced 'jou', meaning woman (m); 'う', pronounced 'u', instead of 'うえ', pronounced 'ue', meaning up (n); 'にい', pronounced 'nii', instead of 'こ', pronounced 'ko', meaning little (o); 'まり', pronounced 'mari', instead of 'もり', pronounced 'mori', meaning 'wood' (p). With permission from Ichikawa, Kawamura, *Brain Nerve* **62**:435–40, 2010

agraphia without dementia or aphasia in patients with ALS (10,56) whose oral language was preserved sufficiently to be comprehended. The patients mainly showed omission of kana with some paragraphia. Satoh *et al.* (57) also reported omission of letters in intellectually normal patients with ALS, and pure agraphia mainly involving syntax has been reported in bulbar-onset ALS by Ferguson and Boller (33). Recently, focal cortical atrophy syndrome with progressive anarthria (63) and single domain cognitive impairment showing isolated agraphia (64,65) have been documented in neurodegenerative disorders.

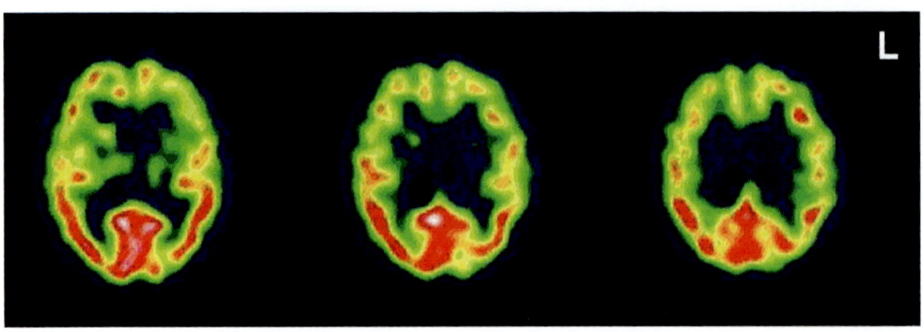

Fig. 6.5 SPECT images of the patient referred to in Figure 6.4. Reduced uptake in the left-side dominant bilateral frontotemporal lobes was observed. SPECT, single-photon emission tomography. With permission from Ichikawa, Kawamura, *Brain Nerve*, **62**:435–40, 2010

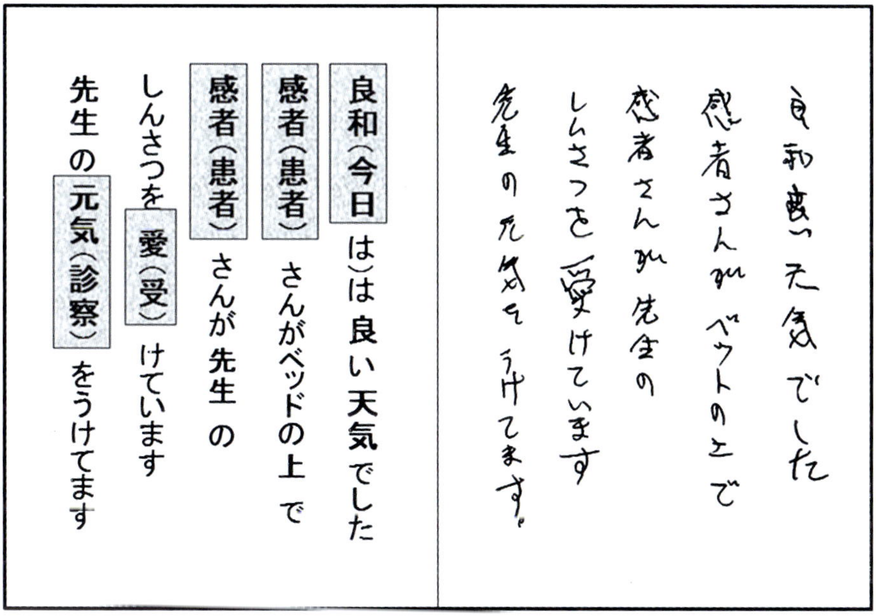

Fig. 6.6 Writing sample of a 50-year-old man with limb-onset ALS. A sample of letters written by the patient (left) and a typed version with corrections (right) are shown. Shadowed characters are kanji and errors are corrected in parentheses in the typed version. Writing errors were observed exclusively in kanji. The patient developed disinhibited behavioural changes and subsequently developed bulbar symptoms.

Interestingly, Luzzi and Piccirilli (66) reported a patient with presumed FTLD without dementia who showed omission of letters for 1 year followed by substitution and insertion of letters and then apraxia of speech.

The involved lesions of pure or isolated agraphia are unclear, but the writing centre is historically considered to be located at the foot of the middle frontal gyrus; the so-called Exner's area (67,69). Recently, functional magnetic resonance imaging studies have also suggested that the left middle frontal region is crucial to writing, along with other regions such as the intraparietal sulcus, cingulate gyrus, supplementary motor cortex, and posterior inferior temporal cortex (70–72). An interesting study of direct cortical stimulation under awake surgery in patients with a brain tumour showed that writing-specific interference was localized in the posterior part of the dominant middle frontal gyrus and that stimulation of this region elicited writing errors such as letter omission and paragraphia (73). We recently described a patient with pathologically proven ALS who showed agraphia without aphasia and preferential involvement of the foot of the middle frontal gyrus (Exner's area) (74). Thus, writing-specific impairment is a problem in patients with ALS, in addition to aphasia, based on the use of the word processor as a communication tool in the clinical domain.

In conclusion, the progressive bulbar symptoms and medical interventions, including artificial ventilation make it difficult to evaluate language function in ALS. Therefore, evaluation of writing is the key to discovery of language problems in patients with ALS. This is supported by unnoticed historical descriptions of this condition. The first account

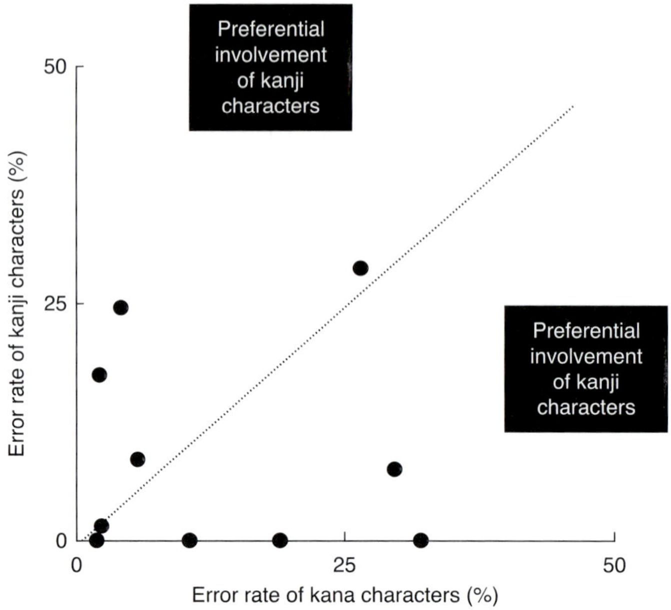

Fig. 6.7 Error rates for kana and kanji characters. Erroneous characters were counted in samples obtained from 14 patients with ALS who showed writing errors, and error rates for kana and kanji were calculated. Dissociation of impairment of kana and kanji is suggested in some patients.

of aphasia in Japan is also the first description of writing errors in a patient with ALS, as reported by Watanabe in 1893. In the literature, these writing errors are described as paraphasia mainly in kana. In alphabetical languages, writing errors in ALS were first described by Ferguson and Boller in 1977, and are now described as spelling and syntactic errors. However, these papers were not referred to in the literature until our documentation of these cases. Thus, it has taken some time for language problems in ALS to be recognized, in association with aphasic dementia with MND and inclusion of the new concepts of PNFA and SD in FTLD. These new concepts have encouraged reports on language problems and writing errors in patients with ALS.

In the recent literature, mainly errors with verbs in patients with ALS or PNFA and with nouns in those with SD have been reported in alphabetical languages. In Japanese, dissociated involvement of kana (Japanese phonogram) and kanji (Japanese morphogram) have been observed, with mainly kana errors in patients with ALS and fewer kanji errors in patients with ALS and SD. These dissociated errors between kanji and kana may be comparable with dissociated involvement of verb and noun errors in alphabetical languages. Such dissociated impairment probably reflects frontal or temporal lobe predominance, and an underlying aphasic condition, including PNFA or SD. In addition to the kanji versus kana problem, isolated writing errors (isolated agraphia) has been reported in ALS, which suggests the presence of focal cortical atrophy. Thus, writing errors require more rigorous exploration to clarify language function in patients with ALS and to provide further understanding of the writing system.

Key points

- ALS is a multisystem disorder that involves the motor system and cognitive factors.
- Language impairment, including PNFA and SD have been overlooked in ALS.
- Patients with ALS often display writing errors, with dissociation between verb and noun processing in English and dissociated errors between kana and kanji characters in Japanese.
- The characteristic features of writing errors may reflect the nature of aphasia and underlying brain locations, including hemispheric dominance and frontal or temporal lobe involvement.

References

1. Meyer A. (1929). Uber eine der amyotrophiscehen Lateralsklerose nahestehende Erkrankung mit psychischen Storungen. *Z Ges Neurol Psychiat*, **121**, 107–138.
2. Wechsler IS, Davison C. (1932). Amyotrophic lateral sclerosis with mental symptoms. *Arch Neurol Psychiat* **27**, 859–880.
3. Yuasa R. (1964). Amyotrophic lateral sclerosis with organic dementia: report of a case. *Clin Neurol (Tokyo)*, **4**, 529–534.
4. Yuasa R. (1970). Amyotrophic lateral sclerosis with dementia. *Clin Neurol (Tokyo)*. **10**, 569–577.
5. Mitsuyama Y, Takamatsu I. (1971). An autopsy case of presenile dementia with motor neuron disease. *Brain Nerve (Tokyo)*, **23**, 409–416.
6. Mitsuyama Y, Takamiya S. (1979). Presenile dementia with motor neuron disease. *Arch Neurol*, **36**, 592–593.
7. Mitsuyama Y. (1984). Presenile dementia with motor neuron disease in Japan: clinico-pathological review of 26 cases. *J Neurol Neurosurg Psychiatry*, **47**, 953–995.
8. Yoshida M, Murakami N, Hashizume Y, Takahashi A. (1992). A clinicopathological study on 13 cases of motor neuron disease with dementia. *Clin Neurol*, **32**, 1193–1202.
9. Ichikawa H, Koyama S, Ohno H, *et al.* (2008). Writing errors and anosognosia in amyotrophic lateral sclerosis with dementia. *Behav Neurol*, **19**, 107–116.
10. Ichikawa H, Takahashi N, Hieda S, *et al.* (2008). Agraphia in bulbar-onset amyotrophic lateral sclerosis: not merely a consequence of dementia or aphasia. *Behav Neurol*, **20**, 91–99.
11. Yuasa M, Inoue T. (2009). Clinical entity of frontotemporal dementia with motor neuron disease. *Neuropathology*, **29**, 649–654.
12. Neary D, Snowden JS, Mann DM, *et al.* (1990). Frontal lobe dementia and motor neuron disease. *J Neurol Neurosurg Psychiatry*, **53**, 23–32.
13. Neary D, Snowden JS, Gustafson L, *et al.* (1998). Frontotemporal lobar degeneration: a consensus on clinical diagnostic criteria. *Neurology*, **51**, 1546–1554.
14. The Lund and Manchester Groups. (1994). Clinical and neuropathological criteria for fronto-temporal dementia. *J Neurol Neurosurg Psychiatry*, **57**, 416–418.
15. Snowden JS, Neary D, Mann DMA. (1996). Fronto temporal lobar degeneration: fronto-temporal dementia. Progressive aphasia, semantic dementia. *Clinical Neurology and Neurosurgery Monographs*. Churchill Livingstone, New York.
16. Okamoto K, Hirai S, Yamazaki T, *et al.* (1991). New ubiquitin-positive intraneuronal inclusions in the extra-motor cortices in patients with amyotrophic lateral sclerosis. *Neurosci Lett*, **129**, 233–236.
17. Jackson M, Lennox G, Lowe J. (1996). Motor neuron disease-inclusion dementia. *Neurodegeneration*, **5**, 339–350.

18. Kertesz A, Kawarai T, Rogaeva E, *et al.* (2000). Familial frontotemporal dementia with ubiquitin-positive, tau-negative inclusions. *Neurology*, **54**, 818–827.
19. Neumann M, Sampathu DM, Kwong LK, *et al.* (2006). Ubiquitinated TDP-43 in frontotemporal lobar degeneration and amyotrophic lateral sclerosis. *Science*, **314**, 130–133.
20. Snowden J, Neary D, Mann D. (2007). Frontotemporal lobar degeneration: clinical and pathological relationships. *Acta Neuropathol*, **114**, 31–38.
21. Arai T, Hasegawa M, Akiyama H, *et al.* (2006). TDP-43 is a component of ubiquitin-positive tau-negative inclusions in frontotemporal lobar degeneration and amyotrophic lateral sclerosis. *Biochem Biophys Res Commun*, **351**, 602–611.
22. Geser F, Martinez-Lage, Robinson J, *et al.* (2009). Clinical and pathological continuum of multisystem TDP-43 proteinopathies. *Ann Neurol*, **66**, 180–189.
23. Geser F, Martinez-Lage M, Kwong LK, Lee VM-Y. (2009). Amyotrophic lateral sclerosis, frontotemporal dementia and beyond: the TDP-43 diseases. *J Neurol*, **256**, 1205–1214.
24. Kwiatkowski TJ, Bosco DA, Leclerc AL, *et al.* (2009). Mutations in the FUS/TLS gene on chromosome 16 cause familial amyotrophic lateral sclerosis. *Science*, **323**, 1205–1208.
25. Vance C, Rogelj B, Hortobágyi T, *et al.* (2009). Mutations in FUS, an RNA processing protein, cause familial amyotrophic lateral sclerosis type 6. *Science*, **323**, 1208–1211.
26. Neumann M, Rademakers R, Roeber S, *et al.* (2009). A new subtype of frontotemporal lobar degeneration with FUS pathology. *Brain*, 132, 2922–2931.
27. Mackenzie IRA, Neumann M, Bigio EH, *et al.* (2010). Nomenclature and nosology for neuropathologic subtypes of frontotemporal lobar degeneration: an update. *Acta Neuropathol*, **119**, 1–4.
28. Kawamura M, Ichikawa H, Koyama S, Ishihara K. (2007). Amyotrophic lateral sclerosis with dementia–neuropsychological aspect. *Brain Nerve*, **59**, 1083–1091.
29. Kawamura M, Hirayama K, Hasegawa K, *et al.* (1987). Alexia with agraphia of kanji (Japanese morphograms). *J Neurol Neurosurg Psychiatry*, **50**, 1125–1129.
30. Soma Y, Yamadori A, Murata S, Imanaga H. (1989). Lexical agraphia in the Japanese language. *Brain*, **112**, 1549–1561.
31. Yokota T, Ishiai S, Furukawa T, Tsukagoshi H. (1990). Pure agraphia of kanji due to thrombosis of the Labbe vein. *J Neurol Neurosurg Psychiatry*, **53**, 335–338.
32. Sakurai Y, Matsumura K, Iwatsubo T, Momose T. (1997). Frontal pure agraphia for kanji or kana: dissociation between morphology and phonology. *Neurology*, **49**, 946–952.
33. Ferguson JH, Boller F. (1977). A different form of agraphia: syntactic writing errors in patients with motor speech and movement disorders. *Brain Lang*, **4**, 382–389.
34. Neary D, Snowden JS, Northern B, Goulding P. (1988). Dementia of frontal lobe type. *J Neurol Neurosurg Psychiatry*, **51**, 353–361.
35. Ferror I, Roig C, Espiano A, Peiro G, Guiu XM. (1991). Dementia of frontotemporal lobe type and motor neuron disease. Golgi study of the frontal cortex. *J Neurol Neurosurg Psychiatry*, **54**, 932–934.
36. Caselli RJ, Windebank AJ, Petersen RC, *et al.* (1993). Rapidly progressive aphasic dementia and motor neuron disease. *Ann Neurol*, **33**, 200–207.
37. Rakowicz W, Hodges JR. (1998). Dementia and aphasia in motor neuron disease: an under-recognized association? *J Neurol Neurosurg Psychiatry*, **65**, 881–889.
38. Doran M, Xuereb J, Hodges JR. (1995). Rapidly progressive aphasia with bulbar motor neuron disease: a clinical and neuropsychological study. *Behav Neurol*, **8**, 169–180.
39. Cavalleri F, De Renzi E. (1998). Amyotrophic lateral sclerosis with dementia. *Acta Neurol Scand*, **89**, 391–394.

40. Strong MJ, Grace GM, Orange JB, *et al.* (1999). A prospective study of cognitive impairment in ALS. *Neurology*, **53**, 1665–1670.
41. Tsuchiya K, Ozawa E, Fukushima J, *et al.* (2000). Rapidly progressive aphasia and motor neuron disease: a clinical, radiological, and pathological study of an autopsy case with circumscribed lobar atrophy. *Acta Neuropathol (Berl)*, **99**, 81–87.
42. Bak TH, O'Donovan DG, Xuereb JH, *et al.* (2001). Selective impairment of verb processing associated with pathological changes in Brodmann areas 44 and 45 in the motor neuron disease–dementia-aphasia syndrome. *Brain*, **124**, 103–120.
43. Hyodo T, Ikeda M, Ueno S, *et al.* (2002). A case of motor neuron disease with progressive aphasia and dementia. *Brain Nerve*, **54**, 713–718.
44. Catani M, Picciirilli M, Geloso MC, *et al.* (2004). Rapidly progressive aphasic dementia with motor neuron disease: a distinctive clinical entity. *Dement Geriatr Cogn Disord*, **17**, 21–28.
45. Lomen-Hoerth C. (2004). Characterization of amyotrophic lateral sclerosis and frontotemporal dementia. *Dement Geriatr Cogn Disord* **17**, 337–341.
46. Hillis AE, Oh S, Ken L. (2004). Deterioration of naming nouns versus verbs in primary progressive aphasia. *Ann Neurol*, **55**, 268–275.
47. Iroi A, Okuma Y, Fukae J, *et al.* (2002). Amyotrophic lateral sclerosis presented with alexia of kanji and word meaning aphasia. *Brain Nerve*, **54**, 903–907.
48. Kanzaki M, Sato M, Ogawa G, *et al.* (2004). A case of dementia with motor neuron disease associated with agraphia the omission of kana letters. *Clin Neurol*, **44**, 673–676.
49. Zago S, Poletti B, Corbo M, *et al.* (2003). Disgraphia as presenting symptom of primary lateral sclerosis. *Amyotroph Lateral Scler Other Motor Neuron Disord*, **4** (Suppl. 1), 205.
50. Lucchelli F, Papagno C. (2005). Slowly progressive anarthria a 'pure' motor-speech disorder? Evidence from writing performance. *Neurocase*, **11**, 234–241.
51. Papagno C, Girelli L. (2005). Writing through the phonological buffer: a case of progressive writing disorder. *Neuropsychologia*, **43**, 1277–1287.
52. Piquard A, Le Forestier N, Baudoin-Madec V, *et al.* (2006). Neuropsychological change in patients with primary lateral sclerosis. *Amyotroph Lateral Scler*, **7**, 150–160.
53. Duffy JR, Peach RK, Strand EA. (2007). Progressive apraxia of speech as a sign of motor neuron disease. *Am J Speech Lang Pathol*, **16**, 198–208.
54. Zago S, Poletti B, Corbo M, *et al.* (2008). Disgraphia in patients with primary lateral sclerosis: A speech-based rehearsal deficit? *Behav Neurol*, **19**, 169–175.
55. Kim SH, Seo AW, Go SM, *et al.* (2009). Semantic dementia combined with motor neuron disease. *J Clin Neurosci*, **16**, 1683–1685.
56. Ichikawa H, Takahashi N, Hieda S, Kawamura M. (2010). Bulbar-onset amyotrophic lateral sclerosis (ALS) with isolated agraphia. *Rinsho Shinkeigaku*, **50**(2), 81–86.
57. Satoh M, Takeda K, Kuzuhara S. (2009). Agraphia in intellectually normal Japanese patients with ALS: omission of kana letters. *J Neurol*, **256**, 1455–1460.
58. Davies RR, Hodges JR, Kril JJ, *et al.* (2005). The pathological bias of semantic dementia. *Brain*, **128**, 1984–1995.
59. Yokota O, Tsuchiya K, Itoh Y, *et al.* (2006). Frontotemporal lobar degeneration with ibiquitin pathology: an autopsy case presenting with semantic dementia and upper motor neuron signs with a clinical course of
19 years. *Acta Neuropathol*, **112**, 739–749.
60. Josephs KA, Stroh A, Dugger B, Dickson DW. (2009). Evaluation of subcortical pathology and clinical correlations in FTLD-U subtypes. *Acta Neuropathol*, **118**, 349–358.
61. Abrahams S, Goldstein LH, Simmons A, *et al.* (2004). Word retrieval in amyotrophic lateral sclerosis: a functional magnetic resonance imaging study. *Brain*, **127**, 1507–1517.

62. Abrahams S, Leigh PN, Goldstein LH. (2005). Cognitive change in ALS: a prospective study. *Neurology*, **64**, 1222–1226.
63. Broussolle E, Bakchine S, Tommasi M, *et al.* (1996). Slowly progressive anarthria with late anterior opercular syndrome: a variant form of frontal cortical atrophy syndrome. *J Neurol Sci*, **144**, 44–58.
64. Heilman KM, Conen A, Kluger B. (2008). Progressive asymmetric apraxic agraphia. *Cogn Behav Neurol*, **21**, 14–17.
65. Fukui T, Lee E. (2008). Progressive agraphia can be a harbinger of degenerative dementia. *Brain Lang*, **104**, 201–210.
66. Luzzi S, Piccirilli M. (2003). Slowly progressive pure agraphia with late apraxia of speech: a further variant of the focal cerebral degeneration. *Brain Lang*, **87**, 355–360.
67. Tohgi H, Saitoh K, Takahashi S, *et al.* (1995). Agraphia and acalculia after a left prefrontal (F1, F2) infarction. *J Neurol Neurosurg Psychiatry*, **58**, 629–632.
68. Anderson SW, Damasio AR, Damasio H. (1990). Troubled letters but not numbers. Domain specific cognitive impairments following focal damage in frontal cortex. *Brain*, **113**, 749–766.
69. Roux FE, Dufor O, Giussani C, *et al.* (2009). The graphemic/motor frontal area Exner's area revised. *Ann Neurol*, **66**, 537–545.
70. Katanoda K, Yoshikawa Y, Sugishita M. (2001). A functional MRI study on the neural substrates for writing. *Hum Brain Mapp*, **13**, 34–42.
71. Matsuo K, Kato C, Ozawa F, *et al.* (2001). Ideographic characters call for extra processing to correspond with phonemes. *Neuroreport*. **12**, 2227–2230.Matsuo K, Kato C, Ozawa F,
72. Sugihara G, Kaminaga T, Sugishita M. (2006). Interindividual uniformity and variety of the 'writing center': A functional MRI study. *Neuroimage*, **32**, 1837–1849.
73. Lubrano V, Roux F-E, Démonet JF. (2004). Writing-specific sites in frontal areas: a cortical stimulation study. *J Neurosurg*, **101**, 787–798.
74. Ichikawa H, Kawamura M. (2009). Symptoms of frontotemporal dementia. *Brain Nerve*, **61**, 1227–1235.

Chapter 7

Amyotrophic lateral sclerosis with dementia: neuropsychological aspects

Mitsuru Kawamura and Hiroo Ichikawa

Previously, the most distinctive feature of amyotrophic lateral sclerosis (ALS) was considered to be the retention of full consciousness until the very end of the patient's life, without development of psychiatric or cognitive (dementia) symptoms. However, in 1964, Yuasa reported clinical cases of ALS manifesting dementia, indicating that dementia and ALS could have a single pathogenic cause (1). Since then, especially in Japan, case reports citing instances of ALS with dementia (ALS-D) have been accumulating. Mitsuyama and colleagues have advocated that ALS-D be distinguished an independent disease entity although some still consider ALS-D to be a subclass of classic ALS (2,3). Furthermore, in terms of dementia, ALS-D is commonly considered to be a subclass of frontotemporal dementia (FTD).

Here, we review previously published case reports (4,5) and describe the key neuropsychological points related to ALS-D as well as the relationship between ALS-D and FTD. Specifically, we will consider the following topics: (a) patients with ALS-D show symptoms of frontal-type dementia consistent with FTD (6); (b) ALS-D can be divided into two categories in terms of its development (dementia preceding ALS-D and ALS preceding ALS-D) and symptoms (bulbar palsy-type and upper-extremity type ALS); (c) computed tomography (CT) and magnetic resonance imaging images show frontal and anterior temporal lobe atrophy in ALS-D, and single-photon emission CT (SPECT) images typically show decreased uptake in the frontal and temporal lobes, which is detectable earlier than morphological changes, and thus, SPECT is an important diagnostic tool for diagnosis of ALS-D; and (d) typical dementia symptoms include paragraphia and anosognosia.

In addition, a case report written by Watanabe in 1893 is presented (7). This is the first case report on aphasia published in Japan, and may be the world's first case report on ALS-D.

Bulbar palsy is commonly found in patients with ALS-D, and disordered speech is usually prominent in the early stages of the disease; thus, it is not easy to evaluate higher brain function in patients with ALS-D (2,8). There have been some cases of ALS in which the patient was first noticed to have an impaired ability to write (dysgraphia) through evaluation of written communication after the disappearance of spontaneous speech (4). Additionally, lack of insight has been described as a core symptom of FTD (6,9,10) and we have noted that anosognosia is similarly an important feature of ALS-D. However, the objectivity of such findings was not investigated in the previously published report on anosognosia in patients with ALS-D (5).

In consideration of the problems related to the evaluation of ALS-D, we analysed the clinical features of ALS-D based on a comprehensive review of the cases we have encountered previously, with a focus on analysis of dysgraphia. In addition, we attempted to quantify the degree of anosognosia by using a Japanese version of the anosognosia questionnaire devised by Deckel and Morrison (11).

Patient descriptions and testing paradigms

Among those who were admitted to the Department of Neurology at our hospital between May 1989 and May 2004, 64 patients clinically and electrophysiologically met the diagnostic criteria for clinically definitive ALS, as described in the Revised Criteria for Diagnosis of Amyotrophic Lateral Sclerosis (12). Of these 64 patients, seven (11%) were diagnosed with ALS-D. During the observation period, dementia was assessed in a comprehensive manner, based primarily on the activities of daily living. The following tests were performed when possible, and their results were used for assessment: Revised Hasegawa's Dementia Scale (HDS-R), the Kana Recognition Test, the Wechsler Adult Intelligence Scales–Revised (WAIS-R), and the Wisconsin Card Sorting Test (WCST).

The seven cases of ALS-D are summarized in Table 7.1. There were four male and three female patients, all of whom were right-handed. The age of onset ranged from 49 years to 80 years (average = 63 years). The upper extremities were affected in one patient, and six patients had bulbar palsy-type ALS. With regard to disease development, three patients showed dementia preceding ALS-D, and four had ALS preceding ALS-D. The duration of the disease was 2–113 months in terms of dementia symptoms and 8–45 months (average = 23 months) in terms of motor symptoms. For the patients who eventually required mechanical ventilation, disease duration was measured as the time from symptom

Table 7.1 Summarized description of the patients with ALS-D

Case no.	Age at onset (years)	Sex	Handedness	ALS type	Preceding symptom
1	49	Male	Right	Upper extremity	Dementia
2	59	Female	Right	Bulbar palsy	Dementia
3	60	Male	Right	Bulbar palsy	Dementia
4	67	Male	Right	Bulbar palsy	ALS
5	51	Female	Right	Bulbar palsy	ALS
6	73	Female	Right	Bulbar palsy	ALS
7	80	Male	Right	Bulbar palsy	ALS

The mean age at the time of symptom onset was 63 years.

*1, For the patients (cases 4, 5, and 6) who eventually required mechanical ventilation, the disease duration was measured as the time from the onset of the disease to the point at which the patient had to be placed on a mechanical ventilator (mean disease duration = 23 months). Cited from reference 5. Reprinted from Behav. Neurol., 19, Ichikawa H, Koyama S, Ohno H et al., Writing errors and anosognosia in amyotrophic lateral sclerosis with dementia, 107-116, Copyright 2008, with permission from IOS Press.

onset to the point at which the patient had to be placed on a mechanical ventilator. The diagnostic imaging findings obtained during the course of the disease were as follows: in all cases, brain CT and magnetic resonance imaging scans showed bilateral atrophy of the frontal and temporal lobes without clear evidence of a cerebrovascular disorder, and SPECT images showed decreased uptake in the bilateral frontal and temporal lobes.

Testing paradigms

The dementia symptoms of the seven patients with ALS-D (Table 7.1) were evaluated in a comprehensive manner based on clinical observation of the activities of daily living. Because many of the patients had speech disorders associated with bulbar palsy, the presence or absence and disease condition of dysgraphia was determined through written communication.

The Anosognosia Scale, devised by Deckel and Morrison (11) for measuring self-assessed bodily functions, was translated to Japanese for use in this study (Table 7.2). The questionnaire contained eight questions regarding a patient's abilities: for example, to 'Walk', 'Accurate and quick use of hands and fingers', and 'Clear speech'. These items were rated on a five-point scale from −2 (Very impaired) to +2 (Excellent). The difference between self-rated scores and non-self-rated scores was considered to be indicative of the severity of anosognosia (maximum difference in score = 32 points). This questionnaire was administered to two patients diagnosed with ALS-D and four patients diagnosed with ALS without dementia. The results were compared among these patients. For each patient, the average non-self-rated score was computed by summing two scores rated by a physician and a nurse and dividing by 2.

SPECT images were obtained for each patient and the results correlated with the patient's clinical features.

Table 7.2 Anosognosia scale of Deckel and Morrison (11)

1	Walk	Very impaired (−2)	Below average (−1)	Average (0)	Above average (+1)	Excellent (+2)
2	Accurate and quick use of hands and fingers	Very impaired (−2)	Below average (−1)	Average (0)	Above average (+1)	Excellent (+2)
3	Clear speech	Very impaired (−2)	Below average (−1)	Average (0)	Above average (+1)	Excellent (+2)
4	Memory retention	Very impaired (−2)	Below average (−1)	Average (0)	Above average (+1)	Excellent (+2)
5	Concentration and attention	Very impaired (−2)	Below average (−1)	Average (0)	Above average (+1)	Excellent (+2)
6	Still and quiet sit	Very impaired (−2)	Below average (−1)	Average (0)	Above average (+1)	Excellent (+2)
7	Expression of thoughts and ideas	Very impaired (−2)	Below average (−1)	Average (0)	Above average (+1)	Excellent (+2)
8	Control of emotions	Very impaired (−2)	Below average (−1)	Average (0)	Above average (+1)	Excellent (+2)

The anosognosia scale was translated into Japanese for use in the study.

Illustrative case histories

Case 1

A 50-year-old, right-handed male patient (case 1 in Tables 7.1, 7.3, and 7.4) presented with a chief complaint of forgetfulness. The past history and family history were unremarkable. Around March 1991, when the patient was 49 years old, his family mentioned the following symptoms: restlessness, inability to solve simple mathematical problems, and marked forgetfulness; weight loss was also observed at about that time. In April 1991, the patient showed decreased speech production and developed muscle contractions (twitches) in the upper limb girdle on both sides. Subsequently, he was admitted to the Department of Neurology at our hospital. He was lucid without restriction on eye movements or disturbance of facial movements. Besides pronounced dysarthria and dysphagia, the patient had decreased soft palatal and gag reflexes, difficulty in protruding the tongue, tongue atrophy, and tongue fasciculation. With regard to the motor system, significant muscular atrophy of the distal extremities and extensive fasciculations were observed; extremity muscle weakness was particularly significant in the distal portion of the limbs. The patient showed increased mandibular reflex and increased tendon reflex of the extremities, but plantar responses were equivocal bilaterally. No sensorimotor disorder, coordination disorder, or bladder and rectal disturbances were observed.

The muscular atrophy and muscle weakness of the extremities gradually worsened, and the symptoms of bulbar palsy also worsened in a piecemeal fashion. In addition, the patient developed respiratory muscle paralysis and subsequently died of respiratory failure 21 months after initial presentation.

On neuropsychological testing, there was pronounced restlessness and disinhibitory behaviour (attempts to escape from the hospital) were observed. In addition, the patient had decreased memory retention, decreased ability to solve mathematical problems (dyscalculia), and decreased decision-making abilities. The following test results were recorded for this

Table 7.3 Summary of dementia symptoms

Dementia symptoms	**Case no.**						
	1	**2**	**3**	**4**	**5**	**6**	**7**
Decrease in the amount of spontaneous speech		+	+	+	+	+	+
Decreased spontaneity		+	+	+	+		+
Disinhibitory behaviours	+	+	+		+	+	
Difficulty in focusing attention	+	+	+	+	+	+	+
Restlessness	+	+	+		+	+	
Attempts to leave	+	+	+	+		+	+
Play antics	+	+	+			+	
Perseveration		+				+	
Imitative behaviour					+		
Decreased ability to solve mathematical problems	+						
Semantic memory impairment	+						

Table 7.4 Summary of dysgraphia and anosognosia observations and SPECT scan results (5)

Clinical findings and SPECT imaging	Case no. 1	2	3	4	5	6	7
Spontaneous speech at the time of evaluation	+	+	–	–	–	–	–
Language comprehension at the time of evaluation	Favourable	Favourable	Favourable	Favourable	Favourable	Favourable	Favourable
Dysphasia	+	*1	+*2	+	+	+	+*3
Paragraphia	+			+	+	+	+
Substitution	+			+	+	+	
Omission				+		+	+
Grammatical error						+	
Predominance of errors in writing kanji and kana	Kanji dominant		Equal	Kana dominant	Kanji dominant	Kana dominant	
Perseveration	+						
Anosognosia	+	+	+	+	+	+	+
SPECT imaging							
Decreased uptake							
Predominance of lesions	F, T –	–	–	–	–	F, T, P Lesions predominantly found on the left side	–

F, frontal, P, parietal, T, temporal.

*1: In case 2, the patient had neither dysgraphia nor aphasic symptoms in the early phase of the disease; subsequently, however, spontaneous speech disappeared, and because the patient's ability to write was not assessed, it was impossible to evaluate dysgraphia.

*2: The predominance of errors was determined according to the following memo written by a speech therapist: 'paragraphia was equally observed in kanji writing and kana writing.' However, we were unable to confirm the contents of the actual text written by the patient.

*3: Omission of kana was observed; for example, the patient wrote 'えんぴ' instead of 'えんぷつ'. However, detailed examination was impossible due to muscle weakness in the upper extremities.

patient: an HDS-R score of 15/30 points; a Mini-Mental State Examination (MMSE) score of 19/30 points; WAIS scores of 62 for intelligence quotient (IQ), 65 for verbal IQ (VIQ), and 67 for performance IQ (PIQ); a WCST score of 31.3% accuracy rate; a Kana Recognition Test score of 18 points; a Raven's Colored Progressive Matrices Test score of 21 points; and a Kohs Block Design Test score of 45 points (equivalent to an IQ of 73). In writing, the patient made many errors, particularly in kanji characters, replacing them with phonologically or morphologically similar characters (Figure 7.1A).

Brain CT showed mild atrophy in the frontal lobes. SPECT images showed decreased uptake in the bilateral frontal lobes and in the anterior temporal lobe.

Case 5

A 54-year-old, right-handed female patient (case 5 in Tables 7.1, 7.3, and 7.4) presented with dysarthria and dysphagia. Both the family history and past history were unremarkable. In January 1987, when the patient was 51 years old, she developed dysarthria and dysphagia, which gradually worsened. Although she was lucid when she first visited our hospital, facial muscle weakness, bulbar palsy, muscular atrophy of the extremities, and muscular fasciculation were observed. The patient showed increased mandibular reflex and increased tendon reflex of the extremities, but plantar responses were equivocal bilaterally. No sensorimotor disorder, coordination disorder, or bladder and rectal disturbances were observed. Dementia became apparent about 3 years after the onset of neurological symptoms. The patient was able to walk without any assistance until the very end of her life; however, she developed aspiration pneumonia concurrent with the above-mentioned symptoms and died 45 months after initial presentation.

On neuropsychological testing, the following symptoms were observed: difficulty in focusing attention, decreased spontaneous speech production, memory disturbance or memory retrieval disturbance, decreased ability to solve mathematical problems, restlessness, personality or behaviour disorders (e.g. disinhibitory behaviour), and incontinence. Her HDS-R score was 17/32.5 points. In writing, the patient made many errors, particularly in kanji characters, replacing them with phonologically or morphologically similar characters (Figure 7.1C) when she was mute and receiving tube feeding due to severe dysphagia (Figure 7.1D).

The brain CT showed mild atrophy in the frontal lobes while the SPECT images showed decreased uptake in the bilateral frontal lobes and in the anterior temporal lobe.

Based on the comprehensive review of all seven of our cases, the following results were obtained:

(1) Table 7.3 summarizes the dementia symptoms observed in this study other than dysgraphia and anosognosia. Behavioural disorders, including the following, were observed in many patients: decreased spontaneous speech production, decreased spontaneity, avolition, and disinhibitory behaviours such as attempts to leave. The following symptoms were observed in some patients: perseveration, imitative behaviour, and decreased ability to solve mathematical problems. In case 1, a factor indicative of semantic memory impairment was observed.

(2) Table 7.4 summarizes the observations of dysgraphia and anosognosia and the results of the SPECT scans. Dysgraphia was confirmed in six cases by observing the patient's

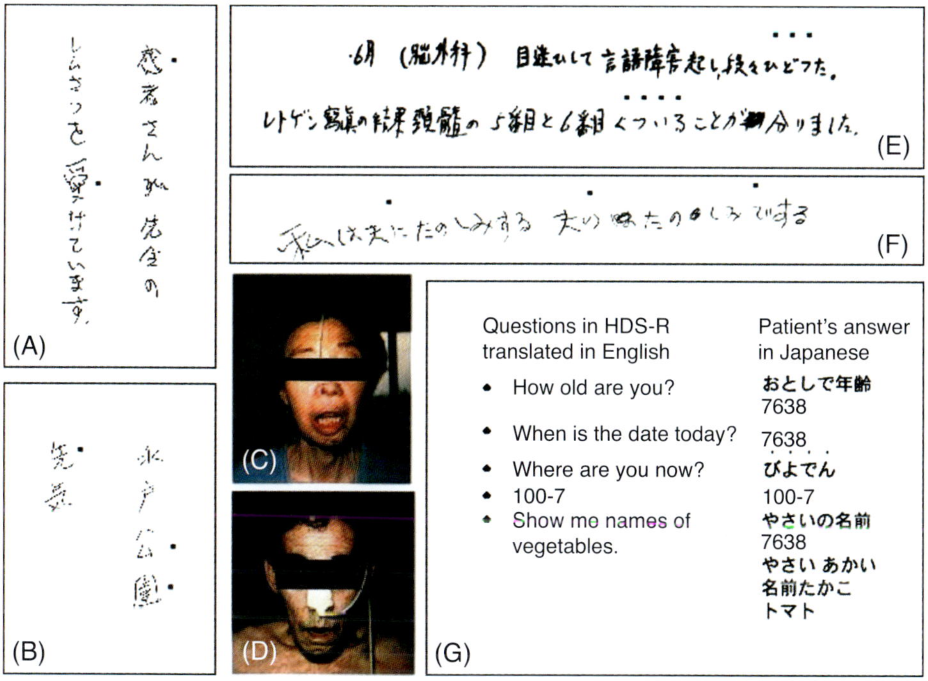

Fig. 7.1 Texts written by the patients. (A) A text written by a patient (case 1) after he was shown an image of an ordinary scene. The patient had spontaneous speech at the time of evaluation; however, he was unaware of his aphasic symptoms. (B) A handwritten medical history brought by a patient (case 4) to the initial visit because of her impaired spontaneous speech production. (C) Texts written by a patient (case 5) while communicating in writing at the bedside; the patient no longer had spontaneous speech at that time. (D) Facial appearance of a patient (case 5). (E) A text voluntarily written by a patient (case 7) at the bedside; the patient no longer had spontaneous speech at that time. Some boxes contain scores of HDS-R test (administered through written communication for the patients with impaired spontaneous speech production) or kana recognition test, which were administered when a patient's ability to write was evaluated. Cited from reference 5. Reprinted from Behav Neurol, 19, Ichikawa H, Koyama S, Ohno H et al, Writing errors and anosognosia in amyotrophic lateral sclerosis with dementia, 107–116, Copyright 2008, with permission from IOS Press.

ability to write or based on medical history. In case 2, the patient had neither dysgraphia nor aphasic symptoms in the early stage of the disease; however, the patient's ability to write had not been assessed in detail. Thus, it was impossible to evaluate dysgraphia in this patient. Marked dysgraphia was observed in all six patients whose ability to write was evaluated. In case 1, the patient still had spontaneous speech at the time of evaluation; however, in cases 3–7, spontaneous speech was absent, and communication was accomplished only through gestures or writing.

Figures 7.1 and 7.2 show the texts written by the patients. In case 1, pronounced paragraphia in writing kanji was observed. The patient wrote '感者' instead of '患者,' meaning patient, and '愛け' instead of '受け,' meaning receive (Figure 7.1A). In case 7, the patient brought a handwritten medical history to the initial visit. This handwritten

A

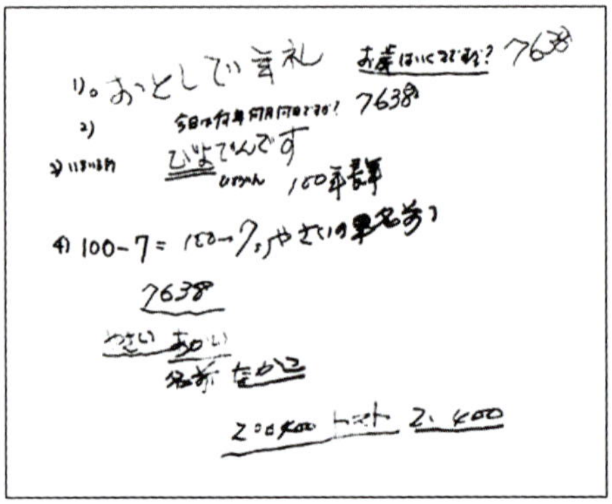

B

HDS-Rにおけるす質問	Patient's answer in Japanese
• お年は？	おとしで年齢 7638
• 今日は何日？	7638
• ここはどこですか？	びよでん
• 100-7	100-7
• 野菜の名前を言って下さい	やさいの名前 7638 やさいあかい 名前たかこ トマト

C

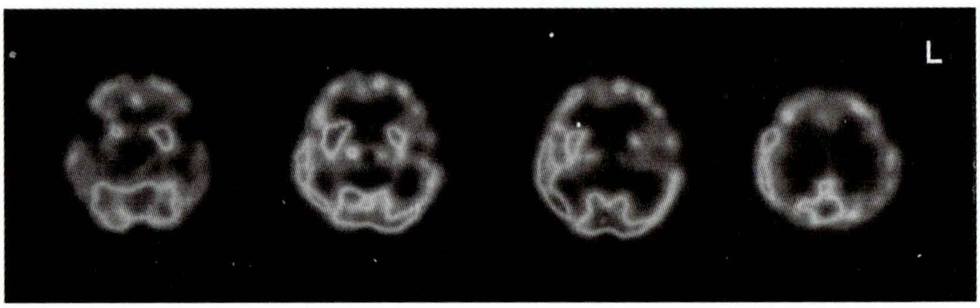

Fig. 7.2 Texts written by a patient (case 7) and SPECT images. (A) Texts written by the patient during HDS-R test. The answers to the questions were obtained in writing because the patient had impaired spontaneous speech production. (B) Typed text of (A). Paraphasia and perseveration are notable. (C) ^{99m}Tc-ethylcysteinate dimer SPECT images. There are areas of decreased uptake in the bilateral frontal and temporal lobes, but predominantly on the left side. Decreased uptake in the left parietal lobe is also notable. With permission from Kawamura et al, Amyotrophic lateral sclerosis with dementia-neuropsychological aspect, *Brain and Nerve* **59**:1083–1091, Igaku-Shoin 2007.

record contained the following features: paragraphia with marked omission of kana characters (e.g. the patient wrote 'ひどつた [hido tsuta]' instead of 'ひどくなった [hidoku natta]') as well as omission of particles (Figure 7.1B). With regard to case 5, the following record of written communication was obtained while the patient stayed at our hospital. When the patient was asked '元気か' (in other words, 'How are you?'), she replied by writing '先気' instead of '元気' (i.e. 'fine'). The patient watched a television programme titled '水戸黄門' every day, but when asked 'What are you watching?,' she replied by writing '水戸公園.' Moreover, although she apparently wanted to visit her ancestor's grave, when asked 'What do you want to do?,' she replied by writing '幕はいりに行きたい [haka hairi ni ikitai],' instead of '墓まいりに行きたい [haka mairi ni ikitai].'(Figure 7.1C). This observation indicated that the patient had paragraphia in writing kanji. In case 6, spontaneous communication in writing showed misuse of particles; for example, the patient wrote '私は夫に楽しみにする [watashi ha otto ni tanosimi ni suru]' instead of '私は夫を楽しみにする [watashi ha otto o tanosimi ni suru]' (i.e. 'I look forward to seeing my husband'), suggesting that she had grammatical deficits (Figure 7.1E). When the HDS-R test was administered to this patient, she responded to the questions in writing as follows: When asked 'How old are you?,' she wrote 'お年で年齢'; when asked 'What is your home telephone number?,' she wrote '7638'; when asked 'What date is it today?,' she wrote '7638'; when asked 'Where are we now?,' she wrote 'びよでん [biyoden]' instead of 'びょういん [byouin],' meaning hospital; and when asked 'What is 100–7?,' she wrote '100–7' (Figure 7.2A, B). Thus, perseveration and paragraphia with marked misuse in writing kana were observed. In this study, similar paragraphia symptoms were observed in six patients although the patterns of omissions, substitutions, and grammatical errors were different among the patients.

Paragraphia was observed predominantly in writing kana in three patients and in writing kanji in two other patients. Equal numbers of errors in writing kanji and kana characters were observed in one patient.

(3) Physicians and nurses noticed anosognosia in all the patients. The Anosognosia Scale Test, devised by Deckel and Morrison (11) was administered to two patients (cases 6 and 7) who had been hospitalized. The patients had no spontaneous speech; thus, when they were asked questions, they answered by using gestures. The differences between the self-rated and non-self-rated scores were 8 points in case 6 and 18 points in case 7; however, these patients denied the existence of their disorders (Figure 7.3). On the other hand, in two other patients without clinically confirmed dementia, the differences between the self-rated and non-self-rated scores were 0 points and 0.5 points.

(4) The SPECT images showed decreased uptake predominantly on the left side in one patient (case 7 shown in Figure 7.1C); however, in many patients, the difference between the right and the left sides was not clear (Table 7.4).

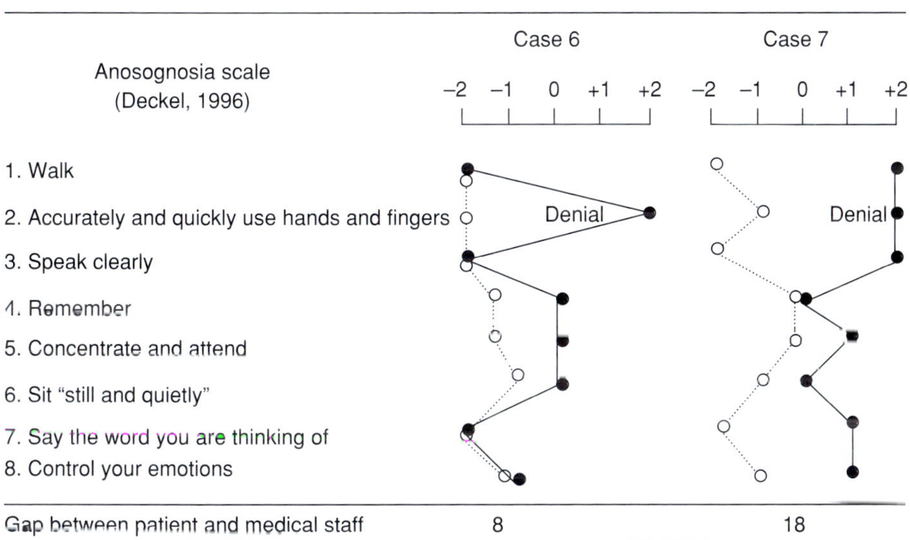

Fig. 7.3 Results of the anosognosia scale test administered to two patients with ALS-D ○:Self-rated score •:Average score computed by summing two scores rated by a physician and a nurse and dividing by 2. *Although the disorder was severe, the patient had an attitude of denying it. Cited from reference 5. Reprinted from Behav Neurol, 19, Ichikawa H, Koyama S, Ohno H et al, Writing errors and anosognosia in amyotrophic lateral sclerosis with dementia, 107–116, Copyright 2008, with permission from IOS Press.

In recent years, in addition to FTD, the concept of frontotemporal lobar degeneration, which encompasses progressive non-fluent aphasia (PA) and subtypes of semantic dementia (SD), has been advocated (6,10). In terms of dementia symptoms, FTD with motor neurone disease (FTD/MND) is considered to be equivalent to MND-D/ALS-D. The pathognomonic features of FTD/MND are said to be the lack of Pick bodies and presence of ubiquitinated inclusion bodies in motor neurones (8,12–14). Moreover, cases of ALS with apparent PA or SD have often been reported in recent years (15–21). The diagnostic criteria of frontotemporal lobar degeneration described in such reports suggest that MND can be complicated with PA or SD (6,9,10). On the other hand, behaviour disorders, such as decreased spontaneity and disinhibitory behaviours, were apparent in the patients examined in the present study; thus, the observed dementia symptoms were considered to belong to the FTD.

We also examined past reports of dysgraphia in patients with ALS. For example, a report written by Ferguson and Boller in 1977 includes a passage stating that dysgraphia is often observed in patients with ALS, which is consistent with our observation (22). Furthermore, this finding suggests that paragraphia may be universally present to a degree greater than we had expected among ALS patients with bulbar palsy and that bulbar palsy, pseudobulbar palsy, and speech disorders can coexist with endophasia disorders. Nevertheless, evaluation of the patient's ability to write is most important for a diagnosis of ALS-D.

There are few reports on dysgraphia in patients diagnosed with ALS-D. Ferguson and Boller reported the autopsy results of patients with ALS in whom agrammatism was observed in addition to paragraphia (22). Recently, Bak and colleagues reported the autopsy results of patients with ALS in whom grammatical errors were observed in addition to a description of a lesion localized in Broca's area (20). Furthermore, the results of a functional imaging study indicate that Broca's area is linked to grammatical function (23). In Japan, reports have been published that describe the differences in mechanisms governing the ability to write kana and kanji (24,25). For example, the left posterior inferior temporal lobe plays an important role in writing and reading kanji. With regard to the dysgraphia observed in the patients examined in the present study, paragraphia and grammatical deficits were suggested; thus, the observed dysgraphia symptoms were considered to be aphasic. However, the differences in the observed symptoms between the cases in the present study and those reported in the literature were probably due to differences in the pattern of lesion(s) in the cerebral hemisphere, primarily in the frontotemporal lobe. Decreased spontaneous speech production (2,3) is typically seen in the early stages of ALS-D. However, considering that aphasic dysgraphia was frequently observed in the patients examined in the present study, it is necessary to re-examine the possibility that in the past, aphasic symptoms were overlooked and described collectively as a decrease in the amount of spontaneous speech production.

Deckel and Morrison (11) devised the Anosognosia Scale Test for numerically quantifying the degree of anosognosia in patients with Huntington's disease. They assessed many patients and obtained the following result: the mean difference between self-rated and non-self-rated scores in patients with Huntington's disease was 5.81 points whereas the mean difference in the control group was 1.2 points; thus, there was a significant difference between the test group (patients with Huntington's disease) and the control group. The authors thereby documented the existence of anosognosia in patients with Huntington's disease. When the Anosognosia Scale Test was administered to two patients with ALS-D in the present study, the difference between the self-rated and non-self-rated scores was large in both cases; in addition, the patients denied their disorders. On the other hand, when the test was administered to patients with ALS without dementia, there was almost no difference between the self-rated and non-self-rated scores. Thus, it is clear that the Anosognosia Scale Test is a useful tool for the objective evaluation of anosognosia. Interestingly, findings indicate that the onset mechanism of anosognosia and/or lack of self-insight is linked to the right frontal lobe (26) as correlated with the amyloid macule in the right subiculum of Alzheimer disease (27) and that the earliest lesions in ALS-D occur in the subiculum. The Anosognosia Scale Test used in the present study can be administered to patients with compromised physical function, and it takes only a few minutes to complete; thus, the test can be administered to patients with advanced-stage ALS.

With regard to hemispheric predominance, disorders occurring predominantly on the left side have been reported in patients who developed ALS with apparent aphasia (28). Thus, agraphia may also suggest left hemispheric involvement in the disease. On the other hand, anosognosia in the disease may indicate right hemispheric involvement.

Significance of the report written by Watanabe (1893)

According to the Collective Bibliography on Aphasia in Japan (Japan Speech Abstracts Publication Committee: Goro Kamiyama [Chairman]), Japan Society for the Promotion of Science, Tokyo, 1972 [published on 30 March in the 47th year of Showa]), the case report written by Eikichi Watanabe, entitled 'One patient who manifested cortical motor aphasia concurrently with bulbar palsy and progressive muscular atrophy', is 'the first case report on aphasia published in Japan', among others found so far.

The year 1893 was the 26th year of the Meiji era. Broca's report on cortical motor aphasia was first published in Paris in 1862. The Watanabe report was published only 30 years or so after Broca's report, which indicates that Broca's discovery may have been rather quickly imported into Japan. However, this is not the only significance of the Watanabe report. A more important fact may be hidden in the report. First, the Watanabe report is summarized as follows.

The patient was 41 years old with a chief complaint of language disorder that had started the previous year. Bulbar palsy symptoms were well described in this report. For example, soft palatal paralysis was discussed based on the following observations: the patient was unable to blow out a candle or match placed in front of him without pinching his nose; moreover, the patient breathed through both the mouth and the nose simultaneously while smoking a cigarette. Tongue atrophy, lip atrophy, and dysphagia were present, but oculomotor nerve palsy was not observed. Moreover, although the motor symptoms in the upper and lower extremities were mild (no atrophy of thenar muscles/superior limb girdle and no increased tendon reflex in the lower extremities), the patient was unable to use chopsticks. However, as the patient's ability to write was mentioned in Watanabe's report (see below), the motor symptoms were probably not so severe as to affect the ability to write. These observations are consistent with the symptoms of ALS with bulbar palsy although, strictly speaking, the possibility of progressive spinal muscular atrophy can probably not be excluded because these symptoms were observed only 1 year after onset of the disease.

The Watanabe report describes the dysphasia symptoms in detail, stating that 'The unique feature of this case is that the patient not only cannot speak but also has a markedly impaired ability to write. Sometimes, the patient cannot write anything, but on other occasions, the patient can write a correct answer after making literal errors and rewriting [a] few times.'

Watanabe further reported that 'The patient had paragraphia in writing kanji: for example, the patient wrote '厚 [atsu]' meaning thick instead of '熱 [netus]' meaning hot. Moreover, when we showed a sake cup (盃) to the patient and asked the patient to write the name of the cup, the patient wrote '盃'; however, when the patient was asked to write the name in kana, the patient wrote 'ヨマ [yoma]' instead of 'サカズキ [sakazuki].' When the patient was shown Japanese sandals (草履), the patient wrote '履草' in kanji and 'ヨウリ [youri]' instead of 'ゾウリ [zouri]' in kana; moreover, the patient was able to write '病院' meaning hospital in kanji correctly but wrote incorrectly 'ビンヒン [bin hin]' instead of 'ビョウイン [byou in]' in kana. These were described as paragraphia, and it was said that the ability to write kana was more severely affected than the ability to write kanji.

On the other hand, the patient's spontaneous speech was severely affected, with the inability to imitate or read out. This probably reflects the dysarthria symptoms associated with bulbar palsy.

Another key point is the psychiatric symptom. According to the report, the patient was always smiling. The word 'always' suggests that this was probably not a forced smile caused by pseudobulbar palsy.

As described before in relation to our observation of patients with ALS, bulbar palsy is very common in patients with ALS-D. There are two distinguishing neuropsychological features in such patients: paragraphia in writing kanji or kana and anosognosia. The paragraphia symptoms observed in this study are consistent with those described in the Watanabe report. In some cases of ALS, patients seem inexplicably unconcerned about their condition even though they are affected by such a calamitous disease and some patients always smile. Thus, the described symptoms might have actually been dementia with paragraphia and anosognosia.

We suspect that the disease described in the Watanabe report may be, in the present terminology, ALS-D. If so, 'the first case report on aphasia published in Japan' may actually be the world's first case report on ALS-D.

Although the clinical nature of aphasia, including PNFA or SD in ALS/MND, has been occasionally documented, as previously mentioned, most of the cases appear to be of PNFA (5,29–32). In most of the reported cases, aphasia preceded or occurred simultaneously with ALS symptoms, and in cases in which ALS symptoms preceded aphasia, the aphasia became evident only through writing (5,29–32). Because motor symptoms progress rapidly in patients with ALS, they may not survive until aphasic symptoms develop. On the other hand, aphasia may be easily masked by severe dysarthria and the use of artificial ventilation. It is of interest that most of the reported cases with aphasia or writing errors exhibit the features of bulbar-onset ALS (5,29–32). Although the reason for this is unclear, we reported a high prevalence of writing errors in bulbar-onset ALS and speculate that the orolingual motor cortex that connects to bulbar areas is adjacent to Broca's area. This may also explain why PNFA is a major type of aphasia in ALS. Bak and colleagues reported cases of bulbar-onset MND that showed PNFA with selective impairment of verb production and comprehension relative to noun understanding and revealed selective involvement of Broca's area (Broadmann 44 and 45) neuropathologically in three patients (20). Hillis and colleagues compared impairment of naming verbs and nouns in patients with fluent primary progressive aphasia (PPA), probably corresponding to SD, to patients with non-fluent PPA, probably corresponding to PNFA, and documented that patients with non-fluent PPA and ALS-FTD were significantly more impaired in verb naming than noun naming and that non-fluent PPA showed the opposite pattern (33).

In the Japanese language, frequent omissions, paragraphia, and syntactic errors in the writing have been observed in patients with ALS (5,29–32). The features of such writing errors are different across patients and the characteristic features of them reflect the nature of the aphasia, such as PA and SD, which are easily masked by dysarthria, or the underlying brain locations, including hemispheric dominance and frontal or temporal involvement. In addition, we have observed dissociated errors between kana and kanji characters (5,7,29–32). Such dissociated impairment may reflect preferentially involved areas of the brain, such as frontal-lobe predominance or temporal-lobe predominance, or an underlying aphasic condition, including PNFA or SD. Otherwise, these dissociated patterns of writing errors in Japanese (i.e. kana versus kanji) may partly correspond to observations in the English language represented by verb versus noun (20,33). Furthermore, we previously reported that atypical language problems could appear as 'isolated agraphia' without aphasia and dementia, and that selective involvement of Exner's writing centre in the frontal lobe may be responsible for such isolated agraphia. Thus, further investigation of the clinical significance of writing errors in ALS and their pathological correlates is warranted.

In conclusion, we have recently visited three patients who were diagnosed with ALS and were receiving nursing care in their homes. The first patient, a middle-aged man, had been placed on a respirator and had typical ALS. The second patient had an approximately 10-year history of ALS with mild bulbar palsy symptoms. According to this patient, the most disturbing symptom was generalized pain. In general, ALS does not cause sensory disturbance; however, pain can be a problem in some cases. The third patient had ALS-D with bulbar palsy. In this patient, the motor symptoms were observed first, followed by paragraphia and other symptoms. The patient was apathetic about the disease. This patient also had valvular heart disease and chronic renal failure, for which the patient received dialysis three times a week. The differing characteristics of these three cases highlight the fact that there are many atypical cases of ALS.

Acknowledgement

M.K. is supported by a grant from the Core Research for Evolutional Science and Technology (CREST, 17022035) and a Grant-in-Aid for Scientific Research on Priority Areas (System Study on Higher-order Brain Functions) from the Ministry of Education, Culture, Sports, Science and Technology (MEXT, 18020027). H.I. is supported by an institutional grant from the Showa University School of Medicine.

References

1. Yuasa R. (1964). Amyotrophic lateral sclerosis with dementia. *Clin Neurol (Japan)*, **4**, 529–534.
2. Mitsuyama Y, Takamiya S. (1979). Presenile dementia with motor neuron disease in Japan. A new entity? *Arch Neurol*, **36**, 592–593.
3. Mitsuyama Y. (1984). Presenile dementia with motor neuron disease in Japan: clinico-pathological review of 26 cases. *J Neurol Neurosurg Psychiatry*, **47**, 953–959.
4. Ichikawa H, Kanda M, Hukui T, *et al.* (1995). Intellectual function and clinical imaging in amyotrophic lateral sclerosis (ALS) with a focus on 123 I-IMP-SPECT imaging findings. *Showa Univ J Med Sci*, **54**, 273–283.
5. Ichikawa H, Koyama S, Ohno H *et al.* (2008). Writing errors and anosognosia in amyotrophic lateral sclerosis with dementia. *Behav Neurol*, **19**, 107–116.
6. Neary D, Snowden JS, Mann DM. (2000). Cognitive change in motor neurone disease/amyotrophic lateral sclerosis (MND/ALS). *J Neurol Sci*, **180**, 15–20.
7. Watanabe E, (1893). One patient who manifested cortical motor aphasia concurrently with bulbar palsy and progressive muscular atrophy, (Hishitsu Undousei Shitsugo-sho to Enzuikyumahi no Shinkousei Kin-ishuku o Gappei-seru Kanja ni tuite [in Japanese]). *J Okayama Med Assoc*, **40**, 138–144.
8. Yoshida M, Murakami N, Hashizume Y, *et al.* (1992). [A clinicopathological study on 13 cases of motor neuron disease with dementia]. *Rinsho Shinkeigaku*, **32**, 1193–1202.
9. Brun AEB, Gustafson L, Passant U, *et al.* (1994). Consensus statement: clinical and neuropathological criteria for frontotemporal dementia. Lund and Manchester groups. *J Neurol Neurosurg Psychiatry*, **57**, 416–418.
10. Neary D, Snowden JS, Mann DMA *et al.* (1990). Frontal lobe dementia and motor neuron disease. *J Neurol Neurosurg Psychiatry*, **53**, 23–32.
11. Deckel AW, Morrison D. (1996). Evidence of a neurologically based 'denial of illness' in patients with Huntington's disease. *Arch Clin Neuropsychol*, **11**, 295–302.
12. Brooks BR, Miller RG, Swash M, *et al.* (2000). El Escorial revisited: revised criteria for the diagnosis of amyotrophic lateral sclerosis. *Amyotroph Lateral Scler Other Motor Neuron Disord*, **1**, 293–299.
13. Lipton AM, White CL, III, Bigio EH. (2004). Frontotemporal lobar degeneration with motor neuron disease-type inclusions predominates in 76 cases of frontotemporal lobar degeneration. *Acta Neuropathol*, **108**, 379–385.
14. Yoshida M. (2004). Amyotrophic lateral sclerosis with dementia: the clinicopathological spectrum. *Neuropathology*, **24**, 87–102.
15. Caselli RJ, Windebank AJ, Petersen RC *et al.* (1993). Rapidly progressing aphasic dementia and motor neuron disease. *Ann Neurol*, **33**, 200–207.
16. Engel PA, Fleming PD. (1997). Primary progressive aphasia, left anterior atrophy, and neurofibrillary hippocampal pathology: observations in an unusual case. *Neuropsychiatry Neuropsychol Behav Neurol*, **10**, 213–218.
17. Iroi A, Okuma Y, Fukae J, *et al.* (2002). [Amyotrophic lateral sclerosis presented with alexia of kanji and word meaning aphasia]. *No To Shinkei*, **54**, 903–907.

18. Hyodo T, Ikeda M, Ueno S, *et al.* (2002). [A case of motor neuron disease with progressive aphasia and dementia]. *No To Shinkei*, **54**, 713–718.
19. Kanzaki M, Sato M, Ogawa G, *et al.* (2004). [A case of dementia with motor neuron disease associated with agraphia—the omission of kana letters]. *Rinsho Shinkeigaku*, **44**, 673–676.
20. Bak TH, O'Donovan DG, Xuereb JH, *et al.* (2001). Selective impairment of verb processing associated with pathological changes in Brodmann areas 44 and 45 in the motor neurone disease-dementia-aphasia syndrome. *Brain*, **124**, 103–120.
21. Tsuchiya K, Ozawa E, Fukushima J, *et al.* (2000). Rapidly progressive aphasia and motor neuron disease: a clinical, radiological, and pathological study of an autopsy case with circumscribed lobar atrophy. *Acta Neuropathol*, **99**, 81–87.
22. Ferguson JH, Boller F. (1977). A different form of agraphia: syntactic writing errors in patients with motor speech and movement disorders. *Brain Lang*, **4**, 382–389.
23. Caplan D. (2001). Functional neuroimaging studies of syntactic processing. *J Psycholinguist Res*, **30**, 297–320.
24. Iwata M. (1984). Kanji versus Kana, neuropsychological correlates of the Japanese writing system. *Trends Neurosci*, **7**, 290–293.
25. Kawamura M, Hirayama K, Hasegawa K, *et al.* (1987). Alexia with agraphia of kanji (Japanese morphograms). *J Neurol Neurosurg Psychiatry*, **50**, 1125–1129.
26. Michon A, Deweer B, Pillon B, *et al.* (1994). Relation of anosognosia to frontal lobe dysfunction in Alzheimer's disease. *J Neurol Neurosurg Psychiatry*, **57**, 805–809.
27. Marshall GA, Kaufer DI, Lopez OL, *et al.* (2004). Right prosubiculum amyloid plaque density correlates with anosognosia in Alzheimer's disease. *J Neurol Neurosurg Psychiatry*, **75**, 1396–1400.
28. Catani M, Piccirilli M, Geloso MC, *et al.* (2004). Rapidly progressive aphasic dementia with motor neuron disease: a distinctive clinical entity. *Dement Geriatr Cogn Disord*, **17**, 21–28.
29. Ichikawa H, Takahashi N, Hieda S, *et al.* (2008). Agraphia in bulbar-onset amyotrophic lateral sclerosis: not merely a consequence of dementia or aphasia. *Behav Neurol*, **20**, 91–99.
30. Ichikawa H, Takahashi N, Hieda S, *et al.* (2010). [Bulbar-onset amyotrophic lateral sclerosis (ALS) with isolated agraphia]. *Rinsho Shinkeigaku*, **50**, 81–86.
31. Ichikawa H, Kawamura M. (2009). [Symptoms of frontotemporal dementia]. *Brain Nerve*, **61**, 1227–1235.
32. Ichikawa H, Kawamura M. (2010). [Language impairment in amyotrophic lateral sclerosis]. *Brain Nerve*, **62**, 435–440.
33. Hillis AE, Oh S, Ken L. (2004). Deterioration of naming nouns versus verbs in primary progressive aphasia. *Ann Neurol*, **55**, 268–275.

Chapter 8

Social cognition in frontotemporal dementia and amyotrophic lateral sclerosis

Sharon Abrahams and Christopher Kipps

Social cognition in frontotemporal dementia

In a series of monographs between 1892 and 1906 Arnold Pick, a neuropathologist working in Prague, described many of the clinical features of the disease, which we now know as Pick's disease or frontotemporal dementia (FTD) (1–4). His account included macroscopic features of the 'circumscribed atrophy', predominantly of the temporal lobe. By 1954, van Mansvelt was able to describe the clinical and pathological features of 196 patients (5). His elegant description of 'essential and fundamental elements' highlighted the dulling of affect, aspontaneity 'mostly preceded by disinhibition', motor restlessness, and disturbance of speech that are well recognized elements of the modern conception of the disease. He identified the pathological predilection for the orbital region of the frontal lobe, temporal pole and insula region, and noted a less commonly reported association with the caudate nucleus, realizing also that the distribution of pathology across the frontal and temporal lobes formed a continuum. His detailed clinico-anatomic correlations yielded the observation that regions within the frontotemporal region were associated with particular clinical features: disinhibition-hyperkinesis was seen in cases with orbitofrontal–thalamic neuronal loss; aspontaneity was linked to maximal atrophy of the polar areas and (dorsolateral) convexity of the frontal lobes; speech deficits were dependent on whether atrophy was predominantly frontal (scantiness of speech), temporal (logorrhea, anomia, and sensory aphasia), or striate (palilalia).

The first attempt to systematically rate the behavioural deficit in Pick's disease, and contrast it with Alzheimer's disease was made by Gustafson and Nilsson (6), who identified the importance of a slow progression, early loss of insight, alterations in speech production, hyperorality, mood changes, and confabulation in clinically diagnosed cases, and verified this against patients with a diagnosis confirmed at post mortem. Collaboration between the Lund and Manchester groups led to the first formal criteria for the disease, and named it FTD (7). Apart from formalizing the diagnostic features of FTD, they drew attention to the fact that the underlying pathology, although distributed identically, is actually heterogeneous, and that it is location, and not pathology that defines the varied behavioural and language presentations.

While the clinical manifestations of FTD clearly involve changes in social interaction and behaviour, this can be difficult to rate objectively. Rating scales in frontal lobe disorders attempt to serve one of two masters. Those that index frontal lobe dysfunction, regardless of aetiology, aim to be sensitive to the range of such deficits, and include the Frontal Systems Behavioral Scale (FrSBe) (8) and the Iowa Rating Scales of Personality Change (IRSPC) (9). These scales were developed for the rating of behavioural symptoms following head injury. Others, particularly those used in dementia, are more clinically oriented, concerned with differential diagnosis, and attempt to balance sensitivity with increased specificity for different disorders. There is inevitably substantial overlap between these two types of scale. Clinical rating scales in common use include the Neuropsychiatric Inventory (NPI) (10), Frontal Behavioural Inventory (FBI) (11–13), Frontal Behavioural Score (FBS) (14), and the Cambridge Behavioural Inventory (CBI). Some are based on direct interview whereas others are rated directly by the carer.

Cognitive performance is markedly affected in behavioural variant FTD (bvFTD), and its assessment may potentially be a more objective marker of deficits than ratings on behavioural inventories. Tests of neuropsychological performance in bvFTD have tended to concentrate on aspects of executive function (15–19): the ability to sustain and redirect attention, inhibit inappropriate responses, and initiate or switch strategy (20). This reflects the perceived role of such tests as measures of frontal lobe function, which are regarded as the source of the disordered conduct. In bvFTD, however, both bedside cognitive assessments and standard formal neuropsychology may be normal (21–23). One explanation is that these tasks may be insensitive to dysfunction of the medial and orbital frontal cortices, the right temporal lobe and amygdala, which have been shown to degenerate early in bvFTD (24,25).

The relative lack of success in delineating a consistent pattern of neuropsychological dysfunction in bvFTD prompted exploration of a range of novel tasks in an attempt to quantify the social cognitive deficit in these patients in the areas of decision-making, insight, emotion processing, empathy, and the Theory of Mind.

Decision-making In view of the prominent impairments shown by patients with bvFTD in the areas of appetite, disinhibition, and impulsivity, there is surprisingly little data on learning for reward in this condition. Rahman and colleagues tested decision-making using a reversal paradigm called the internal dimension/external dimension shift task requiring shifts in discrimination both within (internal dimension) and between (external dimension) set on several stimuli (26). Patients were specifically impaired at the reversal aspects of the task. They could not change their behaviour when a previously rewarded stimulus was no longer rewarded, but had no difficulty in transferring a rule learnt on one set of exemplars to a different, but related set of stimuli. In the same study, the authors used the Cambridge Gamble task to assess risk-taking behaviour. In this task, bets are placed on the likely position of yellow tokens hidden underneath one of two boxes on the screen. Patients with bvFTD showed true risk-taking behaviour in that they bet a larger proportion of their accumulated winnings on the outcome. They did not, however, perform less accurately than controls in this task, even though their deliberation times were significantly longer, a feature seen in other patients with orbitofrontal lesions (27). Their risk taking was not just a reflection of impulsive behaviour, as bets had to be placed in a manner that minimized this possibility.

In a similar study using the Iowa Gambling Task, Torralva and colleagues showed that patients with bvFTD were unable to modify their behaviour in response to changes in reward contingencies (28). Despite obvious monetary losses, these patients continued to bet on risky card decks (i.e. those that gave the chance of big reward, but frequently had much larger losses), while controls realized that betting on safer decks (i.e. less money won each time, but more consistently and with fewer overall penalties) was a better strategy. In other recent work, patients with bvFTD are significantly impaired on a task requiring concurrent visual discriminations and that, unlike controls, their performance is not enhanced by the addition of a genuine, and otherwise motivating, monetary reward (29).

Theory of Mind Demonstration of abnormalities in the ventromedial aspect of the frontal lobes in bvFTD prompted interest in the possibility that aspects of social cognition such as the Theory of Mind, the capacity to ascribe beliefs and intentions to others, might be impaired in these patients. In a comparison with normal controls, and MMSE-matched patients with Alzheimer's disease, Gregory and co-workers (30), showed that in bvFTD, both first- and second-order Theory of Mind was significantly worse than in controls, and that an even greater proportion of patients with bvFTD were impaired on the faux pas task. This task tests the ability to identify socially embarrassing transgressions from story vignettes, and patients made a number of errors, with false positive and false negative endorsements, as well as inappropriately inferring that a faux pas had been caused intentionally. In contrast, performance by patients with Alzheimer's disease was compromised by memory impairment as indicated by their scores on control questions.

In an interesting study, Snowden and colleagues (31) showed that patients with bvFTD were more likely than controls or patients with Huntington's disease to make errors of omission, and to provide inappropriately concrete responses in a cartoon interpretation task. They also used relatively fewer verbs depicting mental states (e.g. thinking, believing) when asked to describe a mental state cartoon. This was not just an effect of poor verbal fluency, as mental state verbs were affected more than physical state verbs. When tested on a story comprehension task, which involved representation of first- and second-order Theory of Mind, the patients with bvFTD performed poorly, although this was with both physical and mental state stories. Verb production overall was impaired relative to controls, and is resonant with findings from studies mentioned earlier that suggest a disproportionate impairment of verbs relative to nouns in bvFTD (32–34). On a test of eye gaze preference, several of the patients persisted in selecting their own personal favourites as the target; such eccentricity highlights one of the potential confounds in testing this particular group.

The role of executive function in performing some of these tasks is controversial. In a recent study, performance on both the Hayling and Brixton tasks was unrelated to the performance of patients with bvFTD on a mental state cartoon interpretation task (35). In fact, it appeared that executive function played a supportive role in processing cartoons and story vignettes rather than being directly involved in mental state representation. Executive impairments, however, have the potential to mask more specific deficits in the theory of mind (31), particularly if they are severe. Furthermore, it seems that the ability to process social rule violations is related to executive function measures; despite this, knowledge of social rules themselves is unaffected (35). The ability to judge the severity of rule violations (moral versus conventional) is compromised in bvFTD, with patients tending to judge all social violations equally severely, and suggests a degree of cognitive inflexibility.

In a further study, patients with bvFTD were impaired in their interpretation of second-order beliefs about characters in story vignettes, where they were required to determine whether a character was lying or joking (36). Despite the fact that they were unimpaired on the factual control question, the vignettes did not contrast mental state questions with non-mental state questions of the same degree of difficulty, and therefore was unable to resolve whether it was truly a problem with mental state representation, or a more general problem with abstract reasoning. These same subjects were also impaired on a task requiring prediction of the consequences of social situations such as a diner finding a fly in his soup, although it could again be argued that this task does not necessarily require mental state processing.

Empathy At least two studies have assessed the characteristic indifference to the emotional concerns of others seen in patients with bvFTD using the interpersonal reactivity index, an instrument with a four-factor structure reflecting cognitive (perspective-taking and fantasy) and emotional (empathic concern and personal distress) aspects of empathy (37,38). In patients with bvFTD, perspective-taking (35,39) and empathic concern were impaired relative to age-matched controls. Patients with semantic dementia were impaired across all four factors, reflecting a more profound cognitive and emotional indifference to others. Interestingly, patients with Alzheimer's disease were not impaired on these measures, suggesting a defined frontotemporal neural substrate for empathy, and not just brain degeneration per se as the reason for empathic changes.

Emotional recognition and regulation The ability of patients with bvFTD to recognize facial emotional expressions in others is particularly impaired for anger, sadness, and disgust (35,40,41). There are, however, inconsistent results when this type of test is applied longitudinally, with Alzheimer's disease, but not bvFTD, patients showing deteriorating performance (42). In two cross-sectional studies, fear recognition was also impaired (35,43). A test of identifying vocal emotion yielded similar results: angry and sad voices were poorly identified, but there were additional deficits in recognizing the sounds of happiness or surprise (41). Both recognition and experience of social emotion appears to be affected: patients with bvFTD subjected to a sudden auditory stimulus show similar defensive reactions to controls, but exhibit far less embarrassment when they review their startled response, a finding consistent with reduced self-referential processing (44). This lack of self-awareness is seen in the failure of insight that is a core feature of the disease (45–47).

Higher order social cognitive deficits Real-world interactions involve dynamic situations, which are not fully captured by static images of emotion expression or morphed facial features, yet there are relatively few studies in bvFTD that use dynamic social exchange as the basis of assessment. The Test of Social Inference uses actors to portray exchanges depicting basic emotions, and more complex exchanges involving sarcasm, deception, and irony (48), and is well validated in controls and brain-injured patients (48,49). Understanding of sarcasm is impaired on this test in bvFTD (50), and is particularly associated with damage to frontotemporal structures, predominantly those on the right (50,51).

Imaging evidence

Recognition that the three major surfaces of the frontal lobes (medial prefrontal (BA 25, 32), dorsolateral prefrontal (BA 9,46), and orbitofrontal (BA 11,12,47)) were not equally involved in the disease process, particularly in the early stages (52–59) has aided the understanding of disease progression, and the relationship of individual symptoms to their underlying neural substrates. Starkstein *et al.* (52) linked behavioural changes in bvFTD to the disproportionate reduction in orbitofrontal cortex blood flow compared with dorsolateral regions, and others have shown that this region degenerates earliest in bvFTD in both imaging (57) and pathological studies (60). Several studies have connected disinhibited behaviour to the orbitofrontal cortex, temporal lobe, and interconnected striatal regions (5,58,61–64).

The adjacent mesial prefrontal region is also involved early in the disease. In a longitudinal PET study, hypometabolism was maximal in the anterior cingulate region in mild disease, with later spread to involve the striatum, thalamus, temporal lobes and ultimately parietal regions (59). Similarly in a structural study using tensor-based morphometry (65), the region with the most rapid progression was the anterior cingulate region, with similar changes in the insula, ventromedial region (BA 11) and amygdala over 1 year. Anterior cingulate hypoperfusion predicts levels of apathy, although this is also associated with dorsolateral and superior frontal regions and even the orbitofrontal cortex in one study (62,63,66). In practice, as already discussed, apathy and disinhibition coexist (67–69); patients are profoundly apathetic until an appropriate environmental stimulus appears that triggers their disinhibited response.

Voxel-based morphometry, used to study the basis for eating disturbance in bvFTD (70) has shown that the orbitofrontal cortex and anterior insula are associated with the pathological 'sweet tooth' seen in this disorder. Other regions within the striatum, temporal poles, inferior and dorsolateral prefrontal regions, principally on the right, appear to form part of a network mediating this behaviour, and were associated at reduced threshold in the analysis. Hyperphagia, another abnormal eating behaviour in bvFTD was also related to the degree of orbitofrontal atrophy, although the local maximum for this association was in a more anterior region of the orbitofrontal cortex, which mediates reward processing of gustatory and olfactory signals (71,72).

There is a frequent bias towards the right hemisphere in these clinico-anatomic associations (73–80) although this is not universally seen (58,61,63,81,82). To some extent, this discrepancy probably reflects differences in the classification of subjects with evidence of right temporal lobe dysfunction. These patients have marked behavioural disturbance (83–86), yet may also have substantial language deficits, and are classed as having semantic dementia, one of the language presentations of frontotemporal dementia (87,88). Although some groups have commented on the behavioural distinctions between frontal and temporal predominant forms of FTD (89), others have found the behavioural disturbance to be quite similar (80,87,90). In one SPECT study, bilateral frontal hypoperfusion was associated with apathy, whereas temporal lobe changes, in both hemispheres, were associated with hypomanic-like behaviour (75). Other neuropsychiatric features such as excessive frivolity, dysthymia, and anxiety are dependent on the degree of hypoperfusion of the right temporal lobe (76). It is worth bearing in mind, however, that while often asymmetric, the disease process in bvFTD is seldom completely unilateral (85,86,91), with simultaneous bi-hemispheric involvement and disease progression (65,88). Thus, correlations with one hemisphere are likely to be reflected in the contralateral hemisphere, although to differing extents.

Two caveats should be noted: behavioural symptoms are rated subjectively by observers, may both fluctuate both in intensity and frequency over time, and may be dependent on other symptoms (e.g. apathy) for their expression. This limits the usefulness of the correlative approach in determining the relative contribution of different structures (or networks) in the genesis of these symptoms. In addition, spurious correlations with simultaneously degenerating structures may be introduced, particularly when using unbiased whole brain correlative techniques (92) (such as statistical parametric mapping), or multiple regions of interest without a priori hypotheses. Conversely, failure to sample sufficient brain regions risks missing a real underlying association and mistakenly associating the cognitive deficit with brain areas simply co-atrophying in tandem with another, unsampled, area, which is truly responsible for the deficit (78).

Fewer studies have attempted to correlate more complex social phenomena such as emotion processing, empathy, and insight (46,79,93) with distinct frontotemporal regions. Perry *et al.* (57), contrasted performance on tasks of facial and emotional prosodic processing, showing right hemispheric dominance for these abilities in a small series of well defined cases. This theme was developed further by Rosen and coworkers (93) who demonstrated impaired emotion recognition for negative emotions (fear, anger, disgust, sadness) in a mixed group of 25 patients with FTD, and correlated this to the volume of inferolateral and anterior temporal regions in the right hemisphere. An additional correlation was seen in the lateral orbitofrontal region (BA 47). The ability to empathize, as rated by carers on the Interpersonal Reactivity Index, is impaired in patients with bvFTD and is dependent on the integrity of right-sided structures involved in emotion processing and Theory of Mind reasoning such as the temporal pole, fusiform gyrus, caudate head, and subcallosal gyrus. In a smaller study, the ability to process faux pas, and thus understand the embarrassment of others, was linearly correlated with the degree of orbitofrontal atrophy (30).

Insight is characteristically poor in bvFTD (7,47,94), and while predictions of a relative's personality were accurate, patients with bvFTD had poor judgement of their own personality traits, and were unable to predict their own behaviour in social and emotional situations (46). A correlation was seen with the degree of hypometabolism of the left temporal pole, which the authors hypothesize results in impaired processing of emotional autobiographical information. Finally, in a task assessing the ability of patients with bvFTD to predict outcomes from social scenarios, performance was associated with the volume of the orbitofrontal cortex, superior temporal gyrus, posterior cingulate, and visual association region (36). While still subject to extraneous factors influencing performance in bvFTD such as disinhibition, distraction, or apathy, performance on objective markers such as these may be more stable for assessing longitudinal change in these patients.

Social cognition in amyotrophic lateral sclerosis

The proposal of a continuum of cognitive change from amyotrophic lateral sclerosis (ALS) to FTD has been primarily driven by the finding of executive dysfunction and corresponding prefrontal (often dorsolateral) changes in a significant proportion of patients with non-demented ALS. The most striking and consistent deficit is found on tests of letter fluency (95–97). This deficit is apparent early on in the disease process (97), is independent of physical disability, can be found in patients without language or working memory dysfunction and has been related to executive dysfunction (96). Evidence of a prefrontal substrate to such dysfunction has strengthened the notion of a continuum with fluency deficits directly related to: dysfunction of the dorsolateral prefrontal cortex and anterior cingulate gyrus through functional neuroimaging (98,99); frontotemporal white matter abnormalities in structural neuroimaging (100) and reduced neuronal receptor binding of Flumazenil in the inferior frontal gyrus (101).

In contrast, evidence of impairments in social and emotional cognition and involvement of more orbital prefrontal pathways typical of bvFTD is in comparison relatively sparse and has only recently become a focus for investigation in ALS. Studies have demonstrated some incidence of behaviour change in ALS (102) with irritability and disinhibition (103) and apathy (104). A recent study investigated a very large (n = 225) cohort of patients with ALS and revealed changes in at least one domain (apathy, disinhibition, executive dysfunction) in up to 39% of cases (105). Moreover Woolley and colleagues revealed that although there was evidence of mild behaviour change in some patients with non-demented ALS, unlike those with FTD, these patients showed insight into these changes with no significant differences between self and carer ratings (106).

However, most of these studies have tended to use questionnaires standardized on the head-injured population. Moreover, measurement of behaviour change in ALS has the additional challenge of accommodating for reactions to the disease or the consequences of physical disability and hence questionnaires designed for other populations may tend to exaggerate dysfunction. In addition, some studies have not considered patients with ALS/FTD and non-demented patients with ALS separately, which is essential to demonstrate a spectrum of change. Gibbons and colleagues reported a detailed case by case investigation of the types of behaviour changes prevalent in bvFTD in a group of patients with ALS, the majority of whom did not have a full dementia syndrome (107). Carers' reports revealed changes in affect and social behaviour with self-centredness/selfishness reported in 11 of 16 patients and loss of interest/apathy in six of 16, while aggression, loss of insight, and social disinhibition were also present, but in only two of 16 cases.

Decision making In terms of the cognitive profile, which may underpin such behaviour change, there is growing evidence of deficits on tasks sensitive to the early stages of bvFTD. A recent study reported by Girardi and colleagues revealed deficits in affective decision making using a modified version of the Iowa Gambling Task (108). A group of 19 patients with non-demented ALS demonstrated dysfunction of reward learning and showed no adjustment of their performance in response to the negative consequences of losing money. Moreover, poor performance related to overall level of behaviour dysfunction in everyday life as measured by the FrSBe. However, caution should be taken when interpreting these findings as although the Iowa task is sensitive to patients with ventromedial lesions (109) and patients with bvFTD (28), performance on this task may also be affected by more dorsal prefrontal dysfunction (110). In accord with this, the performance of patients with ALS remained stable across the task with no evidence of learning; they did not show a tendency to increase selection from disadvantageous decks during the task, which has been shown in bvFTD (28). Hence, the pattern of performance in patients with ALS may therefore indicate a failure to learn (more executive) rather than a tendency to take more risks.

Theory of Mind Two studies have now demonstrated evidence of a deficit on tests of Theory of Mind in patients with ALS. In a study of 16 patients with ALS, Gibbons and colleagues revealed an impairment in a subset all of whom had bulbar signs in interpreting cartoons and stories, which involved understanding a character's mental state and included false beliefs and deception (111). Although no significant group differences were found between patients with ALS and controls a spectrum of scores ranging from normal to abnormal were present. However an analysis of the performance revealed impairments not only in social items, in which the understanding was based on inferring the mental state of another, but also physical scenarios in which humour was based on the physical properties of the scene. A similar pattern of impairment on both social and physical scenarios had been found in patients with FTD (31) and was interpreted as resulting from difficulties with the inferential aspects of the task. Moreover, the types of errors seen in the ALS cases were similar to those found in FTD with a large proportion of concrete responses. Hence, due to the demanding nature of the tasks, which have a strong reasoning and inferential component, executive dysfunction may have been at the root of this deficit in ALS. This was further supported by the finding that poor performance on the Wisconsin Card Sorting Task correlated with deficits on these tasks.

More recently, Girardi and colleagues investigated a group of 14 unselected patients with ALS and demonstrated evidence of impairment on a range of tasks of social and emotional cognition previously shown to be sensitive to impairment in bvFTD (108). The most sensitive of these was a simple Theory of Mind task in which participants had to infer preference judgements about another. The task previously shown to be sensitive to bvFTD (31) has a low and high attentionally demanding condition (involving the presence or absence of a distracter—an arrow near one of the pictures). Although more patients with ALS (64%) showed difficulties on the attentionally demanding (distracter) condition, 36% of patients were in the abnormal range in the condition with low executive demands (no distracter). An analysis of the errors made revealed that patients with ALS were not only influenced by the presence of distracting information, but also showed increased selection of their own favourite object relative to controls. This suggests that on some trials there had been difficulties in inhibiting egocentric responding to stimuli leading to difficulties in using a simple social cue (eye-gaze) to infer the mental state of another. Of note patients with ALS were able to undertake a parallel control task in which the stimuli remained unchanged but the wording was altered from 'Which picture does the face like best?' to 'Which picture is the face looking at?'. This task was also shown to be more sensitive than traditional measures of executive functions, which in comparison detected a deficit in only four of 14 cases. Patients with ALS impaired on this test of social cognition also showed evidence of increased behavioural dysfunction using the FrSBe and changes in apathy were significantly related to poor performance on this task. A more detailed analysis of behaviour change revealed exaggerated emotional display, irritability, loss of emotional insight and embarrassment, selfishness, excessive worrying, inappropriate behaviour, loss of interest, a change in eating behaviour and in sense of smell, and adherence to routine. The presence of behaviour dysfunction strongly overlapped with the social cognition impairment, with 36% showing deficits on the judgement of preference task and behaviour change. However, three cases with social cognition deficits showed no signs of behaviour change, while four cases showed some behaviour dysfunction but no social cognition impairment.

In relation to bulbar involvement, although a relationship appeared strong in the Gibbons study, cognitive deficits and behaviour change in the Girardi study were found in those with and without bulbar involvement. Nevertheless, there was a preponderance of bulbar cases in the cognitively impaired subset at a ratio of approximately 2:1. This finding is supportive of previously reported associations and suggests that those with bulbar involvement are more at risk of developing cognitive change (95,111).

Emotion recognition and regulation Several studies have indicated a deficit in emotional perception in ALS, as has been found in the FTD literature. Some studies have now shown impairments in facial recognition of emotions (108,112), although this has not been consistent (113). Deficits in emotion recognition in faces were found to be more sensitive than emotion recognition in prosody (112). In the study by Girardi and colleagues, complex and simple emotional understanding of expression was investigated using both the Reading the Mind in the Eyes Test and the Facial Expressions of Emotions Test (108). A subset of the patients performed poorly on both of these tasks in addition to the judgement of preference task described above. Further studies that have investigated the social significance of emotional processes have shown that patients with ALS rated faces as more approachable than controls (114). In relation to the processing of socially relevant situation, Lule and colleagues revealed that patients with ALS tended to show a more positive valence towards emotive social situations and demonstrated a more balanced arousal state (rating calm pictures as more exciting and exciting pictures as more calm than controls) (115). In a follow-up study, Lule and colleagues investigated emotional responses using fMRI. Altered activation patterns were observed with increased activation in the right supramarginal area and reduced activation in extrastriate visual areas. Over time patients with ALS showed additional reductions in the anterior insula, which correlated with subjective arousal.

There is evidence of the selectivity of this emotional processing dysfunction rather than it being a manifestation of general cognitive decline or attentional dysfunction. For example, Papps and colleagues demonstrated a failure to show enhanced recognition of emotional words (113). This deficit could not have resulted from a general memory decline as patients with ALS showed superior neutral word recognition. Finally, the relationship between this emotional processing dysfunction and the loss of control of emotional expression (emotional lability), which occurs in 19–49% of patients with ALS in studies, has not yet been investigated, although Palmieri *et al.* (116) demonstrated that lability did not correlate with performance on other cognitive measures indicating differing neuronal pathways.

In conclusion, there is now growing evidence of dysfunction in emotional and social cognition in ALS, which appears parallel to that found in FTD. However, it remains unclear whether these deficits represent more orbitomedial dysfunction as found in bvFTD. The involvement of executive dysfunction in this presentation is contentious, but similar issues are prevalent within the FTD literature. The profile of impairment in ALS resembles that found in FTD and hence appears supportive of a subclinical syndrome in a significant proportion of ALS cases.

These studies have implications for the everyday care for a distinct subset of patients with ALS. The findings predict potential difficulties in social interaction with those around them, with problems using social cues to guide behaviour and understand the emotions and intentions of others. Patients with ALS may have difficulty in attributing to others a mental state that differs from their own. This may manifest as an egocentric perspective, and a lack of concern for partners' views and feelings. Clinicians should be directing appropriate strategies to educate those involved in the direct care of patients with ALS.

References

1. Pick A. (1892). Über die Beziehungen der senilen Hirnatrophie zur Aphasie. *Prager Medizinische Wochenschrift*, **17**(translated in Berrios and Girling 1994), 165–167.
2. Pick A. (1901). Senile Hirnatrophie als Grundlage von Herderescheinungen. *Wien Klin Wochenschr*; **14**(translated in Girling and Marková), 403–404.
3. Pick A. Zur (1904). Symptomatologie der linksseitigen Schläfenlappenatrophie. *Mschr Psychiatr Neurol*, **16**, 378–388.
4. Pick A. (1906). Über einen weiteren Symptomenkomplex im Rahmen der Dementia senilis bedingt durch umschriebene stärkere Hirnatrophie (gemische Apraxie). *Mschr Psychiatr Neurol*, **19**, 97–108.
5. van Mansvelt J. (1954). *Pick's Disease: A Syndrome of Lobar Cerebral Atrophy its Clinico-Anatomical and Histopathological Types*. Enschede, Utrecht.
6. Gustafson L, Nilsson L. (1982). Differential diagnosis of presenile dementia on clinical grounds. *Acta Psychiatr Scand*, **65**, 194–209.
7. Lund and Manchester Groups. (1994). Clinical and neuropathological criteria for frontotemporal dementia. *J Neurol Neurosurg Psychiatry*, **57**, 416–418.
8. Stout JC, Ready RE, Grace J, *et al.* (2003). Factor analysis of the frontal systems behavior scale (FrSBe). *Assessment*, **10**, 79–85.
9. Barrash J, Anderson S, Jones R, and Tranel, D. (1997). The Iowa Rating Scales of Personality Change: Reliability and Validity. *J Int Neuropsychol Soc*, **3**, 27–28.
10. Cummings JL, Mega M, Gray K, *et al.* (1994). The Neuropsychiatric Inventory: comprehensive assessment of psychopathology in dementia. *Neurology*, **44**, 2308–2314.
11. Kertesz A, Davidson W, Fox H. (1997). Frontal behavioral inventory: diagnostic criteria for frontal lobe dementia. *Can J Neurol Sci*, **24**, 29–36.
12. Kertesz A, Davidson W, McCabe P, Munoz D. (2003). Behavioral quantitation is more sensitive than cognitive testing in frontotemporal dementia. *Alzheimer Dis Assoc Disord*, **17**, 223–229.
13. Kertesz A, Nadkarni N, Davidson W, Thomas AW. (2000). The Frontal Behavioral Inventory in the differential diagnosis of frontotemporal dementia. *J Int Neuropsychol Soc*, **6**, 460–468.
14. Lebert F, Pasquier F, Souliez L, Petit H. (1998). Frontotemporal behavioral scale. *Alzheimer Dis Assoc Disord*, **12**, 335–339.
15. Miller BL, Cummings JL, Villanueva-Meyer J, *et al.* (1991). Frontal lobe degeneration: clinical, neuropsychological, and SPECT characteristics. *Neurology*, **41**, 1374–1382.
16. Frisoni GB, Pizzolato G, Geroldi C, *et al.* (1995). Dementia of the frontal type: neuropsychological and (99Tc)-HM-PAO SPET features. *J Geriatr Psychiatry Neurol*, **8**, 42–48.
17. Pachana NA, Boone KB, Miller BL, *et al.* (1996). Comparison of neuropsychological functioning in Alzheimer's disease and frontotemporal dementia. *J Int Neuropsychol Soc*, **2**, 505–510.
18. Kramer JH, Jurik J, Sha SJ, *et al.* (2003). Distinctive neuropsychological patterns in frontotemporal dementia, semantic dementia, and Alzheimer disease. *Cogn Behav Neurol*, **16**, 211–218.
19. Thompson JC, Stopford CL, Snowden JS, Neary D. (2005). Qualitative neuropsychological performance characteristics in frontotemporal dementia and Alzheimer's disease. *J Neurol Neurosurg Psychiatry*, **76**, 920–927.
20. Alvarez JA, Emory E. (2006). Executive function and the frontal lobes: a meta-analytic review. *Neuropsychol Rev*, **16**, 17–42.
21. Gregory CA, Hodges JR. (1996). Frontotemporal dementia: use of consensus criteria and prevalence of psychiatric features. *Neuropsychiatry Neuropsychol Behav Neurol*, **9**, 145–153.
22. Gregory CA, McKenna PJ, Hodges JR. (1998). Dementia of frontal type and simple schizophrenia: two sides of the same coin? *Neurocase*, **4**, 1–6.
23. Lough S, Gregory C, Hodges JR. (2001). Dissociation of social cognition and executive function in frontal variant frontotemporal dementia. *Neurocase*, **7**, 123–130.

24. Kril JJ, Macdonald V, Patel S, *et al.* (2005). Distribution of brain atrophy in behavioral variant frontotemporal dementia. *J Neurol Sci*, **232**, 83–90.
25. Kril JJ, Halliday GM. (2004). Clinicopathological staging of frontotemporal dementia severity: correlation with regional atrophy. *Dement Geriatr Cogn Disord*, **17**, 311–315.
26. Rahman S, Sahakian BJ, Hodges JR, R, *et al.* (1999). Specific cognitive deficits in mild frontal variant frontotemporal dementia. *Brain*, **122** (Pt 8): 1469–1493.
27. Rogers RD, Everitt BJ, Baldacchino A, *et al.* (1999). Dissociable deficits in the decision-making cognition of chronic amphetamine abusers, opiate abusers, patients with focal damage to prefrontal cortex, and tryptophan-depleted normal volunteers: evidence for monoaminergic mechanisms. *Neuropsychopharmacology*, **20**, 322–339.
28. Torralva T, Kipps CM, Hodges JR, *et al.* (2007). The relationship between affective decision-making and theory of mind in the frontal variant of frontotemporal dementia. *Neuropsychologia*, **45**, 342–349.
29. Graham AJ. (2006). *Learning and Memory in Frontotemporal Dementia.* (Thesis Dissertation, University of Cambridge).
30. Gregory C, Lough S, Stone V, *et al.* (2002). Theory of mind in patients with frontal variant frontotemporal dementia and Alzheimer's disease: theoretical and practical implications. *Brain*, **125**, 752–764.
31. Snowden JS, Gibbons ZC, Blackshaw A, *et al.* (2003). Social cognition in frontotemporal dementia and Huntington's disease. *Neuropsychologia*, **41**, 688–701.
32. Rhee J, Antiquena P, Grossman M. (2001). Verb comprehension in frontotemporal degeneration: The role of grammatical, semantic and executive components. *Neurocase*, **7**, 173–184.
33. Bak TH, O'Donovan DG, Xuereb JH, *et al.* (2001). Selective impairment of verb processing associated with pathological changes in Brodmann areas 44 and 45 in the motor neurone disease-dementia-aphasia syndrome. *Brain*, **124**, 103–120.
34. Cappa SF, Binetti G, Pezzini A, *et al.* (1998). Object and action naming in Alzheimer's disease and frontotemporal dementia (see Comment). *Neurology*, **50**, 351–355.
35. Lough S, Kipps CM, Treise C, *et al.* (2006). Social reasoning, emotion and empathy in frontotemporal dementia. *Neuropsychologia*, **4**, 950–958.
36. Eslinger PJ, Moore P, Troiani V, *et al.* (2007). Oops! Resolving social dilemmas in frontotemporal dementia. *J Neurol Neurosurg Psychiatry*, **78**, 457–460.
37. Rankin KP, Kramer JH, Miller BL. (2005). Patterns of cognitive and emotional empathy in frontotemporal lobar degeneration. *Cogn Behav Neurol*, **18**, 28–36.
38. Davis MH. (1980). A multidimensional approach to individual differences in empathy. *JSAS Catalog of Selected Documents in Psychology* 10.
39. Rankin KP, Baldwin E, Pace-Savitsky C, *et al.* (2005). Self awareness and personality change in dementia. *J Neurol Neurosurg Psychiatry*, **76**, 632–639.
40. Lavenu I, Pasquier F, Lebert F, *et al.* (1999). Perception of emotion in frontotemporal dementia and Alzheimer disease. *Alzheimer Dis Assoc Disord*, **13**, 96–101.
41. Keane J, Calder AJ, Hodges JR, Young AW. (2002). Face and emotion processing in frontal variant frontotemporal dementia. *Neuropsychologia*, **40**, 655–665.
42. Lavenu I, Pasquier F. (2005). Perception of emotion on faces in frontotemporal dementia and Alzheimer's disease: a longitudinal study. *Dement Geriatr Cogn Disord*, **19**, 37–41.
43. Rosen HJ, Pace-Savitsky K, Perry RJ, *et al.* (2004). Recognition of emotion in the frontal and temporal variants of frontotemporal dementia. *Dement Geriatr Cogn Disord*, **17**, 277–281.
44. Sturm VE, Rosen HJ, Allison S, *et al.* (2006). Self-conscious emotion deficits in frontotemporal lobar degeneration. *Brain*, **129**, 2508–2516.
45. Eslinger PJ, Dennis K, Moore P, *et al.* (2005). Metacognitive deficits in frontotemporal dementia. *J Neurol Neurosurg Psychiatry*, **76**, 1630–1635.

46. Ruby P, Schmidt C, Hogge M, *et al.* (2007). Social mind representation: where does it fail in frontotemporal dementia? *J Cogn Neurosci*, **19**, 671–683.
47. O'Keeffe FM, Murray B, Coen RF, *et al.* (2007). Loss of insight in frontotemporal dementia, corticobasal degeneration and progressive supranuclear palsy. *Brain*, **130**, 753–764.
48. McDonald S, Flanagan S, Rollins J, Kinch J. (2003). TASIT: a new clinical tool for assessing social perception after traumatic brain injury. *J Head Trauma Rehabil*, **18**, 219–238.
49. McDonald S, Bornhofen C, Shum D, *et al.* (2006). Reliability and validity of The Awareness of Social Inference Test (TASIT): a clinical test of social perception. *Disabil Rehabil*, **28**, 1529–1542.
50. Kipps CM, Nestor PJ, Acosta-Cabronero J, *et al.* (2009). Understanding social dysfunction in the behavioural variant of frontotemporal dementia: the role of emotion and sarcasm processing. *Brain*, **132**, 592–603.
51. Rankin KP, Salazar A, Gorno-Tempini ML, *et al.* (2009). Detecting sarcasm from paralinguistic cues: anatomic and cognitive correlates in neurodegenerative disease. *Neuroimage*, **47**, 2005–2015.
52. Starkstein SE, Migliorelli R, Teson A, *et al.* (1994). Specificity of changes in cerebral blood flow in patients with frontal lobe dementia. *J Neurol Neurosurg Psychiatry*, **57**, 790–796.
53. Varrone A, Pappata S, Caraco C, *et al.* (2002). Voxel-based comparison of rCBF SPET images in frontotemporal dementia and Alzheimer's disease highlights the involvement of different cortical networks. *Eur J Nucl Med Mol Imaging*, **29**, 1447–1454.
54. Salmon E, Garraux G, Delbeuck X, *et al.* (2003). Predominant ventromedial frontopolar metabolic impairment in frontotemporal dementia. *Neuroimage*, **20**, 435–440.
55. Schroeter ML, Raczka K, Neumann J, von Cramon DY. (2006). Neural networks in frontotemporal dementia-A meta-analysis. *Neurobiol Aging*, **29**, 418–426.
56. Schroeter ML, Raczka K, Neumann J, Yves von CD. (2007). Towards a nosology for frontotemporal lobar degenerations-A meta-analysis involving 267 subjects. *Neuroimage,* **36**, 497–510.
57. Perry RJ, Graham A, Williams G, *et al.* (2006). Patterns of Frontal Lobe Atrophy in Frontotemporal Dementia: A Volumetric MRI Study. *Dement Geriatr Cogn Disord*, **22**, 278–287.
58. Borroni B, Grassi M, Agosti C, *et al.* (2007). Latent profile analysis in frontotemporal lobar degeneration and related disorders: clinical presentation and SPECT functional correlates. *BMC Neurol,* **7**, 9.
59. Diehl-Schmid J, Grimmer T, Drzezga A, *et al.* (2007). Decline of cerebral glucose metabolism in frontotemporal dementia: a longitudinal 18F-FDG-PET-study. *Neurobiol Aging*, **8**, 42–50.
60. Broe M, Hodges JR, Schofield E, *et al.* (2003). Staging disease severity in pathologically confirmed cases of frontotemporal dementia. *Neurology*, **60**, 1005–1011.
61. Sarazin M, Pillon B, Giannakopoulos P, *et al.* (1998). Clinicometabolic dissociation of cognitive functions and social behavior in frontal lobe lesions. *Neurology*, **51**, 142–148.
62. Franceschi M, Anchisi D, Pelati O, *et al.* (2005). Glucose metabolism and serotonin receptors in the frontotemporal lobe degeneration. *Ann Neurol*, **57**, 216–225.
63. Peters F, Perani D, Herholz K, *et al.* (2006). Orbitofrontal Dysfunction Related to Both Apathy and Disinhibition in Frontotemporal Dementia. *Dement Geriatr Cogn Disord*, **21**, 373–379.
64. Le B, I, Guedj E, Gabelle A, *et al.* (2006). Demographic, neurological and behavioural characteristics and brain perfusion SPECT in frontal variant of frontotemporal dementia. *Brain*, **129**, 3051–3065.
65. Brambati SM, Renda NC, Rankin KP, *et al.* (2007). A tensor based morphometry study of longitudinal gray matter contraction in FTD. *Neuroimage,* **35**, 998–1003.
66. Rosen HJ, Allison SC, Schauer GF, *et al.* (2005). Neuroanatomical correlates of behavioural disorders in dementia. *Brain,* **128**, 2612–2625.
67. Lebert F, Guedj E, Gabelle A, *et al.* (2006). Demographic, neurological and behavioural characteristics and brain perfusion SPECT in frontal variant of frontotemporal dementia. *Brain*, **129**, 3051–3065.
68. Salmon E, Garraux G, Collette F. (2007). A synthesis of functional neuroimaging in the frontal variant of frontotemporal dementia. *Curr Med Imag Rev*, **3**, 117–121.

69. Kipps CM, Hodges JR. (2005). Frontotemporal dementia syndromes. In: Growdon JH, Rossor MN (eds.), *The Dementias*, Vol. 2. Elsevier, Oxford.
70. Whitwell JL, Sampson EL, Loy CT, *et al.* (2007). VBM signatures of abnormal eating behaviours in frontotemporal lobar degeneration. *Neuroimage*, **35**, 207–213.
71. Kringelbach ML, Rolls ET. (2004). The functional neuroanatomy of the human orbitofrontal cortex: evidence from neuroimaging and neuropsychology. *Prog Neurobiol*, **72**, 341–372.
72. Kringelbach ML. (2005). The human orbitofrontal cortex: linking reward to hedonic experience. *Nat Rev Neurosci*, **6**, 691–702.
73. Miller BL, Chang L, Mena I, *et al.* (1993). Progressive right frontotemporal degeneration: clinical, neuropsychological and SPECT characteristics. *Dementia*, **4**, 204–213.
74. Miller BL, Seeley WW, Mychack P, *et al.* (2001). Neuroanatomy of the self: evidence from patients with frontotemporal dementia. *Neurology*, **57**, 817–821.
75. McMurtray AM, Chen AK, Shapira JS, *et al.* (2006). Variations in regional SPECT hypoperfusion and clinical features in frontotemporal dementia. *Neurology*, **66**, 517–522.
76. Mendez MF, McMurtray A, Chen AK, *et al.* (2006). Functional neuroimaging and presenting psychiatric features in frontotemporal dementia. *J Neurol Neurosurg Psychiatry*, **77**, 4–7.
77. Mychack P, Kramer JH, Boone KB, Miller BL. (2001). The influence of right frontotemporal dysfunction on social behavior in frontotemporal dementia. *Neurology*, **56**, S11–S15.
78. Rankin KP, Rosen HJ, Kramer JH, *et al.* (2004). Right and left medial orbitofrontal volumes show an opposite relationship to agreeableness in FTD. *Dement Geriatr Cogn Disord*, **17**, 328–332.
79. Rankin KP, Gorno-Tempini ML, Allison SC, *et al.* (2006). Structural anatomy of empathy in neurodegenerative disease. *Brain*, **129**, 2945–2956.
80. Liu W, Miller BL, Kramer JH, *et al.* (2004). Behavioral disorders in the frontal and temporal variants of frontotemporal dementia. *Neurology*, **62**, 742–748.
81. Jeong Y, Cho SS, Park JM, *et al.* (2005). 18F-FDG PET findings in frontotemporal dementia: an SPM analysis of 29 patients. *J Nucl Med*, **46**, 233–239.
82. Nakano S, Asada T, Yamashita F, *et al.* (2006). Relationship between antisocial behavior and regional cerebral blood flow in frontotemporal dementia. *Neuroimage*, **32**, 301–306.
83. Edwards-Lee T, Miller BL, Benson DF, *et al.* (1997). The temporal variant of frontotemporal dementia. *Brain*, **120**(Pt 6): 1027–1040.
84. Rosen HJ, Perry RJ, Murphy J, *et al.* (2002). Emotion comprehension in the temporal variant of frontotemporal dementia. *Brain*, **125**, 2286–2295.
85. Thompson SA, Patterson K, Hodges JR (2003). Left/right asymmetry of atrophy in semantic dementia: behavioral-cognitive implications. *Neurology*, **61**, 1196–1203.
86. Seeley WW, Bauer AM, Miller BL, *et al.* (2005). The natural history of temporal variant frontotemporal dementia. *Neurology*, **64**, 1384–1390.
87. Rosen HJ, Allison SC, Ogar JM, *et al.* (2006). Behavioral features in semantic dementia vs other forms of progressive aphasias. *Neurology*, **67**, 1752–1756.
88. Brambati SM, Rankin KP, Narvid J, *et al.* (2007). Atrophy progression in semantic dementia with asymmetric temporal involvement: a tensor-based morphometry study. *Neurobiol Aging*, **30**, 103–111.
89. Snowden JS, Bathgate D, Varma A, *et al.* (2001). Distinct behavioural profiles in frontotemporal dementia and semantic dementia. *J Neurol Neurosurg Psychiatry*, **70**, 323–332.
90. Bozeat S, Gregory CA, Lambon Ralph MA, Hodges JR (2000). Which neuropsychiatric and behavioural features distinguish frontal and temporal variants of frontotemporal dementia from Alzheimer's disease? *J Neurol Neurosurg Psychiatry*, **69**, 178–186.
91. Chan D, Fox NC, Scahill RI, *et al.* (2001). Patterns of temporal lobe atrophy in semantic dementia and Alzheimer's disease. *Ann Neurol*, **49**, 433–442.
92. Williams GB, Nestor PJ, Hodges JR. (2005). Neural correlates of semantic and behavioural deficits in frontotemporal dementia. *Neuroimage*, **24**, 1042–1051.

93. Rosen HJ, Wilson MR, Schauer GF, *et al.* (2006). Neuroanatomical correlates of impaired recognition of emotion in dementia. *Neuropsychologia*, **44**, 365–373.
94. Neary D, Snowden JS, Gustafson L, *et al.* (1998). Frontotemporal lobar degeneration: a consensus on clinical diagnostic criteria. *Neurology*, **51**, 1546–1554.
95. Abrahams S, Goldstein LH, Al-Chalabi A, *et al.* (1997). Relation between cognitive dysfunction and pseudobulbar palsy in amyotrophic lateral sclerosis. *J Neurol Neurosurg Psychiatry*, **62**, 464–472.
96. Abrahams S, Leigh PN, Harvey A, *et al.* (2000). Verbal fluency and executive dysfunction in amyotrophic lateral sclerosis (ALS). *Neuropsychologia*, **38**, 734–747.
97. Abrahams S, Leigh PN, Goldstein LH. (2005). Cognitive change in ALS: a prospective study. *Neurology*, **64**, 1222–1226.
98. Abrahams S, Goldstein LH, Kew JJ, *et al.* (1996). Frontal lobe dysfunction in amyotrophic lateral sclerosis. A PET study. *Brain*, **119** (Pt 6), 2105–2120.
99. Abrahams S, Goldstein LH, Simmons A, *et al.* (2004). Word retrieval in amyotrophic lateral sclerosis: a functional magnetic resonance imaging study. *Brain*, **127**, 1507–1517.
100. Abrahams S, Goldstein LH, Suckling J, *et al.* (2005). Frontotemporal white matter changes in amyotrophic lateral sclerosis. *J Neurol*, **252**, 321–331.
101. Wicks P, Turner MR, Abrahams S, *et al.* (2008). Neuronal loss associated with cognitive performance in amyotrophic lateral sclerosis: an (11C)-flumazenil PET study. *Amyotroph Lateral Scler*, **9**, 43–49.
102. Lomen-Hoerth C, Murphy J, Langmore S, *et al.* (2003). Are amyotrophic lateral sclerosis patients cognitively normal? *Neurology*, **60**, 1094–1097.
103. Murphy J, Henry R, Lomen-Hoerth C. (2007). Establishing subtypes of the continuum of frontal lobe impairment in amyotrophic lateral sclerosis. *Arch Neurol*, **64**, 330–334.
104. Grossman AB, Woolley-Levine S, Bradley WG, Miller RG. (2007). Detecting neurobehavioral changes in amyotrophic lateral sclerosis. *Amyotroph Lateral Scler*, **8**, 56–61.
105. Witgert M, Salamone AR, Strutt AM, *et al.* (2010). Frontal-lobe mediated behavioral dysfunction in amyotrophic lateral sclerosis. *Eur J Neurol*, **17**, 103–110.
106. Woolley SC, Moore DH, Katz JS. (2010). Insight in ALS: awareness of behavioral change in patients with and without FTD. *Amyotroph Lateral Scler*, **11**, 52–56.
107. Gibbons ZC, Richardson A, Neary D, Snowden JS. (2008). Behaviour in amyotrophic lateral sclerosis. *Amyotroph Lateral Scler*, **9**, 67–74.
108. Girardi A, Macpherson SE, Abrahams S. (2011). Deficits in emotional and social cognition in amyotrophic lateral sclerosis. *Neuropsychology*, **25**, 53–65.
109. Bechara A, Damasio AR, Damasio H, Anderson SW. (1994). Insensitivity to future consequences following damage to human prefrontal cortex. *Cognition*, **50**, 7–15.
110. Clark L, Manes F, Antoun N, *et al.* (2003). The contributions of lesion laterality and lesion volume to decision-making impairment following frontal lobe damage. *Neuropsychologia*, **41**, 1474–1483.
111. Gibbons ZC, Snowden JS, Thompson JC, *et al.* (2007). Inferring thought and action in motor neurone disease. *Neuropsychologia*, **45**, 1196–1207.
112. Zimmerman EK, Eslinger PJ, Simmons Z, Barrett AM. (2007). Emotional perception deficits in amyotrophic lateral sclerosis. *Cogn Behav Neurol*, **20**, 79–82.
113. Papps B, Abrahams S, Wicks P, *et al.* (2005). Changes in memory for emotional material in amyotrophic lateral sclerosis (ALS). *Neuropsychologia*, **43**, 1107–1114.
114. Schmolck H, Mosnik D, Schulz P. (2007). Rating the approachability of faces in ALS. *Neurology*, **69**, 2232–2235.
115. Lule D, Kurt A, Jurgens R, *et al.* (2005). Emotional responding in amyotrophic lateral sclerosis. *J Neurol*, **252**, 1517–1524.
116. Palmieri A, Abrahams S, Soraru G, *et al.* (2009). Emotional Lability in MND: Relationship to cognition and psychopathology and impact on caregivers. *J Neurol Sci*, **278**, 16–20.

Chapter 9

Behavioural change in amyotrophic lateral sclerosis

Laura H. Goldstein

In the same way that interest in cognitive change in amyotrophic lateral sclerosis (ALS) developed slowly and challenged the then prevailing view that it was a motor system disorder that left cognitive function intact, research characterizing the potential behavioural change occurring in at least some people with ALS has been relatively slow to gain ground, despite early references to its existence (1). Research into behavioural change in ALS has depended heavily on literature that exists more generally on the syndromes of frontotemporal lobar degeneration (FTLD) (e.g. (2)) and on the view that, as with cognitive change in ALS, there may be a spectrum of behavioural involvement.

In the UK, Neary *et al.*'s (3) early studies of a dementia in ALS identified this as predominantly frontotemporal in nature and helped shape the field, particularly highlighting the role of behavioural and personality change (as well as cognitive impairment) that might occur in advance of, simultaneously with, or after the development of physical signs of ALS. Early accounts by Neary and colleagues documented the prominent cognitive as well as behavioural changes found in people with ALS and dementia (3), and subdivided profiles into disinhibited, apathetic, and stereotypic subtypes. However, the consensus criteria (hereafter referred to as the Neary criteria) (2) that have influenced most of the work looking at behavioural change in ALS were actually developed in the non-ALS field to identify and classify the three main subtypes of FTLD, namely frontotemporal dementia (FTD; often also referred to as frontal or behavioural variant FTD (i.e. fvFTD or bvFTD (4)), semantic dementia (SD) and progressive non-fluent aphasia (PNFA).

Within the Neary criteria, the classification of FTD is based predominantly on personality and behavioural change, characterized either by distractibility and disinhibition or inertia and loss of volition. The core diagnostic features of FTD are as follows: (a) insidious onset and gradual progression; (b) early impairment in social interpersonal conduct; (c) early decline in regulation of personal conduct; (d) early emotional blunting; and (e) early loss of insight. In FTD, speech output is reduced, leading to mutism, although Neary *et al.* indicate that pressure of speech may also occur in patients with a more disinhibited presentation (2). While the diagnosis is based primarily on the presence of behavioural change as described above, supportive evidence is derived from impaired neuropsychological test performance (particularly on measures of executive function). While the core diagnostic features must be present, the existence of a range of other features may also be supportive of a diagnosis of FTD, comprising further aspects of behavioural change, altered speech output, and a range of physical symptoms. Neuropsychological changes, a normal EEG and neuroimaging demonstrating predominantly frontal and/or anterior temporal abnormalities are key results that would further be used to support a diagnosis of FTD. Limitations of these diagnostic criteria have, however, been outlined, although with respect to the diagnosis of bvFTD per se rather than with reference to ALS cases (3).

Two other forms of FTLD have diagnostic criteria described by Neary and colleagues (2). These relate to changes in language processing, and the core diagnostic features reflect impaired cognition (and particularly language) rather than behaviour. PNFA is, as with the other disorders, diagnosed in terms of its insidious onset and gradual progression but its additional core diagnostic features comprise non-fluent spontaneous speech with at least one of the following characteristics: agrammatism; phonemic paraphasia, or anomia. In PNFA, there is early preservation of social skills but later in the illness behavioural changes are seen similar to those characterizing FTD.

A diagnosis of SD (also known as progressive fluent aphasia) requires insidious development and gradual progression. However, here the language disorder is characterized by fluent but empty spontaneous speech, with a loss of word meaning, demonstrated by both impaired naming and comprehension and the presence of semantic paraphasias. There must also be evidence of a perceptual disorder (prosopagnosia and/or impaired recognition of object identity, i.e. associative agnosia). Perceptual matching and drawing reproduction remain intact, as does single-word repetition and the ability to read aloud and write to dictation orthographically regular words. Supportive diagnostic features for SD include behavioural changes characterized by loss of sympathy and empathy, narrowed preoccupations, and parsimony (2). Further details of other supporting diagnostic criteria for both PNFA and SD are to be found in Neary *et al.* (2).

One of the difficulties in applying the above criteria to people with ALS is the need to ensure that any behavioural change is not simply a reaction to the diagnosis of ALS or a result of the physical limitations it imposes. Thus, careful questioning of informants must identify changes that are over and above the person with ALS's reaction to their devastating diagnosis and its resulting physical limitations (1).

Most of the studies that have considered the presence or otherwise of FTLD in people with ALS have applied the Neary criteria as their basis for the diagnosis of FTD, SD, or PNFA. However, Ringholz and colleagues adopted the National Institute of Neurological and Communicative Disorders and Stroke and the Alzheimer's Disease and Related Disorders Association criteria for FTD and Pick's disease (5,6). Here the diagnosis of FTD depends on (a) the development of behavioural or cognitive deficits manifested by either early, progressive change in personality (characterized by difficulty in regulating behaviour), or (b) an early and progressive change in language characterized by problems in the expressive aspects of language, or severe difficulty in naming and impairments in word meaning. In this diagnostic framework, the deficits cause significant impairments in social or occupational functioning and represent a significant deterioration from the person's premorbid level of ability. The deficits must also be progressive and must not be due to other nervous system disease, systemic condition, or drugs/substances, must not occur in a state of delirium, and are not better accounted for by a psychiatric diagnosis. This framework for classifying FTD does not make assumptions about the underlying pathology. Although the McKhann criteria were designed to be useful clinically, they may have less utility for research and may make delineation of disease subtypes in ALS more difficult (4,6).

Very little information is available on the proportions of people who meet criteria for FTD, PNFA, and SD in people with ALS. While Ringholz and colleagues (5) indicated that, of their large sample of 252 people with complete data, 15% met criteria for FTD, Lomen-Hoerth and colleagues (7) classified 18 of 44 patients who underwent neuropsychological assessment as having 'definite' or 'probable' FTLD, with 12 classified as having FTD, four as having PNFA, and two as having SD, according to the Neary criteria. Elsewhere, of 23 patients with ALS, five (21.7%) met criteria for FTLD: two were diagnosed with FTD, two with SD, and one with PNFA (8). The latter two, albeit small, studies currently suggest, therefore, that FTD is the most common form of FTLD likely to be seen in people with ALS.

How should behavioural change in people with amyotrophic lateral sclerosis be measured?

As with the diagnosis of FTD, it has been recommended that less extreme behavioural change in people with ALS should be ascertained via careful interviews with caregivers/other informants to avoid under-reporting of symptoms of change that might occur through lack of insight on the patient's part (1). A limited number of screening questionnaires have been used to quantify behavioural change in people with ALS, namely the Frontal Systems Behavioral Scale (FrSBe) (9), Frontal Behavioral Inventory (10,11), Neuropsychiatric Inventory (12), and Manchester FTD Behavioural Interview (13).

The effective use of questionnaire-based assessments to help identify accurately the presence of significant behavioural change in ALS will depend largely on the psychometric properties of the measure being used and the range of behaviours being assessed. The aim of any such measure would, initially, be to detect difference from an appropriate sample of healthy controls, often using *cut-off* scores to identify impairment in the patient sample. Cut-off scores may be derived from the score just below the control group's lowest scores or below the lowest score made by 95% of the control group (14). Depending on the characteristics of the control sample, cut-off scores derived from one sample may not apply to another.

In general, the metrics of interest for screening measures are their *sensitivity* (i.e. the probability of correctly identifying abnormal functioning in an impaired person) and their *specificity* (i.e. the probability of correctly identifying a normal person or a person from another population who is intact on the measure being used). It is possible, therefore, that cut-off scores may result in patients being misdiagnosed. This may lead to *false positives* (i.e. intact people are diagnosed as impaired) and *false negatives* (i.e. impaired people diagnosed as intact). The decision to use particular cut-off scores will depend on the relative importance and ramifications of minimizing the misclassification of intact people as impaired or of not identifying people who really are impaired. It is very unlikely that it will be possible to identify two groups of people (i.e. impaired and unimpaired) with no false classifications (14). Additionally, the percentage of people who are correctly identified will depend on the base rate of the disorder in the population being studied. Thus, it may be important to consider whether the prevalence of ALS/FTD is being established in a dementia service or in a more general ALS service.

Establishing the validity of a measure of behavioural change requires the existence of an independent means of judging whether or not a score on that measure reflects impairment. That is, the score on the questionnaire is compared with a 'gold standard' against which the sensitivity and specificity of the questionnaire is then evaluated. The sensitivity and specificity of measures can be manipulated by varying the choice of populations or samples being studied (14). Additionally, the use of single as opposed to multiple measures is more likely to lead to misclassification of patients. When trying to decide if a particular measure is assessing the presence of significant behavioural change in patients with ALS, it is therefore going to be important to know whether the 'gold standard' has itself been established in ALS or only in another disorder. If the gold standard being used to diagnose FTD is, for example, that of the Neary criteria, then it is essential that these are applied in a consistent way that takes into account the impact of the physical consequences of ALS on the person's behaviour. It is also important to ascertain that behavioural changes cannot better be accounted for mood changes (particularly depression) and to bear in mind that the measured severity of depressive symptoms may depend on the self-report scale being used (15,16).

Measures used to assess behavioural change in amyotrophic lateral sclerosis

Frontal Systems Behavioral Scale (9)

Perhaps to date the behavioural measure most widely used in ALS studies is the FrSBe (9). This 46-item scale assesses everyday behavioural aspects of executive dysfunction and is subdivided into three domains: apathy, executive dysfunction, and disinhibition. In addition to a patient-completed version, there is a carer/informant version. The questions are used, in ALS studies, to ask about behaviour before and since ALS diagnosis.

Evidence for the validity of the FrSBe comes from studies in other disorders (17–19). In studies of ALS, the predominant change noted using the FrSBe has been increased post-illness-onset scores on the apathy subscale (20,21). Grossman *et al.* (20) relied on carer ratings of the person with ALS and found that post-illness onset, 55.6% of patients had clinically significant scores on the apathy subscale while 46.7% had clinically significant scores on the executive dysfunction scale, and 28.9% of patients with ALS had clinically significant post-illness onset ratings on the disinhibition subscale. Of note was the finding that a percentage of the sample was noted to have premorbidly raised levels of apathy (11%), executive dysfunction (31%), and disinhibition (20%) suggesting that, for some patients at least, behavioural changes may have preceded the onset of the physical aspects of ALS or alternatively may represent pre-existing personality and cognitive characteristics. Grossman and colleagues' data do not permit a distinction to be made between these possibilities (20).

Our study compared 41 patients with sporadic ALS, 10 with familial ALS (fALS) with non-copper/zinc superoxide dismutase (SOD1) mutations, seven patients with fALS with SOD1 mutations, and 35 healthy control participants on the FrSBe and a battery of neuropsychological tests (21). The non-SOD1 and SOD1 fALS groups both had clinically significant post-illness-onset median apathy scores and the non-SOD1 fALS group additionally had clinically significant post-illness-onset median executive dysfunction and total FrSBe scores; in contrast, all median scores for the sporadic ALS group were in the normal range.

Witgert and colleagues examined 225 people with sporadic ALS using the FrSBe and measures of cognitive change (22). Evidence of behavioural change was found in 24.4% of their sample in terms of FrSBe total scores, with changes on the apathy domain being most common (31.1%) followed by changes in executive dysfunction (19.6%) and disinhibition (16.9%); however, none of the group's mean scores were in the clinically impaired range. Where retrospective pre-illness ratings of behaviour were collected (n = 39) there was a significant increase in all FrSBe domain scores following disease onset, although again none of the mean scores were in the clinically impaired range. Of the 141 participants with complete behavioural and cognitive data, nearly 16% of the cognitively-intact patents showed behavioural change, while patients with moderate-to-severe cognitive impairment tended to demonstrate greater levels of behavioural impairment, although this was found only to be significant for apathy scores (22).

Woolley and colleagues used a stringent criterion of a change score of at least two standard deviations between pre-illness and current FrSBe ratings to identify the development of behavioural change; they defined the presence of behavioural abnormality as occurring when current scores were at least 1.5 standard deviations above the average score expected for the normal population (23). They studied behavioural change in 17 people with ALS (ALS-only) and a further four with ALS/FTD (using the Neary criteria). For the patients with ALS-only, premorbid self-ratings of disinhibition were higher than informants' proxy ratings but remained in the normal range. Patients' self-ratings of current apathy, executive dysfunction, and disinhibition were higher than the informants' ratings, although again all ratings were still in the normal range. The patients with ALS only reported greater changes in their behaviour than did their informants but the differences were not significant. For the patients with ALS/FTD, while they described mild increases in apathy scores over time themselves, their informants reported changes in apathy, executive functioning, and disinhibition that approached statistical significance, despite the small sample size, and that were greatest for the apathy domain scores.

The use of the FrSBe in assessing behavioural change in people with ALS is not without its challenges and it is important to ask caregivers, when completing it, to identify behavioural change that has not simply resulted from the person with ALS's limited physical ability (20). This approach needs to be operationalized more widely if findings are to be generalizable across studies of people with ALS. Woolley and colleagues reported that for patients with ALS without FTD, patients' self-ratings of behaviour and carers' proxy ratings did not differ significantly in terms of either premorbid or current behaviour; in contrast carers of (albeit a very small sample of) patients with ALS/FTD rated patients' current behaviour as being more abnormal than did the patients themselves, suggesting loss of insight in the ALS/FTD but not in the patients with ALS only (23). Thus, where ALS/FTD is already suspected, it might be that carer ratings will allow more accurate diagnoses in this respect, although this requires further verification. The latter authors suggest that, overall, the picture may be a complicated one, as it is also possible that in the ALS-only group, carers may under-report patients' behavioural changes, conceivably because the changes have developed very slowly, or they are denying that the person is changing or the emphasis on the motor aspects of ALS makes them less likely to notice other changes. Finally, no information is currently available about the sensitivity and specificity of the FrSBe domain or total scores when considering the diagnosis of FTD in patients with ALS, so this measure should not be used to diagnose FTD in patients with ALS.

Frontal Behavioral Inventory (10,11)

The Frontal Behavioral Inventory (FBI) is a 24-item informant-completed scale. It provides an overall measure of severity of impairment, which can be used to assess change; items can also be classified as representing negative (deficit) and positive behaviours. Those administering the FBI require basic interviewing skills, and the approach is to ask carers about the changes that have occurred in the patient's behaviour from the premorbid state. Scoring reflects the severity rather than the frequency of behaviours; a cut-off score of 30 has been reported to distinguish between patients with FTD, Alzheimer's disease (AD), and depressive disorder (11). In general, the FBI is thought to have high specificity for FTD with the exception of some cases of vascular dementia and manic-depressive psychosis. Different patterns of behaviour measured by the scale may be particularly informative. Thus indifference, perseveration, and utilization behaviour are important for discriminating FTD, while in a low scoring group (<27) verbal apraxia and logopenia may be particularly characteristic of patients with primary progressive aphasia. In other studies, however, different cut-off scores have been reported to yield different measures of sensitivity and specificity (24).

There is relatively little information pertaining to the use of the FBI in ALS. Flaherty-Craig *et al.* considered ratings of moderate-to-severe on the FBI items relating to logopenia and verbal apraxia to be indicative of the presence of PNFA; these ratings were found in 20.4% and 13.6% of their sample of 196 patients with ALS (25). In terms of characteristics considered indicative of what they call 'Social Comportment Dysexecutive subtype of FTD', they reported ratings of moderate-to-severe on items relating to apathy, indifference, perseveration, and utilization behaviour in 13.6%, 4.5%, 9.1%, and 1.1% respectively of their ALS sample.

Gordon and colleagues employed an ALS-carer self-completion version of the FBI questionnaire and found scores to be correlated with measures of cognitive impairment and also scores on the Clinical Dementia Rating Scale. However, no descriptive statistics for FBI scores were presented (26).

Heidler-Gary and colleagues described the use of a self-administered version of the FBI (the FBI-mod) in a study designed to distinguish patients with ALS/FTD from patients with AD (27). They reported data from 15 patients with ALS/FTD and 30 with AD. The FBI-mod comprised two subscales, measuring negative behaviour and disinhibition, but with only one question per item in comparison to the original FBI. The scale was self-administered by the patient's caregiver. Patients also underwent neuropsychological assessment. The authors reported that 10 of 15 (67%) of patients with ALS/FTD and nine of 30 (30%) of patients with AD had total FBI-mod scores of at least 27. In particular, they found the Negative Behaviour Score (reflecting apathy, aspontaneity, indifference, inflexibility, concreteness, personal neglect, disorganization, inattention, loss of insight, verbal apraxia, alien hand syndrome) informative in their study and reported that the best discrimination between patients with ALS/FTD and AD was achieved using a combination of measures; ALS/FTD was best characterized by abnormal FBI scores and impaired verbal fluency in the context of relatively normal MMSE scores and/or delayed verbal recall. They reported that 100% of patients with ALS/FTD and 87% of patients with AD were correctly identified using these measures. While the option of a self-administered and shortened version of the FBI must be attractive for research studies there are, to date, no data on the validation of the FBI-mod against the original FBI.

Neuropsychiatric Inventory (12)

Although the NPI is an informant-administered scale widely used to assess the frequency and severity of behavioural change in dementia, Malloy and Grace (28) reported that no large-scale studies had, at that point, looked at its discriminant validity between patients with frontal lobe dysfunction and healthy groups, although a number of studies have suggested that it is sensitive to behavioural aspects of executive dysfunction (29–31). Elsewhere, Norton and colleagues reported significant correlations between NPI total scores and FrSBe total scores and between the NPI apathy and disinhibition and the FrSBe apathy and disinhibition scores (32).

Although Olney and colleagues used the NPI in their assessment of patients with ALS they present no data on this scale (33). Murphy and colleagues defined the presence of behavioural impairment in people with ALS as an NPI domain score (the product of measures of severity × frequency) of at least three on at least two domains (8). Of their sample of 23 patients, five had FTLD according to the Neary criteria while a further four were classified as showing milder evidence of behavioural change. The latter authors reported that the patients with ALS in their sample with both cognitive and behavioural impairment showed more disinhibition and irritability than those patients with ALS showing neither behavioural nor cognitive change. The authors also acknowledged the need for validation of their criterion for presence of behavioural impairment in people with ALS.

The study by Murphy and colleagues raises the possibility that the NPI may add to the knowledge of the spectrum of behavioural change in ALS. Some doubt, however, has been cast on whether the administration of the NPI has been uniform in many other studies and on how those obtaining the NPI ratings are trained (34); such doubts may affect the generalizability of findings across studies.

Manchester Frontotemporal Dementia Behavioural Interview (13,35)

Gibbons and colleagues used this informant-administered measure to assess changes in behaviour in 16 people with ALS in the domains of affect and social behaviour; sensory behaviour; eating oral and vegetative behaviours; behaviours that are ritualistic, repetitive, and compulsive in nature; environmentally dependent behaviours such as hoarding; behaviours that reflect cognitive change such as misplacing objects, using the wrong word and the failure to recognize faces (36). Elsewhere, this scale has been found to distinguish between patients with AD and FTLD (13) and can detect different patterns of behaviour change in patients with either FTD or SD (35). Gibbons and colleagues reported a range of signs of behavioural change in 14 of their sample of 16 people with ALS (see Table 9.1) (36).

Behaviour change was more common in patients with bulbar palsy. The most frequently reported examples of behaviour change were in the realm of affect and social behaviour, which are commonly reported in patients with FTD, although Gibbons and colleagues caution over the interpretation of some of the changes, such as in irritability, as necessarily reflecting frontal changes in ALS, in view of the generally devastating impact

Table 9.1 Informant-reported behaviour change in people with ALS (36)

Behaviour	*n* (% of sample) showing change
Self-centredness/selfishness	19 (69)
Irritability	10 (63)
Altered sensory behaviour (exaggerated sensory/heat/cold response and/or reduced pain awareness)	8 (50)
Apathy/reduced interest in activities	6 (38)
Blunting of emotion	4 (25)
Loss of embarrassment	3 (19)
Loss of concern for hygiene	3 (19)
Repetitive behaviours, compulsions, rituals	3 (19)
Socially disinhibited behaviour	2 (13)
Lack of awareness of/concern for own illness	2 (13)
Increased aggression	2 (13)
Altered eating habits	1 (6)

of the physical aspects of the illness for the patient. None the less, the prevalent finding of loss of interest in and concern for others was felt to mirror the egocentric behaviour seen in FTD. It was also considered that the reported change in terms of apathy was unlikely to have occurred as a result of depression.

The spectrum of behavioural change reported in these patients was further highlighted by the observation that the sensory changes reported were largely characterized by increased sensory responsiveness and this was considered to be similar to the overreaction to sensory stimuli seen in SD. This was also the case for the repetitive, ritualistic, and compulsive behaviours reported by informants. Although Gibbons and colleagues acknowledged that inevitability of dietary changes in people with ALS, only one patient, who it was felt met criteria for FTD, demonstrated the major changes in food preferences and eating behaviour seen in FTD (36).

Summary of findings of behavioural change in amyotrophic lateral sclerosis

Although measured indifferent ways, the research summarized above indicates that the possibility of behavioural change in people with ALS should, as with cognitive change, be considered (1). The most prominent feature appears to be characterized by changes in affect and social functioning (36) and, when measured using scales as the FrSBe, in the domain of apathy. Nonetheless, other aspects of behavioural change such as disinhibition and everyday executive dysfunction may occur, as may features more typically characteristic of SD.

Implications of behavioural change in amyotrophic lateral sclerosis

In terms of pronounced behavioural change, it is generally accepted that FTD is accompanied by a poor prognosis. Thus, for example patients with autopsy-confirmed FTD were found to have a worse prognosis than patients with AD; FTD with associated ALS further reduces survival (37). It has also been shown that survival is significantly shorter in patients with ALS/FTLD than with classic ALS (33). In the latter study, however, the adverse effect of FTLD on survival was not independent of site of disease onset, and bulbar onset was significantly associated with development of FTLD. In addition, the effect of FTLD on survival in patients with bulbar onset was found to be independent of age. Of further relevance for survival was the finding that non-compliance with non-invasive ventilation and percutaneous endoscopic gastrostomy feeding was about twice as high for people with ALS/FTLD than for those with classical ALS, suggesting that where bulbar patients are non compliant with these interventions, the possibility of behavioural and/or cognitive change should be considered as explanatory factors.

It has been shown that behavioural change predicts carer burden in several neurodegenerative diseases. In FTD, caregiver distress has been related to agitation and psychosis, followed by mood disturbance (as measured by the NPI) (38). Behavioural change in people with FTD can lead to distress in carers (39). Behavioural change is also likely to impact on carers of people with ALS. Indeed, our group's early study of patients with ALS (who had not received a diagnosis of FTD/FTLD) indicated that carers' self-reported strain was predicted by both communication and behavioural changes in the person with ALS (40). Elsewhere, carers rating the person with ALS as above cut-off for impairment (i.e. showing significantly changed behaviour) on the FrSBe had lower quality of life and higher depression scores (41). Gordon and colleagues reported that carer-rated behavioural changes in the person with ALS (using the FBI) were correlated with carers' depression scores (26). A further behavioural change that may be found in ALS, that of emotional lability, was one of a number of factors shown to be predictive of carer distress (42).

Management of behaviour change in amyotrophic lateral sclerosis

Information on how to manage behavioural change that may occur in people with ALS is even scarcer than for the management of behavioural change in people with FTLD/FTD. When considering behavioural management for patients with ALS/FTD, there is the additional complication of dealing with the physical symptoms that may be taking priority in the person's care and which may make the overall issues to be dealt with more complex than when dealing with FTLD alone. Even in the latter case, key issues for a multidisciplinary team (MDT) will be educational, over and above the initial diagnosis of cognitive (and behavioural) impairment (43). Thus, there will be the need to fulfil an educational role for both the patient (depending on their level of cognitive impairment) and for the family, and to assist patients and their carers to adjust to the diagnosis. While lack of knowledge can contribute to caregiver stress (44), different information may be needed at different stages, with people varying in their patterns of information seeking and information requirements (45). Relatives may also require assistance in adjusting to new aspects of their caring role. In a number of areas, male and female carers have been shown to experience different levels of burden and use different coping strategies with respect to their caring role (46,47) and this may need to be borne in mind when considering carers of people with ALS. The MDT should also take an active role in addressing the ability of carers to cope with these changes and in liaising with other organizations to arrange state financial benefits and the provision of aids. This will already be a key role of service provision for people with ALS when dealing with the impact of physical symptoms on everyday life. In the case of families of people with FTLD, Lough and Garfoot also highlight the importance of working with children of affected patients and indeed there is increasing focus on issues of child safety/protection and professionals' statutory obligations in this respect (43).

Working with carers

A major role of the MDT should be to implement interventions to manage both cognitive and behavioural change. However, a number of writers have emphasized that where patients' behaviour cannot be altered, the team may need to work to change carers' attributions about, and their own emotional responses, to such changes. Thus, for example, Lomen-Hoerth and Murphy (48) suggested that it may be helpful to educate caregivers about the biological basis of behavioural changes (e.g. brain changes underlying aggression, irritability, and impulsivity, as well as emotional lability). Lough and Garfoot suggested that carers might find it easier to attribute, for example, a partner's inappropriate sexual behaviour or apparent change in personality to brain pathology rather than to a change in the relationship between them (43). Day programmes specialized for people with FTDs (but without physical disabilities) exist, where education can be provided to families and caregivers about behaviour modification techniques, features of FTLD, home safety, and stress management; they may provide models for ALS services (49). The importance of education for carers of people with ALS has been highlighted elsewhere: Wicks and Frost in an online survey of people with ALS as well as their carers, found that the majority of responding carers indicated that they would have wanted to have been told by professionals about the likelihood of cognitive dysfunction (73% of carers) and of the potential occurrence of emotional lability (80% of carers) in the person with ALS (50).

Lough and Garfoot (43) have described the use of a number of established psychological models to assist in the formulation of how carers deal with FTLD patients' presentations, most notably cognitive-behavioural therapy and the Stress-Process Model of Caregiving (43,51). Litvan recommended consideration of caregiver burden as a factor predicting caregiver distress and healthcare use and costs (52). The latter author recommended educating caregivers about the disease process as well as options for care, but also emphasized the identification of psychiatric morbidity in carers and providing appropriate emotional support and where helpful, respite care. Additionally, the author highlighted the role of social support in modulating caregivers' immune function, and indeed social support has been found to be important in predicting carers' psychological well-being in a study of spouse carers of people with ALS (42).

Managing behavioural change in the person with amyotrophic lateral sclerosis

The use of pharmacological agents to alter behaviour in FTD cases has received some attention (e.g. (52,53) although there is insufficient evidence to judge whether neurotransmitter replacement therapies will be of value in people with ALS to manage behaviour. Perry and Miller discussed the possible use of selected serotonin reuptake inhibitors for compulsions and carbohydrate cravings in FTD (53). Selected serotonin reuptake inhibitors have been used in case studies to treat, in a single case of ALS/FTD, inappropriate sexual behaviour (54) as well as more generally in ALS to treat emotional lability (55). In addition, a combination of dextromethophan and quinidine has been reported to reduce the frequency and severity of pathological laughter and crying and improve quality of life ratings (56).

For the non-pharmacological management of behavioural problems in FTLD, Lough and Garfoot suggested an approach that incorporates advances from learning theory, cognitive-behavioural therapy, and neuropsychological rehabilitation, among others (43). Talerico and Evans had previously highlighted the fact that in FTLD, behavioural changes of aggression and disinhibition might place the person at risk of injury (57). They also noted the potential importance of communication difficulties, socially inappropriate behaviour, and compulsions as posing challenges in the care and management of patients with FTLD. While the main focus of their recommendations is to ensure safety of the person with FTLD, many of the principles they advocated, such as careful behavioural monitoring and dealing with the most challenging behaviour first, would be equally applicable to people with ALS where behavioural change is posing care and safety issues, such as in feeding or the use of non-invasive ventilation.

Advice and suggestions concerning behavioural management for aspects of behavioural change in FTLD comes from a variety of sources (e.g. (43,57–59)). In the case of apathy, management might include encouraging the person to undertake activities while constructing a plan for their execution. Thus, help might be given in breaking complex tasks down into smaller and simple steps, monitoring the completion of each one. Assistance might also be given in providing guidance or redirection of the person with ALS to facilitate performance of these activities. Apathy might also be countered by providing a clear structure to the person's day. In the case of perseverative behaviour, if cognitive deterioration is not too advanced then instruction in self-monitoring of behaviour may be implemented. Otherwise, distraction or the removal of environmental targets/triggers for perseverative behaviour may be of assistance. Lough and Garfoot suggested that one might chose to avoid situations that provoke unwanted or disinhibited behaviour in the person with FTLD (43). Thus, for example, they suggest that if crowded places or large family gatherings provoke confusion or agitation in the patient then it might be advisable for the person only to attend smaller gatherings or avoid crowded situations. Other interventions might also include training the person to use self-control statements or to employ flashcards with commands if the person can only generate self-control statements with difficulty. The same authors highlight the importance of using positive commands rather than negative ones in such instances. Examples of how such approaches might be used might include the encouragement of more considered approaches to chewing and swallowing food in patients with bulbar ALS if behaviour might otherwise be impulsive; here self-instruction or flashcards might, for example, remind the person to count the number of times they have chewed their food and to stop before swallowing to ensure that the food has been chewed sufficiently. Environmental manipulation might also be incorporated, for example, to ensure that the person with ALS is not distracted during eating.

To provide a model to account for symptoms and to facilitate interventions in patients with FTD, Gregory and Lough (58) and Lough and Garfoot (43) adopted Eslinger *et al.*'s (60,61) Social Executors model to explain changes in social behaviour following frontal lobe damage. This relies heavily on the premise that the frontal lobes operate to control a complex functional system from which social behaviour emanates. Trauma- or disease-related dysfunction of frontal structures (as may occur in ALS) is held within this model to lead to possible personality and social behavioural change. Eslinger and colleagues model outlines a range of processes that would normally produce context-appropriate interpersonal behaviours (60,61). As they are interlinked with cognitive aspects of executive function, these Social Executors are viewed as distinct from other emotional and reactive processes such as depression, anxiety, and low self-esteem, which themselves may be found in ALS (e.g. (15,16,62)). Although the model was derived for people who have experienced head trauma, the concept of Social Executors may be applicable in the case of behavioural change in ALS as they can mediate how the cognitive, neuropsychiatric, and reactive psychological sequelae of the disease are expressed, with premorbid characteristics (including family and social systems as well as individual personality and cognitive characteristics) acting as moderators (see Figure 9.1). Although a little researched area, findings relating to a possible premorbid personality characteristic in people with ALS, associated with reduced intensity in experiencing emotions may be relevant within this model (63).

Within Eslinger and colleague's model there are four putative Social Executors (60,61).

(1) **Social self-regulation.** This Executor is considered to provide the ability to control the initiation, rate, intensity, and duration of social interaction, and when impaired may lead to social withdrawal (perhaps underpinning the apathetic presentation seen in ALS, discussed earlier) as well as difficulties in appreciating interpersonal boundaries and recognizing the cues to signal the termination of an interaction, being manifest in disinhibited behaviour.

(2) **Social self-awareness.** This Executor provides the person with the ability to have knowledge and insight about themselves in social situations. This allows them to

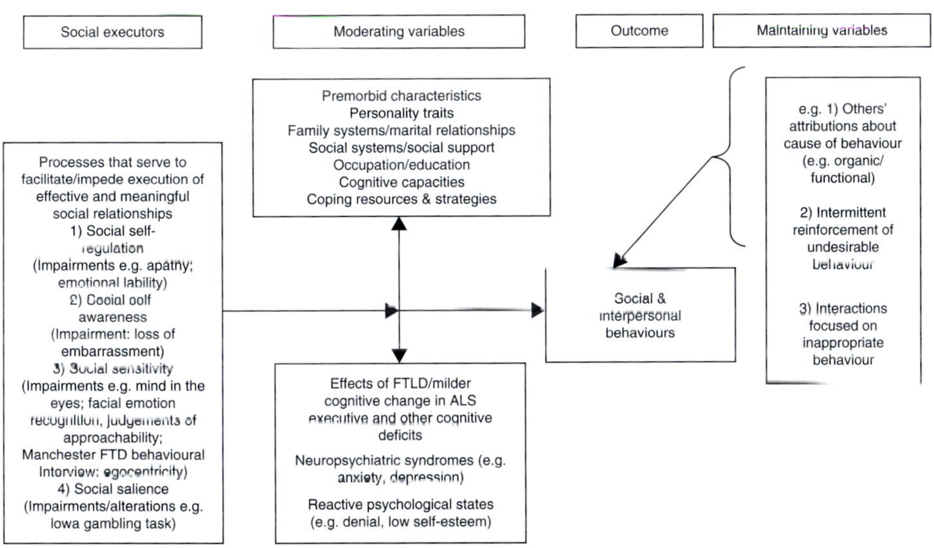

Fig. 9.1 Social Executors Model applied to behavioural change in ALS (adapted from (43,58,60,61)).

perceive accurately their own emotional state, regulate their emotions, and to understand how their behaviour affects others. Deficits in this Executor can lead the person to misjudge the impact of their emotional or social behaviour on others. Gibbons and colleagues described loss of embarrassment as one of the behavioural changes carers reported in people with ALS (36).

(3) **Social sensitivity.** Lough and Garfoot indicate that this Executor is the closest to the constructs of Theory of Mind and empathy (43). This Executor provides the person with the ability to take someone else's point of view and to understand another person's emotional state. Loss of empathy has been reported in FTD (64) while in ALS, self-centredness/selfishness as a relatively common feature (36). It is conceivable that the deficits in recognition and interpretation of facial emotion (65–67), subtle alterations in identification of emotional tone in speech (prosody; (66)), alterations in interpreting emotions from eye expressions ((67); and see Abrahams and Kipps, Chapter 8) and inappropriate judgements of the approachability of people from their photographs (65,68) may all reflect impairment of this Executor.

(4) **Social salience.** Eslinger and colleagues defined this Executor as representing the combination of the cognitive, autonomic, and visceral processes that regulate somatic and emotional states (60,61). It was suggested that dysfunction of this Executor would result in reduced autonomic responsiveness to the social environment and would be accompanied by an inability to share the emotional experiences of others. It would also result in the neutralization of social salience whereby all interpersonal and social stimuli would be judged to be similar. This might lead the person to pay insufficient attention to certain emotional situations and have less autonomic information available to be able to interpret their own and others' emotional states. Dysfunction of this Executor was thought also possibly to reduce the information available to the person to mediate social reinforcement.

In studies in ALS, alterations in the processing of emotional material have examined the effect of the emotional valence of material on memory and the level of arousal produced by emotionally laden visual stimuli. In support of impairment in this Social Executor, Papps and colleagues found that an ALS sample showed altered processing of normally emotionally salient material in a recognition memory task (68). However, data concerning the possibility of altered salience of visual socio-emotional stimuli are not entirely consistent. Verbal descriptions by people with ALS of the arousability of visual stimuli suggested an overall neutralization of perceived emotional salience; however, this occurred in the absence of significantly different patterns of autonomic responding between patients with ALS and healthy controls when viewing emotional stimuli (69). Additionally, the finding of a trend towards faster and more pronounced heart deceleration and delayed but stronger and more persistent galvanic skin responses in patients with ALS in response to emotional stimuli, was interpreted as suggesting, if anything, a more attentive response by patients to emotional material. As with controls, patients with ALS showed more pronounced deceleration for unpleasant than pleasant stimuli. However, further tentative support for dysfunction of this Executor comes from Girardi *et al.*'s ((67) and see Abrahams and Kipps, Chapter 8) findings of impaired performance on the Iowa Gambling Task) suggesting altered responsiveness to reward schedules.

In summary it would appear possible that dysfunction in these Social Executors might contribute to alterations in behaviour found in interview/questionnaire studies or people with ALS. The inability to recognize correctly emotions in others might be expected to result in altered family dynamics, perhaps unexpected responses to clinicians and to others; such changes might also render patients more vulnerable than they might otherwise have been in a given social context (65). Alterations in assigning valence to events might also produce unexpected responses to disease-imposed restrictions (69).

Lough and Garfoot provide examples of how the Social Executors model can be applied in the formulation and treatment of behavioural complications of FTLD (64). Effectiveness depends on intervening at the level of the correct Social Executor. While this model has not been applied explicitly to deal with behavioural complications in ALS it offers a potentially useful framework for clinicians to use in such cases, both in terms of devising interventions and to serve as an explanatory model to help carers understand why behavioural change has occurred in the person with ALS in the way it has.

Conclusions

In much the same way as it is now accepted that cognitive change may occur in about 50% of people with ALS (5), some of whom will have a full-blown dementia, behavioural change is now being viewed as an important potential aspect of ALS even if patients only meet partial criteria for FTD (8). Just as patients and carers wish to be told about the possibility of cognitive change in ALS the importance of acknowledging and explaining (as well as then managing) behavioural change is likely to be welcomed by patients and carers, particularly given the potential impact of behavioural change in the person with ALS on carers (50). Clinicians might, however, need to be mindful of the possibility that knowledge about potential behavioural change (as opposed to cognitive change—see Silverstein *et al* (70)) might lead patients to make different decisions about their future care. Wicks and Frost suggest that clinicians may be wary of burdening patients and their carers with information but warn that the absence of such information might also create additional burden for those affected by ALS, either directly or indirectly (49). Nonetheless, such imparting of information has to allow for the fact that patients and carers may have different information-seeking preferences (45). To address the clinical ramifications of behavioural as well as cognitive aspects of ALS, clinical teams will need sufficient resources to be able to involve the family/carers of people with ALS in assessing the challenging behaviour and implementing strategies, and to provide support for carers. Of considerable importance also will be a consistent MDT approach to the individual's management both within and across clinical services.

References

1. Strong MJ, Grace GM, Freedman M, *et al.* (2009). Consensus criteria for the diagnosis of frontotemporal cognitive and behavioural syndromes in amyotrophic lateral sclerosis. *Amyotroph Lateral Scler*, **10**, 131–146.
2. Neary D, Snowden JS, Gustafson L, *et al.* (1998). Frontotemporal lobar degeneration. A consensus on clinical diagnostic criteria. *Neurology*, **51**, 1546–1554.

3. Neary D, Snowden JS, Mann DMA, *et al.* (1990). Frontal lobe dementia and motor neuron disease. *J Neurol Neurosurg Psychiatry*, **53**, 23–32.
4. Rascovsky K, Hodges JR, Kipps CM, *et al.* (2007). Diagnostic criteria for the behavioral variant of frontotemporal dementia (bvFTD): current limitations and future directions. *Alzheimer Dis Assoc Disord*, **21**, S14–S18.
5. Ringholz GM, Appel SH, Bradshaw M, *et al.* (2005). Prevalence and patterns of cognitive impairment in sporadic ALS. *Neurology*, **65**, 586–590.
6. McKhann GM, Albert MS, Grossman M, *et al.* (2001). Clinical and pathological diagnosis of frontotemporal dementia. *Arch Neurol*, **58**, 1803–1809.
7. Lomen-Hoerth C, Murphy J, Langmore S, *et al.* (2003). Are amyotrophic lateral sclerosis patients cognitively normal? *Neurology*, **60**, 1094–1097.
8. Murphy JM, Henry RG, Langmore S, *et al.* (2007). Continuum of frontal lobe impairment in amyotrophic lateral sclerosis. *Arch Neurol*, **64**, 530–534.
9. Grace J, Malloy P. (2002). *Frontal Systems Behavior Scale.* Psychological Assessment Resources Inc., Florida.
10. Kertesz A, Davidson W, Fox H. (1997). Frontal behavioral inventory: diagnostic criteria for frontal lobe dementia. *Can J Neurol Sci*, **24**, 29–36.
11. Kertesz A, Nadkarni N, Davidson W, *et al.* (2000). The frontal behavioral inventory in the differential diagnosis of frontotemporal dementia. *JINS*, **6**, 460–468.
12. Cummings JL, Mega M, Gray K, *et al.* (1994). The neuropsychiatric inventory: comprehensive assessment of psychopathology in dementia. *Neurology*, **44**, 2308–2314.
13. Bathgate D, Snowden JS, Varma A, *et al.* (2001). Behaviour in frontotemporal dementia, Alzheimer's disease and vascular dementia. *Acta Neurol Scand*, **103**, 367–378.
14. Lezak MD, Howieson DB, Loring DW. (2004). *Neuropsychological Assessment.* Oxford University Press, Oxford.
15. Wicks P, Abrahams S, Masi F, *et al.* (2007). Prevalence of depression in a 12-month consecutive sample of patients with ALS. *Eur J Neurol*, **14**, 993–1001.
16. Taylor L, Wicks P, Leigh PN, *et al.* (2010). Prevalence of depression in amyotrophic lateral sclerosis and other motor disorders. *Eur J Neurol*, **17**, 1047–1053.
17. Grace J, Stout JC, Malloy PF. (1999). Assessing frontal lobe behavioral syndromes with the Frontal Lobe Personality Scale. *Assessment*, **6**, 269–284.
18. Malloy P, Tremont G, Grace J, *et al.* (2007). The Frontal Systems Behavior Scale discriminates frontotemporal dementia from Alzheimer's disease. *Alzheimers Dement*, **3**, 200–203.
19. Chiaravalloti ND, Deluca J. (2003). Assessing the behavioral consequences of multiple sclerosis: an application of the Frontal Systems Behavior Scale (FrSBe). *Cogn Behav Neurol*, **16**, 54–67.
20. Grossman AB, Woolley-Levine S, Bradley WG, *et al.* (2007). Detecting neurobehavioural changes in amyotrophic lateral sclerosis. *Amyotroph Lateral Scler*, **8**, 56–61.
21. Wicks P, Abrahams S, Papps B, *et al.* (2009). SOD1 and cognitive dysfunction in familial amyotrophic lateral sclerosis. *J Neurol*, **256**, 234–241.
22. Witgert M, Salamone AR, Strutt AM, *et al.* (2010). Frontal-lobe mediated behavioral dysfunction in amyotrophic lateral sclerosis. *Eur J Neurol*, **17**, 103–110.
23. Woolley SC, Moore DH, Katz JS. (2010). Insight in ALS: Awareness of behavioral change in patients with and without FTD. *Amyotroph Lateral Scler*, **11**, 52–56.
24. Kertesz A, Blair M, McMonagle P, *et al.* (2007). The diagnosis and course of frontotemporal dementia. *Alzheimer Dis Assoc Disord*, **21**, 155–163.
25. Flaherty-Craig C, Brothers A, Dearman B, *et al.* (2009). Penn State screen exam for the detection of frontal and temporal dysfunction syndromes: application to ALS. *Amyotroph Lateral Scler*, **10**, 107–112.

26. Gordon PH, Wang Y, Doorish C, *et al.* (2007). A screening assessment of cognitive impairment in patients with ALS. *Amyotroph Lateral Scler*, **8**, 362–365.
27. Heidler-Gary J, Gottesman R, Newhart M, *et al.* (2007). Utility of behavioral versus cognitive measures in differentiating between subtypes of frontotemporal lobar degeneration and Alzheimer's disease. *Dement Geriatr Cogn Disord*, **23**, 184–193.
28. Malloy P, Grace J. (2005). A review of rating scales for measuring behavior change due to frontal systems damage. *Cogn Behav Neurol*, **18**, 18–27.
29. Levy ML, Miller BL, Cummings JL, *et al.* (1996). Alzheimer disease and frontotemporal dementias. *Arch Neurol*, **53**, 687–690.
30. Tekin S, Mega MS, Masterman DM, *et al.* (2001). Orbitofrontal and anterior cingulate cortex neuro-fibrillary tangle burden is associated with agitation in Alzheimer disease. *Ann Neurol*, **49**, 355–361.
31. Srikanth S, Nagaraja AV, Ratnavalli E. (2005). Neuropsychiatric symptoms in dementia-frequency, relationship to dementia severity and comparison in Alzheimer's disease, vascular dementia and frontotemporal dementia. *J Neurol Sci*, **236**, 43–48.
32. Norton LE, Malloy PF, Salloway S. (2001). The impact of behavioral symptoms on activities of daily living in patients with dementia. *Am J Geriatr Psychiatry*, **9**, 41–48.
33. Olney RK, Murphy J, Forshew D, *et al.* (2005). The effects of executive and behavioral dysfunction on the course of ALS. *Neurology*, **65**, 1774–1777.
34. Connor DJ, Sabbagh MN, Cummings JL. (2008). Comment on administration and scoring of the Neuropsychiatric Inventory in clinical trials. *Alzheimers Dement*, **4**, 390–394.
35. Snowden JS, Bathgate D, Varma A, *et al.* (2001). Distinct behavioural profiles in frontotemporal dementia and semantic dementia. *J Neurol Neurosurg Psychiatry*, **70**, 323–332.
36. Gibbons ZC, Richardson A, Neary D, *et al.* (2008). Behaviour in amyotrophic lateral sclerosis. *Amyotroph Lateral Scler*, **9**, 67–74.
37. Rascovsky K, Salmon DP, Lipton AM, *et al.* (2005). Rate of progression differs in frontotemporal dementia and Alzheimer disease. *Neurology*, **65**, 397–403.
38. Mourik JC, Rosso SM, Niermeijer MF, *et al.* (2004). Frontotemporal dementia: behavioral symptoms and caregiver distress. *Dement Geriatr Cogn Disord*, **18**, 299–306.
39. De Vugt ME, Riedijk SR, Aalten P, *et al.* (2006). Impact of behavioural problems on spousal caregivers: a comparison between Alzheimer's disease and frontotemporal dementia. *Dement Geriatr Cogn Disord*, **22**, 35–41.
40. Goldstein LH, Adamson M, Jeffrey L, *et al.* (1998). The psychological impact of MND on patients and carers. *J Neurol Sci*, **160**, S114–S121.
41. Vignola A, Palmariello V, Pedone V *et al.* Influence of frontotemporal dementia on ALS patients and caregivers' quality of life and depression. *Amyotroph Lateral Scler* **9**(Suppl 1), 36. 2008.
42. Goldstein LH, Atkins L, Landau S, *et al.* (2006). Predictors of psychological distress in carers of people with amyotrophic lateral sclerosis: a longitudinal study. *Psychol Med*, **36**, 865–875.
43. Lough S, Garfoot V. (2007). Psychological interventions in frontotemporal dementia. In: Hodges JR (ed.), *Frontotemporal Dementia Syndromes*, pp. 277–326. Cambridge University Press, Cambridge.
44. Wald C, Fahy M, Walker Z, *et al.* (2003). What to tell dementia caregivers—the rule of threes. *Int J Geriatr Psychiatry*, **18**, 313–317.
45. O'Brien MR. (2004). Information-seeking behaviour among people with motor neurone disease. *Br J Nurs*, **13**, 964–968.
46. Zarit SH, Todd PA, Zarit JM. (1986). Subjective burden of husbands and wives as caregivers: a longitudinal study. *Gerontologist*, **26**, 260–266.
47. Bookwala J, Schulz R. (2000). A comparison of primary stressors, secondary stressors, and depressive symptoms between elderly caregiving husbands and wives: the Caregiver Health Effects Study. *Psychol Aging*, **15**, 607–616.

48. Lomen-Hoerth C, Murphy J. (2005) The neuropsychology of ALS. First International Research Workshop on Frontotemporal Dementia in ALS, May. London Ontario, Canada.
49. Grinberg A, Lagunoff J, Phillips D, *et al.* (2007). Multidisciplinary design and implementation of a day program specialized for the frontotemporal dementias. *Am J Alzheimers Dis Other Demen*, **22**, 499–506.
50. Wicks P, Frost J. (2008). ALS patients request more information about cognitive symptoms. *Eur J Neurol*, **15**, 497–500.
51. Pearlin LI, Mullan JT, Semple SJ, *et al.* (1990). Caregiving and the stress process: an overview of concepts and their measures. *Gerontologist*, **30**, 583–594.
52. Litvan I. (2001). Therapy and management of frontal lobe dementia patients. *Neurology*, **56**, S41–S45.
53. Perry RJ, Miller BL. (2001). Behavior and treatment in frontotemporal dementia. *Neurology*, **56**, S46–S51.
54. Anneser JM, Jox RJ, Borasio GD. (2007). Inappropriate sexual behaviour in a case of ALS and FTD: successful treatment with sertraline. *Amyotroph Lateral Scler*, **8**, 189–190.
55. Leigh PN, Abrahams S, Al-Chalabi A, *et al.* (2003). The management of motor neurone disease. *J Neurol Neurosurg Psychiatry*, **74** (Suppl 4), iv32–iv47.
56. Brooks BR, Thisted RA, Appel SH, *et al.* (2004). Treatment of pseudobulbar affect in ALS with dextromethorphan/quinidine: a randomized trial. *Neurology*, **63**, 1364–1370.
57. Talerico KA, Evans LK. (2001). Responding to safety issues in frontotemporal dementias. *Neurology*, **56**, S52–S55.
58. Gregory CA, Lough S. (2001). Practical issues in the management of early onset dementia. In: Hodges JR (ed.), *Early Onset Dementias: A Multidisciplinary Approach*, pp. 449–468. Oxford University Press, Oxford.
59. Massimo L, Grossman M. (2008). Patient care and management of frontotemporal lobar degeneration. *Am J Alzheimers Dis Other Demen*, **23**, 125–131.
60. Eslinger PJ, Grattan LM, Geder L. (1996). Neurologic and neuropsychiatric aspects of frontal lobe impairments in postconcussive syndrome. In: Rizzo M, Tranel D (eds.), *Head Injury and Postconcussive Syndrome*, pp. 415–440. Churchill Livingstone, New York.
61. Eslinger PJ, Grattan LM, Geder L. (1995). Impact of frontal lobe lesions on rehabilitation and recovery from acute brain injury. *NeuroRehabiliation*, **5**, 161–182.
62. Hogg KE, Goldstein LH, Leigh PN. (1994). The psychological impact of motor neurone disease. *Psychol Med*, **24**, 625–632.
63. Grossman AB, Levin BE, Bradley WG. (2006). Premorbid personality characteristics of patients with ALS. *Amyotroph Lateral Scler*, **7**, 27–31.
64. Lough S, Kipps CM, Treise C, *et al.* (2006). Social reasoning, emotion and empathy in frontotemporal dementia. *Neuropsychologia*, **44**, 950–958.
65. Schmolck H, Mosnik D, Schulz P. (2007). Rating the approachability of faces in ALS. *Neurology*, **69**, 2232–2235.
66. Zimmerman EK, Eslinger PJ, Simmons Z, *et al.* (2007). Emotional perception deficits in amyotrophic lateral sclerosis. *Cogn Behav Neurol*, **20**, 79–82.
67. Girardi A, Macpherson SE, Abrahams S. (2011). Deficits in emotional and social cognition in amyotrophic lateral sclerosis. *Neuropsychology*, **25**, 53–65.
68. Papps B, Abrahams S, Wicks P, *et al.* (2005). Changes in memory for emotional material in amyotrophic lateral sclerosis (ALS). *Neuropsychologia*, **43**, 1107–1114.
69. Lule D, Kurt A, Jurgens R, *et al.* (2005). Emotional responding in amyotrophic lateral sclerosis. *J Neurol*, **252**, 1517–1524.
70. Silverstein MD, Stocking CB, Antel JP, *et al.* (1991). Amyotrophic lateral sclerosis and life-sustaining therapy: patients' desires for information, participation in decision making, and life-sustaining therapy. *Mayo Clin Proc*, **66**, 906–913.

Chapter 10

Cognition in amyotrophic lateral sclerosis

Jennifer Murphy, Fizaa Ahmed, and
Catherine Lomen-Hoerth

This publication is a testament to the now wide acceptance that amyotrophic lateral sclerosis (ALS) is a multisystem disorder affecting extra-motor cerebral areas. The overlap of frontotemporal dementia (FTD) and ALS has been well documented in both patients with FTD with comorbid motor neurone deterioration (1) and patients with ALS with frontotemporal dysfunction (2–4). In this chapter the nature and prevalence of frontotemporal dysfunction in ALS is described in a historical context, followed by a review of recent consensus criteria intended to unify the measurement and diagnosis of the overlapping syndromes. Lastly, clinical mimics, effects on survival, and treatment considerations are discussed.

The subtle features of amyotrophic lateral sclerosis with frontotemporal dysfunction

There are two reasons why the ALS field and individual families have been rather slow to identify and treat the cognitive and behavioural deficits in ALS. The neuropsychological deficits seen in ALS are sometimes subtle, and range across a continuum into the moderate and severe dementia category for only a small proportion of patients. Secondly, because dementia is popularly conceived as being synonymous with memory loss, families and clinicians are prone to miss the frontotemporal dysfunction symptoms present in ALS. As a result, the cognitive and behavioural changes in ALS are interpreted as psychiatric in nature.

It is estimated that up to 30% of patients with ALS experience mild cognitive and behavioural changes that affect their daily functioning, relationships, and clinical care. This subgroup of patients has been underidentified in part because neurologists specializing in ALS have focused on the more salient motor neurone pathology. Additionally, families and patients are not prone to report personality and cognitive change to their physicians, because they often attribute the changes to emotional reactions to the disease, and do not view the ALS physician-visit as a place to report what they perceive as psychological symptoms. Typically, those patients with ALS with a comorbid, full-blown dementia syndrome have behavioural and emotional changes that precede their motor neurone symptoms, and have been seen in psychiatric or dementia clinics before the ALS clinic. As a result, patients with advanced dementia are commonly cotreated in dementia clinics by behavioural neurologists.

Because the nature of cognitive change in ALS is different than that seen in Alzheimer's disease, with its preponderance of episodic memory loss, word-finding difficulty, and spatial confusion, the family are frequently not cognisant of the frontotemporal cognitive-behavioural changes seen in ALS. The memory and visuospatial awareness of the patient with ALS may be quite intact, but their executive functioning capacity and interpersonal skills may be reduced from their baseline level of functioning.

The nature of frontotemporal dysfunction in amyotrophic lateral sclerosis

Executive functioning is a term used to describe the complex cognitive processing the frontal lobe performs, to integrate input from multiple cortical systems. Planning, organizing information, shifting attention, inhibiting behaviour, and negotiating social–emotional relationships are all examples of executive functioning. A proportion of patients with non-demented ALS display a pattern of mild but statistically measurable executive functioning deficits, which are not present in age-matched controls, and are not accounted for by disease progression, dysarthria, or motor slowing. Documented deficits consist of verbal and design fluency loss, poorly sustained attention, inflexibility in thinking, poor abstract reasoning, impaired set shifting, poor response inhibition, loss of visual attention, decreased initiation of random movements on a joystick task, and poor problem solving and judgement on tests such as the Wisconsin Card Sorting Test (5). The most common deficit documented in patients with ALS with and without a dementia diagnosis is a deficit in verbal fluency (6,7). The presence of episodic memory impairment remains questionable, in part due to variations in how the skill is measured (8).

Social disinhibition refers to the inability to control one's egocentric, sexual, or aggressive impulses, and it expresses itself socially as a reduction in interpersonal skills. Disinhibited patients fail to attend to the emotional needs of others, and do not adjust their behaviour to changing environments. Such patients may make child-like or off-colour jokes, dominate conversations, or show a general unwillingness to take into account the needs and feelings of family members. A loss of insight or self-awareness can accompany this syndrome, making it difficult for the patient to monitor their own physical changes as much as they fail to monitor how the demands of the illness affect their caregiver (9). An increasing number of investigations have documented the underlying cognitive deficits involved in social disinhibition, including recent studies of theory of mind (10) and emotional processing of facial stimuli. ALS patients without dementia fail to show the normal pattern of enhanced memory for emotional words as compared with neutral words (11) and abnormal arousal on functional magnetic resonance imaging for emotional images (12) suggesting that emotion-processing in general may play a role in interpersonal deficits.

Prevalence rates of amyotrophic lateral sclerosis with frontotemporal dysfunction

Historically, the prevalence rate of cognitive change in ALS was reported as very low, in part because of the widely circulated assumption that motor neurone disease (MND) spares cognitive functioning. Early investigations documenting very low prevalence rates were based on Alzheimer's disease-based neuropsychological measures using tests of intelligence and memory, excluding tests of executive functioning and verbal fluency (13). Widely cited studies in the 1990s suggested rates as low as 5% (5,14–16), in part because the focus of these investigations was on the association between ALS and advanced fronto-temporal lobar dementia.

The widely discrepant prevalence rates reported in the past 15 years are due to varying selection criteria, the specific measures used, and the cut-off criteria to define impairment. The consensus criteria established in 2009 (4) address these problems, suggesting uniform practices to help clinicians compare across investigations and agree upon more uniform principles of measurement and diagnosis (see 'Consensus criteria' in this chapter).

Investigations enrolling patients referred to the dementia clinic are bound to underestimate the prevalence of the syndrome and to overestimate the severity of the deficits, because enrolment is typically biased towards patients with advanced dementia. Only studies enrolling an unreferred, unselected sample of patients attending the ALS clinic will give a true representation of cognitive-impairment prevalence rates. A consensus has been reached that effective prevalence investigations should employ neuropsychological batteries with a representation of executive functioning measures and careful controls of clinical variables. The following literature review of prevalence rates meets these three criteria: unreferred sample selection, proper neuropsychological measures, and clinical controls of important variables (e.g. depression, hypoxia, and disease progression).

Literature review of cognitive functioning in amyotrophic lateral sclerosis

Prevalence rates of cognitive impairment have ranged between 17% (8) and 50–60% (2,17–19) based upon the cut-off stringency and measures used, yet the range of 28–35% has been a persistent finding across many independent investigations.

Massman *et al.* (20) found that 28% of non-demented patients performed at or below the 10th percentile on five or more neuropsychological tests, with dysarthric patients performing almost twice as poorly as non-dysarthric patients when using a more stringent 5th percentile cut-off. Gordon *et al.* (21) reported a rate of 28% as cognitively impaired, with impairment correlating with older age and longer disease progression. Rakowicz and Hodges identified five of 18 patients (28%) with measurable aphasia syndromes, each performing in the impaired range on more than one neuropsychological measure (22). Robinson *et al.* (23) reported 36.8% of a sample had neuropsychological impairment, and Rippon *et al.* (24) documented prevalence rates of 30% with measurable cognitive impairment, and 23% with ALS dementia. Rusina *et al.* (25) documented that 25% of a sample of 67 patients had cognitive impairment, with equal rates of impairment across the bulbar and limb onset groups. Our group at University of California, San Francisco (26) reported a continuum of cognitive and behavioural abnormalities varying in severity, with 22% meeting Neary criteria for frontotemporal lobar degeneration, 17% demonstrating subtle behavioural disturbances, and 9% exhibiting subtle cognitive dysfunction.

Whether or not patients with familial versus sporadic ALS have different rates of prevalence of cognitive impairment is yet undetermined. In one large sample, comparing the neuropsychological functioning of patients with familial and sporadic ALS, and prevalence and pattern of cognitive impairment was similar across the two groups (19). This sample of familial patients was heterogeneous in terms of their superoxide dismutase 1 status and they were not screened for other mutations.

The 2009 consensus criteria

Strong *et al.*'s 2009 consensus criteria address important disparities that had been identified by practising neuropsychologists in the ALS field. The criteria establish uniformity in the diagnosis of the range of cognitive change in ALS and highlight the specific neuropsychological measures, clinical control variables, and clearly defined cut-off criteria needed to advance the field and direct clinical interventions.

Diagnostic categories of cognitive impairment in amyotrophic lateral sclerosis

Clear criteria now exist to subtype the range of cognitive impairment in patients with ALS (4). Table 10.1 illustrates the consensus criteria for six subtypes of MND-related cognitive impairment. The western Pacific variant ALS/parkinsonism–dementia complex subtype is distinguished from the FTD/ALS variant, and the three subtypes of FTD are described, including ALS with the behavioural variant of FTD (ALS/bvFTD), ALS with progressive non-fluent aphasia (ALS/PNFA), and ALS with semantic dementia (ALS/SD). The details of the three FTD subtypes, ALS/parkinsonism–dementia complex, and FTD/MND-like

Table 10.1 Subtypes of frontotemporal impairment in ALS*

ALS/FTD	ALS/bvFTD	Patient with ALS meeting either the Neary criteria or Hodge's criteria for FTD
	ALS/PNFA	Patient with ALS meeting Neary criteria for PNFA
	ALS/SD	Patient with ALS meeting Neary criteria for SD
ALS with behavioural impairment		Patient with ALS meeting at least 2 non-overlapping supportive diagnostic features from either the Neary criteria or Hodge's criteria for FTD
ALS with cognitive impairment		Evidence of cognitive impairment at or below the 5th percentile on at least two distinct tests of cognition that are sensitive to executive functioning
FTD/MND-like		A neuropathological diagnosis with a primary frontotemporal lobar degeneration diagnosis with evidence of MND-type degeneration, but insufficient to be classified as ALS
ALS/dementia		ALS with dementia, not typical of FTD
ALS/parkinsonism dementia complex		ALS concurrent with dementia and/or parkinsonism occurring in hyperendemic foci of the western Pacific

Adapted from Strong 2009.

are discussed in other chapters in this publication. FTD/MND-like is characterized by a primary diagnosis of FTD with mild MND symptoms, and ALS/dementia is defined as the presence of non-FTD dementia co-occurring with ALS. The most notable advancement in the field of the overlapping syndromes is the addition of two subtypes of impairment that do not meet full threshold for FTD/dementia status. The continuum of frontotemporal impairment in ALS is highlighted with the creation of these new subtypes, and they provide clinicians, families, and patients with a valuable tool to characterize a syndrome that had been largely undocumented and thus invisible.

Amyotrophic lateral sclerosis with cognitive impairment

Amyotrophic lateral sclerosis with cognitive impairment (ALSci) describes those patients who do not meet full criteria for FTD dementia, but who perform at or below the 5th percentile on at least two distinct neuropsychological tests that are sensitive to executive functioning or language processing. Clinically, patients may have difficulty executing complex recommendations involving equipment and medication changes, and families may report the patient is having difficulty with financial and household responsibilities they once managed well. Patients often display no behavioural or personality change, despite their new difficulty with executive functioning.

Amyotrophic lateral sclerosis with behavioural impairment

Amyotrophic lateral sclerosis with behavioural impairment (ALSbi) characterizes patients who do not meet full criteria for the frontal variant of FTD dementia, but who are rated by caregivers as having at least two non-overlapping behavioural disturbances, as measured by either the Neary criteria (14) or Hodge's criteria (27) for FTD. Frequently reported symptoms include new troublesome behaviours such as social disinhibition or irritability (26) or, conversely, they may lack expected behaviours (negative behaviours), such as apathy and poor emotional responsiveness to others.

The three-tiered system of patient identification

Use of a three-tiered system of patient-identification has been identified as a goal (4) because expedient, validated measures are needed by busy clinic staff who do not have a neuropsychologist available to conduct in depth evaluations during busy clinic days.

Routine clinic visits provide the best opportunity to identify patients who may require additional support because of cognitive or behavioural involvement. A 5-minute screen is the most expedient method of identifying patients, as the exam can take place as part of the neurological exam, or can be administered by any trained staff. Clinics with the resources to administer a 30-minute exam will have a greater opportunity to understand the nature and severity of the cognitive and/or behavioural change. Table 10.2 shows the most commonly used 5-minute and 30-minute exams in current use.

The gold standard of diagnosing cognitive and behavioural impairment in ALS is the administration of a neuropsychological exam by a PhD level neuropsychologist who is

Table 10.2 Screening exams—strengths and weaknesses

5–10 minute exams	Targeted population	Strengths	Weaknesses	Length
ALS–Cognitive Behavioral Screen (ALS/CBS; (32))	ALS-specific Public domain	Specifically designed for ALS population; Some controls for dysarthria, motor weakness	Early in the standardization process	<10 min
Montreal Cognitive Assessment (33)	General population Public domain for non-commercial use	Well-standardized; in common use; measures frontal lobe functioning	Not specifically designed to tap ALS-specific deficits; no controls for dysarthria, motor weakness	10 min
Written fluency (35)	ALS-specific Public domain	Specifically designed for ALS population Controls for dysarthria, motor weakness	Early stages of standardization; no behavioural component	10 min
30-minute exams				
Penn State Exam (57)	General population Copyrighted	National norms, including measure of judgement and problem solving	Not specifically designed to tap ALS-specific deficits; no controls for dysarthria, motor weakness	20–30 min
Addenbrooke's (34)	General population Copyrighted	Well-standardized; in common use; measures frontal lobe functioning	Not specifically designed to tap ALS-specific deficits; no controls for dysarthria, motor weakness	30 min
UCSF Screening Exam (58)	ALS-specific Public domain	Specifically designed for ALS population; controls for dysarthria, motor weakness; includes in-depth behaviour interview	Behavioural measure requires staff time to interview caregiver. Early in the standardization process	30 min

familiar with frontotemporal dysfunction. Patients identified using the two tiers of screening exams should be referred to a neuropsychologist for a full examination.

Screening exam advancement

Screening exams for use in identifying cognitive impairment in ALS have been explored for decades (8,28), with success at identifying short batteries that identify neuropsychological deficits (29). Since the consensus on useful screening exams has been established in the mid-2000s, at least five screening exams have been well-used in the ALS community, and they have been successful in identifying those patients with ALS in need of further examination. There are three types of screening exams in use: (a) compilations of previously standardized tests specifically selected for use with ALS; (b) tests taken from standardized neuropsychological exams; and (c) a newly constructed exam that is specifically designed for ALS cognition. Table 10.2 shows some of the strengths and weaknesses of each exam.

Penn State rapid screening battery

The Penn State rapid screening battery (30) employs sections of the Neurobehavioral Cognitive Status Examination (31), letter fluency, category fluency (animals), and the New Adult Reading Test (NART). The COGNISTAT measures several important executive functions, including, but not limited to: reasoning, orientation, auditory attention span, language, and verbal memory. Cut-off scores at 1.5 standard deviations below the mean have successfully identified executive functioning deficits.

Amyotrophic lateral sclerosis–Cognitive Behavioral Screen

The ALS–Cognitive Behavioral Screen (32) (ALS/CBS) is a new, independently created 5-minute screening tool tailored to measure a wide range of tasks known to be involved in cognitive impairment with ALS. Attention, concentration, tracking/monitoring, and verbal fluency subscores are generated, in addition to the total score. A separate behavioural questionnaire is administered to the caregiver, to identify behavioural changes.

Dementia Rating Scale-2

The Dementia Rating Scale (DRS-2) is a well standardized, widely used measure to identify mental status in cognitively impaired adults. The DRS-2 measures cognitive functioning on five subscales: attention, initiation-perseveration, construction, conceptualization, and memory. The test employs 32 stimulus cards, and is particularly sensitive to the lower levels of functioning.

Montreal Cognitive Assessment

The Montreal Cognitive Assessment (MoCA) (33) was designed as a rapid screening instrument for mild cognitive dysfunction, for use in the general population. Eight cognitive domains are measured: attention and concentration, executive functions, memory, language, visuoconstructional skills, conceptual thinking, calculations, and orientation. The exam is well standardized, and the administration time is approximately 10 minutes.

Addenbrooke's Cognitive Examination Revised

The Addenbrooke's Cognitive Examination Revised (ACE-R) is a brief battery for dementia screening, commonly used in the UK. Five subdomain scores (orientation/attention, memory, verbal fluency, language, and visuospatial) are generated with this well-standardized, general use, copyrighted tool (34).

The UCSF Screening Battery

The 30-minute UCSF screening battery consists of one cognitive measure and one behavioural interview with a caregiver. Both the phonemic verbal fluency and the Frontal Behavioral Inventory (FBI) are standardized, widely used measures in the field of neuropsychology, yet each have been altered to fit the clinical needs of patients with ALS. The written fluency test (35) employs an additional timed feature to adjust scores for patients with hand weakness, while also removing the bias of dysarthria. A revised version of the FBI (FBI–ALS) was developed as a behavioural interview with the caregiver, which disentangles the behaviour and emotional changes due to dementia from clinical symptoms due to the MND.

Neuropsychological test selection

Uniformity of neuropsychological measures and proper clinical control variables has been established as a second goal for the field (4), to ensure valid diagnoses of cognitive impairment and facilitate cross-comparison studies to advance the field. The past decade has seen a significant increase in the number of MND clinics employing cognitive screening and full-scale neuropsychological exams to identify patients with cognitive impairment. The field has made some progress in achieving uniformity of measures, as shown in Table 10.3. Although there is no consensus across groups in the measure of memory and visuospatial skills, there is a growing consensus in the use of tools to measure the two primary abilities that are affected in ALS (i.e. executive functioning and language ability).

The selection of neuropsychological measures to diagnose cognitive deficits in ALS should be weighted towards the measurement of executive functioning, and should include a verbal fluency measure, and a caregiver interview that measures changes in behavioural and emotional functioning. Efforts should be made to minimize the effects of dysarthria and motor weakness. Measures of disease progression, breathing function, and intellectual functioning should be administered to statistically control for variables that may influence cognitive functioning. Measures of pseudobulbar affect (PBA) and depression should be included, to rule out the possibility that emotional and behavioural changes are due to these commonly co-occurring clinical syndromes.

Evidence for a continuum of cognitive impairment in amyotrophic lateral sclerosis

Although the recently published consensus criteria identify distinct categories of cognitive impairment, evidence from fields as broad as pathology, structural imaging, positron

Table 10.3 Standardized neuropsychological measures used in peer reviewed studies of ALS–dementia

Frequency of use	Exec Functioning	Language	Memory	IQ	Visuospatial
Used in >5 studies	WCST; Digits Bkwds; Category fluency; Stroop Int	FAS/COWAT; Written verbal fluncy test; BNT		NART/ AMNART; Ravens Colored Matrices; WAIS-III	
Used in 2–5 studies	Symbol Digit Modalities Test;VSAT; Trails A&B; Design Fluency	Pyramids and Palm Trees Test; Graded Naming Test	Kendrick Object Learning Test; Rey Aud Verbal Learning Test; CVLT-II; RMT; Logical Memory Test		Benton Judgment of Line Orientation; MfVPT; Block Design; Rey figure

WCST, Wisconsin Card Sort (59); Digits Backwds, Digits Backwards subtest of the Wechsler Adult Intelligence test (60); Category fluency subtest of the DKEFS (61); Stroop Interference subtest of the Dellis–Kaplan Executive Functioning Test (61); Symbol Digit Modalities Test (62); VSAT: Verbal Serial Attention Test (63); BNT, Boston Naming Test (64); FAS/COWAT, Controlled Oral Word Association Test (65); Written Verbal Fluency Test (35); Category Fluency, Subtest of Dellis–Kaplan Executive Functioning Test (61); WAIS, Wechsler Adult Intelligence test (60); Trails subtest of the Dellis–Kaplan Executive Functioning Test (61); VSAT, Visual; NART, National Adult Reading Test (66); AMNART, American version of the National Adult Reading Test (67); CVLT-II, California Verbal Learning Test (68); RMT, Warrington Recognition Memory Test (69); MfVPT, Motor Free Visual Perception Test (70); Rey Complex Figure Test (71); Rey Auditory Verbal Lerning Test (72); Kendrick Object Learning Test (73); Block Desing Subtest of the WAIS(60); Design Fluency, Subest of the Dellis–Kaplan Executive Functioning Test (61); Stroop Int, Stroop Interference subtest of the Dellis–Kaplan Executive Functioning Test (61); Trails A and B Subtest of the Dellis–Kaplan Executive Functioning Test (61); Logical Memory Test, Subtest of the Wechsler Memory Scale (74); Pyramids and Palmtrees (75); Graded Naming Test (76); Ravens Colored Matrices (77); Benton Judgment of Line Orientation (78).

emission tomography, single photon emission computed tomography, and neuropsychology suggest that the frontotemporal impairment in patients with ALS lies on a broad spectrum, with approximately half of the patients displaying at least mild abnormalities. A consistent finding has emerged: the pathological signs (36), cerebral atrophy (5), blood flow decrements, electroencephalography (37), neurotransmitter decrease, and neuropsychological impairment (18,20,22,26,38–44) are present in a sizeable number of patients with ALS. These investigations reveal the same pattern: patients with ALS display the same neurological, pathological, and neuropsychological characteristics, despite their mild, moderate, or full-blown dementia status, suggesting that a frontotemporal degenerative process in patients with ALS exists on a continuum. The new diagnostic categories (i.e. ALS cognitive impairment and ALS with behavioural impairment) enable the field to move forward to more closely investigate the aetiology and treatment of frontotemporal dysfunction in ALS.

Survival

Physicians caring for patients with ALS often question the importance of identifying cognitive and behavioural impairments in ALS. Besides the impact on caring for the patient and on the family, these impairments impact survival. In the FTD field, comorbid ALS clearly has a dramatic impact on survival. Roberson *et al.* (45) have shown that patients with FTD and comorbid ALS on average live only 2 years after diagnosis compared with patients with FTD who live 10–12 years after diagnosis. This is in comparison with Alzheimer's disease where patients may live 20 years or more after the diagnosis. Similar findings were found by Hu *et al.* (46), in a cohort of 87 patients with FTD/ALS. Even with mild disease, where patients with ALS have cognitive and behavioural impairments not severe enough to qualify as a diagnosis of FTD, survival is impacted. Olney *et al.* (47) showed a survival difference of more than a year between patients with comorbid disease versus ALS alone. He determined that this difference was likely due to compliance with treatment recommendations such as percutaneous endoscopic gastrostomy (PEG) and bilevel positive airway pressure (BiPAP), as these recommendations were followed only one-third of the time compared with two-thirds of the time with patients who were cognitively and behaviourally normal, as seen in Table 10.4.

Since the Olney publication, subsequent authors have demonstrated similar findings with a shortened survival in patients with ALS with comorbid disease for both mildly impaired and moderately impaired patients (21). Site of onset does not correlate with cognitive changes, but the presence of dysarthria has been shown to correlate with cognitive deterioration (17). Conversely, Rusina *et al.* (25) studied patients with ALS prospectively with single-photon emission computed tomography and neuropsychological testing. They found no correlation between cognitive impairment and survival, but there was also no correlation between performance on neuropsychological testing and single-photon emission computed tomography findings. The lack of correlation with survival in this study as opposed to those cited above might be because patients were not tested for behavioural dysfunction, which can significantly influence compliance with treatment recommendations and presumably influence survival.

Treatable mimics of cognitive and behavioural function

It is absolutely critical to exclude mimics of cognitive and behavioural dysfunction. Most mimics are treatable, and even reversible with therapy. For example, severe depression is uncommon in ALS, but when present, does improve with antidepressant therapy and/or counselling. Importantly, survival is impacted when depression, stress, or other measures of psychological distress are measured (48), because patients with ALS with high comorbid

Table 10.4 Survival impact in ALS with FTLD

NPPV and PEG compliance		
	NPPV	**PEG**
ALS/FTLD	5 of 18 (28%)	4 of 16 (25%)
ALS only	14 of 23 (61%)	8 of 12 (67%)
Z	2.22	2.01
P (one-tail)	<0.2	<0.03

ALS, amyotrophic lateral sclerosis; FLTD, frontotemporal lobar degeneration; NPPV, non-invasive positive pressure ventilation; PEG, percutaneous endoscopic gastrostomy.

psychological distress have greater mortality than those with low psychological distress. Screening with the depression screen of choice, such as the Beck Depression Inventory (49) or Geriatric Depression Scale (50) is important whenever there are concerns about cognitive and behavioural function.

It is important to exclude and treat PBA (easy laughing and crying), which is sometimes confused with depression but is a very different condition. Patients with PBA do not necessarily feel depressed but they do have trouble with excessive emotional expression that they are unable to control. The Center for Neurologic Study-Lability Scale is a common screen used to diagnosis this condition and is a simple series of seven questions (51). Other, more in-depth measures of PBA also exist (49,52,53). The treatments most typically used include low-dose amitriptyline or a serotonin reuptake inhibitor. More recently, the combination of dextromethorphan and quinidine, approved by the Food and Drug Administration in the USA in late 2010, has demonstrated positive results in an ALS clinical trial (54).

Many of the medications to treat symptoms of ALS can cause sedation and confusion such as the antispasticity medications of valium, baclofen, and zanaflex. Sleep aids and sedating antidepressants may have unwanted sedating after-effects the next day. Riluzole, which is the only FDA-approved drug to slow disease progression in ALS, causes sleepiness and confusion in some patients, particularly older patients. It is recommend to reduce the dose of any potentially offending medication, and to consider a drug holiday for a week or two to see if improvement is noted.

Retaining carbon dioxide or having low oxygenation can dramatically affect both behaviour and cognition (55). A sleep study or home nocturnal oximetry study is helpful to diagnose this problem. Typically, BiPAP is recommended once the forced vital capacity falls below 50% predicted. Obtaining a sleep study before and after BiPAP can identify desaturations and prompt necessary changes in BiPAP settings. Testing maximal inspiratory force during spirometry testing can help identify diaphragm weakness, which contributes to difficulty breathing at night when lying flat and can qualify a patient for BiPAP even when the forced vital capacity is still above 50% predicted.

Fatigue is a difficult problem with ALS and can impact cognition and behaviour if sleep is disrupted. Energy conservation and good sleep hygiene are common recommendations. Troubleshooting the underlying cause of fatigue is important, to identify sedating medications, over exertion in the setting of worsening weakness, breathing difficulties, etc. It is important to also exclude any premorbid condition affecting cognition or behaviour such as a psychiatric condition, head injury, stroke, or other CNS condition.

Once these mimics have been excluded and the problem still persists, further testing is warranted. Anxiety, hypochondria, and stress can impact test performance, and it is important that testing be given in a manner to minimize the impact of these problems as well as to accommodate patients with difficulty speaking or using their hands to write. Other diseases that mimic ALS can cause cognitive problems such as certain hereditary conditions such as Tay Sachs disease, infectious conditions such as Creutzfeld–Jacob disease, and paraneoplastic syndromes due to cancer. Neuropsychological testing, neuroimaging, and blood testing can help distinguish among these conditions.

Treatment

The cognitive and behavioural impairments in ALS are very difficult to treat. In part, this is due to the lack of effective treatments for FTD. Treatment is approached with behavioural and medication management. Effective behavioural treatments include the simplification of communication, limiting access in the patient's environment, recognizing the patient's inability to have insight, and supervision of eating and other activities of daily living to maintain patient safety. These tools can be applied in the medical setting and may help to ensure patients' compliance (56).

Medication management is a goal aimed at managing the most prominent symptoms troubling the patient. If the patient is apathetic, for example, an activating serotonin reuptake inhibitor is recommended. Hallucinations may be treated with one of the newer neuroleptics, such as Seroquel, and insomnia and poor appetite may be addressed with Remeron. In terms of slowing the rate of cognitive and behavioural decline, memantine may be somewhat effective but does have significant side effects such as nausea and stomach upset, which could be a problem for a patient with ALS, where avoiding weight loss is critical.

When cognitive and behavioural impairments are present, special considerations need to be taken in managing the ALS symptoms. For example, simple tools are needed for communicating when patients are no longer able to speak, as patients may not be able to learn how to use a sophisticated computer system to speak for them. A power wheelchair with caregiver controls rather than patient controls may be needed if patients are impulsive and demonstrate poor wheelchair control themselves. Patients are often resistant to PEG and BiPAP recommendations, which are essential to help prolong both quality and quantity of life. While the wishes of the patient need to be respected, if they continue to deny these treatments, it may help to present the information simply, start to discuss early on in the disease progress, and make sure the patient is reassured that whatever they decide will be respected. The severity of the cognitive and behavioural changes rarely worsens to the degree that they are considered incapable of making major medical decisions, but poor judgement and reduced decision-making skills may require them to have more involvement from caregivers. Simplifying medical treatment for conditions such as excess saliva or spasticity may also help with compliance (e.g. Botox injections every 3 months rather than daily pills or a baclofen pump rather than taking multiple baclofen pills three or four times per day). It is critical to involve hospice early so patients with rigid thinking and irritability learn to feel comfortable with the personnel. Particularly for those patients having trouble swallowing without a PEG tube, comfort and safety can be more difficult to manage. Hospital admission to administer intravenous pain control near the end of life may be required. Lastly, respite and counselling are critical for the caregiver and family members to help cope with the devastating effects of ALS and the cognitive and behavioural problems that often limit family communication about end of life issues.

References

1. Lomen-Hoerth C, Anderson T, Miller B. (2002). The overlap of amyotrophic lateral sclerosis and frontotemporal dementia. *Neurology*, **59**, 1077–109.

2. Lomen-Hoerth C, Murphy J, Langmore S, *et al.* (2003). Are amyotrophic lateral sclerosis patients cognitively normal? *Neurology*, **60**, 1094–1097.
3. Strong MJ. (2008). The syndromes of frontotemporal dysfunction in amyotrophic lateral sclerosis. *Amyotroph Lateral Scler*, **9**, 323–338.
4. Strong MJ, Grace GM, Freedman M, *et al.* (2009). Consensus criteria for the diagnosis of frontotemporal cognitive and behavioural syndromes in amyotrophic lateral sclerosis. *Amyotroph Lateral Scler*, **10**, 131–146.
5. Frank B, Haas J, Heinze HJ, *et al.* (1997). Relation of neuropsychological and magnetic resonance findings in amyotrophic lateral sclerosis: evidence for subgroups. *Clin Neurol Neurosurg*, **99**, 79–86.
6. Abrahams S, Leigh PN, Kew JJ, *et al.* (1995). A positron emission tomography study of frontal lobe function (verbal fluency). in amyotrophic lateral sclerosis. *J Neurol Sci*, **129** (Suppl), 44–46.
7. Abrahams S, Goldstein LH, Suckling J, *et al.* (2005). Frontotemporal white matter changes in amyotrophic lateral sclerosis. *J Neurol*, **252**, 321–331.
8. Gallassi R, Montagna P, Morreale A, *et al.* (1989). Neuropsychological, electroencephalogram and brain computed tomography findings in motor neuron disease. *Eur Neurol*, **29**, 115–120.
9. Woolley SC, Moore DH, Katz JS. (2010). Insight in ALS: awareness of behavioral change in patients with and without FTD. *Amyotroph Lateral Scler*, **11**, 52–56.
10. Adenzato M, Cavallo M, Enrici I. (2010). Theory of mind ability in the behavioural variant of frontotemporal dementia: an analysis of the neural, cognitive, and social levels. *Neuropsychologia*, **48**, 2–12.
11. Papps B, Abrahams S, Wicks P, *et al.* (2005). Changes in memory for emotional material in amyotrophic lateral sclerosis (ALS). *Neuropsychologia*, **43**, 1107–1114.
12. Lule D, Kurt A, Jurgens R, *et al.* (2005). Emotional responding in amyotrophic lateral sclerosis. *J Neurol*, **252**, 1517–1524.
13. Poloni M, Capitani E, Mazzini L, Ceroni M. (1986). Neuropsychological measures in amyotrophic lateral sclerosis and their relationship with CT scan-assessed cerebral atrophy. *Acta Neurol Scand*, **74**, 257–260.
14. Neary D, Snowden JS, Mann DM, *et al.* (1990). Frontal lobe dementia and motor neuron disease. *J Neurol Neurosurg Psychiatry*, **53**, 23–32.
15. Kew J, Leigh N. (1992). Dementia with motor neurone disease. *Baillieres Clin Neurol*, **1**, 611–626.
16. Gubbay SS, Kahana E, Zilber N, *et al.* (1985). Amyotrophic lateral sclerosis. A study of its presentation and prognosis. *J Neurol*, **232**, 295–300.
17. Ringholz GM, Appel SH, Bradshaw M, *et al.* (2005). Prevalence and patterns of cognitive impairment in sporadic ALS. *Neurology*, **65**, 586–590.
18. David AS, Gillham RA. (1986). Neuropsychological study of motor neuron disease. *Psychosomatics*, **27**, 441–445.
19. Wheaton MW, Salamone AR, Mosnik DM, *et al.* (2007). Cognitive impairment in familial ALS. *Neurology*, **69**, 1411–1417.
20. Massman PJ, Sims J, Cooke N, *et al.* (1996). Prevalence and correlates of neuropsychological deficits in amyotrophic lateral sclerosis. *J Neurol Neurosurg Psychiatry*, **61**, 450–455.
21. Gordon PH, Goetz RR, Rabkin JG, *et al.* (2010). A prospective cohort study of neuropsychological test performance in ALS. *Amyotroph Lateral Scler*, **11**, 312–320.
22. Rakowicz WP, Hodges JR (1998). Dementia and aphasia in motor neuron disease: an underrecognised association? *J Neurol Neurosurg Psychiatry*, **65**, 881–889.
23. Robinson KM, Lacey SC, Grugan P, *et al.* (2006). Cognitive functioning in sporadic amyotrophic lateral sclerosis: a six month longitudinal study. *J Neurol Neurosurg Psychiatry*, **77**, 668–670.
24. Rippon GA, Scarmeas N, Gordon PH, *et al.* (2006). An observational study of cognitive impairment in amyotrophic lateral sclerosis. *Arch Neurol*, **63**, 345–352.

25. Rusina R, Ridzon P, Kulist'ak P, *et al.* (2010). Relationship between ALS and the degree of cognitive impairment, markers of neurodegeneration and predictors for poor outcome. A prospective study. *Eur J Neurol*, **17**, 23–30.
26. Murphy JM, Henry RG, Langmore S, *et al.* (2007). Continuum of frontal lobe impairment in amyotrophic lateral sclerosis. *Arch Neurol*, **64**, 530–534.
27. Gregory CA, Serra-Mestres J, Hodges JR. (1999). Early diagnosis of the frontal variant of frontotemporal dementia: how sensitive are standard neuroimaging and neuropsychologic tests? *Neuropsych Neuropsychol Behav Neurol*, **12**, 128–135.
28. Gallassi R, Lenzi P, Stracciari A, *et al.* (1986). Neuropsychological assessment of mental deterioration: purpose of a brief battery and a probabilistic definition of 'normality' and 'non-normality'. *Acta Psychiatr Scand*, **74**, 62–67.
29. Caltagirone C, Gainotti G, Masullo C, Miceli G. (1979). Validity of some neuropsychological tests in the assessment of mental deterioration. *Acta Psychiatr Scand*, **60**, 50–56.
30. Flaherty-Craig C, Eslinger P, Stephens B, Simmons Z. (2006). A rapid screening battery to identify frontal dysfunction in patients with ALS. *Neurology*, **67**, 2070–2072.
31. Kiernan RJ, Mueller J, Langston JW, Van Dyke C. (1987). The Neurobehavioral Cognitive Status Examination: a brief but quantitative approach to cognitive assessment. *Ann Intern Med*, **107**, 481–485.
32. Woolley SC, York MK, Moore DH, *et al.* (2010). Detecting frontotemporal dysfunction in ALS: utility of the ALS Cognitive Behavioral Screen (ALS-CBS). *Amyotroph Lateral Scler*, **11**, 303–11.
33. Nasreddine ZS, Phillips NA, Bedirian V, *et al.* (2005). The Montreal Cognitive Assessment, MoCA: a brief screening tool for mild cognitive impairment. *J Am Geriatr Soc*, **53**, 695–699.
34. Mioshi E, Dawson K, Mitchell J, *et al.* (2006). The Addenbrooke's Cognitive Examination Revised (ACE-R): a brief cognitive test battery for dementia screening. *Int J Geriatr Psychiatry*, **21**, 1078–1085.
35. Abrahams S, Leigh PN, Harvey A, *et al.* (2000). Verbal fluency and executive dysfunction in amyotrophic lateral sclerosis (ALS). *Neuropsychologia*, **38**, 734–747.
36. Wilson CM, Grace GM, Munoz DG, *et al.* (2001). Cognitive impairment in sporadic ALS: a pathologic continuum underlying a multisystem disorder. *Neurology*, **57**, 651–657.
37. Ogawa T, Tanaka H, Hirata K. (2009). Cognitive deficits in amyotrophic lateral sclerosis evaluated by event-related potentials. *Clin Neurophysiol*, **120**, 659–664.
38. Murphy J, Henry R, Lomen-Hoerth C. (2007). Establishing subtypes of the continuum of frontal lobe impairment in amyotrophic lateral sclerosis. *Arch Neurol*, **64**, 330–334.
39. Moretti R, Torre P, Antonello RM, *et al.* (2002). Complex cognitive disruption in motor neuron disease. *Dement Geriatr Cogn Disord*, **14**, 141–150.
40. Ludolph AC, Langen KJ, Regard M, *et al.* (1992). Frontal lobe function in amyotrophic lateral sclerosis: a neuropsychologic and positron emission tomography study. *Acta Neurol Scand*, **85**, 81–89.
41. Kew JJ, Leigh PN, Playford ED, *et al.* (1993). Cortical function in amyotrophic lateral sclerosis. A positron emission tomography study. *Brain*, **116**, 655–680.
42. Kew JJ, Goldstein LH, Leigh PN, *et al.* (1993). The relationship between abnormalities of cognitive function and cerebral activation in amyotrophic lateral sclerosis. A neuropsychological and positron emission tomography study. *Brain*, **116**, 1399–1423.
43. Kilani M, Micallef J, Soubrouillard C, *et al.* (2004). A longitudinal study of the evolution of cognitive function and affective state in patients with amyotrophic lateral sclerosis. *Amyotroph Lateral Scler Other Motor Neuron Disord*, **5**, 46–54.
44. Abrahams S, Goldstein LH, Al-Chalabi A, *et al.* (1997). Relation between cognitive dysfunction and pseudobulbar palsy in amyotrophic lateral sclerosis. *J Neurol Neurosurg Psychiatry*, **62**, 464–472.
45. Roberson ED, Hesse JH, Rose KD, *et al.* (2005). Frontotemporal dementia progresses to death faster than Alzheimer disease. *Neurology*, **65**, 719–725.

46. Hu WT, Seelaar H, Josephs KA, *et al.* (2009). Survival profiles of patients with frontotemporal dementia and motor neuron disease. *Arch Neurol*, **66**, 1359–1364.
47. Olney RK, Murphy J, Forshew D, *et al.* (2005). The effects of executive and behavioral dysfunction on the course of ALS. *Neurology*, **65**, 1774–1777.
48. McDonald ER, Wiedenfeld SA, Hillel A, *et al.* (1994). Survival in amyotrophic lateral sclerosis. The role of psychological factors. *Arch Neurol*, **51**, 17–23.
49. Beck AT, Steer RA. (1984). Internal consistencies of the original and revised Beck Depression Inventory. *J Clin Psychol*, **40**, 1365–1367.
50. Yesavage JA, Brink TL, Rose TL, *et al.* (1982). Development and validation of a geriatric depression screening scale: a preliminary report. *J Psychiatr Res*, **17**, 37–49.
51. Moore SR, Gresham LS, Bromberg MB, *et al.* (1997). A self report measure of affective lability. *J Neurol Neurosurg Psychiatry*, **63**, 89–93.
52. Robinson RG, Parikh RM, Lipsey JR, *et al.* (1993). Pathological laughing and crying following stroke: validation of a measurement scale and a double-blind treatment study. *Am J Psychiatry*, **150**, 286–293.
53. Newsom-Davis IC, Abrahams S, Goldstein LH, Leigh PN. (1999). The emotional lability questionnaire: a new measure of emotional lability in amyotrophic lateral sclerosis. *J Neurol Sci*, **169**, 22–25.
54. Brooks BR, Thisted RA, Appel SH, *et al.* (2004). Treatment of pseudobulbar affect in ALS with dextromethorphan/quinidine: a randomized trial. *Neurology*, **63**, 1364–1370.
55. Miller RG, Jackson CE, Kasarskis EJ, *et al.* (2009). Practice parameter update: the care of the patient with amyotrophic lateral sclerosis: multidisciplinary care, symptom management, and cognitive/behavioral impairment (an evidence-based review): report of the Quality Standards Subcommittee of the American Academy of Neurology. *Neurology*, **73**, 1227–1233.
56. Merrilees J, Klapper J, Murphy J, *et al.* (2010). Cognitive and behavioral challenges in caring for patients with frontotemporal dementia and amyotrophic lateral sclerosis. *Amyotroph Lateral Scler*, **11**, 298–302.
57. Flaherty-Craig C, Brothers A, Dearman B, *et al.* (2009). Penn State screen exam for the detection of frontal and temporal dysfunction syndromes: application to ALS. *Amyotroph Lateral Scler*, **10**, 107–112.
58. Murphy J. (2010). The University of California San Francisco Cognitive Screening Exam. Verbal communication.
59. Heaton R, Chelune G, Talley J, *et al.* (1993). *Wisconsin Card Sorting Test (WCST). Manual: Revised and Expanded.* Psychological Assessment Resources, Odessa, FL.
60. Wechsler D. (1997). *Wechsler Adult Intellectual Scale*, (3rd edn). The Psychological Corporation, San Antonio, TX.
61. Dellis, Kaplan E, Kramer JH. (2001). *Dellis-Kaplan Executive Functioning System Technical Manual.* The Psychological Corporation, San Antonio, TX.
62. Smith A. (1991). *Symbol Digit Modalities Test.* Western Psychological Services, Los Angeles, CA.
63. Lezak M (ed.). (1995). *Neuropsychological Assessment*, (3rd edn). Oxford University Press, New York.
64. Goodglass H, Kaplan E. (1983). *Boston Diagnostic Aphasia Examination*, (2nd edn). Lea and Febiger, Malvern, PA.
65. Benton AL, Hamsher KD, Sivan AB. (1994). *Multilingual Aphasia Examination: manual of instructions.* AJA Associates, Iowa City.
66. Bright P, Jaldow E, Kopelman MD. (2002). The National Adult Reading Test as a measure of premorbid intelligence: a comparison with estimates derived from demographic variables. *J Int Neuropsychol Soc*, **8**, 847–854.
67. Uttl B. (2002). North American Adult Reading Test: age norms, reliability, and validity. *J Clin Exp Neuropsychol*, **24**, 1123–1137.

68. Dellis D, Kramer JH, Kaplan E, Ober B. (2000). *California Verbal Learning Test-Adult Version*, (2nd edn). New York, Pearson Education, San Antonio, USA.
69. Warrington E. (1984). *Recognition Memory Test.* NFER-Nelson, Windsor, UK.
70. Colarusso R, Hammill D. (1996). *Motor-Free Visual Perception Test-Revised.* Academic Therapy Publications, Novato, CA.
71. Meyers J, Meyers K. (2003). *Rey Complex Figure Test and Recognition Trial: Professional manual.* PAR, Inc. Lutz, Florida, USA.
72. Rey A. (1941). A psychological examination of traumatic encephalopathy. *Arch Psychol*, **28**, 286–340.
73. Kendrick DC, Gibson AJ, Moyes IC. (1979). The Revised Kendrick Battery: clinical studies. *Br J Soc Clin Psychol*, **18**, 329–340.
74. Wechsler D. (1997). *Wechsler Memory Scales*, (3rd edn). *Administration and Scoring Manual.* The Psychological Corporation, San Antonio, TX.
75. Howard D, Patterson K. (1992). *Pyramids and Palm Trees.* Suffolk: Thames Valley Test Company, Bury St Edmonds.
76. McKenna P, Warrington E. (1983). *The Graded Naming Test.* NFER-Nelson, Windsor.
77. Raven J, Court JH. (2003). *Manual for Raven's Progressive Matrices and Vocabulary Scales.* Section 1: *General Overview.* Harcourt Assessment, San Antonio, TX.
78. Woodard JL, Benedict RH, Roberts VJ, *et al.* (1996). Short-form alternatives to the Judgment of Line Orientation Test. *J Clin Exp Neuropsychol*, **18**, 898–904.

Chapter 11

Frontotemporal syndromes of primary lateral sclerosis

Vincenzo Silani, Barbara Poletti, and Stefano Zago

The term primary lateral sclerosis (PLS) implies the presence of a rare motor neurone disease that causes a slowly progressive spinobulbar spasticity with weakness, eventually accompanied by dysarthria and dysphonia due to upper motor neurone disturbance. PLS is differentiated from amyotrophic lateral sclerosis (ALS) by the absence of lower motor neurone involvement, a cardinal feature of ALS (see Rosenfeld, Chapter 2). First signalled by Türck (1) and Charcot (2), it was Erb (3) who refined the concept of 'PLS' to indicate a selective degeneration of the lateral columns of the cord. Ever since, long-standing sceptical discussion has arisen from the observation that many patients with PLS seemed ultimately to have different diseases such as ALS, spinal multiple sclerosis, or cervical spondylotic myelopathy (4–6).

In 1945, Stark and Moersch proposed the first clinical diagnostic criteria for PLS. These included insidious onset, slow progression, dysfunction limited to the pyramidal tracts, and a course lasting more than 5 years (7). Revisions of pathological observations with modern techniques (8) and the documented presence of speech and swallowing impairments led to new established clinical and laboratory criteria (9). Gordon and colleagues noted that development of lower motor neurone signs inevitably follow electromyographic findings of denervation in 77% of cases within 4 years of symptom onset (10). They, therefore argued that a 4-year span should be a component of the diagnostic criteria, and proposed a more specific nomenclature based on the constellation of clinical and electromyographic features. In the more detailed set of diagnostic categories for the PLS spectrum disorders, complicated PLS (PLS plus) has been considered, inclusive of predominant upper motor neurone signs plus pathological evidence of dementia (10,11). According to these revisions, at present PLS is considered to be part of the range of motor neurone diseases consisting of PLS, ALS, and progressive spinal muscular atrophy. PLS is now considered a dysfunction of the corticospinal pathway with or without very mild lower motor neurone involvement but with clinical features of prominent spasticity and pseudobulbar symptoms (dysarthria and compulsive laughing or crying). The diagnosis is usually made after the exclusion of other diseases with a similar clinical spectrum. In fact, failure to develop signs of lower motor neurone dysfunction, either clinically or electrophysiologically within 4 years of symptom onset, differentiates this entity from the more common ALS disorder. Thus, the diagnosis of PLS needs a careful clinical and laboratory investigation and an adequate follow-up. The aetiology of PLS and the genetic trait have not been identified yet, even if a family with three affected brothers has been reported (12) and, more recently, an autosomal dominant PLS described (13).

Cognitive impairment in primary lateral sclerosis and its substrate

As there was a widely held belief that PLS did not affect higher cognitive functions (9), neuropsychological investigations in patients with PLS have received attention only in the last two decades. Advances in our understanding and classification of this condition have taken place over a diverse range of disciplines: from neuropsychology testing, imaging studies, neuropathological, and genetic data. Table 11.1 summarizes the patients' data reported in literature in which cognitive damage has been observed.

Patients with primary lateral sclerosis and dementia

Since the mid-1990s, there have been a number of PLS single case reports in which late-onset dementia is described. In a fraction of these cases, the evidence of progressive degeneration of the frontotemporal regions, along with absence of pathological lower motor neurone involvement, prompted the hypothesis of a new separate disease entity named frontotemporal lobar degeneration with primary lateral sclerosis (FTLD/PLS) (14). Although in the majority of these reports histopathological data were present the results must be interpreted with caution as they were obtained before the recognition of Bunina bodies and ubiquinated inclusions as being neuropathological hallmarks of ALS.

Given this limitation, however, there have been a number of informative clinicopathological case descriptions. Hainfellner and colleagues described a PLS case with intellectual decay, perseverations and disorientation in which neuropathology demonstrated abundant Lewy body disease as an almost ubiquitous disorder of the neuronal cytoskeleton (15). Sugihara and colleagues described a case of PLS with progressive dementia with a diffuse cerebral atrophy, more marked in the striatum and thalamus. An unusual ballooning of dendrites was observed in both the molecular and Purkinje cell layers of the cerebellum, as well as in the anterior horn of the spinal cord (16). Engel and Grunnet reported the occurrence of progressive spastic paraplegia and frontal system dementia in a patient with post-mortem features of PLS combined with moderate Alzheimer-like changes in the neocortex and hippocampus (17). Tan and colleagues reported a case of PLS in which a progressive dementia with FTLD was characterized by microvacuolation, and ubiquinated neuronal inclusion (18) (see Figure 11.1). The authors, in reviewing the literature, asserted that at least seven similar autopsy cases were reported in Japanese literature (16,19–24). However, Josephs and Dickson pointed

Table 11.1 PLS studies reported in literature in which a neuropsychological analysis have been performed

Reference	Examined patients (*n*)	Neuropsychological tests performed	Neuropsychological impairment detected	Neuroradiological (CT/MRI findings)	Neuropathological findings	Neurofunctional (SPECT, PET, fMRI, findings)
Lewis (1991)	2	WAIS-R and Halstead Reitan battery	Impairment on some tests of the Halstead Reitan battery (e.g. Category Test, TPT not dominant hand trial, TPT memory, Seashore Rhythm Test, Finger Oscillation, Grip Strength measures)	NR	NR	NR
Hainfellner *et al.* (1995)	1	Only clinical examination of cognitive abilities without detailed neuropsychological test assessment	Cognitive impairment with perseveration and disorientation	Cerebral atrophy at MRI with ventricular enlargement and normal spinal structures	Diffuse Lewy body disease as an ubiquitous disorder of the neuronal cytoskeleton	NP
Caselli, Smith, Osborne (1995)	9	Brief Mental Status tool (Kokmen Short Test of Mental Status), temporal orientation (Benton orientation questionnaire), intelligence (WAIS-R), memory (WMS), verbal Associative fluency and psychomotor speed (COWA), frontal abilities (WCST, TMT, Stroop Colour-Word Test), verbal memory (AVLT). constructional praxis (CFT), visual naming (Boston Naming Test), oral comprehension (Token Test)	None was demented but 8 patients had mild cognitive impairment. Primary impairment on neuropsycholgical tests sensitive to frontal lobe functions, followed by test tests sensitive to memory	Focal pericentral atrophy was evident in 2 patients	NP	6 patients underwent HMPAO-SPECT: bilateral posterior frontal hypoperfusion was evident in all; 2 patients showed additional hypoperfusion in temporal areas

(Continued)

Table 11.1 (continued) PLS studies reported in literature in which a neuropsychological analysis have been performed

Reference	Examined patients (*n*)	Neuropsychological tests performed	Neuropsychological impairment detected	Neuroradiological (CT/MRI findings)	Neuropathological findings	Neurofunctional (SPECT, PET, fMRI, findings)
de Konig, van Doorn, van Dongen (1997)	1	Follow-up with non-verbal intelligence test (Raven's CPM); clinical examination without tests	Mild frontal lobe deficits at clinical examination (concept shifting, generation of new ideas, planning and impulsive behaviour)	MRI showed one lacunar infarct in the right cerebral peduncle	NP	At SPECT bilaterally reduced activity preferentially in the basal motor cortex with normal activity at the level of the brainstem nuclei
Konagaya *et al.* (1998)	1	Cognitive abilities could not be investigated because of severe anarthria and motor disorders	Character change, obstinacy	CT and MRI disclosed bilateral frontotemporal atrophy	Remarkable bilateral atrophy of the frontal and temporal lobes, degeneration in Ammon's horn, amygdala marked neuronal loss and gliosis, presence of ubiquitin-immunoreactive neurones in the frontotemporal cortex	NP
Sugihara *et al.* (1999)	1	Follow-up with Hasegawa Dementia Scale (HDS)	From moderate to severe dementia	CT revealed a moderate to remarkable degree of cerebral atrophy. Head circumference smaller than normal. Increased thickness of cranial bone	Unusual clear ballooning of dendrites observed in the molecular and Purkinjie cell layers of the cerebellum, and the anterior horn of the spinal cord	NP
Engel, Grunnet (2000)	1	Follow-up with neuropsychological formal assessment	Mild frontal dementia. Impaired reasoning and abstraction, difficulty initiating, planning, and implementing effective problem-solving strategies, very poor hypothesis testing during the Wisconsin Card Sorting Test, perseveratives responses, impoverished word list generation	No abnormalities at MRI 3 years later disease onset	Mild atrophy. Degeneration of the lateral corticospinal and dorsal spinocerebellar tracts; numerous beta/A4 amyloid positive diffuse plaques in neocortex and neurofibrillary tangles in hippocampus	NP

Kuipers-Upmeijer *et al.* (2001)	10	Clinical follow-up without any neuropsychological formal assessment	NR clinical signs of cognitive deterioration	At MRI conspicuous precentral atrophy and in the frontal and parietal–occipital regions	NP	NP
Tan *et al.* (2003)	1	Clinical follow-up without any neuropsychological formal assessment	Progressive cognitive deterioration inferred by inability and slowness in responding orders	At MR bilateral frontotemporal atrophy with dilatation of ventricular system	Microvacuolation and ubiquitin-positive neuronal inclusions and presence of dystrophic neuritis in cortical layer II. Ubiquitin-positive structures in the striatum	NP
Mochizuki *et al.* (2004)	1	Clinical follow-up without any neuropsychological formal assessment.	Behavioural abnormality and character change (apathy, uncooperative). Cognitive assessment NR	At CT severe atrophy of the frontal and temporal lobes	Marked atrophy of the frontal and temporal lobes with Betz cell completely absent and moderate atrophy of the neostriatum. Ubiquitin-positive but tau-negative intraneuronal inclusions were found in the frontal and temporal cortices, including the precentral cortex and the hyppocampal dentate gyrus and the neostriatum	NP
Mackenzie, Feldman (2004)	1	Clinical assessment without any neuropsychological formal assessment	Problems with verbal comprehension and fluency. Inappropriate, apathetic and abulic behaviour, impaired judgement and poor short-term memory	MRI demonstrated moderate frontal lobe atrophy	Numerous neuronal cytoplasmic inclusions in many regions. Some inclusions were immunoreactive for ubiquitin while others showed strong positivity for neurofilament proteins. Intranuclear neuronal inclusions were also present	NP

(Continued)

Table 11.1 (continued) PLS studies reported in literature in which a neuropsychological analysis have been performed

Reference	Examined patients (*n*)	Neuropsychological tests performed	Neuropsychological impairment detected	Neuroradiological (CT/MRI findings)	Neuropathological findings	Neurofunctional (SPECT, PET, fMRI, findings)
Gordon *et al.* (2006)	29	NR	Only one subject had symptomatic cognitive deterioration (PLS plus)	NR	NP	NR
Piquard *et al.* (2006)	20	Memory (WAIS-R forward and backword Digit Span, Grober and Buschke word list and recall test), language (DO80), written language (three sentence phrases extracted from the French version of the BDAE) attention (Stroop Colour-Word Test), visual-constructional ability (Rey-Ostrierreth complex figure), praxis (Symbolic gestures and pantomimes), prefrontal functions (Word fluency task, TMT, Stroop Colour-Word Test, Similarities subtest of WAIS-R, WCST), premotor functions (Graphic test, Finger Tapping Test, Repetition of series of words)	None was demented but they all presented memory deficits reflecting an executive dysfunction. All patients but three had signs of premotor and/or prefrontal cortex deficits	Absence of high signal lesions outside the cortical tract on brain MRI	NP	NP

Grace *et al.* (2006)	18	Executive skills (Controlled Oral Word Fluency, Thurstone Written Word Fluency, Delayed Alteration Test, Wisconsin Card Sorting Test), attention and concentration (Consonant Trigrams Test), visual–perception/visual–construction (Block Design WAIS-III, Motor Free Visual Perception Test–Revised), memory (Recognition Memory Test, Rey Auditory Verbal Learning Test). Language (Modified 30-item Boston Naming Test (BNT); 55-item Action Naming Test (ANT). Neurobehavioural symptoms investigated with Geriatric Depression Scale (GDS), Neuropsychiatric Inventory (NPI). Frontal Behavioural Inventory (FBI)	None was demented but on 18 patients 22% were cognitively impaired (PLSci) consisting with a frontotemporal lobar dysfunction (executive dysfunction, oral word fluency most frequently impaired measure); production of fewer items than controls on verbal fluency for category; 18% of patients had depressive symptoms at GDS; 57% of relatives identified neuropsychiatric symptoms; none scored in the FTD range.	CT perfusion head scan showed haemodynamic changes in PLSci globally extended throughout cortices and underlying white and grey matter. Frontotemporal region most prominent perfusion deficit with cortical decreases in cerebral blood volume and with Associated frontal lobe changes in mean transit time in both cortical and subcortical region	NP	Patients with PLSci revealed an increased cerebral blood volume and mean transit time with a reduced cerebral blood flow. Mean transit time as a sensitive indicator correlated with cognitive change in PLS
Josephs and Dickson (2007)	2	Clinical observation without testing	Case 1: Cognitive impairment with executive dysfunction and later aphasia. Case 2: Cognitive impairment with expressive aphasia and ideomotor apraxia	NR	In both cases neuronal loss and gliosis in frontotemporal cortices, also parietal for case 2. Ubiquitin and TDP-43 positive cytoplasmic inclusions and neuritis in the frontal and temporal neocortices and in the dentate granule cells of the hippocampus	NR

(Continued)

Table 11.1 (continued) PLS studies reported in literature in which a neuropsychological analysis have been performed

Reference	Examined patients (*n*)	Neuropsychological tests performed	Neuropsychological impairment detected	Neuroradiological (CT/MRI findings)	Neuropathological findings	Neurofunctional (SPECT, PET, fMRI, findings)
Zago *et al.* (2008)	16	Writing examination consisting in three tasks (dictation, copy, composing preformed letters) Token Test, Raven's CPM	Only writing errors (omissions, transpositions, insertions, letter substitutions suggesting) a pattern of central dysgraphia	Absence of high signal lesions outside the cortical tract on brain MRI	NP	NP
Murphy *et al.* (2008)	18	Executive skills (Controlled Oral Word Fluency, Thurstone Written Word Fluency, Delayed Alteration Test, Wisconsin Card Sorting Test), attention and concentration (Consonant Trigrams Test), visual–perception/visual–construction (Block Design WAIS-III, Motor Free Visual Perception Test–Revised), memory (Recognition Memory Test, Rey Auditory Verbal Learning Test)	None was demented but on 18 patients 22% were cognitively impaired (PLSci) consisting with a frontotemporal lobar dysfunction (executive dysfunction, oral word fluency most frequently impaired measure)	CT perfusion head scan showed haemodynamic changes in PLSci globally extended throughout cortices and underlying white and grey matter. Frontotemporal region most prominent perfusion deficit with cortical decreases in cerebral blood volume and with associated frontal lobe changes in mean transit time in both cortical and subcortical region	NP	Patients with PLSci revealed an increased cerebral blood volume and mean transit time with a reduced cerebral blood flow. Mean transit time as a sensitive indicator correlated with cognitive change in PLS

Tomik *et al.* (2008)	4	Clinical assessment with neuropsychological formal assessment NR	One patient showed discrete cognitive impairment without features of dementia	All but one showed normal MRI. Only one patient showed a single, small hypertensive focus in white matter inferior to the precentral gyrus on the right side	NP	NP
Grace *et al.* (2011)	18	Neuropsychological test battery performed (Wisconsin Card Sorting Test -WCST, Controlled Oral Word Fluency - COWAT, Thurstone Written Word Fluency -TWWF, Delayed Alternation Test - DAT, Consonant Trigrams Test - CTT, Motor-Free Visual Perception Test - MFVPT-R, Block Design (WAIS-III), Rey Auditory Verbal Learning Test - RAVLT, Warrington Recognition Memory Test - WRMT). Also behavioural scales performed (Geriatric Depression Scale - GDS, Neuropsychiatric Inventory - NPI, Frontal Behavioral Inventory - FBI).	39% patients met criteria for cognitive impairment	NR	NR	NR

fMRI, Functional magnetic resonance imaging; HMPAO-SPECT, hexamethylpropylene amine oxime single-photon emission computed tomography; MRI, magnetic resonance imaging; NP, not performed; NR, not reported.

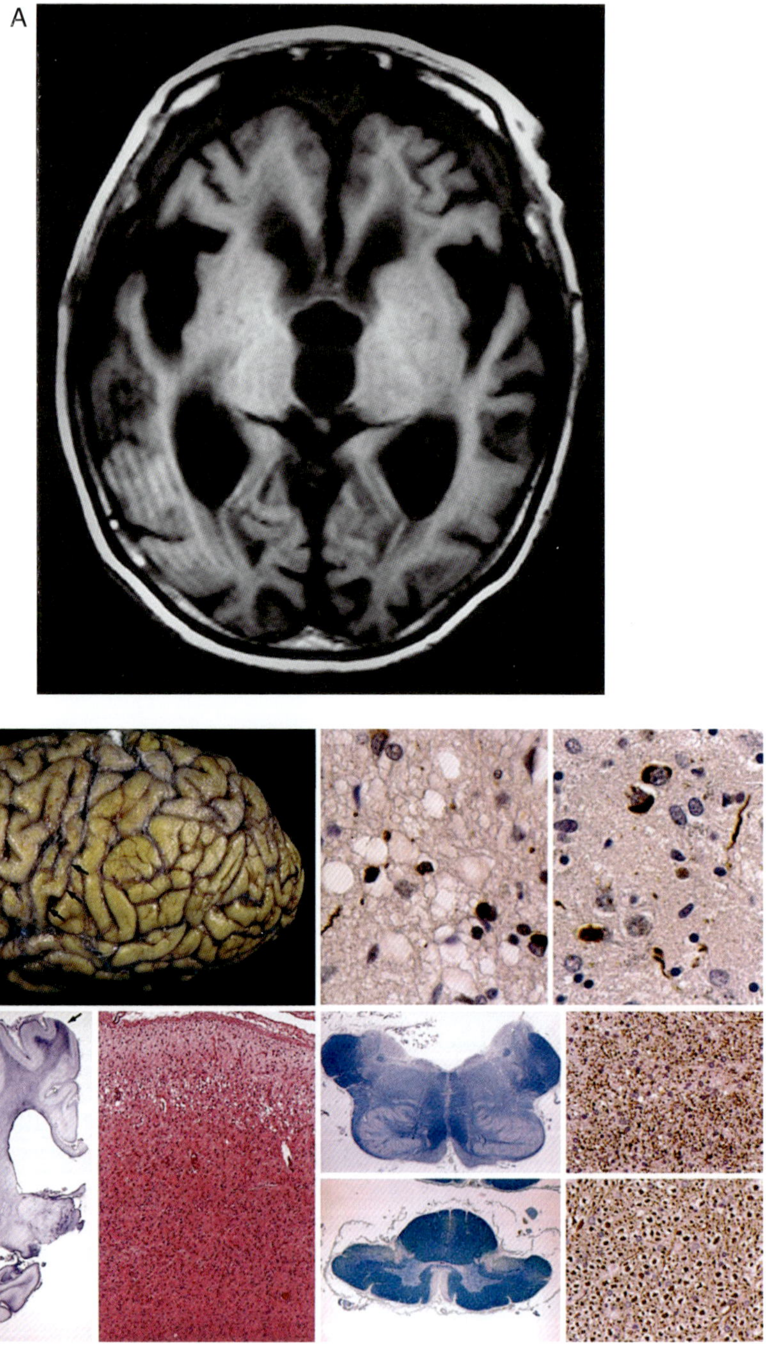

Fig. 11.1 PLS case presented by Tan *et al*. (2003). (a) Magnetic resonance imaging showed extensive frontotemporal atrophy with marked ventricular dilatation; (b) autopsy of the brain with histological data. With kind permission from Springer Science+Business Media: Acta Neuropathologica, Primary lateral sclerosis: a rare upper-motor-predominant form of amyotrophic lateral sclerosis often accompanied by frontotemporal lobar degeneration with ubiquitinated neuronal inclusions? Report of an autopsy case and review of the literature, **105**(6), 2003, 615–620, Tan *et al*., Figure 1 and 2.

out that only a single patient in this series could be considered a possible true case of FTLD/PLS (14).

More recently, Mackenzie and Feldman described a young woman who suffered from rapidly progressive frontal cortical dysfunction leading to dementia along with features of PLS who died aged 29 (25). Magnetic resonance imaging (MRI) demonstrated moderate frontal lobe atrophy. At autopsy, numerous cytoplasmatic inclusions were observed throughout the CNS, although most prominently in the neocortex and hippocampus. The inclusions varied in morphology with some being immunoreactive for ubiquitin while others showed strong positivity for neurofilament proteins.

Mochizuki and colleagues reported a PLS case that, in addition to signs of upper motor neurone dysfunction, displayed parkinsonism and behavioural abnormalities (26). At autopsy, marked degeneration of the precentral cortex, neostriatum, and frontotemporal lobes was observed. Ubiquitinated neuronal inclusions were prominent. This case could be considered a behavioural variant (bvFTD) of FTLD/PLS, even if the parkinsonian symptoms render the case spurious.

Josephs and Dickson analysed two patients with PLS in whom clinical features of frontotemporal dementia (FTD), including aphasia in one case, were congruent with FTLD/PLS (14). The histological findings included neuronal loss and gliosis in frontotemporal areas in both cases, and the parietal neocortices only in case 2. Interestingly, there were ubiquitin and transactive response DNA-binding protein of 43 kDa (TDP-43) immunoreactive cytoplasmic inclusions and neurites in both frontal and temporal neocortices and in the dentate granule cells of the hippocampus. Case 1 also had neuropathological features typical of Alzheimer's disease. The authors concluded that further genetic studies are necessary to determine if FTLD/PLS is a variant of typical FTLD/MND or a separate disease entity.

More recently, a single case of bvFTD of FTLD/PLS has been reported ante mortem, supported by clinical features and MRI evidence of frontotemporal atrophy (27).

To summarize, at present the more interesting results regarding the PLS/dementia relationship is the PLS and FTD overlap with ubiquitin-positive inclusions. In two cases, TDP-43 has been identified as a constituent of the ubiquitin inclusions.

Cognitive frontal deficits in patients with non-demented primary lateral sclerosis

There have been a number of reports that support the occurrence of subtle cognitive impairment, prevalently in frontal executive functions, in a number of patients with PLS. Lewis, in a preliminary report on two patients with PLS (mother and son), found a reduced ability on cognitive tasks of the Halstead Reitan Battery sensitive to frontal lobe damage (Category Test, TDP non-dominant hand trial, TPT Memory, Seashore Rhythm Test, Finger Oscillation, and Grip Strength measures) (28).

Caselli and colleagues (29) first systematically investigated this aspect in a retrospective review of nine patients who met the criteria for PLS and had also been assessed with formal neuropsychological tests. They found that none was demented but eight showed mild cognitive impairment. Deficits were most consistently evident on neuropsychological tests sensitive to frontal lobe function, followed by tests sensitive to memory. Interestingly, six patients underwent hexamethylpropylene amine oxime single-photon emission computed tomography, and bilateral posterior frontal hypoperfusion was displayed in all. In two patients, areas of hypoperfusion were observed: left temporal in one and right greater than left inferomedial temporal in another. These findings indicate that patients with PLS without dementia show cognitive deficits escaping detection using a brief mental status tool as well as with a well-standardized Wechsler Adult Intelligence Scale-Revised (WAIS-R). The most sensitive test was the Controlled Oral Word Association Test (COWA), a brief test of verbal associative fluency and psychomotor speed sensitive to frontal lobe function. The authors concluded that the evaluation of cognitive impairment in ALS requires a specific battery of tests (29). Consistent with this conclusion, it is noteworthy that in studies in which no formal assessment was applied, no cognitive deficit was detectable (4,30). The Caselli *et al.* study would suggest that, in the absence of detailed neuropsychological testing, this conclusion could not be reached.

de Koning *et al.* (31) reported a 72-year-old woman with PLS in whom a slowly progressive isolated dysarthria was the first and only sign for 5 years. Serial neuropsychological examination demonstrated an IQ within the normal range, with intact memory, speech, and praxis. However, behaviour at testing was slightly impulsive and mild frontal cognitive deficits (e.g. concept shifting, generating new ideas, planning), were evident.

Le Forestier and colleagues observed that in 20 patients with PLS, 16 made significantly more errors in the frontal lobe and/or the premotor function tests than age- and education-matched controls (32). In all cases, abnormalities were moderate. In a follow-up paper, the authors noted that while none of the patients developed dementia, they all developed memory deficits consistent with an executive dysfunction (33). All but three patients developed signs of premotor and/or prefrontal cortex deficits. Gordon *et al.* (10) noted on 29 patients that only one had symptomatic cognitive deterioration (PLS plus). Tomik *et al.* describe four PLS patients one of which showed discrete cognitive impairment without features of dementia.

Murphy and colleagues, in a study on the relationship between cognitive decline and cerebral haemodynamics in 18 patients with PLS, observed that 22% of patients were cognitively impaired (named PLSci) (34). Deficits were consistent with frontotemporal lobar dysfunction (executive dysfunction and oral word fluency being the most frequently impaired measure). The authors also observed an alteration in cerebral blood flow in patients with PLS, marked predominantly by an increased cerebral blood volume and mean transit time with a reduced cerebral blood flow in absence of an overt FTD. Recently, Grace *et al.* in a comparative study found no differences in cognitive test scores and overall/behavioural symptoms between PLS and ALS patients (36).

Support for the assumption that cortical degeneration is more extensive than previously believed in PLS derives from a body of research evidence on MRI. Smith presented a single case report of serial MRI performed over 8.5 years (37). The imaging showed progressive atrophy during the course of the disease, extending to the premotor and prefrontal, superior parietal, and primary sensorimotor cortex, but sparing the temporal and occipital lobes and cerebellum. Kuipers-Upmeijer and colleagues examined brain MRI images in 10 patients with PLS over a period of 15 years and observed cortical atrophy in the precentral gyrus extending to the frontal and parietal–occipital regions (30). More recently, Tartaglia *et al.* (38) acquired MRI high-resolution axial three-dimensional T1-weighted images to quantify regional and global brain volumes in 11 patients with PLS and 10 age-matched healthy controls. Compared with controls, patients with PLS displayed significant focal atrophy in the precentral cortex, frontal lobe, and corpus callosum.

Oral and written language in primary lateral sclerosis

In addition to dysarthria and anarthria, PLS is characterized by the development of language disturbance. Grace *et al.* (39) administered some lexical tests (modified 30-item Boston Naming Test, 55-Action Naming Test, Verbal Fluency task with living and non living things) to 17 patients with PLS. No significant differences between patients with PLS versus controls were observed for naming pictured nouns and pictured verbs, while patients with PLS produced significantly fewer items than controls on verbal fluency per category. However, the impairment was statistically significant only for the living category and no difference emerged within the PLS for living versus non living categories.

Of particular interest is the impairment in written language in PLS due to possible writing/spelling impairment (33,40–42). Piquard and colleagues clinically observed spelling errors in PLS during a dictation task declaring that: '*Grammatical errors found in writing language in PLS patients might be a consequence of a frontal lobe dysfunction*' (33). The authors concluded that '*Further studies with a more systematic analysis of written language are needed in order to verify the existence of dysorthographia in PLS and possibly in ALS*'. Zago and colleagues reported that relative to controls, patients with PLS made a greater number of spelling errors but an equivalent performance on a copy task (40,41). The error type included omissions, transpositions, insertions, and letter substitutions, equally distributed on the writing task and composing words with a set of preformed letters. At the most peripheral level, the writing graphic details were always recognizable if not well specified, a pattern of performance adherent to a central written impairment. The greatest number of errors was observed in those patients in whom the degree of dysarthria was the greatest. In particular, deficits were prominent in those patients with PLS with an absence of movements, suggesting the possibility that a defective overt articulation could impair subvocal articulation. The authors hypothesized that frontal regions (Brodmann's 44/45 areas) would be recruited during writing for refreshing the orthographic representation and that in PLS, the patient's limited subvocal rehearsal opportunity would prevent the correct sequencing/assembly of letter and syllables in writing.

Therefore, the past decade has seen a rapid growth of interest in PLS. Our knowledge of cognition in patients with PLS is continually evolving, being enriched by the attempt to apply molecular pathology and genetic evidence to support clinical neuropsychology and neuroimaging features. As seen with ALS, extensive extra-motor system involvement has also been documented in patients with PLS using both neuroradiological and brain perfusion studies. A mild cognitive impairment that is most consistent with prefrontal cortex involvement (PLSci) has been observed. In addition, a small subset of patients with PLS developed a pattern of frontotemporal lobar atrophy with overt cognitive decline and behavioural abnormalities consistent with FTD.

The presence of TDP-43 immunoreactive inclusions (see Highley and Ince, Chapter 19) lends significant support to the concept that PLS, like ALS, has significant non-motor pathology with prominent involvement of the frontal and temporal neocortices (14). It can be anticipated that genetic studies will further support this and, specifically, the continuum between PLS and FTD, similar to that proposed for ALS.

Furthermore, it is clear that patients with PLS need to be better characterized for the clinical phenotypes to permit the molecular correlations. For this reason, there is the need to conduct preliminary systematic studies with formal neuropsychological testing on patients with PLS. It is important to bear in mind that the neuropsychological assessment of PLS is complicated by the same testing issues that arise for ALS. As commented upon by Phukan and colleagues, standard testing and psychometric methods may underestimate or exaggerate the presence of cognitive impairment (43). The use of specific frontal batteries that minimize the impact of speech and motor dysfunction on testing outcomes, using untimed tests or tests requiring no speech production or minimal motor requirements, is crucial. Moreover, new tools for assessing neuropsychological performances, using advanced technologies, such as eye-tracking, could allow a more sensitive detection of minimal cognitive changes and longitudinal testing even in the presence of speech or motor impairments, thus fully understanding the impact of cognitive changes along the course of the disease (44, 45, 46).

A great deal of cognitive heterogeneity exists in patients with PLS, similar to that observed in ALS. Neuropsychology seems to play an important role in distinguishing between mild forms of cognitive impairment and cases with overt FTD, but converging evidence of genetics, molecular pathology, and neuroimaging is needed to further characterize the frontotemporal involvement of PLS. Advances in genetics and molecular pathology make the prospect of biologically driven, disease-specific therapies for PLS the most promising approach for the future after accurate characterization of the frontotemporal syndromes accompanying PLS.

References

1. Türck L. (1855). Über das Leitungsvermog. des menschl. *Ruckemmarkes.* Sitz der Kais. Acad.
2. Charcot JM. (1865). Sclérose des cordons latéraux de la moelle épinière chez une femme hystérique, atteinte de contracure permanente des quatre members. *Bull Mém Soc Méd Hôp Paris*, second series, **2**, 24–42.
3. Erb WH. (1875). Uber einen wenig bekannten spinalen Symptomencomplex. *Berliner Klin Wochenschr*, **12**, 357–359.
4. Swash M, Desai J, Misra VP. (1999). What is primary lateral sclerosis? *J Neurol Sci*, **170**(1), 5–10.
5. Sotaniemi KA, Myllylä VV. (1985). Primary lateral sclerosis. A debated entity. *Acta Neurol Scand*, **71**(4), 334–336.
6. Pearce JMS. (2004). Primary lateral sclerosis and Pierre Marie. *J Neurol Neurosurg Psychiatry*, **75**(4), 897.
7. Stark FM, Moersch FP. (1945). Primary lateral sclerosis. *J Nerv Ment Dis*, **102**, 332–333.

8. Younger DS, Chou S, Hays AP, *et al.* (1988). Primary lateral sclerosis. A clinical diagnosis reemerges. *Arch Neurol*, **45**(12), 1304–1307.
9. Pringle CE, Hudson AJ, Munoz DG, *et al.* (1992). Primary lateral sclerosis. Clinical features, neuropathology and diagnostic criteria. *Brain*, **115**(2), 495–520.
10. Gordon PH, Cheng B, Katz IB, *et al.* (2006). The clinical natural history of primary lateral sclerosis. *Neurology*, **66**(5), 647–653.
11. Singer MA, Statland JM, Wolfe GI, Barohn RJ. (2007). Primary lateral sclerosis. *Muscle Nerve*, **35**(3), 291–302.
12. Lerman-Sagie T, Filiano J, Simth DW, Korson M. (1996). Infantile onset of hereditary ascending spastic paralysis with bulbar involvement. *J Child Neurol*, **11**(1), 54–57.
13. Dupré N, Valmanis PN, Bouchard JP, Rouleau GA. (2007). Autosomal dominant primary lateral sclerosis. *Neurology*, **68**(14), 1156–1157.
14. Josephs KA, Dickson DW. (2007). Frontotemporal lobar degeneration with upper motor neuron disease/primary lateral sclerosis. *Neurology*, **69**(18), 1800–1801.
15. Hainfellner JA, Pilz P, Lassman H, *et al.* (1995). Diffuse Lewy body disease as substrate of primary lateral sclerosis. *J Neurol*, **242**(2), 59–63.
16. Sugihara H, Horiuchi M, Kamo T, *et al.* (1999). A case of primary lateral sclerosis taking a prolonged course with dementia and having an unusual dendritic ballooning. *Neuropathology*, **19**(1), 77–84.
17. Engel PA, Grunnet M. (2000). Atypical dementia and spastic paraplegia in a patient with primary lateral sclerosis and numerous neocortical beta amyloid plaques: new disorder or Alzheimer's disease variant? *J Geriatr Psychiatry Neurol*, **13**(2), 60–64.
18. Tan C-F, Kakita A, Piao Y-S, *et al.* (2003). Primary lateral sclerosis: a rare upper-motor-predominant form of amyotrophic lateral sclerosis often accompanied by frontotemporal lobar degeneration with ubiquitinated neuronal inclusions? Report of an autopsy case and review of the literature. *Acta Neuropathol*, **105**(6), 615–620.
19. Imai H, Furukawa Y, Sumino S, *et al.* (1995). A 65-year-old woman with dysarthria, dysphagia, weakness, and gait disturbance (in Japanese with English abstract). *No to Shinkei*, **47**(4), 399–410.
20. Watanabe R, Iino M, Honda M, *et al.* (1997). Primary lateral sclerosis. *Neuropathology*, **17**(3), 220–224.
21. Konagaya M, Sakai M, Matsuoka Y, Hashizume Y. (1998). Upper motor neuron predominant de generation with frontal and temporal lobe atrophy. *Acta Neuropathol*, **96**(5), 532–536.
22. Tsuchiya K, Arai M, Matsuya S, *et al.* (1999). Sporadic amyotrophic lateral sclerosis resembling primary lateral sclerosis: report of an autopsy case and a review of the literature. *Neuropathology*, **19**(1), 71–76.
23. Yamazaki M, Yamazaki MM, Mori O, *et al.* (2000). An autopsy case of amyotrophic lateral sclerosis with upper motor neuron (UMN) predominant degeneration presenting slowly progressive aphasia: a subtype of ALS with dementia (ALS-D)? *Neuropathology*, **20**, Suppl, A18.
24. Mochizuki A, Komatsuzaki Y, Shoji S. (2002). A case of frontotemporal atrophy with ubiquitin inclusions presenting with upper motor neuron signs at onset follow by extrapyramidal signs and dementia (abstract in English). *Neuropathology*, **22**(Suppl), 1C 4.
25. Mackenzie, IRA, Feldman H. (2004). Neurofilament inclusion body disease with early onset frontotemporal dementia and primary lateral sclerosis. *Clin Neuropathol*, **23**(4), 183–193.
26. Mochizuki A, Komatsuzaki Y, Iwamoto H, Shoji S. (2004). Frontotemporal dementia with ubiquinated neuronal inclusions presenting with primary lateral sclerosis and parkinsonism: clinicopathological report of an autopsy case. *Acta Neuropathol*, **107**(4), 377–380.
27. Suvendrini L, Tang-Wai D. (2010). Fronto-temporal dementia associated with primary lateral sclerosis in the antemortem. *Neurology*, **74**(Suppl 2), A132.

28. Lewis GP. (1991). Neuropsychological findings in primary lateral sclerosis. *Arch Clin Neuropsychol*, **6**(3), 203.
29. Caselli RJ, Smith BE, Osborne D. (1995). Primary lateral sclerosis: a neuropsychological study. *Neurology*, **45**(11), 2005–2009.
30. Kuipers-Upmeijer J, de Jager AE, *et al.* (2001). Primary lateral sclerosis: clinical, neurophysiological, and magnetic resonance findings. *J Neurol Neurosurg Psychiatry*, **71**(5), 615–620.
31. de Koning I, van Doorn PA, van Dongen HR. (1997). Slowly progressive isolated dysarthria: longitudinal course, speech features, and neuropsychological deficits. *J Neurol*, **244**(10), 664–667.
32. Le Forestier N, Maisonobe T, Piquard A, *et al.* (2001). Does primary lateral sclerosis exist? A study of 20 patients and a review of the literature. *Brain*, **124**(10), 1989–1999.
33. Piquard A, Le Forestier N, Baudoin-Madec V, *et al.* (2006). Neuropsychological changes in patients with primary lateral sclerosis. *Amyotroph Lateral Scler*, **7**(3), 150–160.
34. Murphy MJ, Grace GM, Tartaglia MC, *et al.* (2008). Cerebral haemodynamic changes accompanying cognitive impairment in primary lateral sclerosis. *Amyotroph Lateral Scler*, **9**(6), 359–368.
35. Tomik B, Zur KA, Szczudlik A. (2008). Pure primary lateral sclerosis–Case reports. *Clin Neurol Neurosurg*, **110**(4), 387–391.
36. Grace GM, Orange JB, Rowe A, Findlater K, Freedman M, Strong MJ. (2011). Neuropsychological functioning in PLS: a comparison with ALS. *Can J Neurol Sci.*, **38**(1), 88–97.
37. Smith CD. (2002). Serial MRI findings in a case of primary lateral sclerosis. *Neurology*, **57**(4), 647–649.
38. Tartaglia MC, Laluz V, Rowe A, *et al.* (2009). Brain atrophy in primary lateral sclerosis. *Neurology*, **72**(14), 1236–1241.
39. Grace GM, Orange JB, Murphy MJ, *et al.* (2006). Primary lateral sclerosis: cognitive, language, and cerebral hemodynamic findings. In: Strong MJ (eds), *Dementia and Motor Neuron Disease*, pp. 87–97. Informa healthcare, UK Ltd.
40. Zago S, Poletti B, Corbo M, *et al.* (2003). Dysgraphia as the presenting symptom of primary lateral sclerosis. *Amyotroph Lateral Scler*, **4**(Suppl 1), 205.
41. Zago S, Poletti B, Corbo M, *et al.* (2008). Dysgraphia in patients with primary lateral sclerosis: A speech-based rehearsal deficit? *Behav Neurol*, **19**(4), 169–175.
42. Silani V, Poletti B, Zago S. (2009). Dysgraphia in Primary Lateral Sclerosis (PLS). *Oral Presentation at the Third International Research Workshop on Frontotemporal Dementia in ALS.* June 21–25, 2009, London, Ontario, Canada.
43. Phukan J, Pender NP, Hardiman O. (2007). Cognitive impairment in amyotrophic lateral sclerosis. *Lancet Neurol*, **6**(11), 994–1003.
44. Poletti B, Maringelli F, Meriggi P, *et al.* (2009). Cognitive frontal assessment in Amyotrophic Lateral Sclerosis: the Anti-Saccade Paradigm. *J Neurol Sci*, Suppl **30**, S257.
45. Poletti B, Maringelli F, Lafronza A, *et al.* (2009). Anti-saccade paradigm in the cognitive frontal assessment of amyotrophic lateral sclerosis. *Amyotroph Lateral Scler*, **10** (Suppl 1), 45.
46. Donaghy C, Pinnock R, Abrahams S, Cardwell C, Hardiman O, Patterson V, McGivern RC, Gibson JM. (2010). Slow saccades in bulbar-onset motor neurone disease. *J Neurol*, **257**(7), 1134–1140.

Chapter 12

Electrophysiological evaluation of lower motor neurone loss in amyotrophic lateral sclerosis

Jeremy M. Shefner

Motor neurone loss has been recognized as an intrinsic component of amyotrophic lateral sclerosis (ALS) since its original description by Charcot. In current practice, clinicians seek evidence for this loss both from the clinical neurological examination and from clinical neurophysiological studies. Physiological signs of ongoing nerve or axon loss include the presence of fibrillation potentials and positive sharp waves on needle electromyography; fasciculation potentials also suggest irritability or damage to the lower motor neurone (1). The compensatory reinnervation that occurs as a consequence of denervation was elegantly described by Erminio *et al.* in the 1950s and has not been significantly refined since that time (2). Motor unit potentials become enlarged, prolonged, polyphasic, and unstable as terminal axons reinnervate muscle fibres that have lost their original nerve supply. However, while the presence of ongoing denervation and reinnervation can be well documented by classical techniques, disease progression has been more difficult to assess accurately. The extent of fibrillation potential activity waxes and wanes with progression, and a quantitative index has never been established. Similarly, while aspects of motor unit changes can be measured, they do not clearly change in ways that allow an accurate and reproducible index of progression. Progressive motor unit loss is a critical event related to disability in ALS, and an attractive target for treatment. For these reasons, investigators have actively sought a measure of motor unit loss that is reproducible, non-invasive, rapidly obtained, and amenable to repeated evaluation over time.

Motor unit number estimation (MUNE) refers to a group of techniques that share the goal of estimating the number of intact motor units innervating a single muscle being studied. A secondary goal is to estimate that size of individual motor units within that muscle. All techniques share a common framework; a maximum response generated by activation of all motor units is recorded, and an estimate of individual motor unit size is generated. The motor unit estimate is arrived at by dividing the amplitude of the maximum response by an estimate of the individual motor unit amplitude. The validity of the motor unit estimate is thus impacted by several factors. First, it is assumed that maximum response is a linear summation of individual motor units.

This assumption is unlikely to be completely valid, as most motor units recorded with surface electrodes have both positive and negative components, allowing for the possibility of phase cancellation impacting the sum. However, the negative component of motor units predominates, so that the requirement of linear summation is approximately met. Second, variability of motor axon conduction velocities create dispersion of the summed response. In the absence of a superimposed demyelinating process, however, motor axon conduction velocities are quite uniform compared with sensory fibres, so that dispersion is not a significant confounder. Third, and most important, the estimate of individual motor unit size must be valid and reproducible. The method for obtaining this estimate is different for the different techniques, and no clear standard has emerged.

Despite the lack of consensus regarding how individual motor units should be measured and average amplitude estimated, MUNE has been used effectively to follow patients with ALS, to assess disease progression in animal models, and as a secondary outcome measure in ALS clinical trials. In this review, the most commonly employed techniques will be described and evaluated, and the use of MUNE in ALS will be discussed.

Review of techniques

The incremental technique

In 1971, McComas and colleagues described an attractively simple method for counting motor units (3). Initially recording from a small intrinsic foot muscle, a maximal compound motor action potential (CMAP) was obtained in a manner identical to standard nerve conduction studies. Then, starting from subthreshold stimulation levels and recording at a high amplifier gain, stimulus intensity was gradually increased until a small all or nothing response was seen, representing the first motor unit activated. With further stimulus intensity increases, quantal increases in the response were recorded. Up to 11 discrete increments were recorded, with each increment assumed to represent the addition of one motor unit (see Figure 12.1). The amplitude of the final response was divided by the number of increments and taken as the estimate of average single unit amplitude for that muscle; this value was divided into the maximum CMAP to calculate MUNE. The incremental MUNE technique was soon applied to upper extremity muscles supplied by median, ulnar, and radial nerves (4–6), with motor unit counts in young subjects averaging between approximately 250 and 420.

Several theoretical and practical objections to this technique were immediately obvious. Only motor units activated with low stimulus intensities are sampled; there are a number of reasons to suggest that these motor units might not be representative of the entire population, Second, it is clear that the activation thresholds of motor axons overlap to a significant degree, so that a constant stimulus presented repeatedly may evoke responses from different motor units at different times. Thus, an incremental response could represent alternation of one smaller motor unit with another unit of larger amplitude. Treating the difference in amplitude between two units as a separate unit would lead to an underestimate of motor unit size and an overestimate of MUNE. Motor unit instability due to neuromuscular transmission defects also has the potential to increase MUNE values, as

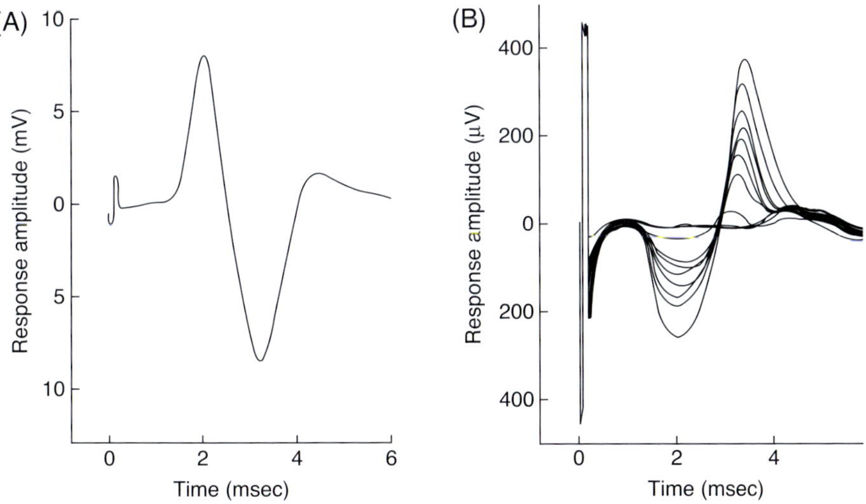

Fig. 12.1 Example of incremental MUNE. (A) Maximum compound muscle action potential is shown. (B) Incremental responses to small, graded stimuli are displayed. With permission from Shefner JM, Reaume AG, Flood DG, Scott RW, Kowall NW, Ferrante RJ, et al. (1999) Mice lacking cytosolic copper/zinc superoxide dismutase display a distinctive motor axonopathy. *Neurology*. 1999; 53,(6): 1239–46.

small changes in motor unit morphology could be interpreted as the addition of very small motor units.

The incremental method has been modified in several ways since its original inception. Ballantyne and Hansen subtracted successive responses from each other so that individual motor units could be evaluated (7,8). This technique has the advantage that errors due to phase cancellation can be avoided, but does not address any of the issues mentioned above. An automated method that included an algorithm to detect and remove alternating responses has been developed (9); as expected, this method produced smaller MUNEs than the manual method performed on the same patient, but intersubject variability was not reduced.

Multiple point stimulation

The major problems inherent in the incremental technique have to do with the analysis of waveforms that result from the activation of multiple motor units. The multiple point stimulation technique (MPS) was developed to avoid this difficulty. In MPS MUNE, the nerve is stimulated at very low intensities just sufficient to elicit an initial all or none response (10–13). The stimulating electrode is then moved some distance along the nerve and the process repeated; quite often, a response of differing morphology and amplitude can be recorded. For median and ulnar innervated intrinsic hand muscles, 15–20 morphologically distinct units can usually be recorded. From this sample, mean amplitude is calculated and used as the estimate for single unit potential amplitude; this value is divided into the maximum response to yield the MUNE. Similar to incremental MUNE, the MPS technique assumes that the responses recorded do in fact represent single unit responses, and that the single units recorded are representative of the entire motor unit population.

The assumption that threshold motor do represent the entire population of units present in a muscle is indirectly addressed by studies showing that threshold fibres spanned a wide range of conduction velocities, suggesting an equally wide range of axon diameters (11).

Although voluntary recruitment of motor units clearly follows a pattern of small units recruited before large, it appears that the primary determinant of relative sensitivity to electrical stimulation is the position of the axon in the nerve bundle, with axons situated close to the stimulus more likely to be activated than those farther away.

The MPS technique has been modified in several ways since its initial introduction. To increase the speed of data acquisition, Wang and Delwaide recorded incremental responses to increasing stimulus intensity in a fashion similar to the incremental technique, but limited recording to only 2 ± 3 increments at each stimulus location (13). They reasoned that alternation could more easily be perceived and eliminated if only 2 ± 3 units were being stimulated at a time. With a computer program that performed point by point subtraction of successive increments, they were able to limit testing to 4 ± 10 stimulation sites and still record 10 ± 20 units. Porter and colleagues showed that the modified technique produced slightly higher test–retest reliability than traditional MPS (14).

Spike-triggered averaging

The preceding methods use responses evoked by electrical stimulation at low stimulus intensities to provide estimates of single motor unit amplitude. A systematic bias is therefore possible because of the tendency of low amplitude stimuli to evoke responses in larger diameter axons (15). In addition, the necessity of using electrical stimuli makes it difficult to apply MUNE techniques to proximal muscles, whose nerves are often relatively inaccessible. The spike-triggered averaging (STA) technique avoids these problems by studying voluntarily activated motor units (16,17). The subject voluntary activates the muscle being studied at a low level. The response to a single motor unit is recorded with either a concentric or single fibre electromyography needle, and the electrode is positioned so that only that single motor unit response is recorded. Concurrently, surface potentials are recorded; the single motor unit spike is used as a trigger to time lock the surface recorded potentials so that an average surface response can be calculated corresponding to the needle recorded spike. By altering needle position to record from different motor units, a sample of surface motor unit potentials can be generated, and average motor unit amplitude calculated. MUNE is then generated in the typical way, by dividing the average single unit response into the maximum CMAP.

The STA method is practical to perform only with software available on certain electromyographs. It is technically more difficult than some other MUNE methods, as it requires a needle electrode insertion and is critically dependent on the operator's ability to trigger only on the intended motor unit. In addition, just as there is bias inherent in the units preferentially evoked by electrical stimulation, voluntary motor unit activation is not random, but occurs according to the Henneman size principle. Thus, smaller motor units are activated before large units, potentially leading to an overestimation of MUNE. The STA technique has been applied to proximal as well as distal muscles; in general, reproducibility for this technique is significantly worse than for other commonly used methods. Other limitations are the significant discomfort subjects experience with multiple needle movements, as well as the high degree of cooperation required by the subject.

Recent advances in computational power have led to a promising extension of the STA method. By using a decomposition-based method of identifying individual motor units from a muscle being activated, surface recorded potentials from multiple motor units can be identified. Depending on the degree of effort, a 30-second train of action potentials may yield five or more motor units. Thus, an adequate number of single motor unit potentials can be recorded from a small number of needle movements (18). The single motor units generated in this way may be averaged and divided into the maximum compound motor action potential in a manner similar to the previously discussed techniques.

MUNE using decomposition-based electromyography shows excellent test–retest reliability. However, the estimate of single motor unit potential amplitude is directly related to the level of voluntary activation. With minimal effort, small motor units are recruited and recorded, with progressively larger motor units firing as effort increases. Thus, the MUNE also changes, showing a clear decline with increasing effort (19). Given that the true number of functional motor units in a muscle is a static number, the dependence of decomposition MUNE on effort limits its potential application.

The statistical method

All of the MUNE techniques so far discussed sample motor units near either the electrical or voluntary threshold. This introduces the potential for systematic bias, although it is unclear how significant such bias may be. The statistical technique avoids such bias by sampling motor units over a wider response range (20,21). The method of estimation of single motor unit potentials is fundamentally different in the statistical method than other MUNE methods. The entire response range of a muscle is first evaluated by presenting graded stimuli that evoke a full range of motor responses. From this stimulus–response function, certain response ranges are chosen, and a constant intensity stimulus producing a response within a given range is presented repeatedly. The responses to this repeated constant intensity stimulus would vary in amplitude; it is assumed that this variability reflects variable firing of units close to their activation threshold. If certain assumptions are fulfilled, this variability directly estimates the size of the variably firing motor units. Four stimulus intensities are chosen, and estimates of motor unit size at each intensity are obtained; these estimates are averaged to produce a single motor unit potential amplitude, which can be divided into the maximum CMAP response to yield the MUNE.

The validity of this technique depends on a number of assumptions; the most critical is that the variability of response to a constant stimulus depends only on motor units that are near their threshold and thus firing variably to the stimulus. This assumption may hold for normal subjects; however, it is clear that motor units from patients with ALS are unstable, and variability in the amplitude of single units produces variability that artefactually lowers the estimated amplitude of single units and thus increases the motor unit estimate (22,23). Jillapalli and Shefner showed that single motor units of patients with ALS are significantly more variable in their response amplitude than motor units from normal subjects (24). In two multicentre studies, various methods were employed to filter this excess variability, but estimates of single motor unit potential amplitude derived using the statistical method were much smaller than would be expected, resulting in MUNE values that were inappropriately large. Moreover, over 6 or 12 months of study, there was no change in the average single motor unit potential values, a finding at odds with the known natural history of the disease.

Modified incremental motor unit number estimation

In an attempt to reduce the variability inherent in both incremental and MPS techniques, a technique that combines the two with standardization of stimulus locations was recently described (25). With this technique, three standard stimulus locations are established, and three incremental responses are obtained at each location. Thus, nine motor units are estimated; these are averaged to generate an estimate of single motor unit potential amplitude. This estimate is divided into the maximum response to yield the motor unit estimate.

Preliminary studies on both normal subjects and those with ALS have shown excellent test–retest reliability, and expected changes in subjects with ALS. In a natural history study performed at 10 sites, motor unit potential amplitude increased over time, and MUNE fell at a rate greater than that observed using the statistical technique. This technique is now being used in a multicenter clinical trial.

Use in patients and animal models of amyotrophic lateral sclerosis

Despite the limitations of the methods discussed above, MUNE has been successfully employed to gain insight into disease progression in both patients with ALS and animal models.

Human studies

In theory, ALS is a disease perfectly suited to study with MUNE. It is purely motor, uniformly progressive, and weakness occurs in large measure because of dropout of motor units. For all these reasons, investigators employed MUNE techniques on patients with ALS soon after its original development. Using the incremental technique, Hansen and Ballantyne (26) compared MUNE in intrinsic foot muscles of normal subjects and 32 patients with ALS. As expected MUNE in patients with ALS was reduced while individual motor unit potential amplitude increased. Carleton and Brown (27) performed MPS studies of hand muscles of patients with ALS and found much the same pattern. Because of this compensatory increase in motor unit size, compound motor action potential amplitude was within normal limits until MUNE dropped below 10% of normal numbers. These findings suggest that simply following changes in compound motor action potential amplitude will be less sensitive than measuring MUNE. Clinical atrophy was apparent at about the same level of motor unit loss. The time course of motor unit loss in patients with ALS was first studied by Dantes and McComas (28); their data suggested that motor unit loss occurred more rapidly early in the disease, with the slope of motor unit decline levelling off after the first year. Using a variation of the MPS technique, Arasaki and Tamaki (29) also found that MUNE dropped by 70% in the first year after diagnosis. Coupled with data showing that muscle strength declines quite linearly in ALS during most of the course of the disease (30,31) it appears that the early rapid decline in motor unit numbers is compensated for by increases in individual motor unit force generating capacity (Figure 12.2). Consistent with this idea is the finding that isometric strength in elbow flexors and biceps and STA MUNE are only minimally correlated over a wide range of muscle strength (32) although correlations between strength and MUNE are somewhat higher in more distal muscles (33).

Motor unit dropout is a hallmark of progression in ALS and virtually all force and electrophysiological measures show declines with time after diagnosis. Hence, the fact that MUNE behaves similarly does not confer upon it any unique utility. However, if MUNE declines to a greater extent than either quantitative strength measures or compound motor action potential amplitude, it may have use as an outcome measure in clinical trials. Mitsumoto and colleagues performed a single site longitudinal study evaluating the change of a variety of outcome measures including manual muscle testing, MUNE using the MPS method, and the ALS functional rating scale (34). The rate of decline over time was similar for all three measures; however, the variability of MUNE suggested that it was less sensitive than the other measures in detecting change over time. In another single site study performed in the context of a multicentre clinical trial, MUNE generated using MPS, compound motor action potential amplitude, hand grip, strength testing, and vital capacity were all measured at regular intervals for 1 year (35); in this study, the decline in MUNE was greater than any of the other measures. Liu and colleagues performed a

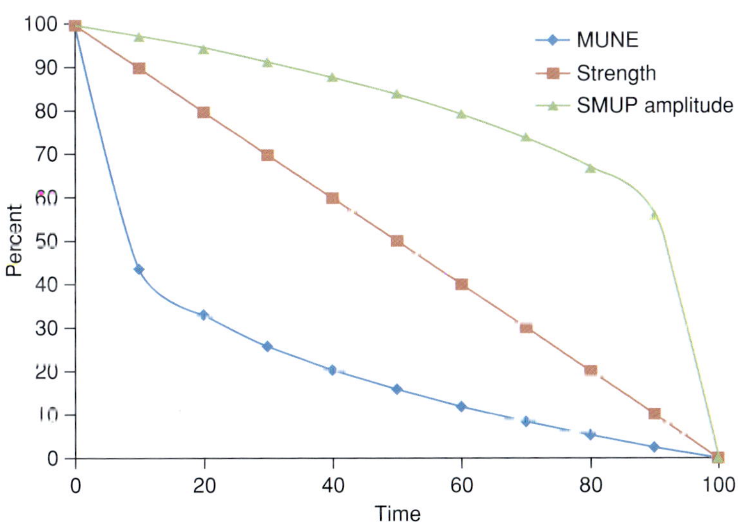

Fig. 12.2 Hypothesized relationship between MUNE, single motor unit action potential amplitude, and muscle strength.

longitudinal study of patients with ALS in China; using incremental MUNE, they found that the percentage change in MUNE over 12 months was greater than the ALS functional rating scale, manual muscle testing, vital capacity, or compound motor action potential amplitude (36). Over a shorter period of study, MUNE performed using the statistical method declined statistically significantly over 3 months but grip strength and compound motor action potential amplitude did not (37).

Another important use of MUNE would be to stratify patients according to rate of progression. This would be critical both for the design of clinical trials, and to provide prognostic information to patients in a clinical setting. In a recent study, the rate of change in statistical MUNE was shown to be a strong predictor of survival in patients with ALS. Using a single MUNE evaluation and extrapolation to normal values assumed to be present just before disease onset, incremental MUNE predicted patient survival, and provided a means of stratification into slowly progressing and rapidly progressing groups (38).

MUNE has been employed in two multicentre clinical trials as a secondary outcome measure (22,23). The statistical technique was chosen for use as it was felt that it was more amenable to standardization across sites than either the incremental or MPS methods. With extensive training and validation, clinical trial sites were able to reach a criterion of 20% for maximum test–retest variability. In both trials, MUNE declined monotonically over the duration of the trials, with an average decline over 12 months of 46%. This decline was less than that noted in other trials, and approximately corresponded to the decline noted in both strength and compound motor action potential amplitude. The failure of MUNE to decline at a faster rate was shown to be due to the fact that in both trials, single motor unit amplitude remained stable over time, contrary to the expected progressive increase as a function of compensatory reinnervation. This was felt to be an artefact of the statistical method, which attributed variability due to unstable motor units to the presence of inappropriately small motor units. For this reason, trials now underway are employing alternate methods to estimate motor unit number.

One such method is the modified incremental technique described above; this technique has been employed as one measure in a natural history study of subjects with ALS at 10 centres. Although the study is ongoing, preliminary results from 40 normal subjects and 56 subjects with ALS followed for up to 500 days, showed that test–retest variability was 9% and mean decline in MUNE was 9.5% per month when scaled according to baseline value at study entry (25). As expected in ALS, single motor unit amplitude increased as MUNE decreased. These attributes suggest that this method may be superior to previously described methods for use as an outcome measure in clinical trials.

Animal studies

Shortly after the discovery that point mutations in the gene encoding Cu/Zn superoxide dismutase (SOD) were responsible for some forms of familial ALS, a mouse model overexpressing mutant SOD1 was developed (39). These mice develop a syndrome that clinically and pathologically closely resembles human ALS. Incremental MUNE studies performed on these animals (40,41) show loss of motor units that begins before the onset of clinical signs (41) and proceeds throughout the course of the disease. Although the disease course is too rapid for extensive reinnervation to occur, single motor unit amplitude also increases with time, albeit to a lesser extent than that seen in human disease. MUNE has also been shown to correlate with behavioural indices in the transgenic mouse (42). When incremental MUNE was performed at regular intervals starting at 80 days of age, disease onset was highly correlated with the initial MUNE value. Similarly, the rate of decline of MUNE correlated well with the total disease duration in these animals. In contrast, motor unit estimate at day 120 of life did not significantly correlate with the length of survival. As death in these animals is primarily a respiratory event and motor unit estimates were performed in the distal hind limb, this lack of correlation is not surprising. The pattern is much different in SOD1 knockout mice, who develop without detectable levels of murine SOD1 (43). These latter animals were initially thought not to have a phenotype that included motor neurone loss, as they live a nearly normal lifespan and do not display obvious weakness. However, incremental MUNE performed over time demonstrated a progressive loss of units at a much slower rate than that seen in the transgenic overexpressing mice. Motor unit size remained normal despite dropout of motor units, suggesting a defect in reinnervation (41).

MUNE abnormalities in the absence of a behavioural phenotype were also found in a transgenic mouse model overexpressing the ALS-2/Alsin gene (44). ALS-2 is the cause of a rare autosomal recessive form of motor neurone disease, which begins in childhood and results in a slowly progressive spastic paraplegia with modest motor neurone loss. Mice with homozygous disruption of the ALS-2 genes were developed. However, they appeared phenotypically normal and by 21 months, no obvious developmental, reproductive, or motor abnormalities were noted. For this reason, MUNE was used to determine whether a subtle motor neurone phenotype could be identified. At 12 months of age, MUNE in wild-type control animals was 275 while in the ALS-2 knockout animals the average MUNE was 200. This difference was statistically significant. Thus, even in the absence of behavioural phenotype, MUNE is able to show a subtle loss of motor neurones in a genetic model that is expected to demonstrate only a modest lower motor neurone phenotype.

Thus, MUNE can provide insight into the pathophysiology of novel genetic abnormalities. Similarly, the mechanism of novel therapeutics can be elucidated by MUNE; a recent study evaluating the therapeutic effect of neurophilin ligands in transgenic mice showed that motor unit size was preferentially enhanced, while the rate of motor unit dropout was unchanged (45). This result suggests that MUNE studies may aid in the design of rational polydrug therapies for ALS based on increased knowledge of mechanisms of drug action.

A more dramatic example of changes in MUNE related to therapeutic intervention was noted in a study of adult rats treated with embryonic stem cells after being subjected to a viral motor neurone disease (46). These rats were infected with *Sindbis* virus, which induces a poliomyelitis-like drop out of spinal motor neurones. Animals infected with *Sindbis* virus showed varying levels of weakness either resulting in death or predominately lower extremity paralysis. Embryonic stem cells were directed down a motor neurone lineage and surgically implanted at multiple levels of the spinal cord 12 days after disease onset, when survival was assured and maximal weakness was evident. There was clear anatomical evidence of transplant survival. With a variety of interventions to provide trophic support and directional guidance, transplanted cells extended axons through the ventral root and towards previously denervated muscle fibres, where neuromuscular junctions were established. At day 120 after transplantation, MUNE values increased from an average of 44 at day 12 shortly after the disease was at its maximum to 92 at day 120. Animals treated with sham transplantations showed no increases over this time. Behaviourally, animals showed functional behaviour of the lower extremities at day 120 with some having a nearly normal gait.

Summary

Although still being refined, MUNE has provided important information about disease course in patients with ALS, and has served as a sensitive marker of motor neurone loss in animal models. Modifications in current techniques have the potential to reduce variability of measurement and improve ease of use. As a surrogate outcome measure in phase II clinical trials, MUNE may reduce sample size required to show a meaningful effect of therapy as compared with other commonly used measures.

References

1. Carvalho MD, Swash M. (2009). Awaji diagnostic algorithm increases sensitivity of El Escorial criteria for ALS diagnosis. *Amyotroph Lateral Scler*, **10**, 53–57.
2. Erminio F, Buchthal F, Rosenfalk P. (1959). Motor unit territory and muscle fiber concentration in paresis due to peripheral nerve injury and anterior horn involvement. *Neurology*, **9**, 657–671.
3. McComas A, Fawcett P, Campbell M, Sica R. (1971). Electrophysiological estimation of the number of motor units within a human muscle. *J Neurol Neurosurg Psychiatry*, **34**, 121–131.
4. Brown WF. (1972). A method for estimating the number of motor units in thenar muscles and the changes in motor unit count with ageing. *J Neurol Neurosurg Psychiatry*, **35**, 845–852.
5. Defaria CR, Toyonaga K. (1978). Motor unit estimation in a muscle supplied by the radial nerve. *J Neurol Neurosurg Psychiatry*, **41**, 794–797.
6. Sica RE, McComas AJ, Upton AR, Longmire D. (1974). Motor unit estimations in small muscles of the hand. *J Neurol Neurosurg Psychiatry*, **37**, 55–67.
7. Ballantyne JP, Hansen S. (1974). New method for the estimation of the number of motor units in a muscle. 2. Duchenne, limb-girdle and facioscapulohumeral, and myotonic muscular dystrophies. *J Neurol Neurosurg Psychiatry*, **37**, 1195–1201.
8. Hansen S, Ballantyne JP. (1977). Axonal dysfunction in the neuropathy of diabetes mellitus: a quantitative electrophysiological study. *J Neurol Neurosurg Psychiatry*, **40**, 555–564.
9. Galea V, de Bruin H, Cavasin R, McComas AJ. (1991). The numbers and relative sizes of motor units estimated by computer. *Muscle Nerve*, **14**, 1123–1130.
10. Brown WF, Milner-Brown HS. (1976). Some electrical properties of motor units and their effects on the methods of estimating motor unit numbers. *J Neurol Neurosurg Psychiatry*, **39**, 249–257.
11. Doherty TJ, Stashuk DW, Brown WF. (1993). Determinants of mean motor unit size: impact on estimates of motor unit number. *Muscle Nerve*, **16**, 1326–1331.
12. Felice KJ. (1995). Thenar motor unit number estimates using the multiple point stimulation technique: reproducibility studies in ALS patients and normal subjects. *Muscle Nerve*, **18**, 1412–1416.

13. Wang FC, Delwaide PJ. (1995). Number and relative size of thenar motor units estimated by an adapted multiple point stimulation method. *Muscle Nerve*, **18**, 969–979.
14. Porter CL, Alvarez A, Jones KE, Ming Chan K. (2008). Test–retest reliability of a modified multiple point stimulation technique for motor unit number estimation. *Clin Neurophysiol*, **119**, 2287–2290.
15. Erlanger J, Gasser H. (1937). *Electrical Signs of Nervous Activity*. University of Pennsylvania Press, Philadelphia.
16. Brown WF, Strong MJ, Snow R. (1988). Methods for estimating numbers of motor units in biceps-brachialis muscles and losses of motor units with aging. *Muscle Nerve*, **11**, 423–432.
17. Strong MJ, Brown WF, Hudson AJ, Snow R. (1988). Motor unit estimates in the biceps-brachialis in amyotrophic lateral sclerosis. *Muscle Nerve*, **11**, 415–422.
18. Boe SG, Stashuk DW, Doherty TJ. (2004). Motor unit number estimation by decomposition-enhanced spike-triggered averaging: control data, test-retest reliability, and contractile level effects. *Muscle Nerve*, **29**, 693–699.
19. Boe SG, Stashuk DW, Doherty TJ. (2007). Motor unit number estimates and quantitative motor unit analysis in healthy subjects and patients with amyotrophic lateral sclerosis. *Muscle Nerve*, **36**, 62–70.
20. Daube JR (2003). MUNE by statistical analysis. *Clin Neurophysiol*, **55** (Suppl), 51–82.
21. Lomen-Hoerth C, Slawnych MP. (2003). Statistical motor unit number estimation: from theory to practice. *Muscle Nerve*, **28**, 263–272.
22. Shefner JM, Cudkowicz ME, Zhang H, *et al.* (2004). The use of statistical MUNE in a multicenter clinical trial. *Muscle Nerve*, **30**, 463–469.
23. Shefner JM, Cudkowicz ME, Zhang H, *et al.* (2006). Revised statistical motor unit number estimation in the celecoxib/ALS trial. *Muscle Nerve*, **35**, 228–234.
24. Jillapalli D, Shefner JM. (2004). Single motor unit variability with threshold stimulation in patients with amyotrophic lateral sclerosis and normal subjects. *Muscle Nerve*, **30**, 578–584.
25. Shefner JM, Watson ML, David W, *et al.* (2009). *Modified Incremental MUNE in a Multicenter Natural History Study of Subjects with ALS*. International Symposium of MND/ALS, Berlin, Germany.
26. Hansen S, Ballantyne JP. (1978). A quantitative electrophysiological study of motor neurone disease. *J Neurol Neurosurg Psychiatry*, **41**, 773–783.
27. Carleton SA, Brown WF. (1979). Changes in motor unit populations in motor neurone disease. *J Neurol Neurosurg Psychiatry*, **42**, 42–51.
28. Dantes M, McComas A. (1991). The extent and time course of motoneuron involvement in amyotrophic lateral sclerosis. *Muscle Nerve*, **7**, 416–421.
29. Arasaki K, Tamaki M. (1998). A loss of functional spinal alpha motor neurons in amyotrophic lateral sclerosis. *Neurology*, **51**, 603–605.
30. Andres P, Hedlund W, Finison L, *et al.* (1986). Quantitative motor assessment in amyotrophic lateral sclerosis. *Neurology*, **36**, 937–941.
31. Andres PL, Finison LJ, Conlon T, *et al.* (1988). Use of composite scores (megascores) to measure deficit in amyotrophic lateral sclerosis. *Neurology*, **38**(3), 405–408.
32. Bromberg MB. (1993). Motor unit estimation: reproducibility of the spike-triggered averaging technique in normal and ALS subjects. *Muscle Nerve*, **16**, 466–471.
33. Bromberg MB, Larson WL. (1996). Relationships between motor-unit number estimates and isometric strength in distal muscles in ALS/MND. *J Neurol Sci*, **139** (Suppl.), 38–42.
34. Mitsumoto H, Ulug AM, Pullman SL, *et al.* (2007). Quantitative objective markers for upper and lower motor neuron dysfunction in ALS. *Neurology*, **68**, 1402–1410.
35. Felice KJ. (1997). A longitudinal study comparing thenar motor unit number estimates to other quantitative tests in patients with amyotrophic lateral sclerosis. *Muscle Nerve*, **20**, 179–185.
36. Liu XX, Zhang J, Zheng JY, *et al.* (2009). Stratifying disease stages with different progression rates determined by electrophysiological tests in patients with amyotrophic lateral sclerosis. *Muscle Nerve*, **39**, 304–309.

37. Yuen EC, Olney RK. (1997). Longitudinal study of fiber density and motor unit number estimate in patients with amyotrophic lateral sclerosis. *Neurology*, **49**, 573–578.
38. Armon C, Brandstater ME. (1999). Motor unit number estimate-based rates of progression of ALS predict patient survival. *Muscle Nerve*, **22**, 1571–1575.
39. Gurney ME, Pu H, Chiu AY, *et al.* (1994). Motor neuron degeneration in mice that express a human Cu, Zn superoxide dismutase mutation [see comments]. *Science*, **264**, 1772–1775. [Published erratum appears in Science 1995, **269**, 149.]
40. Azzouz M, Leclerc N, Gurney M, *et al.* (1997). Progressive motor neuron impairment in an animal model of familial amyotrophic lateral sclerosis. *Muscle Nerve*, **20**, 45–51.
41. Shefner JM, Reaume AG, Flood DG, S *et al.* (1999). Mice lacking cytosolic copper/zinc superoxide dismutase display a distinctive motor axonopathy. *Neurology*, **53**, 1239–1246.
42. Shefner JM, Cudkowicz M, Brown RH, Jr (2006). Motor unit number estimation predicts disease onset and survival in a transgenic mouse model of amyotrophic lateral sclerosis. *Muscle Nerve*, **34**, 603–607.
43. Reaume A, Elliot J, Hoffman E, *et al.* (1996). Motor neurons in Cu/Zn superoxide dismutase-deficient mice develop normally but exhibit enhanced cell death after axonal injury. *Nature Genetics*, **13**, 43–47.
44. Hadano S, Benn SC, Kakuta S, *et al.* (2006). Mice deficient in the Rab5 guanine nucleotide exchange factor ALS2/alsin exhibit age-dependent neurological deficits and altered endosome trafficking. *Hum Mol Genet*, **15**, 233–250.
45. Shefner J, Brown R, Cole D, *et al.* (2000). Neurophilin ligands enhance motor unit size in the FALS mouse. *Neurology*, **54**(Suppl. 3), A155.
46. Deshpande DM, Kim YS, Martinez T, *et al.* (2006). Recovery from paralysis in adult rats using embryonic stem cells. *Ann Neurol*, **60**, 32–44.

Chapter 13

Multimodality approach to neuroimaging in amyotrophic lateral sclerosis/frontotemporal dementia

Jan Kassubek and Albert C. Ludolph

At the London (Ontario) conference in June 2009, one of us (ACL) was asked to tell the story of how he got into touch with the fact that, at that time contrary to beliefs in many parts of the neurological world, amyotrophic lateral sclerosis (ALS) may not be a disease in which cognition, behaviour, and affection remains always intact and why we had already been using imaging studies in ALS since the mid-1980s.

In 1984, I was in my residency at the Department of Neurology, University of Münster, when my respected colleague and friend Dr Christian Elger (later the Chair of the Department of Epileptology, University of Bonn, Germany) approached me and asked my opinion on a 47-year-old patient who had developed asymmetric, pure motor paralysis of the legs. After we both had simultaneously examined a rich and successful businessman, we came to the unanimous conclusion that he had ALS. When we told him about the diagnosis and his likely prognosis, he was not very impressed and expressed the wish that we allow him to sell his sail boat because he had learnt that he would not need it any more. Of course, we agreed and 36 hours later the man came back to the hospital telling us that he successfully sold the boat for a good price at a place at the North Sea. However, this place was 250 km away from Münster and we asked how he had transported this middle-sized boat. He told us, without hesitation, that he used his powerful BMW, borrowed a trailer for the boat and he had built a rope system so he could handle the gas and brakes with his hands, without using his paralysed legs. In addition, he was proud to tell us that he made the trip within 2 hours, both ways.

We both came to the conclusion that this disease could therefore not be textbook ALS. And, as the *N*-isopropyl-*p*-^{123}I-amphetamine (IMP) single-photon emission computed tomography (SPECT) technique had just been made available, out of curiosity we tried to measure blood flow using this technique (Figure 13.1). We were surprised to see (although we could not quantify the IMP binding at that time) a depressed binding that we had never seen before—not seen in any other disease. This was the start of a study of normal and disease controls and patients with ALS, which was eventually published in 1989 (1). However, we still did not completely trust our results, as when we compared IMP SPECT

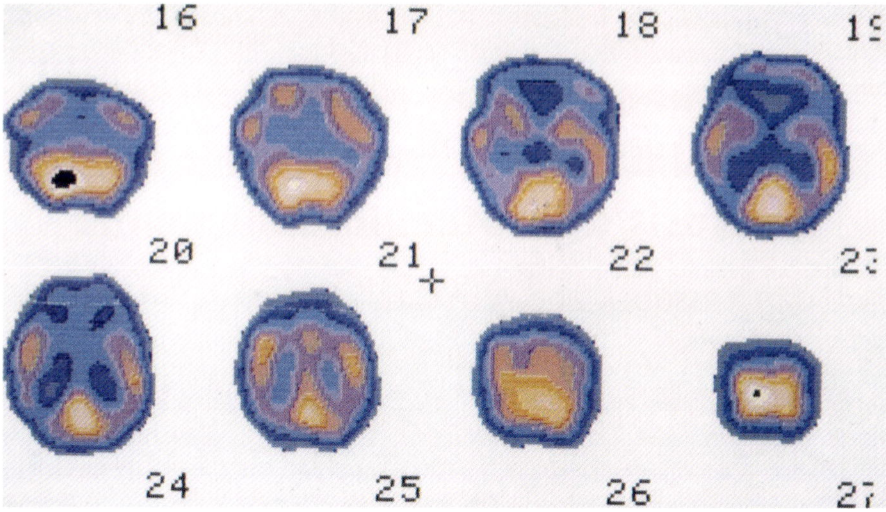

Fig. 13.1 The first IMP SPECT of a patient with ALS with clinical evidence of frontal lobe impairment (see text). Although the quality of the scans was poor and they could not be quantified, the difference to an image in a control subject was obvious.

imaging with ^{99m}Tc-hexamethylpropylene amine oxime (^{99m}TcHMPAO) imaging (unpublished) we noticed differences. The changes in ^{99m}TcHMPAO SPECT studies were also detectable but restricted to the frontal lobes or parts of it and seemingly—no methods for quantification existed—less severe.

To clarify these issues, in 1986 we teamed up with the K-J Langen group at the Department of Nuclear Medicine in Jülich to perform quantifiable glucose positron emission tomography (PET) studies and looked for support from neuropsychologists to study, in parallel, the cognition of patients with ALS, in particular frontal lobe function. Several authorities in the field declined as they thought our enterprise would turn out to be fruitless, as the cognition of patients with ALS was believed to be intact. However, we were delighted to hear that a young neuropsychologist from Freiburg, Dr Marianne Regard, liked the idea of this study. She also suggested using a new tool to study non-verbal fluency that she recently developed (later widely known as the Regard test). We followed her methodological advice, and in 1987 had obtained the complete results: at a group level, there was clear-cut evidence for deficits in glucose metabolism of the brain, which clearly exceeded the motor areas and we saw convincing deficits in tests that were thought to mirror frontal lobe function. This was particularly evident in tests that measured verbal and non-verbal fluency. In addition, both deficits—neuropsychological and imaging—seemed to correlate with each other!

We were excited about this series of findings; however, when we wanted to publish the results in one of the major neurology journals, the responses were quite unfavourable. For example, one editor wrote back: 'Dr Ludolph, I regret to say that I cannot send out your paper for review since your hypothesis seems to be wrong'. Frustrated by these responses, the results disappeared in a drawer and in a final attempt—after 4 years—the study was sent to *Acta Neurologica Scandinavica* where it was published without major objections (2). Ten years later, Herbert Schreiber showed that neuropsychological deficits were present at the beginning of the disease (at a group level) in patients with non-demented ALS and that it did not progress as fast as the motor deficits of the patients (3).

Single-photon emission computed tomography and positron emission tomography imaging in amyotrophic lateral sclerosis and amyotrophic lateral sclerosis/frontotemporal dementia

With respect to the *in vivo* investigation, patients with motor neurone disorders/ALS and the diagnosis of frontotemporal dementia (FTD)/frontotemporal lobar degeneration (FTLD), or at least neuropsychological (frontal) abnormalities at the time of clinical presentation, neuroimaging techniques have proven to be very helpful in visualizing pathological functional and/or structural findings beyond mere neuropsychological studies. The initial approaches were mostly performed using functional techniques such as PET and SPECT, both of which record the distribution of isotopic substances in the human brain administered to a subject. Here, a radiotracer marks activity in the brain, accumulating in areas of high oxygen or glucose consumption depending on the type of radionuclides, so that PET or SPECT may be used to display the basic metabolic turnover in the human brain in different pathologies. From the historical point of view, these were the first techniques to investigate the association of ALS and FTD, as described above.

For the assessment of ALS-related regional abnormalities of cerebral perfusion, the early study by use of N-isopropyl-*p*-^{123}I-amphetamine SPECT and blinded qualitative assessment in 17 non-selected ALS patients without detailed neuropsychological characterization found varying lesion patterns, i.e. global cortical reduction, multifocal reduction (including frontal/temporal areas), and frontotemporal reduction (1). These early neuroimaging studies of frontotemporal dysfunction correlates in association with motor neurone disease (MND) were supported by further SPECT studies. Ohnishi and coworkers described flow deficits by IMP SPECT in the bilateral frontal and temporal cortices in three patients with MND and progressive dementia, but no flow deficits in the parietal association cortex in contrast to eight patients with Alzheimer's disease (4). Waldemar and colleagues assessed regional cerebral blood flow (rCBF) using ^{99m}Tc-*d*, l-HMPAO SPECT, and observed reduced rCBF primarily in the frontal lobes in eight of 14 consecutive patients with ALS, of whom three had mild to moderate dementia (5). These results were in agreement with the observations of Talbot and colleagues in which 'classical' MND and FTD/MND were compared using ^{99m}Tc-HMPAO SPECT (6). In this study, reductions in rCBF were observed in both frontal and anterior temporal lobes in patients with both the 'classical' MND and FTD/MND compared with neurologically normal controls, with the findings being more pronounced in patients with FTD/MND.

While these early studies confirmed the impression of frontal or frontotemporal atrophy or dysfunction in patients with MND, they were insufficient to clearly demonstrate a true pathological association. This changed with the advent of PET. In 1992, an investigation of cerebral glucose metabolism using fluorodeoxyglucose (FDG) PET was reported in 18 patients with ALS whose neuropsychological performance with respect to frontal lobe function was studied in detail (2). Glucose metabolism was significantly reduced not only in the frontal cortex, but in the entire cortex compared with controls. The mild frontal dysfunction (impaired word and design fluency) observed as a group effect in patients with ALS in part significantly correlated with this reduced glucose metabolism in the cortex and subcortical structures. These observations were seminal in supporting the rCBF studies in providing substantive evidence of a more widespread involvement of the brain in MND.

FDG PET is still used to explore the continuum between MND and FTD and to characterize the functional cerebral lesion pattern in more detail. Here, also familial forms of ALS/MND were investigated by FDG PET, such as the finding of markedly reduced glucose uptake in both frontal and temporal lobes in a family with ALS/FTD and heterozygous R1101K mutation of the DCTN1 gene (7). In these later FDG PET studies, largely automatic postprocessing techniques mainly based upon statistical parametric mapping were taken advantage of. For example, Jeong and colleagues compared the glucose metabolism of eight patients with FTD/MND with that of 29 patients with FTD and observed regional hypometabolism circumscribed to the frontal lobe in a symmetric fashion in FTD/MND, sparing the temporal lobe, while the patients with FTD without signs of MND showed hypometabolism both in the frontal and the anterior temporal lobes (8). These data were at odds with a previous FDG PET study by Garraux and colleagues who described statistically comparable frontal and lateral temporal hypometabolism in both FTD ($n = 10$) and FTD/MND ($n = 3$), but greater impairment of medial temporal lobe activity in FTD/MND (9). However, the small samples limited generalization of results in both studies. A more recent statistical parametric mapping-based analysis of 99m Tc-ethylcysteinate perfusion SPECT by the French Research Network on FTD or FTD/MND (9), performed in 24 patients with FTD/MND versus 28 controls and 54 patients with FTD without MND, showed that both patients with FTD/MND and FTD, compared with healthy subjects, had the same pattern of predominantly symmetric and anterior hypoperfusion, involving association frontal, temporal, cingular, and insular cortices (10).

Overall, these functional imaging studies of ALS/FTD have supported the neuropsychological observations that frontal and temporal regions are consistently involved in the disease process of ALS, augmenting further the concept that ALS is a multisystem disorder. The notion that the lesion pattern is more symmetric and more pronounced in frontal areas in MND-associated FTD in contrast to other FTLD variants is heterogeneous among studies.

Later studies exploited the development of activation protocols using ^{15}O-based tracers that allowed correlation with neuropsychological measures, and the refinement of mapping techniques to delineate the extra-motor areas involved in the disease process. For example, rCBF abnormalities were specifically investigated in patients with ALS with verbal fluency deficits in two early functional PET activation studies. A group of five patients with ALS who were impaired on a verbal fluency test showed abnormalities in the medial prefrontal cortex, anterior cingulate gyrus, parahippocampal gyrus and anterior thalamus in a motor activation task while such dysfunction was less marked in patients with ALS with unimpaired verbal fluency (11). In a later investigation, verbal fluency was directly employed as the activating PET paradigm, and a group of six patients with ALS with deficits on the Written Verbal Fluency Test displayed reduced activation in extensive prefrontal regions, including the dorsolateral prefrontal cortex, medial prefrontal cortex, premotor cortices, insular cortex, and anterior thalamus, in contrast to patients with ALS who were cognitively unimpaired (12).

PET studies have, for the most part, been replaced by functional magnetic resonance imaging (fMRI). The exception, however, is the more recent focus on the use of PET-based imaging in MND/FTD using novel tracers and ligands that might identify changes in specific neurochemical and cellular systems. As one approach, PET with the benzodiazepine $GABA_A$ marker ^{11}C flumazenil was used to investigate cerebral extramotor regions (i.e. frontal and temporal areas), in addition to motor regions, as $GABA_A$ receptors are widely distributed in the cerebral cortex and are located both on pyramidal cells and interneurones. In 17 non-demented ALS patients significant decreases in relative flumazenil volumes of distribution were found in several areas, most pronounced in the prefrontal cortex (13). Additional regions with relative reductions included both the prefrontal and temporal cortex. Using the same technique, 10 patients with ALS homozygous for the *D90A SOD1* gene mutation were shown to have decreased flumazenil binding in the left frontotemporal junction, including a small cluster of regional reduction in the same area in two pre-symptomatic *D90A SOD1* mutation carriers (14). Unfortunately, other than being documented as not being demented according to DSM-IV criteria, no details on neuropsychological status were provided and thus the true clinical relevance of these findings remains uncertain.

Using ^{11}C-WAY100635 PET, a sensitive marker of *in vivo* serotonin 5-HT_{1A} receptor binding, the greatest differences were observed between patients with sporadic ALS and controls with involvement of frontotemporal regions, in addition to cingulate and lateral precentral gyri (15). However, the functional correlate of this finding in this sample of 21 ALS patients who had neither dementia nor anxiety/depressive symptoms according to DSM-IV remains unclear. The authors postulated that the impairment in ^{11}C-WAY100635 binding reflected neuronal damage but could not rule out alterations in receptor expression/function. PET with ^{11}C-labelled PK11195 as a ligand for the peripheral benzodiazepine binding site that is expressed by activated microglia demonstrated widespread cerebral microglial activation in 10 patients with ALS, including increased activity in the dorsolateral prefrontal cortex according to VOI positioning in the frontal lobe (16).

These latter studies lack a clear-cut clinical correlate in the neuropsychological domain. As discussed by others within this text, neuropsychological and language phenomenon in ALS can be subtle and are deserving of detailed assessment before their presence or absence can be confirmed. The strength of these studies, however, is that they do, as indicated, provide substantive evidence of the non-motor pathology of ALS. Efforts to augment this by combining detailed neuropsychological testing and imaging have proven fruitful. Among these, ^{11}C-flumazenil PET study was performed in 10 patients with ALS in whom mild neuropsychological deficits were observed (17). Deficits included impaired verbal fluency, a finding that correlated with decreased flumazenil binding in the inferior frontal gyrus, superior temporal gyrus, and anterior insula. Impaired performance in confrontation naming correlated with decreased ^{11}C-flumazenil binding in the left middle frontal gyrus and left cuneus, indicating cortical regions associated with cognitive deficits in ALS.

In summary, PET has provided valuable neuroimaging support for the frontotemporal involvement in the cerebral alteration pattern associated with ALS in the conceptual evolution of the MND/FTD complex. The statement in an early review on the role of PET in ALS, however, that PET studies do not provide a reliable surrogate measure for disease progression is still valid also for the MND/FTD complex (18). The potential of multimodal approaches using multitracer PET together with multiparametric MRI techniques remains to be explored.

Magnetic resonance imaging in amyotrophic lateral sclerosis

Currently, MRI has become the most widely applied neuroimaging technique in analysing brain structure and function in association with FTD/MND. In the clinical diagnostic examination of patients with ALS and cognitive or behavioural abnormalities, visual assessment of conventional MRI scans is often able to reveal volume reductions of the frontal and/or temporal lobes, which might be either symmetric or asymmetric.

Voxel-based morphometry (VBM) has been extensively used in evaluating patients with ALS with either subtle neuropsychological deficits or those with ALS/FTD. This technique compares neuroanatomical differences on a voxel by voxel basis to analyse changes in grey or white matter volumes of the brain in groups of three-dimensional MRI data sets of patients, upon the basis of automated postprocessing and standardized parametric statistics in comparison with a normal data base (19). Using this technique, Chang and colleagues contrasted 10 patients with ALS with normal cognitive and behavioural functions, 10 patients with ALS meeting clinical criteria for ALS/FTD, and 22 healthy controls (20). The authors observed large regional volume decreases in the analysis of all 20 patients with ALS versus controls. The most significant areas of atrophy were in the bilateral motor/premotor cortices and anterior portion of the superior frontal gyrus bilaterally. In addition, atrophy was also observed in the left middle and inferior frontal gyri, left posterior thalamus, bilateral superior temporal gyri, and right temporal pole. When patients with ALS/FTD were compared with patients with ALS, a greater degree of atrophy in the former was observed in the left middle frontal gyrus, left inferior frontal gyrus, and medial premotor cortex. In addition, the middle and inferior frontal gyri both showed more significant or more extended involvement in the ALS/FTD group. Thus, a frontotemporal pattern of brain atrophy in ALS/FTD but also frontal atrophy in ALS without dementia was demonstrated, in accordance with the hypothesis of a pathoanatomic continuum between the two syndromes.

Similarly, Whitwell and coworkers used VBM to contrast the MRI data of seven patients with pathologically confirmed ALS/FTLD and 11 patients with FTLD with ubiquitin-only-immunoreactive neuronal changes without signs of MND (i.e. the analysis was performed from the MRI database after the neuropathological investigation) (21). Compared with controls, the FTLD group showed grey matter volume reduction affecting bilateral frontal and temporoparietal regions, whereas the ALS/FTLD sample showed bilateral grey matter decreases mainly in the frontal lobes with minor temporal lobe atrophy. This study thus revealed a predominantly frontal lobe pattern of structural volume decrease in ALS/FTLD, whereas the more widespread pattern of atrophy in FTLD included the frontal, temporal, and parietal lobes. However, a direct comparison of ALS without dementia, ALS/FTLD, and FTLD without MND with respect to frontal and temporal affection is not possible across these two studies due to differences in the study samples and methodological differences.

In the application of VBM to ALS without dementia, a sample of 22 patients with clinically definite ALS without any signs of FTD as assessed by a standardized neuropsychological test battery showed, besides motor areas, only small regional volume decreases in the grey matter of the medial frontal gyrus (22). In another application of optimized VBM to 17 patients with probable or definite ALS, it was observed that regional cortical volume decreases in the bilateral pre- and postcentral gyrus extended to premotor, parietal, and frontal areas bilaterally (23). Although the patients in this study had no overt cognitive abnormalities, no formal neuropsychological testing was performed, which might have revealed abnormalities in that respect. This latter result was supported by another VBM study by Mezzapesa and colleagues who described grey matter reductions in extramotor areas, including the bilateral frontal and temporal lobes in 16 patients with ALS (24). Remarkably, no significant white matter atrophy was found in the ALS and ALS/FTLD groups when compared with controls and with each other by Chang and coworkers (20).

Abrahams and colleagues performed a morphometric MRI analysis of 12 patients with definite ALS with normal results in the Written Verbal Fluency Test, 11 patients with definite ALS and impaired verbal fluency, and controls (25). The authors reported extensive white matter changes that correlated with test performance and concluded that involvement of frontotemporal association fibres may underlie the cognitive abnormalities in non-demented ALS patients.

In summary, the morphometric MRI studies in ALS/FTD and ALS with cognitive/behavioural abnormalities demonstrate a pattern of widespread non-motor area changes in the sense of frontal atrophy in addition to sensorimotor cortical volume decreases, in further support of the continuum of the ALS- and FTD/MND-associated pathoanatomy. These frontal/temporal volume alterations were only observed in patients with ALS and not in other motor neurone disorders such as hereditary spastic paraparesis (26).

Another valuable modality in the study of ALS/FTD is that of diffusion tensor imaging (DTI), a MR modality that provides directional information on white matter orientation *in vivo* based upon the degree of freedom of molecular motion in nerve fibre bundles. To date, DTI has been applied mainly to visualize the fibre tracts of the motor system in ALS (27). However, two recent DTI-based studies in patients with ALS have also reported white matter changes in frontal areas. Sage and colleagues observed white matter alterations within the (pre)frontal areas and the insula (28), while Müller and colleagues reported areas of reduced white matter integrity in the frontal lobe adjacent to the middle and inferior frontal gyrus (29). Studies in patients with ALS/FTD combining MRI techniques prone to analyse white matter tract and grey matter alterations will help in an improved understanding of the pathoanatomy of the entity.

In view of this, fMRI as a non-invasive technique, to investigate dynamic processing in the human brain by measuring mainly blood flow-related effects, has supported the clinical findings of frontal cortical involvement not only in patients with ALS/FTD but also in patients with ALS and subclinical cognitive impairment (30). Findings from fMRI studies support the association of reduced frontal executive function and reduced activity in frontoparietal areas, and confirm the findings from the above-named neuroimaging studies. In 22 non-demented ALS patients, a correlation between reduced verbal fluency and reduced activity in middle and inferior frontal gyrus, anterior cingulate cortex, and parietal and temporal lobe has been observed in a fMRI study (31). There is no evidence of additional recruitment in other areas to compensate the functional loss in the frontal cortex, as has been shown for the motor system. Further differences in cortical pattern activation were observed in patients with ALS without significant cognitive impairments during the processing of socio-emotional stimuli. In this latter study, pictures of people in emotional situations were presented to 13 patients with ALS and healthy controls at an initial measurement and to 10 of these patients with ALS and controls after 6 months. Patients with ALS presented an increased activity in the right-sided supramarginal area, which is part of the social–information processing network. This difference in social–information processing pattern increased over the 6 months (32). The increased activity in the social–information processing pathway might represent an altered sensitivity to social–emotional cues in patients with ALS without cognitive deficits. Further (longitudinal) fMRI studies of different cognitive functions in patients with ALS with and without dementia might improve our understanding of the cognitive deficits associated with ALS (29).

In summary, each of the methodologies applied to imaging the brain in ALS have provided discrete bundles of information that have enhanced our understanding of the non-motor manifestations of the disease process. In general, they have provided clear evidence of pathological involvement of the frontal and temporal lobes, particularly the anterior cingulate and anterior temporal lobes, while also delineating a more widespread impairment of rCBF, discrete regions of neuronal loss (or loss of neuronal receptors) and activation of glia. The promise of MR spectroscopy (not discussed here, but see (33)) and DTI to further define the neuroanatomical substrate of the frontotemporal syndromes of ALS is as yet not fully tapped. Combining these techniques with rigorous neuropsychological evaluations will be critical. Indeed, we have come a long way from reviewers believing that we were simply wrong—the neuropsychological manifestations of ALS are indeed significant and can be clearly linked to neuroimaging correlates.

References

1. Ludolph AC, Elger CE, Böttger IW, *et al.* (1989). N-isopropyl-*p*-^{123}I-amphetamine single photon emission computer tomography in motor neuron disease. *Eur Neurol*, **29**, 255–260.
2. Ludolph AC, Langen KJ, Regard M, *et al.* (1992). Frontal lobe function in amyotrophic lateral sclerosis: a neuropsychological and positron emission tomography study. *Acta Neurol Scand*, **85**, 81–89.

3. Schreiber H, Gaigalat T, Wiedemuth-Catrinescu U, *et al.* (2005). Cognitive function in bulbar- and spinal-onset amyotrophic lateral sclerosis. *J Neurol*, **252**, 772–781.
4. Ohnishi T, Hoshi H, Nagamachi S, *et al.* (1991). Regional cerebral blood flow study with ^{123}I-IMP in patients with degenerative dementia. *Am J Neuroradiol*, **12**, 513–520.
5. Waldemar G, Varstrup S, Jensen TS, *et al.* (1992). Focal reductions in cerebral blood flow in amyotrophic lateral sclerosis: A [^{99m}Tc]-*d*, l-HMPAO SPECT study. *J Neurol Sci*, **107**, 19–28.
6. Talbot PR, Goulding PJ, Lloyd JJ, *et al.* (1995). Inter-relation between 'classic' motor neuron disease and frontotemporal dementia: neuropsychological and single photon emission computed tomography study. *J Neurol Neurosurg Psychiatry*, **58**, 541–547.
7. Münch C, Rosenbohm A, Sperfeld A-D, *et al.* (2005). Hetereozygous R1101K mutation of the *DCTN1* gene in a family with ALS and FTD. *Ann Neurol*, **58**, 777–780.
8. Jeong Y, Park KC, Cho SS, *et al.* (2005). Pattern of glucose hypometabolism in frontotemporal dementia with motor neuron disease. *Neurology*, **64**, 734–736.
9. Garraux G, Salmon E, Degueldre C, *et al.* (1999). Medial temporal lobe metabolic impairment in dementia associated with motor neuron disease. *J Neurol Sci*, **168**, 145–150.
10. Guedj E, Le Ber I, Lacomblez I, *et al.* (2007). Brain spect perfusion of frontotemporal dementia associated with motor neuron disease. *Neurology*, **69**, 488–490.
11. Kew JJM, Goldstein LH, Leigh PN, *et al.* (1993). The relationship between abnormalities of cognitive function and cerebral activation in amyotrophic lateral sclerosis. *Brain*, **116**, 1399–1423.
12. Abrahams S, Goldstein LH, Kew JJM, *et al.* (1996). Frontal lobe dysfunction in amyotrophic lateral sclerosis. A PET study. *Brain*, **119**, 2105–2120.
13. Lloyd CM, Richardson MP, Brooks DJ, *et al.* (2000). Extramotor involvement in ALS: PET studies with the $GABA_A$ ligand [^{11}C]flumazenil. *Brain*, **123**, 2289–2296.
14. Turner MR, Hammers A, Al-Chalabi A, *et al.* (2005). Distinct cerebral lesions in sporadic and 'D90A' *SOD1* ALS: studies with [^{11}C]flumazenil PET. *Brain*, **128**, 1323–1329.
15. Turner MR, Rabiner EA, Hammers A, *et al.* (2005). [^{11}C]-WAY100635 PET demonstrates marked 5-HT_{1A} receptor changes in sporadic ALS. *Brain*, **128**, 896–905.
16. Turner MR, Cagnin A, Turkheimer FE, *et al.* (2004). Evidence of widespread cerebral microglial activation in amyotrophic lateral sclerosis: an [^{11}C](R)-PK11195 positron emission tomography study. *Neurobiol Dis*, **15**, 601–609.
17. Wicks P, Turner MR, Abrahams S, *et al.* (2008). Neuronal loss associated with cognitive performance in amyotrophic lateral sclerosis: an [11C]-flumazenil PET study. *Amyotroph Lateral Scler*, **9**, 43–49.
18. Turner MR, Leigh PN. (2000). Positron emission tomography (PET)—its potential to provide surrogate markers in ALS. *Amyotroph Lateral Scler Other Motor Neuron Disord*, **1**, S17–S22.
19. Grosskreutz J, Peschel T, Unrath A, *et al.* (2008). Whole brain-based computerized neuroimaging in ALS and other motor neuron disorders. *Amyotroph Lateral Scler*, **9**, 238–248.
20. Chang JL, Lomen-Hoerth C, Murphy J, *et al.* (2005). A voxel-based morphometry study of patterns of brain atrophy in ALS and ALS/FTLD. *Neurology*, **65**, 75–80.
21. Whitwell JL, Jack CR, Jr, Senjem ML, *et al.* (2006). Patterns of atrophy in pathlogically confirmed FTLD with and without motor neuron degeneration. *Neurology*, **66**, 102–104.
22. Kassubek J, Unrath A, Huppertz HJ, *et al.* (2005). Global brain atrophy and corticospinal tract alterations in ALS, as investigated by voxel-based morphometry of 3-D MRI. *Amyotroph Lateral Scler*, **6**, 213–220.
23. Grosskreutz J, Kaufmann J, Fradrich J, *et al.* (2006). Widespread sensorimotor and frontal cortical atrophy in amyotrophic lateral sclerosis. *BMC Neurol*, **6**, 17.
24. Mezzapesa DM, Ceccarelli A, Dicuonzo F, *et al.* (2007). Whole-brain and regional brain atrophy in amyotrophic lateral sclerosis. *Am J Neuroadiol*, **28**, 255–259.
25. Abrahams S, Goldstein LH, Suckling J, *et al.* (2005). Frontotemporal white matter changes in amyotrophic lateral sclerosis. *J Neurol*, **252**, 321–331.

26. Kassubek J, Juengling FD, Baumgartner A, *et al.* (2007). Different regional brain volume loss in pure and complicated hereditary spastic paraparesis: a voxel-based morphometric study. *Amyotroph Lateral Scler*, **8**, 328–336.
27. Turner MR, Kiernan MC, Leigh PN, *et al.* (2009). Biomarkers in amyotrophic lateral sclerosis. *Lancet Neurol*, **8**, 94–109.
28. Sage CA, Van HW, Peeters R, *et al.* (2009). Quantitative diffusion tensor imaging in amyotrophic lateral sclerosis: revisited. *Hum Brain Mapp*, **30**, 3657–3675.
29. Müller HP, Lule D, Unrath A, *et al.* (2011). Complementary image analysis of diffusion tensor imaging and 3-dimensional t1-weighted imaging: white matter analysis in amyotrophic lateral sclerosis. *J Neuroimaging*, **21**, 24–33.
30. Lule D, Ludolph AC, Kassubek J. (2009). MRI-based functional neuroimaging in ALS: an update. *Amyotroph Lateral Scler*, **10**, 258–268.
31. Abrahams S, Goldstein LH, Simmons A, *et al.* (2004). Word retrieval in amyotrophic lateral sclerosis: a functional magnetic resonance imaging study. *Brain*, **127**, 1507–1517.
32. Lule D, Diekmann V, Anders S, *et al.* (2007). Brain responses to emotional stimuli in patients with amyotrophic lateral sclerosis (ALS). *J Neurol*, **254**, 519–527.
33. Strong MJ, Grace GM, Orange JB, *et al.* (1999). A prospective study of cognitive impairment in ALS. *Neurology*, **53**, 1665–1670.

Chapter 14

Using neuroimaging to understand brain–behaviour relationships in the context of motor neurone disease

Sandra E. Black and Yana Yunusova

Traditionally, amyotrophic lateral sclerosis (ALS) was considered a lethal single-system disease that destroyed upper (UMN) and lower motor neurones (LMN). However, it is very clinically heterogeneous in the motor signs first manifested, the extent of extramotor involvement, and progression rate. Cognitive-behavioural syndromes such as behavioural variant frontotemporal lobar degeneration (bvFTLD), or primary progressive aphasia, may initiate, predominate, or emerge as the disease progresses. Rapid motor decline, including severe dysarthria can make cognitive assessment difficult, when motor symptoms manifest first, and the shortened lifespan may prevent expression of cognitive deficits. Now recognized to be a multisystem disease, its variety of endophenotypes are being elucidated through genetic, biochemical, neuroimaging, and pathological studies (1).

Advances in neuroimaging, including computational analysis, are increasingly important in capturing in vivo patterns of brain degeneration not readily apparent by qualitative interpretation of structural scans. In particular, functional imaging using single-photon emission computerized tomography (SPECT) or ^{18}fluorodeoxy glucose positron emission tomography (PET), magnetic resonance spectroscopy (MRS), diffusion tensor imaging (DTI), and quantitative structural magnetic resonance imaging (MRI) analysis, can be used to quantify distribution and severity of neuropathology in life. DTI provides a means to map microstructural change in motor projections and association tracts that may prove useful not only in correlation with symptomatology but also in predicting progression patterns and guiding treatment.

An important landmark study of 42 patients with sporadic ALS demonstrated that neuropathology was more widespread than the motor neurone system in the 27 post-mortem cases, eight of whom had parkinsonism–ALS dementia, seven had substantia nigra degeneration, and one had Alzheimer's disease (AD). Many had vacuolation in specific areas of the frontal cortices (2) The multisystem nature of ALS has been validated in subsequent studies (3,4). Subsequent studies have also confirmed cognitive deficits in about 30% of patients with sporadic ALS and 15% of familial ALS cases. Moreover, new insights have been gained into the molecular neuropathology within the family of frontotemporal lobar degeneration with transactive response DNA-binding protein of 43 kDa and fused in sarcoma proteinopathies accounting for many cases of FTLD-ubiquitin/ALS (5).

This chapter will summarize neuroimaging advances pioneered in the study of AD exemplified by the Alzheimer's Disease Neuroimaging Initiative (ADNI) and show how different imaging modalities can be applied to ALS, such as SPECT and PET, with new ligands on the horizon, and multimodal MRI, ranging from tissue volumetrics, DTI, MEG to resting-state and activation functional (MRI) fMRI. We will show how clinical imaging can help diagnosis in a case example. We will review how neuroimaging can provide diagnostic biomarkers to detect early disease and document heterogeneity, follow course and monitor therapy (6), and understand the brain–behaviour relationship in neurodegenerative disorders using different MR modalities, with an emphasis on DTI, which has been the most widely applied advance technique in ALS.

Case example

Ascertainment of neurocognitive-behavioural deficits in ALS may depend on how the patient presents. Usually with motor presentations, the patient is seen in neuromuscular clinics where the focus is on management of motor deficits, whereas patients presenting with cognitive-behavioural symptomatology are often seen in memory clinics, where subtle motor deficits may initially go unnoticed, though as they emerge they may dominate and accelerate the terminal stages. An illustrative case in point is a 55-year old man with a 2-year history of memory loss and anomia, who was still working as an accountant and jogging 10 miles daily. His mother was diagnosed with AD, at age 64, as were a maternal uncle and cousin. He was initially thought to have AD, but started to demonstrate subtle changes in personality. He was becoming irritable, temperamental, and disinhibited. He began to make sexual propositions to his sister-in-law when she and her family came to visit from out of town. He was less empathetic and became emotionally distant from his wife and sons. He enjoyed speeding through stop signs for excitement in the rural area where they lived. One day, when the small family dog nipped his finger while being bathed, he proceeded to beat the dog almost to death, and was unapologetic when the family managed to rescue the poor creature and expressed dismay at this aggressive behaviour.

On initial examination, he was neurologically normal with a Mini Mental State exam of 27/30 and on more detailed testing, he showed poor short-term memory, decreased phonemic fluency, concreteness in proverbs and similarities, and impairments in many other executive functions. Visuospatial skills and speech were intact, though he was circumlocutory. On the Frontal Behavioral Inventory, he scored 17, with 26 being the usual cut-off for frontotemporal dementia (FTD) (7).

His baseline scans are shown in Figures 14.1(a) and 14.2(a). The MR was interpreted to be normal, but the SPECT scan, using ethylcysteinate dimer SPECT with a triple-head camera, showed subtle decreased perfusion bilaterally in the inferior and dorsolateral frontal regions and left temporal region. A diagnosis of bvFTLD was made. Over the next year, he showed more anomia and paraphasias, more mental rigidity and concreteness. He had to stop working. His scans showed more frontal atrophy and worsening frontal–temporal hypoperfusion (Figures 14.1b and 14.2b and Tables 14.1 and 14.2). At home he began to wander, became aggressive and agitated, and soon required placement in a locked psychogeriatric facility. Over the next few months he became mute and developed swallowing difficulties with leg weakness and reduced mobility, which solved his exiting behaviour. He had both UMN and LMN signs and was diagnosed with FTLD/ALS. He died of aspiration 30 weeks after his first memory clinic visit. Autopsy showed ubiquitin-positive, tau-negative neuropathology with nuclear inclusions, consistent with FTLD-ubiquitin. He demonstrates that functional imaging can help support an FTD diagnosis and can track the clinical and neurobehavioural decline.

Structural imaging

CT has played a minor role in the diagnosis of ALS, although when bvFTLD or primary progressive aphasia occurs early, frontal and temporal atrophy may be perceived even on CT. In disturbed patients or those with marked dysphagia who may find lying supine too difficult for MRI, CT can be useful to rule out other pathologies and screen for atrophy patterns.

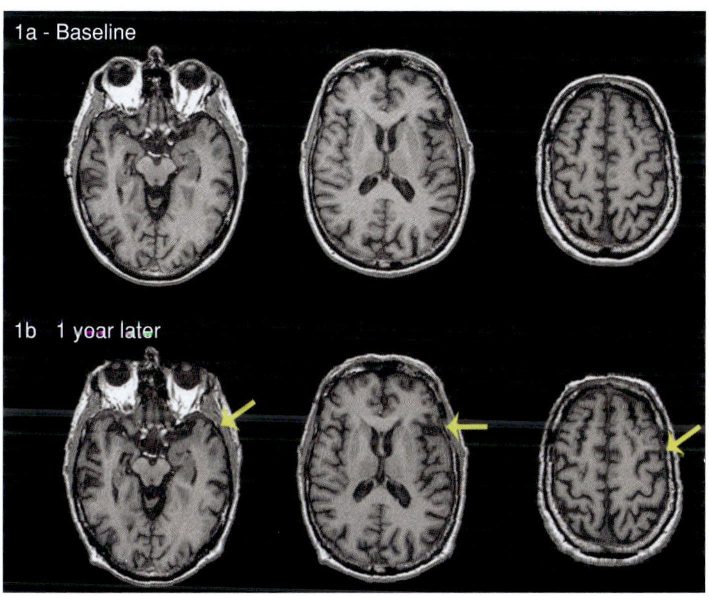

Fig. 14.1 Structural changes detectable by SABRE in a 56-year-old man with FTD/ALS. (a) T1-weighted scan at baseline. (b) Co-registered T1-weighted scan at 1-year follow-up, with arrows indicating regions of increased atrophy.

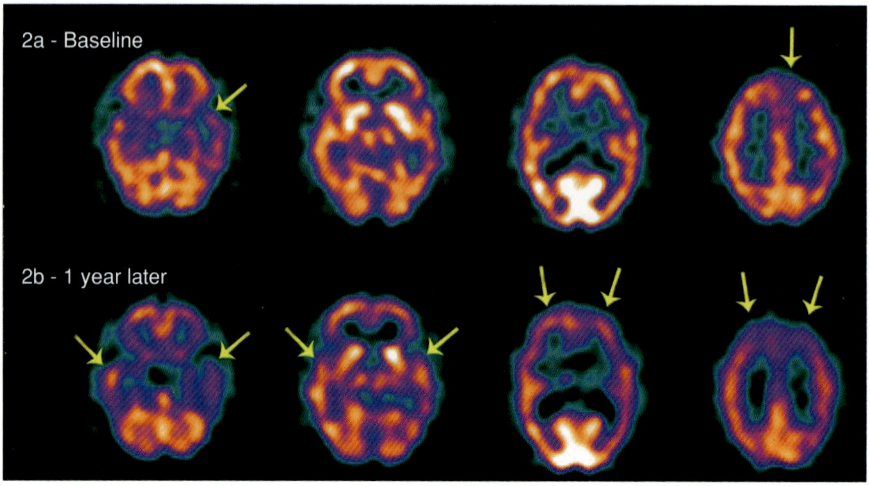

Fig. 14.2 SPECT perfusion changes in a 56-year-old man with FTD/ALS, with arrows indicating regions of decreased perfusion.

Conventional MR techniques are relatively insensitive to detection of UMN abnormalities in ALS (8,9). A recent study, combining proton density/T2-weighted, and FLAIR imaging, showed they are 62% sensitive in detecting hyperintensities along the corticospinal tract (CST) in patients with ALS (10). Conventional MRI, however, remains an essential screening tool to rule out ALS mimics such as cervical spondylosis or cerebral lesions.

Table 14.1 Volumetric changes over 1 year, with corresponding normal values, from subject shown in Figure 14.1

	GM % change–baseline to 1 year	WM % change–baseline to 1 year	Volume change (cm^3)–baseline to 1 year
FTD/ALS subject shown in Figure 14.1			
Left inferior frontal	–4.84	–16.98	–1.89
Left medial inferior frontal	–10.10	–8.24	–1.35
Left anterior temporal	–10.48	–8.52	–2.14
Right inferior frontal	–5.64	–20.75	–1.82
Right medial inferior frontal	–1.97	–13.00	–1.17
Right anterior temporal	–8.97	–4.15	–2.08
Mean of 45 age-matched controls			
Left inferior frontal	2.82	–1.13	0.02
Left medial inferior frontal	–5.00	–1.40	–0.33
Left anterior temporal	–1.57	0.19	–0.06
Right inferior frontal	–3.52	–2.94	–0.40
Right medial inferior frontal	–3.33	–0.98	–0.25
Right anterior temporal	0.22	–1.65	–0.26

Table 14.2 FTD+ALS subject–% SPECT perfusion change–baseline to 1 year, from subject shown in Figure 14.2

	Dorsal inferior frontal gyrus	Ventral inferior frontal gyrus	Dorsal middle frontal gyrus	Ventral middle frontal gyrus	Orbitofrontal gyrus	Dorsal superior frontal gyrus	Ventral superior frontal gyrus	Temporal pole
Left	–20.2	–17.8	–12.1	–11.7	–13.4	–14.2	–13.7	–28.0
Right	–7.2	–24.2	–15.9	–15.7	–15.1	–9.3	–14.1	–23.0

The Alzheimer's Disease Neuroimaging Initiative (ADNI), in which patients with possible prodromal AD ($n = 398$), mild AD ($n = 192$), healthy age-matched controls ($n = 229$) are being followed every 6 months for 2–5 years, has been a major catalyst for the use of structural imaging in neurodegenerative diseases (http://www.adni-info.org/). The project has broken new ground by developing cross-platform standardized phantom-corrected protocols permitting valid comparison across 50 North American sites (11). It has driven progress in developing automatic brain imaging analyses with the major goals being early diagnosis and development of reliable, pragmatic imaging biomarkers as surrogate outcomes for proof of concept studies and for reducing sample size in phase I–II clinical trials of disease-modifying therapies.

There are many lessons from this project for ALS. In AD, there is a 20-year lead in quantitative brain imaging analysis focused on focal atrophy of the hippocampus, a major target of the disease, as well as posterior cingulate and parietal–temporal atrophy, which are also known to be hypometabolic on glucose PET for almost 30 years. AD subjects show more rapid rates of brain volume loss, making the disease amenable to the use of quantitative structural imaging measures for early detection, prognostication, and monitoring disease course. Well over 250 papers have been published in the last 5 years since the project began, the majority relating to structural imaging techniques in AD using computational methodologies, such as co-registration to detect progression changes, tensor-based and voxel-based morphometry (VBM), automatic segmentation and shape analysis of the hippocampus, cortical thickness mapping, quantification of white matter (WM) disease, etc. (11).

Subsets of ADNI participants have also undergone 18-fluorodeoxyglucose PET to examine glucose metabolism and amyloid labelling PET with Pittsburgh Compound (12,13) and ^{18}F florbetapir, an ^{18}F-amyloid label, is being used in the ADNI extensions (14). This is relevant not only for AD but other disorders, as the ADNI study provides comparative data on normal controls and patients with AD, which is publicly available for download. New ^{18}F-amyloid labels, ^{18}F-flutemetemol and ^{18}F-florbetaben are also in development. These labelled compounds are more useful in a clinical setting because they do not require an on site cyclotron as does ^{11}C-labelled Pittsburgh Compound-B Molecular Imaging as well as multiple MR acquisition techniques allow multimodal imaging, which may prove valuable in diagnosis and management of other neurodegenerations, such as ALS ± FTD. Apart from individuals in whom FTD may appear early in the course, ALS cases typically presenting to ALS clinics may show no obvious focal brain atrophy. Computationally aided imaging analysis techniques, such as cortical thickness mapping, might be able to show differences between patients with ALS and controls. Whether these analyses will be clinically meaningful need to be explored in ALS populations. We will highlight studies applying these different techniques as well as MRS, fMRI, and DTI to understand brain–behavioural relationships in ALS.

Computational structural analysis in amyotrophic lateral sclerosis/frontotemporal dementia shows extramotor involvement

As mentioned, the topographical selectivity of typical AD, preferentially involving parietal posterior and medial temporal regions versus typical FTD, in which frontal and anterior temporal changes predominate, has been the basis for using metabolic (glucose PET) and cerebral blood flow (SPECT) for differential diagnosis of these two dementias for a few decades. Region of interest (ROI) (15) as well as statistical parametric mapping methods (16) can be used to compare and contrast groups as well as correlate findings with clinical findings. Similar approaches can be applied to three-dimensional, high-resolution T1-weighted images. Figure 14.3 (and Table 14.3a,b) demonstrates the ROI approach, a semiautomatic technique to analyse MRI scans called SABRE (17–20). A different automatic parcellation using Freesurfer (http://surfer.nmr.mgh.harvard.edu/), has been applied to 10 cases of primary lateral sclerosis (PLS), and showed that the frontal lobes, precentral cortex, corpus callosum, and total brain volume were smaller than in controls (21). Whole-brain approaches such as VBM are also becoming popular in ALS (22–24). When applied to AD and FTD populations, the contrasting posterior and anterior predilections can be shown, but there is topographical overlap in the medial and lateral temporal and dorsolateral frontal regions (25). Using this technique, Seeley *et al.* mapped out the anatomically dissociable neuronal systems targeted by AD and different subtypes of FTD, noting the right insula as a focal target of bvFTD (26). The selective topographies of nonfluent and fluent primary progressive aphasia have been demonstrated, (27) and more grey matter atrophy has been shown in FTLD-tau versus FTLD-ubiquitin cases in the caudate and genu of the corpus callosum (28). Rosen *et al.* showed specific brain atrophy correlations between various cingulate regions and disinhibition, apathy, and aberrant motor behaviours (29). Specifically in ALS, relative grey matter atrophy was shown in and around the central gyrus extending towards the parietal region, and in spinal muscular atrophy there were widespread WM changes (30). One study showed cortical thinning in the primary motor cortex and conjunction with decreased fractional anisotropy (FA) and increased apparent diffusion coefficient (ADC) in the CST in a small sample of ALS (31).

^{1}H Magnetic resonance spectroscopy can monitor change and possible treatment effects in amyotrophic lateral sclerosis

MRS studies in ALS have shown decreased *N*-acetyl aspartate/choline ratios in the mid-cingulate cortex (32), and *N*-acetyl aspartate measures in the motor cortex correlated with disease progression over time in other series (33,34), suggesting it may be a useful

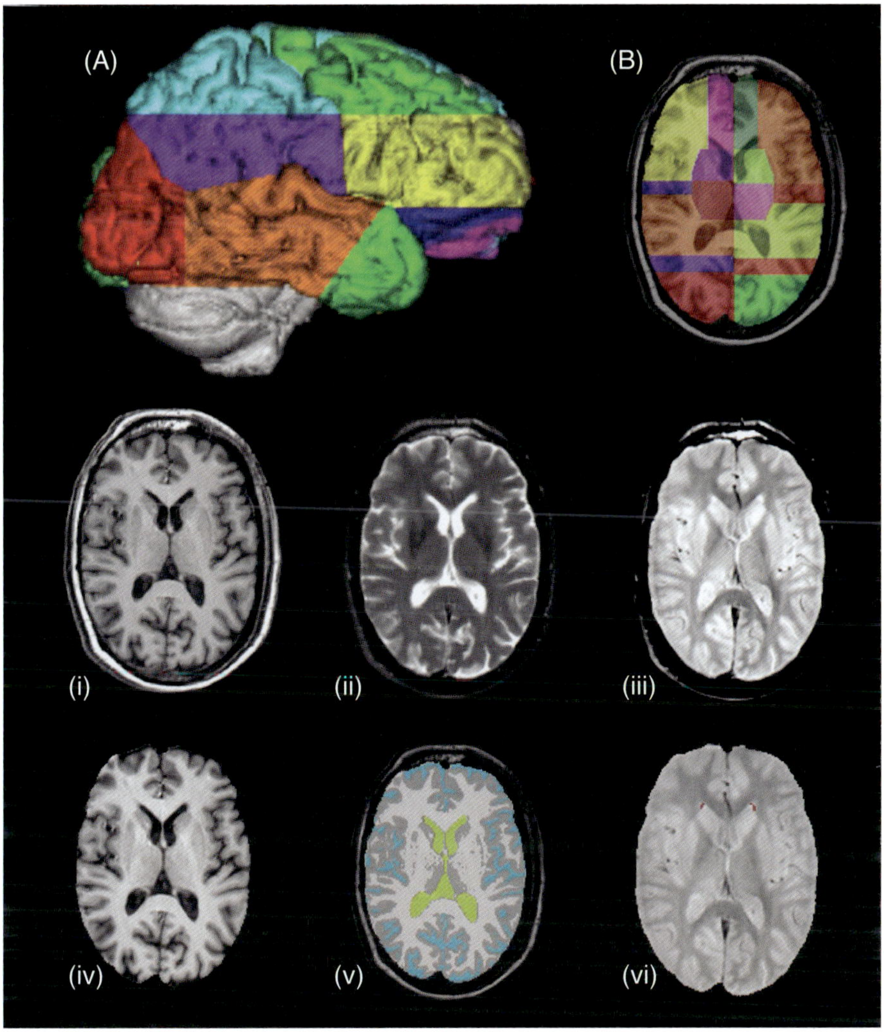

Fig. 14.3 MRI pipeline using SABRE and Lesion Explorer on a 58-year-old woman with ALS. (A) Three-dimensional, surface cerebrospinal fluid (CSF) eroded, T1-weighted brain with SABRE parcellated regions overlayed with different colours denoting different brain regions. (B) Axial view showing same as in (A). (i) T1-weighted image; (ii) T2-weighted image; (iii) proton density image; (iv) skull-stripped T1; (v) T1-segmentation showing gray matter, white matter, sulcal CSF, and ventricular CSF; and (vi) skull-stripped proton density with white matter hyperintensity (WMH) overlay in red.

progression marker. In fact, feasibility studies have used ^{1}H-MRS to monitor changes with treatment with riluzole (35,36), brain-delivered neurotrophic factor (37), and gabapentin therapy (38). Specifically, Kalra and colleagues found that riluzole treatment, the only intervention proven to prolong survival in patients with ALS, was associated with less reduction in *N*-acetyl aspartate/choline ratio in the primary and supplementary motor areas, but not in the post-central gyrus or parietal lobe.

Table 14.3 Tissue Compartment Volumes ALS Patient Compared to Controls

	Total intracranial capacity	Ventricular CSF	Sulcal CSF	Gray matter	White matter	WMH
(a) Sample tissue compartment volumes from the subject shown in Figure 14.3 (in cm^3)						
Volume (cm^3)	1138.3	24.8	179.6	527.7	404.3	1.9
% of total intracranial capacity		2.2	15.8	46.3	35.5	0.2
(b) Comparison mean tissue compartment volumes from eight cognitively normal women (mean age 60.5)						
Volume (cm^3)	1176.2	22.4	180.1	549.3	421.9	2.4
% of total intracranial capacity		1.9	15.3	46.7	35.9	0.2

CSF, cerebrospinal fluid.

Functional magnetic resonance imaging reveals compensatory changes in early amyotrophic lateral sclerosis

fMRI studies have also been undertaken in ALS. One ALS series found increasing bold activation patterns in ALS, paralleling severity of decline, in imagery for right hand movement with recruitment of the premotor regions. In response to emotional stimuli, there was increased activation of the right supramarginal region, suggesting compensatory recruitment (39). Li *et al.* used both DTI and fMRI to study swallowing in patients with ALS with and without dysphagia, and found that patients without dysphagia showed increased activation involving the primary sensory, inferior parietal, and middle cingulate regions, whereas those with dysphagia showed marked decreased activation in the postcentral, anterior, and medial frontal, and supplementary motor areas. FA on DTI was decreased in both groups, more so with dysphagia, but in different regions (40). The study demonstrated the complementary information offered by the two techniques, and that fMRI shows recruitment of nearby regions in the pre-symptomatic phase.

Diffusion tensor imaging may be sensitive for early detection and monitoring disease progression

DTI measures the diffusion of water molecules along a predetermined axis, using direction-dependent anisotropic diffusion, which occurs when water molecules encounter barriers such as axonal membranes, microtubules, and myelin sheathes (41). A commonly used DTI metric is FA, defined as the degree of directionality of diffusion, ranging from 0, representing the most direction-independent FA, to 1, indicating a direction along a single axis. The magnitude of diffusion is called mean diffusivity (MD), and the measure of bulk diffusion is the ADC. These measures can be taken at specific sites (ROIs) or across multiple regions. They show inconsistent results across studies with respect to between-group differences and correlations between the imaging parameters and measures of disease severity and progression. As an alternative to these traditional measures, which is independent of the direction of water diffusion, axial (DA) and radial diffusivity (DR) have

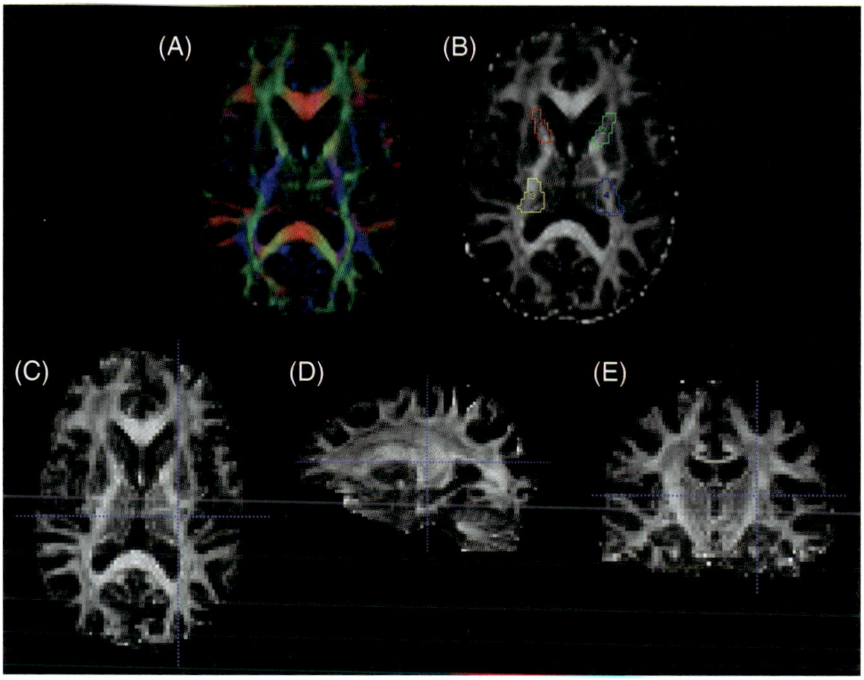

Fig. 14.4 Fractional anisotropy (FA) measures on a 58-year-old woman with ALS. (A) Colourized FA map showing tract directionality. (B) Axial FA map through anterior and posterior limbs of the internal capsule, showing ROIs from which to sample FA. (C) Axial FA map. (D) Sagittal FA map. (E) Coronal FA map.

been used more recently (42). DA represents the largest eigenvalue in the direction parallel to the fibre bundles, while DR represents the average of the two smallest eigenvalues, perpendicular to the direction of the axons.

One of the most unique features of DTI is tractography and colour maps, based on pixel by pixel analysis of fibre track orientation combined into a cohesive representation. Although specific fibres cannot be identified using DTI, tract-specific quantitative studies can be conducted, particularly with relatively prominent tracts. These maps can also be used to identify ROI for more detailed regional analyses of DTI parameters (see Figure 14.4 and Table 14.4a,b).

Changes in these measures relative to normal values are attributed to neuronal loss, axonal changes, including demyelination, glial cell proliferation, as well as extracellular matrix expansion (43,44). However, the specific mechanisms changing DTI parameters remain. A detailed description of WM neuroanatomy and integrity provided by DTI is relevant to many neurodegenerative diseases, particularly the ones that might be associated with damage to specific WM tracts (e.g. ALS, FTD, multiple sclerosis).

Diffusion tensor imaging and amyotrophic lateral sclerosis

DTI has generated a lot of excitement in ALS imaging as it affects specific tracts, such as the pyramidal tract (CST and cortical bulbar tract), probably the largest and most coherent

Table 14.4 (a) Sample fractional anisotropy values from the four ROIs shown in Figure 14.4(B); (b) Comparison fractional anisotropy values from a group of 10 normal controls (mean age 65)

	(1) Right anterior limb internal capsule	(2) Left anterior limb internal capsule	(3) Right posterior limb internal capsule	(4) Left posterior limb internal capsule
(a) Fractional anisotropy values, mean (SD)	0.41 (0.16)	0.41 (0.16)	0.49 (0.17)	0.42 (0.16)
(b) Mean fractional anisotropy values, mean (SD)	0.43 (0.15)	0.43 (0.16)	0.50 (0.15)	0.49 (0.16)

tract in the brain (Figure 14.5). DTI provides an index for UMN disease by quantifying integrity of the pyramidal and other tracts (45), applications of which are discussed below.

Regional differences between patients and normal controls

Early studies showed significant reduction in FA and increase in MD in the internal capsule of ALS patients (46). Further studies revealed mixed results, however, with inconsistencies in the regional distribution of abnormalities and measures affected (45–48). Across studies, the posterior limb of the internal capsule, cerebral peduncles, and corona radiata have emerged as most consistently revealing UMN pathology in ALS (23,46,47,49,50). Graham and colleagues showed reduction in FA in patients with ALS compared with controls in the posterior third of the posterior limb of the internal capsule, composed of the densely packed

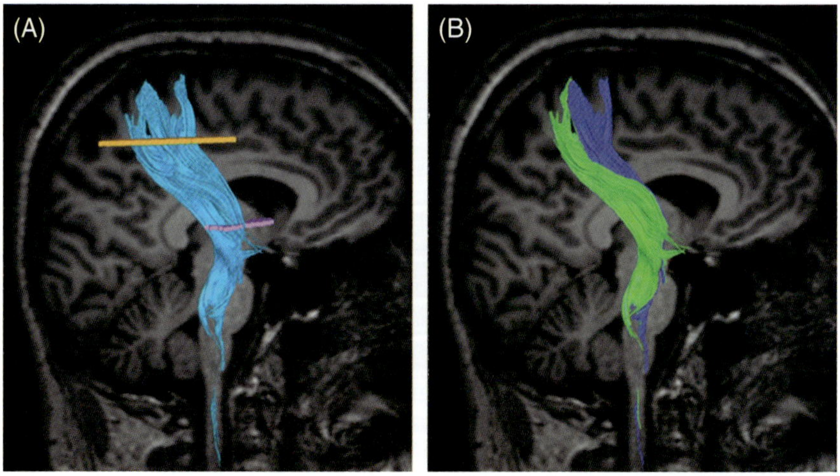

Fig. 14.5 (A) Representative example of fibre tracking of the mean CST. This tract was reconstructed by tracking through a ROI containing the pre- and postcentral gyrus (orange) and a ROI placed on the posterior limb of the internal capsule (purple). (B) Separation of mean CST was done by limiting the upper ROI to the precentral gyrus for reconstruction of the precentral CST (blue) and to the postcentral gyrus for the reconstruction of the postcentral CST (green) and using the same ROI in the internal capsule as used for reconstruction of mean CST. The reconstructed tracts are overlaid on a sagittal view of a 3D-TFE image for anatomical reference. Reprinted with permission from *Neuroimage* 2007: **34**: 486–499. ©2007. Elsevier Ltd.

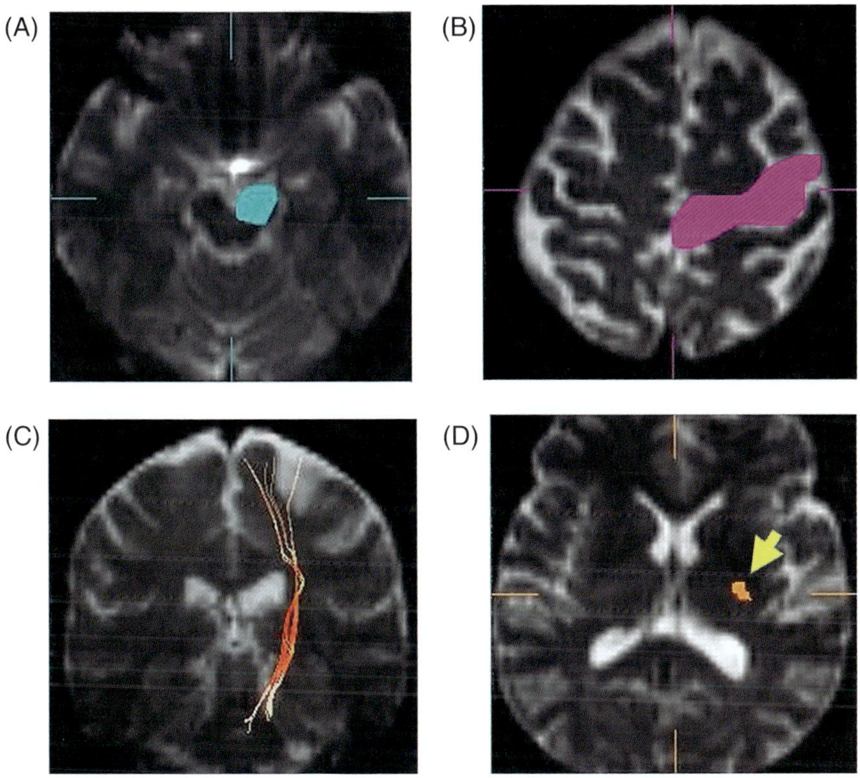

Fig. 14.6 ROI for internal capsule. T2-weighted images showing the seed area to be the cerebral peduncle (A), and the target area to be the precentral gyrus (B). The entire pyramidal tract is shown (C). The ROI in the internal capsule is enclosed within closed curves drawn to define the visualized pyramidal tracts (yellow arrow) (D). With permission from Informa healthcare, Joe Senda, Mizuki Ito, Hirohisa Watanabe et al, Correlation between pyramidal tract degeneration and widespread white matter involvement in amyotrophic lateral sclerosis: A study with tractography and diffusion-tensor imaging, *Amyotrophic Lateral Sclerosis* 2009, Vol. **10**, No. 5–6 , Pages 288–294.

fibres of the CST (47) (see Figures 14.6 and 14.7). Hong and colleagues studied FA along the CST in the brainstem and found that the most consistent group differences were observed at the cerebral peduncles (see Figure 14.6) (50). The authors concluded that due to the high values and consistency of FA across slices in this region, the cerebral peduncles would be an ideal region to investigate UMN pathology in ALS. Filippini and colleagues studied the corpus callosum in patients with ALS and found significant FA differences in the region of the corpus callosum where fibres link the motor and premotor cortices (23,51).

Limited attempts have been made to detect changes in DTI measures in the cortical bulbar tract, implicated in approximately 30% of patients with bulbar-onset ALS, the fastest progressing form of the disease. Cortical bulbar tract is difficult to study due to its size and non-distinctive nature. However, despite the difficulties, successful attempts have been made to localize the tract and compute its DTI indices (52,53). Both studies revealed a significant reduction in FA in patients with bulbar as compared with limb-onset ALS, with both patient subgroups showing reduction relative to controls.

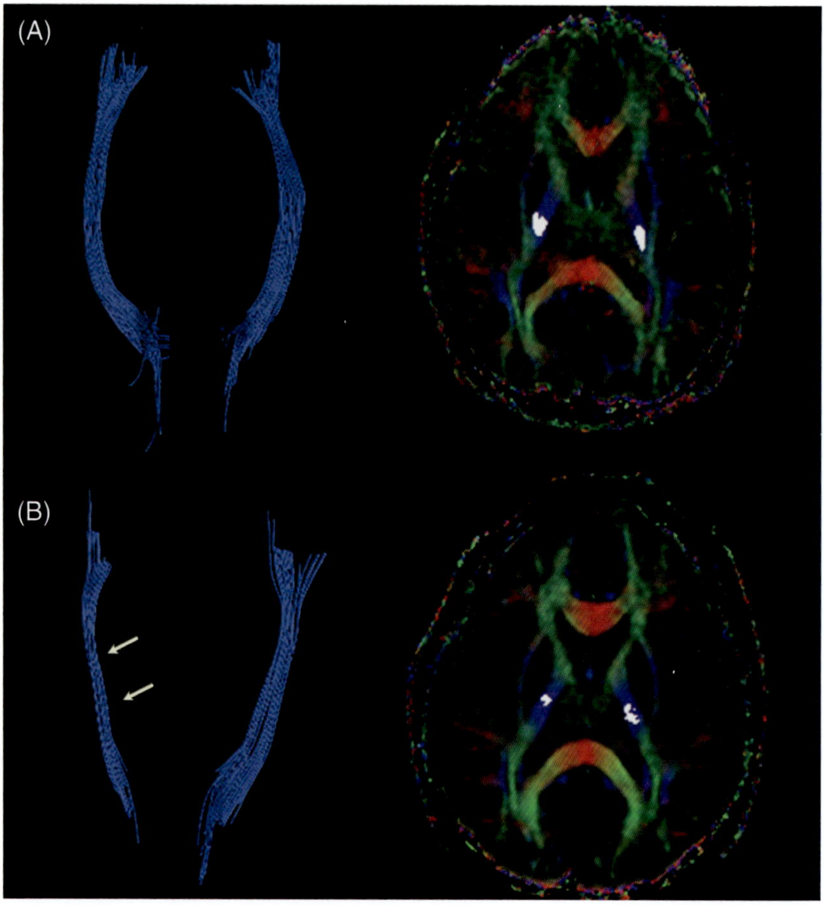

Fig. 14.7 CST in normal volunteers and patients with ALS. CST analysed by fibre tractography displayed as three-dimensional fibre bundles (left) and overlaid on conventional axial colour maps (right) from a normal volunteer (A) and a patient with ALS (B). The right CST in the patient with ALS shows decreased fibre bundles (arrows) compared with the normal volunteers. With permission from Hong Yin, Sandy HT Cheng, Jian Zhang, Lin Ma, Yuangui Gao, Dejun Li, CC Tchoyoson Lim, Corticospinal Tract Degeneration in Amyotrophic Lateral Sclerosis: A Diffusion Tensor Imaging and Fibre Tractography Study, *Ann Acad Med Singapore* 2008; **37**:411–5.

Comparative sensitivity of diffusion tensor imaging measures

There are inconsistencies in the literature regarding the most sensitive DTI metrics to detect abnormalities in WM in patients with ALS. FA and MD commonly emerged as sensitive, yet location-dependent, indices (46,54,55). However, Karlsborg and colleagues found that ADC was most consistently different at various levels in the CST compared with FA and deemed it more sensitive (45). Considering the differences in the DTI measures across different subject samples in various studies, as well as the differences in their associations with clinical findings (e.g. Amyotrophic Lateral Sclerosis Functional Rating Scale (ALSFRS), disease duration), these DTI measures may be probing different pathological effects (49). FA may be sensitive to axonal degeneration and changes at the earlier phases of the disease, whereas changes in MD may reflect astrocytic gliosis and demyelination, occurring later in the course (46,47). An increase in DR but not DA along the CST in patients with ALS was reported in a number of studies (56–59). This finding has been interpreted as evidence of dysmyelination as well as changes in axonal size (diameter) and the composition of the axonal wall in ALS (43,44). Noteworthy correlations of DR with clinical measures of UMN involvement were observed in CST (59) and cervical spinal cord (60). FA differences might be masked by simultaneous changes in DR and DA. Recently, DR and DA were shown to be more sensitive to disease-related changes compared with FA in a group of patients with ALS (61).

Early detection and differential diagnosis

Ideally, a diagnostic imaging marker should be able to detect changes in the brain as early as possible and to be able to distinguish ALS from other conditions. Early detection of UMN involvement is important because LMN symptoms often mask UMN pathology, which confounds the diagnosis of ALS. Preliminary evidence suggests DTI might reveal UMN pathology in the absence of the clinical signs and symptoms. Sach and colleagues examined a small group of patients without clinical UMN signs at the time of the MRI examination and found reduced FA in the corona radiata and the posterior half of the posterior limb of the internal capsule. Their patients developed UMN signs later as the disease progressed (54). Similarly, four patients with predominantly LMN signs exhibited lower FA scores compared with controls, suggesting underlying undetected UMN pathology (47). However, these patients were not tracked over time, so the evidence is still too limited to pronounce definitively on the potential role of DTI in early diagnosis.

At present, DTI, although useful, has not been specific enough to provide a diagnostic marker. In one study, FA obtained in the posterior limb of the internal capsule was estimated to be 95% sensitive, but only 71% specific (47). Only preliminary work has been done on comparing patients diagnosed with ALS, PLS (in which only UMN signs are present), and LMN-predominant subtypes such as Kennedy's disease (62,63). FA was reduced in the corpus callosum and in the WM adjacent to the right primary motor cortex in patients with PLS as compared with those with ALS (62). Reduced FA in the WM adjacent to the superior frontal gyrus also distinguished the ALS group.

Correlations with clinical measures of upper motor neurone involvement

The majority of existing studies report moderate but significant correlations between the DTI parameters and clinical measures of UMN involvement (e.g. Ashworth spasticity scale; UMN burden score) in patients with a range in severity of clinical UMN involvement (48–50). Wong *et al.* showed an association between the modified Ashworth scale and ADC, but not other measures of diffusivity (59). However, a number of studies have shown disassociation between clinical measures of UMN integrity and DTI measures (46,59), which might indicate that DTI is more sensitive in detecting UMN abnormalities compared with clinical tests (see above). However, not enough is known to establish the time course of changes in DTI measures and clinical measures of UMN involvement.

Longitudinal studies where DTI and clinical observations are collected prospectively in the same group of individuals are minimal (24,64,65). Blain *et al.* showed no change in FA obtained along the CST over the course of 6 months in 11 patients with ALS, who also showed no change in clinical UMN burden score in the seven patients who returned for a second scan (64). In this subgroup, however, global WM FA decreased significantly, while mean FA in CST showed only a trend in the same direction. A clinical measure of UMN disease was not used in this study. However, an association was observed between the decline in FA and the change in ALSFRS score for these patients.

Correlations with disease severity and progression

Significant correlations have been reported between FA and ALS severity scales such as ALSFRS (66). However, these correlations have been observed much less consistently compared with correlations with clinical UMN involvement scales (24,46,48,59,64,67). The lack of relationship is not surprising because these severity scales are focused on functional daily performance of patients, which is affected by both UMN and LMN abnormalities, albeit the LMN component (i.e. muscle weakness and atrophy) may be the most detrimental for daily functioning (48).

Although DTI measures are often the most affected in the bulbar subgroup of patients (40,49), the extent of bulbar disability is rarely evaluated independently of the overall severity of motor disability. As an exception moderate association was found between FA and functional bulbar scores (31).

Correlations with measures of motor performance

There have been no detailed studies quantifying and comparing motor performance and brain neuroanatomy. However, Wong *et al.* measured finger and foot tapping speeds (number of taps in 10 seconds averaged over two attempts) and found no correlation between the motor measure and FA (59). A number of studies employed the Medical Research Council scale, a subjective measure of muscle strength (47). Graham *et al.* found a moderate correlation between the scores obtained using the Medical Research Council scale and FA in the posterior limb of the internal capsule and the WM of the precentral gyrus (47). Expanding on the recent work of Ciccarelli *et al.*, it would be interesting to link the behavioural profiles characteristic of primarily UMN versus LMN damage to understand the effect of both on motor—limb and bulbar function—outcomes (62). (For example, see DePaul and Brooks, who showed that primary tongue impairment was associated with significant UMN deficits in patients with bulbar ALS (68).)

Diffusion tensor imaging and the assessment of cognitive function in amyotrophic lateral sclerosis

With increasing recognition of ALS as a multisystem disorder (3,4,69,70), DTI has been used as a predictor of cognitive performance. A DTI voxel-based analysis revealed changes in FA in the (pre)frontal lobe, orbitofrontal WM, hippocampal formation and insula bilaterally, as well as the left parietal lobe (24). Directionally averaged MD (D_{av}) was increased in the hippocampal formation and right insula. Similar results were found with addition of reduced FA in the thalamus and right parietal cortex co-occurring with the increase in MD in the opercular regions of the frontal lobe and centrum semiovale (66). Sach *et al.* reported DTI evidence for extramotor involvement in ALS in the corpus callosum, thalamus, and the frontal lobe underneath the left inferior and medial frontal gyri (54). Sato *et al.* examined the uncinate fasciculus, which connects the frontal and temporal lobes and is thought to mediate retrieval of names and autobiographical memories in FTD and ALS (71–73). The authors found differences in FA between a group of 15 patients with ALS and nine normal controls, but did not perform any cognitive behavioural measures.

Although neuroanatomical changes were observed, these studies did not report results of neuropsychological assessment. Considering that the DTI provides a superior basis for the analyses of WM, the lack of behavioural findings is a significant limitation of current research and should be addressed in the future.

Diffusion tensor imaging and therapeutic interventions

When identified, a reliable biomarker can be used to establish efficacy of neuroprotective therapeutics, but so far, DTI has not been used in such a context.

Issues with diffusion tensor imaging

There have been many discrepancies between studies with respect to specific sites and measures sensitive to ALS. These discrepancies can be explained in part by the heterogeneity of this clinical population. Extensive variability of the CST architecture across individuals and the variability of the disease effects along the tract contribute to inconsistent results as well (46,74). Additional variability is introduced by differences in MR scanners, acquisition parameters (image resolution and signal-to-noise ratio) and measurement methods between different research groups. These challenges must be addressed to standardize DTI methods, which might lead in the future to the use of DTI for diagnostic purposes. As an example, the majority of studies published to date use a Region of Interest (ROI) approach to identify anatomical regions, where diffusion indices are calculated. One of the limitations of this approach is that it is prone to partial contamination from adjacent tracts. Hong and colleagues compared the FA values in the brainstem derived using seed/target ROIs with those obtained using tractography derived ROI and showed that with the latter approach the ALS group showed more robust differences in FA relative to normal controls (75). Tractography, however, has its own limitations such as dependency on threshold values (FA and angle) and the length of the vector step and seed ROI (76). Improved methodology is of great importance in implementing approaches such is DTI into clinical practice.

A promising whole-brain method is tract-based spatial statistics (TBSS), which overcomes some challenges of more established DTI analyses such as the subjectivity and focus on individual tracts using ROI methods, as well as issues with image alignment from multiple subjects in VBM approaches (77). At the core of TBSS is the development of the tract skeleton, representing the centre of all WM fibre tracts common across study participants. Each subject's FA image is aligned to the skeleton by finding the local tract centre. Voxel-based statistics is performed on these data. Sage *et al.* compared TBSS with the traditional VBM approach conducted on the same group of patients and found a similar pattern of changes in FA and additional differences in MD when using TBSS (24,78). They observed strong correlations between the measures of FA and MD across WM and clinical indicators of disease severity and progression. They deemed TBSS superior to the other method, avoiding the co-registration problem and differences due to the selection of smoothing parameters. TBSS was used by Ciccarelli *et al.* to distinguish the patterns of WM damage in ALS and PLS, a condition affecting UMNs only (62). The authors reported that DTI and TBSS were successful in showing different patterns of WM damage in these two diseases. A single study reported the results of a voxel-based analysis using TBSS on skeletonized axial and radial diffusivity images obtained for a group of patients with ALS and controls (42). The authors found that directional diffusivity measures were most extensively affected than the more standard FA and MD measures, suggesting that DR in particular might be most sensitive to neurodegeneration in ALS. However, the changes in these measures were not associated with clinical indices of disease severity or progression.

Conclusions

In this chapter, we have attempted to highlight how structural and functional neuroimaging techniques can be used as biomarkers in neurodegenerative disease for early detection, differential diagnosis, monitoring progression, and potential response to therapies. These methods are also used to investigate brain–behaviour relationships, giving insight into presymptomatic stages, including compensatory phases or alterations in connectivity captured by fMRI. While neuroimaging biomarker development is more advanced in AD, we have illustrated how this is being increasingly used in ALS, providing concrete evidence that ALS has extramotor, multisystem involvement, particularly of frontotemporal regions implicated in the broader family of FTLD. Different types of structural imaging analysis, such as VBM, cortical thickness mapping, and ROI analysis are being applied, as well as MRS and activation/resting state fMRI.

The greatest interest, however, has been DTI, which probes microstructural integrity when the brain superficially looks normal, as is often the case in ALS. However, the group sizes have been small in these studies, so the results are preliminary, and it is still not clear how these techniques can be reliably used to monitor progression and response to therapy. Numbers are often <20, making it difficult to detect reproducible significant change. In DTI, for example, a number close to 50 is estimated to be necessary to detect significant longitudinal change in FA at the 95% level with 80% power (64). As scanning protocols and analyses vary, it is difficult to compare between studies, and more work is needed to ensure cross-platform comparability for different MRI vendors, if these techniques are to be used in multisite studies. Patients are often inadequately described and subtypes are not sufficiently delineated. Cognitive and behavioural measures are seldom collected. Longitudinal studies correlating brain and clinical measures are also lacking.

Harmonized standardized assessments, such as that undertaken for vascular cognitive impairment (79) should be developed and validated, if not already available, including relatively motor-free cognitive measures to allow assessment when speech and motor function is severely compromised.

Clinicians and researchers need to work together to create a core set of imaging, clinical, functional, and cognitive and behavioural measures, which can be repeated over time. Then an ALS neuroimaging initiative could be undertaken, built on the progress already made in cross-platform comparison and in use of more advanced neuroimaging techniques. This is very important if disease-modifying therapies do emerge, so that candidate drugs can be tested in proof-of-concept studies that may use neuroimaging as a surrogate measure to determine quickly if the intervention is promising, and also if multisite phase 2 and 3 studies are to be undertaken. Neuroimaging tools have never been more promising and now the goal must be to use them responsibly and efficiently in ALS to understand heterogeneity in presentation and progression and design appropriate clinical trials to address this devastating neurodegenerative disorder.

Acknowledgements

SEB acknowledges the Canadian Institutes of Health Research MT-13129 for operational financial support. In addition, she is grateful for personnel support from the Departments of Medicine at Sunnybrook Health Sciences Centre and University of Toronto, the Sunnybrook Research Institute, the Heart and Stroke Foundation Centre for Stroke Recovery, and the Brill Chair of Neurology. YY acknowledges the financial support of the NIH-NIDCD Grant no. 1R01DC009890 as well as the Bernice Ramsay Discovery Grant from ALS Society of Canada.

References

1. Strong MJ. (2008). The syndromes of frontotemporal dysfunction in amyotrophic lateral sclerosis. *Amyotroph Lateral Scler*, **9**, 323–338.
2. Hudson AJ. (1981). Amyotrophic lateral sclerosis and its association with dementia. parkinsonism and other neurological disorders: a review. *Brain*, **104**, 217–247.
3. Ringholz GM, Appel SH, Bradshaw M, *et al.* (2005). Prevalence and patterns of cognitive impairment in sporadic ALS. *Neurology*, **65**, 586–590.
4. Wilson CM, Grace GM, Munoz DG, *et al.* (2001). Cognitive impairment in sporadic ALS: a pathologic continuum underlying a multisystem disorder. *Neurology*, **57**, 651–657.
5. Cairns NJ, Bigio EH, Mackenzie IR, *et al.* (2007). Neuropathologic diagnostic and nosologic criteria for frontotemporal lobar degeneration: consensus of the Consortium for Frontotemporal Lobar Degeneration. *Acta Neuropathol*, **114**, 5–22.
6. Turner MR, Kiernan MC, Leigh PN, *et al.* (2009). Biomarkers in amyotrophic lateral sclerosis. *Lancet Neurol*, **8**, 94–109.
7. Kertesz A, Davidson W, Fox H. (1997). Frontal behavioral inventory. diagnostic criteria for frontal lobe dementia. *Can J Neurol Sci*, **24**, 29–36.
8. Hecht MJ, Fellner F, Fellner C, *et al.* (2001). MRI-FLAIR images of the head show corticospinal tract alterations in ALS patients more frequently than T2-, T1- and proton-density-weighted images. *J Neurol Sci*, **186**, 37–44.

9. Ishikawa K, Nagura H, Yokota T, *et al.* (1993). Signal loss in the motor cortex on magnetic resonance images in amyotrophic lateral sclerosis. *Ann Neurol*, **33**, 218–222.
10. Charil A, Corbo M, Filippi M, *et al.* (2009). Structural and metabolic changes in the brain of patients with upper motor neuron disorders: a multiparametric MRI study. *Amyotroph Lateral Scler*, **10**, 269–279.
11. Weiner MW, Aisen PS, Jack CR, Jr, *et al.* (2010). The Alzheimer's disease neuroimaging initiative: progress report and future plans. *Alzheimers Dement*, **6**, 202–211.
12. Jagust WJ, Bandy D, Chen K, *et al.* (2010). The Alzheimer's Disease Neuroimaging Initiative positron emission tomography core. *Alzheimers Dement*, **6**, 221–229.
13. Rowe CC, Ng S, Ackermann U, *et al.* (2007). Imaging beta-amyloid burden in aging and dementia. *Neurology*, **68**, 1718–1725.
14. Clark CM, Schneider JA, Bedell BJ, *et al.* (2011). Use of florbetapir-PET for imaging beta-amyloid pathology. *JAMA*, **19**;305, 275–283.
15. Lobaugh NJ, West R, McIntosh AR. (2001). Spatiotemporal analysis of experimental differences in event-related potential data with partial least squares. *Psychophysiology*, **38**, 517–530.
16. Friston KJ, Holmes AP, Worsley KJ, *et al.* (1995). Statistical parametric maps in functional imaging: A general linear approach. *Hum Brain Mapping*, **2**, 189–210.
17. Dade LA, Gao F, Kovacevic N, *et al.* (2004). Semiautomatic brain region extraction (SABRE): A method of parcellating brain regions from structural magnetic resonance images. *Neuroimage*, **22**, 1492–502. Medical Image Computing and Computer Assisted Intervention - MICCAI 2003, Lecture Notes in Computer Science, 2003, Volume 2879/2003, 949–950.
18. Ramirez J, Gibson E, Quddus A, et al. (2011). Lesion Explorer: a comprehensive segmentation and parcellation package to obtain regional volumetrics for subcortical hyperintensities and intracranial tissue. *Neuroimage*, **54**, 963–973.
19. Bocti C, Rockel C, Roy P, *et al.* (2006). Topographical pattern of lobar atrophy in frontotemporal dementia and Alzheimer's disease. *Dement Geriatr Cogn Disord*, **21**(5–6), 364–72.
20. Kovacevic N, Lobaugh N, Bronskill MJ, *et al.* (2002). A robust method for extraction and automatic segmentation of brain images. *Neuroimage*, **17**, 1087–1100.
21. Tartaglia MC, Laluz V, Rowe A, *et al.* (2009). Brain atrophy in primary lateral sclerosis. *Neurology*, **72**, 1236–1241.
22. Abe O, Yamada H, Masutani Y, *et al.* (2004). Amyotrophic lateral sclerosis: diffusion tensor tractography and voxel-based analysis. *NMR Biomed*, **17**, 411–416.
23. Filippini N, Douaud G, Mackay CE, *et al.* (2010). Corpus callosum involvement is a consistent feature of amyotrophic lateral sclerosis. *Neurology*, **75**, 1645–1652.
24. Sage CA, Peeters RR, Gorner A, *et al.* (2007). Quantitative diffusion tensor imaging in amyotrophic lateral sclerosis. *Neuroimage*, **34**, 486–499.
25. Rabinovici GD, Seeley WW, Kim EJ, *et al.* (2007). Distinct MRI atrophy patterns in autopsy-proven Alzheimer's disease and frontotemporal lobar degeneration. *Am J Alzheimers Dis Other Demen*, **22**, 474–488.
26. Seeley WW, Crawford RK, Zhou J, *et al.* (2009). Neurodegenerative diseases target large-scale human brain networks. *Neuron*, **62**, 42–52.
27. Gorno-Tempini ML, Dronkers NF, Rankin KP, *et al.* (2004). Cognition and anatomy in three variants of primary progressive aphasia. *Ann Neurol*, **55**, 335–346.
28. Kim EJ, Rabinovici GD, Seeley WW, *et al.* (2007). Patterns of MRI atrophy in tau positive and ubiquitin positive frontotemporal lobar degeneration. *J Neurol Neurosurg Psychiatry*, **78**, 1375–1378.
29. Rosen HJ, Allison SC, Schauer GF, *et al.* (2005). Neuroanatomical correlates of behavioural disorders in dementia. *Brain*, **128**, 2612–2625.

30. Grosskreutz J, Peschel T, Unrath A, *et al.* (2008). Whole brain-based computerized neuroimaging in ALS and other motor neuron disorders. *Amyotroph Lateral Scler*, **9**, 238–248.
31. Roccatagliata L, Bonzano L, Mancardi G, *et al.* (2009). Detection of motor cortex thinning and corticospinal tract involvement by quantitative MRI in amyotrophic lateral sclerosis. *Amyotroph Lateral Scler*, **10**, 47–52.
32. Sudharshan N, Hanstock C, Hui B, *et al.* (2011). Degeneration of the mid-cingulate cortex in amyotrophic lateral sclerosis detected *in vivo* with MR spectroscopy. *AJNR Am J Neuroradiol*, **32**, 403–407.
33. Unrath A, Ludolph AC, Kassubek J. (2007). Brain metabolites in definite amyotrophic lateral sclerosis. A longitudinal proton magnetic resonance spectroscopy study. *J Neurol*, **254**, 1099–1106.
34. Pyra T, Hui B, Hanstock C, *et al.* (2010). Combined structural and neurochemical evaluation of the corticospinal tract in amyotrophic lateral sclerosis. *Amyotroph Lateral Scler*, **11**, 157–165.
35. Kalra S, Cashman NR, Genge A, *et al.* (1998). Recovery of N-acetylaspartate in corticomotor neurons of patients with ALS after riluzole therapy. *Neuroreport*, **9**, 1757–1761.
36. Kalra S, Tai P, Genge A, *et al.* (2006). Rapid improvement in cortical neuronal integrity in amyotrophic lateral sclerosis detected by proton magnetic resonance spectroscopic imaging. *J Neurol*, **253**, 1060–1063.
37. Kalra S, Genge A, Arnold DL. (2003). A prospective, randomized, placebo-controlled evaluation of corticoneuronal response to intrathecal BDNF therapy in ALS using magnetic resonance spectroscopy: feasibility and results. *Amyotroph Lateral Scler Other Motor Neuron Disord*, **4**, 22–26.
38. Kalra S, Cashman NR, Caramanos Z, *et al.* (2003). Gabapentin therapy for amyotrophic lateral sclerosis: lack of improvement in neuronal integrity shown by MR spectroscopy. *AJNR Am J Neuroradiol*, **24**, 476–480.
39. Lule D, Ludolph AC, Kassubek J. (2009). MRI-based functional neuroimaging in ALS: an update. *Amyotroph Lateral Scler*, **10**, 258–268.
40. Li S, Chen Q, Yu B, *et al.* (2009). Structural and functional changes mapped in the brains of amyotrophic lateral sclerosis patients with/without dysphagia: a pilot study. *Amyotroph Lateral Scler*, **10**(5–6), 280–287.
41. Basser PJ, Mattiello J, LeBihan D. (1994). MR diffusion tensor spectroscopy and imaging. *Biophys J*, **66**, 259–267.
42. Metwalli NS, Benatar M, Nair G, *et al.* (2010). Utility of axial and radial diffusivity from diffusion tensor MRI as markers of neurodegeneration in amyotrophic lateral sclerosis. *Brain Res*, **1348**, 156–164.
43. Sasaki S, Maruyama S. (1992). Increase in diameter of the axonal initial segment is an early change in amyotrophic lateral sclerosis. *J Neurol Sci*, **110**, 114–120.
44. Song SK, Sun SW, Ramsbottom MJ, *et al.* (2002). Dysmyelination revealed through MRI as increased radial (but unchanged axial) diffusion of water. *Neuroimage*, **17**, 1429–1436.
45. Karlsborg M, Rosenbaum S, Wiegell M, *et al.* (2004). Corticospinal tract degeneration and possible pathogenesis in ALS evaluated by MR diffusion tensor imaging. *Amyotroph Lateral Scler Other Motor Neuron Disord*, **5**, 136–140.
46. Toosy AT, Werring DJ, Orrell RW, *et al.* (2003). Diffusion tensor imaging detects corticospinal tract involvement at multiple levels in amyotrophic lateral sclerosis. *J Neurol Neurosurg Psychiatry*, **74**, 1250–1257.
47. Graham JM, Papadakis N, Evans J, *et al.* (2004). Diffusion tensor imaging for the assessment of upper motor neuron integrity in ALS. *Neurology*, **63**, 2111–2119.
48. Iwata NK, Aoki S, Okabe S, *et al.* (2008). Evaluation of corticospinal tracts in ALS with diffusion tensor MRI and brainstem stimulation. *Neurology*, **70**, 528–532.

49. Ellis CM, Simmons A, Jones DK, *et al.* (1999). Diffusion tensor MRI assesses corticospinal tract damage in ALS. *Neurology*, **53**, 1051–1058.
50. Hong YH, Lee KW, Sung JJ, *et al.* (2004). Diffusion tensor MRI as a diagnostic tool of upper motor neuron involvement in amyotrophic lateral sclerosis. *J Neurol Sci*, **227**, 73–78.
51. Bartels C, Mertens N, Hofer S, *et al.* (2008). Callosal dysfunction in amyotrophic lateral sclerosis correlates with diffusion tensor imaging of the central motor system. *Neuromuscul Disord*, **18**, 398–407.
52. Aoki S, Iwata NK, Masutani Y, *et al.* (2005). Quantitative evaluation of the pyramidal tract segmented by diffusion tensor tractography: feasibility study in patients with amyotrophic lateral sclerosis. *Radiat Med*, **23**, 195–199.
53. Iwata NK, Aoki S, Masutani Y, *et al.* (2005). Corticospinal tract and corticobulbar tract dysfunction in ALS: combined study using transcranial magnetic stimulation and diffusion tensor tractography. *Int Congr Ser*, **1278**, 181–184.
54. Sach M, Winkler G, Glauche V, *et al.* (2004). Diffusion tensor MRI of early upper motor neuron involvement in amyotrophic lateral sclerosis. *Brain*, **127**, 340–350.
55. Sato K, Aoki S, Iwata NK, *et al.* (2010). Diffusion tensor tract-specific analysis of the uncinate fasciculus in patients with amyotrophic lateral sclerosis. *Neuroradiology*, **52**, 729–733.
56. Agosta F, Pagani E, Petrolini M, *et al.* (2010). Assessment of white matter tract damage in patients with amyotrophic lateral sclerosis: a diffusion tensor MR imaging tractography study. *AJNR Am J Neuroradiol*, **31**, 1457–1461.
57. Cosottini M, Giannelli M, Siciliano G, *et al.* (2005). Diffusion-tensor MR imaging of corticospinal tract in amyotrophic lateral sclerosis and progressive muscular atrophy. *Radiology*, **237**, 258–264.
58. Ng MC, Ho JT, Ho SL, *et al.* (2008). Abnormal diffusion tensor in nonsymptomatic familial amyotrophic lateral sclerosis with a causative superoxide dismutase 1 mutation. *J Magn Reson Imaging*, **27**, 8–13.
59. Wong JC, Concha L, Beaulieu C, *et al.* (2007). Spatial profiling of the corticospinal tract in amyotrophic lateral sclerosis using diffusion tensor imaging. *J Neuroimaging*, **17**, 234–240.
60. Nair G, Carew JD, Usher S, *et al.* (2010). Diffusion tensor imaging reveals regional differences in the cervical spinal cord in amyotrophic lateral sclerosis. *Neuroimage*, **53**, 576–583.
61. Metwalli NS, Benatar M, Usher S, *et al.* (2009). Sensitivity of axial and radial diffusivity to the neuropathology of amyotrophic lateral sclerosis. *Neuroimage*, **47**, S39-S41.
62. Ciccarelli O, Behrens TE, Johansen-Berg H, *et al.* (2009). Investigation of white matter pathology in ALS and PLS using tract-based spatial statistics. *Hum Brain Mapp*, **30**, 615–624.
63. Nelles M, Block W, Traber F, *et al.* (2008). Combined 3T diffusion tensor tractography and 1H-MR spectroscopy in motor neuron disease. *AJNR Am J Neuroradiol*, **29**, 1708–1714.
64. Blain CR, Williams VC, Johnston C, *et al.* (2007). A longitudinal study of diffusion tensor MRI in ALS. *Amyotroph Lateral Scler*, **8**, 348–355.
65. Jacob S, Finsterbusch J, Weishaupt JH, *et al.* (2003). Diffusion tensor imaging for long-term follow-up of corticospinal tract degeneration in amyotrophic lateral sclerosis. *Neuroradiology*, **45**, 598–600.
66. Thivard L, Pradat PF, Lehericy S, *et al.* (2007). Diffusion tensor imaging and voxel based morphometry study in amyotrophic lateral sclerosis: relationships with motor disability. *J Neurol Neurosurg Psychiatry*, **78**, 889–892.
67. Schimrigk SK, Bellenberg B, Schluter M, *et al.* (2007). Diffusion tensor imaging-based fractional anisotropy quantification in the corticospinal tract of patients with amyotrophic lateral sclerosis using a probabilistic mixture model. *AJNR Am J Neuroradiol*, **28**, 724–730.
68. DePaul R, Brooks BR. (1993). Multiple orofacial indices in amyotrophic lateral sclerosis. *J Speech Hear Res*, **36**, 1158–1167.

69. Turner MR, Scaber J, Goodfellow JA, *et al.* (2010). The diagnostic pathway and prognosis in bulbar-onset amyotrophic lateral sclerosis. *J Neurol Sci*, **294**, 81–85.
70. Witgert M, Salamone AR, Strutt AM, *et al.* (2010). Frontal-lobe mediated behavioral dysfunction in amyotrophic lateral sclerosis. *Eur J Neurol*, **17**, 103–110.
71. Abrahams S, Goldstein LH, Simmons A, *et al.* (2004). Word retrieval in amyotrophic lateral sclerosis: a functional magnetic resonance imaging study. *Brain*, **127**, 1507–1517.
72. Matsuo K, Mizuno T, Yamada K, *et al.* (2008). Cerebral white matter damage in frontotemporal dementia assessed by diffusion tensor tractography. *Neuroradiology*, **50**, 605–611.
73. Levine B, Black SE, Cabeza R, *et al.* (1998). Episodic memory and the self in a case of isolated retrograde amnesia. *Brain*, **121**, 1951–1973.
74. Virta A, Barnett A, Pierpaoli C. (1999). Visualizing and characterizing white matter fiber structure and architecture in the human pyramidal tract using diffusion tensor MRI. *Magn Reson Imaging*, **17**, 1121–1133.
75. Hong YH, Sung JJ, Kim SM, *et al.* (2008). Diffusion tensor tractography-based analysis of the pyramidal tract in patients with amyotrophic lateral sclerosis. *J Neuroimaging*, **18**, 282–287.
76. Wang S, Melhem ER. (2005). Amyotrophic lateral sclerosis and primary lateral sclerosis: The role of diffusion tensor imaging and other advanced MR-based techniques as objective upper motor neuron markers. *Ann N Y Acad Sci*, **1064**, 61–77.
77. Smith SM, Jenkinson M, Johansen-Berg H, *et al.* (2006). Tract-based spatial statistics: voxelwise analysis of multi-subject diffusion data. *Neuroimage*, **31**, 1487–1505.
78. Sage CA, Van HW, Peeters R, *et al.* (2009). Quantitative diffusion tensor imaging in amyotrophic lateral sclerosis: revisited. *Hum Brain Mapp*, **30**, 3657–3675.
79. Hachinski V, Iadecola C, Petersen RC, *et al.* (2006). National Institute of Neurological Disorders and Stroke-Canadian Stroke Network vascular cognitive impairment harmonization standards. *Stroke*, **37**, 2220–2241.

Chapter 15

Amyotrophic lateral sclerosis and the frontotemporal dementias: using neuroimaging to quantitate disease progression

S. Kalra

Introduction

After decades of clinical trials, there remains a lack of effective disease-modifying therapies for amyotrophic lateral sclerosis (ALS). In addition to the complex pathogenic mechanisms that are not fully understood, other important factors contributing to this deficiency include the lack of a sensitive and objective biomarker and the biological heterogeneity of ALS.

Diagnosis is dependent on physical signs emanating from the cardinal feature of ALS: combined upper motor neurone (UMN) and lower motor neurone (LMN) degeneration. However, these signs are crude and insensitive. Additionally, UMN signs may be lacking or attenuate over time as LMN degeneration progresses. Thus, typical outcome measures in clinical trials have been composite measures of strength (e.g. manual muscle testing, maximum voluntary isometric contraction) or disability (Amyotrophic Lateral Sclerosis Functional Rating Scale-Revised (ALSFRS-R)), respiratory function (forced vital capacity), and survival. Drug trials based on such endpoints require hundreds of patients per study arm and are lengthy and expensive. This is a major impediment to early drug development programmes, as achieving such numbers in a timely fashion is difficult given the low prevalence of ALS. Furthermore, disability scales and survival in particular are only indirectly related to the true biological lesion (motor neurone dysfunction/death) and do not discriminate between UMN and LMN function.

The heterogeneity of ALS is evident in the simple clinical observations of varied age of onset, site of symptoms onset, progression rate, and survival. This is compounded by the variable presence of frontotemporal lobar degeneration (FTLD), necessitating the designation of ALS as a spectrum rather than a single disease entity (1). Cognitive impairment secondary to FTLD is highly prevalent and detectable by focused neuropsychometric testing in upwards of 50% of patients (2,3). Thus, variability in the clinical phenotype of ALS extends beyond that resulting from motor neurone degeneration (UMN versus LMN predominant versus mixed UMN and LMN, limb versus bulbar onset, slow versus rapid progression) to include a spectrum of cognitive and behavioural dysfunction. (4)

There have been important recent developments in elucidating the overlap of FTLD with ALS from a pathological and molecular perspective, as delineated elsewhere in this text. The clinical syndrome is better understood with consensus-based criteria now published to guide clinical evaluation (5,6). However, varying prevalence rates, conflicting reports regarding its natural history and an unclear relationship between FTLD and motor neurone degeneration make clinical measures of cognitive impairment unsuitable for monitoring disease progression. A biomarker is required to address these issues of biological and clinical heterogeneity and lack of optimal outcome measures (Table 15.1).

Serum, cerebrospinal fluid, and neuroimaging biomarkers have been investigated in ALS (7), and are areas of intense research. Brain imaging is an obvious candidate as a biomarker of disease because: (a) it is *objective*; (b) it provides *in vivo* data; (c) it allows assessment *repeatedly* during the course of the disease; and (d) it allows assessment of *specific regions* of the brain, which is vital in understanding the impact of degeneration on behaviour. Magnetic resonance imaging techniques, in particular, are advantageous because, unlike positron emission tomography and single-photon emission tomography, they are non-invasive and do not require exposure to ionizing radiation.

This chapter will review the potential role, experience, limitations, and future directions of neuroimaging in monitoring disease progression in ALS and ALS/FTLD. Discussion will be largely limited to magnetic resonance (MR) technology as longitudinal studies with other imaging modalities are scarce, most recent developments are in advanced MR methods, and MR imaging (MRI) installations are becoming ubiquitous.

Imaging modalities

Conventional MRI may reveal signal changes in ALS, including hypointensity in the pre-central gyral cortex and hyperintensity of the corticospinal tract (CST) on T2-weighted and

Table 15.1 Potential roles of biomarkers in ALS and FTLD

Explore biological basis of phenotypic heterogeneity in ALS and FTLD	Neuroimaging markers: neuronal, glial, neurotransmitters, atrophy, functional cortical adaptation, etc. Cerebrospinal fluid and serum markers: neuronal, glial, inflammatory, tau, neurofilament, etc.
Quantify disease burden	Stage disease
	Assist in diagnosis
	Monitor progression
	Monitor differential rate of degeneration of discrete systems (e.g. UMN, LMN, frontotemporal, neuronal, glial)
Evaluate therapeutic efficacy	Phase II trials of novel compounds
	Increase efficiency, reduce sample size, trial duration, cost
	Select homogeneous group (e.g. pure motor)
	Confirm drug is having desired biological effect
	Optimize treatment in individuals

fluid-attenuated inversion recovery (FLAIR) sequences. Focal atrophy may be observed in the motor cortex or frontotemporal regions. However, these changes are neither sensitive nor specific to ALS and thus conventional MRI remains essentially a means to rule out other disorders that may mimic ALS rather than confirm diagnosis (8). Longitudinal studies are scarce; one study systematically evaluated signal changes in 17 patients on T1-weighted, T2-weighted, and FLAIR images 15.7 months after a baseline scan (9). Visually apparent changes in hyperintensity were not evident; however, quantitative analysis revealed an increase in precentral gyrus subcortical hyperintensity on FLAIR; these changes did not correlate with clinical progression.

Advanced neuroimaging techniques have superseded conventional MRI to study specific pathobiological elements related to neurodegeneration (Table 15.2). Their utility in diagnosing ALS/FTLD and understanding pathophysiology is covered elsewhere in this text [see Chapter 13]. They differ in regards to what pathological elements they can monitor, and over what time course changes can be detected in response to treatment. All have the capacity to detect long-term changes, for example, due to slowing of neuronal loss by a neuroprotective agent. Short-term changes, presumably due to functional recovery, would be amenable to detection with MR spectroscopy (MRS), PET, and functional MRI (fMRI).

Magnetic resonance volumetry

Quantification of the volume of different central nervous system compartments is possible to determine the extent of atrophic changes (Table 15.1). A relatively simple automated technique is to 'segment' the grey matter (GM) or white matter (WM) in a defined region. This was done bilaterally in the motor cortex and subjacent WM of the CST in a longitudinal MRS study (see MRS section for additional details) (10). GM decreased in the more affected hemisphere after 6 months and WM increased in the less affected hemisphere after 3 months.

Voxel-based morphometry (VBM) allows for a voxel-wise comparison of MRI to detect differences in GM or WM. It has the advantage of providing an unbiased whole-brain

Table 15.2 Biological processes and pathologies that can be detected with neuroimaging

Biological correlate	Imaging modality	Imaging parameter
Neuronal loss	MRV	Compartmental volumes: whole brain, lobes (e.g. frontal, temporal), ventricles, cortical thickness, GM, WM
	DTI	Fractional anisotropy, mean diffusivity
	MRS*	*N*-acetylaspartate
	PET*	Perfusion, glucose metabolism, receptor binding
	fMRI*	Cerebral activation
Astrogliosis	MRS	Myo-inositol, choline
Metabolic processes	MRS	Neurotransmitters, amino acids
Cortical functional adaptation	fMRI PET	Cerebral activation

*Changes may reflect neuronal dysfunction in absence of neuronal loss.

DTI, diffusion tensor imaging; fMRI, functional magnetic resonance imaging; GM, grey matter; MRS, magnetic resonance spectroscopy; MRV, magnetic resonance volumetry; PET, positron emission tomography; WM, white matter.

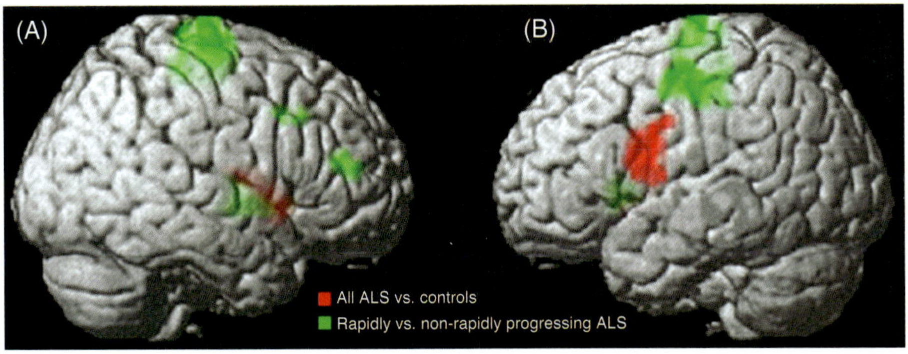

Fig. 15.1 Progressive grey matter atrophy occurs in motor and non-motor regions in cognitively intact patients with ALS. The right (A) and left (B) hemisphere of a three-dimensional surface rendering shows regions of significantly progressing atrophy over 9 months in all patients compared with healthy controls (red) and in rapidly progressing compared with non-rapidly progressing patients (green). Agosta F, Gorno-Tempini ML, Pagani E, Sala S, Caputo D, Perini M, et al. Longitudinal assessment of grey matter contraction in amyotrophic lateral sclerosis: A tensor based morphometry study. *Amyotroph Lateral Scler* 2009. Reproduced with permission of Informa Medical and Pharmaceutical Science–Journals.

analysis and thus has been useful to demonstrate atrophy in and beyond the motor cortex, including frontotemporal areas (11–13). Tensor-based morphometry, a technique incorporating VBM, was used to measure longitudinal GM changes in 16 patients with ALS (14). Each subject underwent two scans with a mean interval of 9 months. GM decreased in the left premotor cortex and right caudate and putamen (Figure 15.1). A subgroup analysis was done with patients dichotomized according to rate of progression. The rapidly progressing group (progression rate above the median rate of the group) additionally showed GM atrophy of the left motor cortex, bilateral supplementary motor areas, right inferior and middle frontal gyri, and left caudate. This study demonstrates that ongoing volume loss in cognitively unimpaired patients with ALS is not restricted to the motor cortex, but includes premotor, prefrontal, and subcortical regions and thus likely reflects elements of both motor neurone degeneration and FTLD.

Tensor-based morphometry was used to assess progressive atrophy in patients with ALS with frontotemporal dementia (ALS/FTD) (15). In this study of four patients, GM volume decline was noted after 5 months in the premotor cortex, primary motor cortex, and parietal lobe. It is unclear why prefrontal GM atrophy did not occur; though the small sample size and relatively short observation interval may partly explain this. However, it is interesting to note that there was partial overlap in regions with declining GM as observed in the patients with ALS without cognitive impairment (14) described above.

When TBM was applied to study patients with FTD (16), progressing GM volume loss was seen in different regions compared with the studies of ALS and ALS/FTD. In the standard whole-brain analysis, this was demonstrated in limbic regions (anterior cingulate and paracingulate gyri) (Figure 15.2), rather than motor and premotor regions as seen in ALS or ALS/FTD. An a priori region-specific analysis additionally showed atrophy of specific prefrontal and mesial and anterior temporal structures.

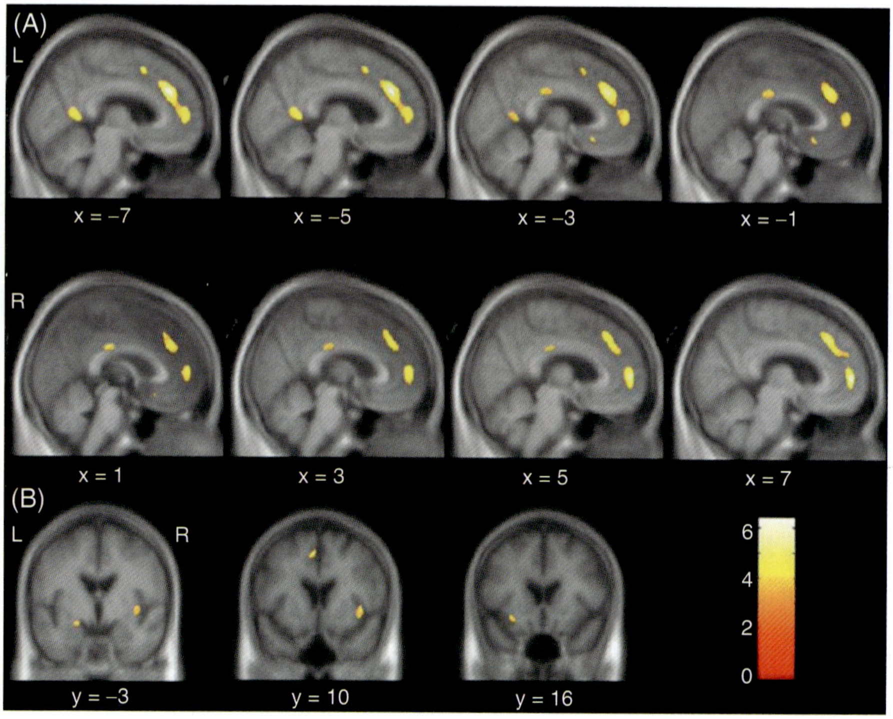

Fig. 15.2 Sagittal (A) and coronal (B) images showing regions of progressive atrophy in patients with FTD. The colour scale indicates the statistical level of significance, where white is most significant. Reproduced with permission from Brambati *et al.* (16).

Whole-brain and ventricular volume changes occurring over 1 year were reported by Knopman in a multicentre study of 76 patients with FTLD (17). The degree of whole brain volume loss (1.62%) and ventricular volume increase (11.6%) were comparable in patients with behavioural variant FTD, progressive non-fluent aphasia, and semantic dementia. Changes were slightly more prominent in patients with progressive logopenic aphasia compared with the rest of the group. The volumetric change correlated with decline in cognitive performance. Sample size calculations were performed based on the results: 139 or 55 patients would be required respectively to detect a small (25%) or medium (50%) effect in a randomized placebo-controlled trial of a drug. Others have reported similar rates of change of whole brain and ventricular volume in FTLD. Of note, rates are generally faster in FTLD compared with other dementias though with overlap between groups (18–20).

In summary, topographical patterns and rates of progressive atrophy may assist in differentiating FTLD from other degenerative dementia. Additionally, whole brain atrophy and ventricular volume expansion rates show promise as potential biomarkers in clinical trials.

Magnetic resonance spectroscopy

Proton MRS permits non-invasive quantification of cerebral metabolites *in vivo*. Studies in ALS have consistently demonstrated impaired neuronal integrity based on the finding of decreased levels of the neuronal marker *N*-acetyl aspartate (NAA) (and its ratio to choline or creatine) in the motor cortex (21–30), frontal lobe (23,26), and brainstem (31,32). A number of studies have demonstrated declining NAA indices in the motor cortex (Table 15.3). Correlations of the rate of decline were observed for disease severity as assessed by the Jablecki score (25) and with the ALSFRS (10).

Two longitudinal studies examined extramotor regions. Strong *et al.* reported a 3.5% decline in NAA/creatine over 6 months in the anterior cingulate cortex (23). Patients had mild and progressive impairment in various cognitive domains. However, correlation analysis between NAA/creatine and cognitive measures was not reported. Rule studied motor cortex and non-motor (frontal and parietal) cortex regions in 45 patients every 3 months for a year and found a different pattern of spectroscopic change depending on the initial diagnosis (29). In patients with suspected or possible ALS, NAA declined in and outside the motor cortex at 3 months but not beyond this time period. In those with probable or definite ALS a decline in NAA was only observed outside the motor cortex and at 9 months. The cognitive status of the patients was not reported.

In summary, MRS shows promise as a tool to monitor degeneration given the detectability of short and long-term changes in cerebral neurochemicals. The variability in reported rates of NAA decline is likely a result of differing patient characteristics and methodologies. The development of guidelines for standardized MRS acquisition protocols, as have been done for multiple sclerosis (33), will be useful to reduce variability from experimental factors and help move MRS into the clinical trials arena.

Diffusion tensor imaging

DTI has revealed abnormalities in axonal integrity by the finding of decreased fractional anisotropy (FA) or increased mean diffusivity (MD). These are most apparent in the CST (34–42). Studies revealing changes beyond the motor system, including frontotemporal areas, have been scarce (41,43). Three (30,44,45) of four longitudinal studies (Table 15.3) were unable to reveal progressive changes in DTI. The remaining study (41) revealed a significant decline in whole-brain WM FA, which correlated with a drop in ALSFRS, and a trend to a decreasing FA in the CST (41).

Emerging studies of quantitative neuroimaging of the spinal cord are important developments given the heterogeneous motor systems pathology of ALS (UMN, LMN, brain, brainstem, spinal cord). In addition to FA and MD measurements of the CST in the brain, Agosta *et al.* assessed cervical cord FA, MD, and cross-sectional area with longitudinal follow-up (45). Cord FA declined and cross-sectional declined, and MD increased over a mean of 9 months. This was in contrast to the brain CST FA and MD, which did not change as noted above.

Functional magnetic resonance imaging

Lulé *et al.* studied cortical activation in response to a motor task and motor imagery in 14 patients with ALS. (46) With either task, activation was stronger in premotor areas compared with controls. Eleven patients returned for follow-up after 6 months: activation now extended into the precentral and frontoparietal areas. These topographical changes

Table 15.3 Select studies reporting the use of neuroimaging parameters to monitor disease progression in ALS

	Technique	Patients	Scans	Interval	Region	Findings
	Magnetic resonance spectroscopy					
Kalra (48)	MRSI	12 probable/definite	2	21 days	MC	NAA/Cr ↓ 4% (*P* <0.1)
Block (22)	SVS	9 (4 without UMN signs)	2–3	4–22 mo	MC	↓ NAA/Cho Smaller changes: ↓ NAA/Cr, ↑ Cho/Cr, ↑mI/Cr
Strong (23)	SVS	6 definite	2	6 mo	MC AC	NAA/Cr ↓ 16% NAA/Cr ↓ 4%
Pohl (25)	SVS	16 (3 without UMN)	2–4	12 ± 8 mo	MC	NAA/Cho ↓ 9% Cho/Cr ↑ 7%
Suhy (27)	MRSI	6 suspected/possible 3 probable/definite	3	Scans at 0, 1, 3 mo	MC	At 1 mo: NAA/Cr ↓ 7.4%, NAA/(Cr+Cho) ↓ 7.4% At 3 mo: NAA ↓ 14.5%, Cr ↓ 11.8%, Cho ↓ 18.8%
Rule (29)		21 suspected/ possible 24 probable/definite	5	3 mo	MC Non-MC (frontal, parietal)	NAA ↓ in MC and non-MC in more affected hemisphere at 3 months. No significant changes beyond 3 months. With patients stratified according to diagnosis: -suspected/possible: NAA↓ MC at 3 months -probable/definite: NAA ↓ non-MC at 9 months No change in ratios, though these were abnormal at baseline and absolute values were not.
Unrath (10)	SVS	11 definite	3	3 mo	MC CST	NAA/Cho ↓ in GM of less affected side NAA ↓ in most and less affected side at 6 months. No significant change in Cho+Cr, mI, Glu+Gln, and their ratios
Mitsumoto (30)	MRSI	30	Every 3 mo (mean 3)	6–15 mo	MC	NAA/Cr ↓ 0.44 per month (p=0.06)

	Diffusion tensor imaging					
Blain (44)	ROI	8 possible, probable, definite 3 progressive muscular atrophy	2	6 mo	CST	FA and MD no change
Sage (41)	Tractography	7 probable/definite	2	5–11 mo	CST Whole brain	FA ↓ 1.9% (NS) FA ↓ 8.5%.
Mitsumoto (30)	ROI	30	Every 3 mo (mean 3)	6–15	IC	FA and MD no change
Agosta (45)	Tractography and ROI	17 probable/ definite	2	6–12 mo, mean 9 mo	CST Cervical cord	FA and MD no change Cord FA ↓, MD ↑
	Magnetic resonance volumetry					
Unrath (10)	Segmentation of SVS voxels	11 definite	3	3 mo	MC CST	GM ↓ at 6 mo in more affected hemisphere WM ↑ at 3 mo in less affected hemisphere
Agosta (14)	TBM	16 probable/ definite	2	6–12 mo, mean 9 mo	Whole brain	GM ↓ in left premotor cortex, right putamen and caudate GM↓ in rapidly progressing group in left MC, bilateral SMA, right inferior and middle frontal gyri
Avants (15)	TBM	4 ALS/FTD	2	5 mo	Whole brain	Premotor, primary motor, parietal
Agosta (45)	ROI	17 probable/ definite	2	6–12 mo, mean 9 mo	Cervical cord	Cross-sectional area ↓
	Functional MRI					
Lule (46)	fMRI (BOLD) Motor task	11	2	6 mo		Extension of cortical activation into precentral gyrus and frontoparietal areas
Lule (47)	fMRI (BOLD) Emotional processing task	10	2	6 mo		Enhancement of right supramarginal activation

AC, anterior cingulate; BOLD, blood oxygen level-dependent; BSI, boundary shift integral; bvFTD, behavioural variant frontotemporal dementia; Cho, choline; Cr, creatine; CST, corticospinal tract; DTI, diffusion tensor imaging; FA, fractional anisotropy; fMRI, functional magnetic resonance imaging; GM, grey matter; IC, internal capsule; MC, motor cortex; MD, mean diffusivity; mo, month(s); MRSI, magnetic resonance spectroscopic imaging; NAA, *N*-acetylaspartate; PLA, progressive logopenic aphasia; PNFA, progressive non-fluent aphasia; ROI, region of interest; SD, semantic dementia; SMA, supplementary motor area; SVS, single voxel spectroscopy; TBM, tensor based morphometry; WM, white matter.

Suspected, possible, probable, definite: categories of ALS diagnosis according to El Escorial Criteria.

suggest ongoing adaptation to progressing weakness. Lule *et al.* (47) also studied emotional processing in 13 patients, 10 of whom had follow-up assessment after 6 months. Patients had increased cortical activity in the right supramarginal area at baseline; at follow-up this activity increased and reduced activation appeared in the left anterior insula.

Evaluating drug effect

Whereas there has been considerable progress in the use of brain imaging markers in clinical trials in other neurological disorders such as multiple sclerosis and Alzheimer's disease, to date there have only been a few pilot studies assessing drug efficacy in ALS. Studies using MRS have detected an increase in motor cortex NAA/creatine soon following the commencement of riluzole therapy (48,49). Similarly, 1 month of creatine treatment in ALS showed favourable NAA/creatine trends (50). These observations infer the existence of dysfunctional neurones amenable to therapy resulting in increased NAA production. MRS did not reveal similar changes with gabapentin (51), brain-derived neurotrophic factor (28), and TCH346 (Kalra, unpublished).

A phase II clinical trial of memantine in ALS is underway that, in addition to conventional functional outcome measures and motor unit number estimation, incorporates MRS to monitor the progress of motor and prefrontal cortex degeneration and response to treatment (ClinicalTrials. gov Identifier NCT00409721).

Animal studies

The G93A superoxide dismutase-1 transgenic mouse has contributed significantly as an animal model to study pathogenesis in ALS. A series of experiments from the University of Magdeburg have been conducted to study advancing neurodegeneration in this animal model using several MR parameters. Sequential conventional MRI done at 50, 90, 112, and 130 days postpartum revealed the progressive appearance of hyperintensities in cranial nerve motor nuclei on T2-weighted images (52). The signal changes first appeared at 90 days, near the onset of first clinical signs of disease. They then measured quantitative MR parameters to generate spin–spin relaxation (T2) and diffusion weighted (apparent diffusion coefficient) maps at 70, 90, and 110 days postpartum. T2 values progressively increased in cranial nerve motor nuclei and upper cervical spinal cord. Apparent diffusion coefficient values were increased at 90 days; no change was seen in the spinal cord or for either parameter in the motor cortex and thalamus (53). In a subsequent experiment, MRS was used to quantify metabolites in tissue extracts of the brain and spinal cord (54). Although this was not an *in vivo* study, it sampled mice at serial ages (34, 75, 90, and 120 days post-partum). Spinal cord NAA levels were decreased at 34 days, as were and glutamine and gamma-aminobutyric acid levels at 75 days. The brainstem was involved at 75 days. Metabolic changes were progressively more marked in older mice who had more advanced disease. Changes appeared late in the cortex at 90 days and consisted of increased taurine.

Andreassen *et al.* examined the behavioural effects of creatine supplementation in G93A mice and additionally measured treatment effect in the brain using *in vivo* MRS (55).

Compared with healthy wild-type mice, transgenic mice had an elevated Glx (glutamate + glutamine) signal in the sensorimotor cortex. Mice fed a creatine-supplemented diet beginning at 4 weeks of age showed improved behavioural indices (rotarod performance and survival). At 80 days (but not at 110 days towards end-stage) these mice had a reduced Glx signal compared with G93A mice that had not been receiving creatine.

In summary, neuroimaging studies in the transgenic mouse provide a controlled environment where pathology can be detected before the appearance of clinical signs and how it progresses topographically over time. It affords the ability to assess the regional response to treatment in a quantitative fashion.

Experience from other diseases

Studies in other neurological disorders such as Alzheimer's disease and multiple sclerosis suggest that: (a) atrophy of the brain and spinal cord may be an important and relevant measure given it represents neuronal loss (56,57) (this comes with the proviso in ALS/FTLD that volume loss is largely regional and probably a late event); (b) multicentre studies are feasible; (c) valuable experience and insight into the utility of imaging in ALS will be gained with its inclusion in clinical trials; and (d) a consortium, similar to the Alzheimer's Disease Neuroimaging Initiative (http://www.adni-info.org/), to establish imaging standards and co-ordinate the systematic collection of imaging data would be of significant benefit to ALS research.

Challenges and limitations

Neuroimaging in ALS/FTLD is faced with several challenges. Difficulty in handling oral secretions, respiratory impairment, discomfort due to reduced mobility, and impaired cognition can decrease tolerability and preclude lengthy scans. Longitudinal studies are challenging given the rapid accrual of disability. Thus, healthier subjects with slower progression rates may be overrepresented in some studies. Imaging studies monitoring disease progression in ALS usually exclude patients with concurrent FTD; and few report cognitive testing in subjects. Cognitive and behavioural testing will be a critical component in future studies to reduce variability due to biological heterogeneity and so that such studies can be more informative towards understanding the ALS/FTLD syndrome. Furthermore, studies should incorporate validation by pathological diagnosis.

Future directions

Structural changes, neuronal integrity, metabolic function, and cortical adaptation can be monitored with current neuroimaging techniques in ALS. The field continues to evolve rapidly with improvement in sensitivity of the techniques expected with the use of higher field magnets and improved acquisition and data processing protocols. Standardization of the methods will be important to reduce experimental variability, allow for comparison of data from different centres, and pave the way for multicentre studies. The inclusion of neuroimaging parameters in clinical trials as exploratory outcome measures would assist in their evaluation as biomarkers of disease progression and aid in understanding pathophysiology, particularly regarding the biological heterogeneity of the ALS/FTLD syndrome.

References

1. Strong MJ. (2001). Progress in clinical neurosciences: the evidence for ALS as a multisystems disorder of limited phenotypic expression. *Can J Neurol Sci*, **28**(4), 283–298.
2. Lomen-Hoerth C, Murphy J, Langmore S, Kramer JH, Olney RK, Miller B. (2003). Are amyotrophic lateral sclerosis patients cognitively normal? *Neurology*, **60**(7), 1094–1097.
3. Ringholz GM, Appel SH, Bradshaw M, Cooke NA, Mosnik DM, Schulz PE. (2005). Prevalence and patterns of cognitive impairment in sporadic ALS. *Neurology*, **65**(4), 586–590.
4. Strong MJ. (2008). The syndromes of frontotemporal dysfunction in amyotrophic lateral sclerosis. *Amyotroph Lateral Scler*, **9**(6), 323–338.
5. Strong MJ, Grace GM, Freedman M, *et al.* (2009). Consensus criteria for the diagnosis of frontotemporal cognitive and behavioural syndromes in amyotrophic lateral sclerosis. *Amyotroph Lateral Scler*, **10**(3), 131–146.
6. Miller RG, Jackson CE, Kasarskis EJ, *et al.* (2009). Practice parameter update: The care of the patient with amyotrophic lateral sclerosis: multidisciplinary care, symptom management, and cognitive/behavioral impairment (an evidence-based review): report of the Quality Standards Subcommittee of the American Academy of Neurology. *Neurology*, **73**(15), 1227–1233.
7. Turner MR, Kiernan MC, Leigh PN, Talbot K. (2009). Biomarkers in amyotrophic lateral sclerosis. *Lancet Neurol*, **8**, 94–109.
8. Filippi M, Agosta F, Abrahams S, *et al.* (2010). EFNS guidelines on the use of neuroimaging in the management of motor neuron diseases. *Eur J Neurol*, **17**, 526–533.
9. Hecht MJ, Fellner F, Fellner C, Hilz MJ, Neundorfer B, Heuss D. (2002). Hyperintense and hypointense MRI signals of the precentral gyrus and corticospinal tract in ALS: a follow-up examination including FLAIR images. *J Neurol Sci*, **199**(1–2), 59–65.
10. Unrath A, Ludolph AC, Kassubek J. (2007). Brain metabolites in definite amyotrophic lateral sclerosis: a longitudinal proton magnetic resonance spectroscopy study. *J Neurol*, **254**(8), 1099–1106.
11. Chang JL, Lomen-Hoerth C, Murphy J, *et al.* (2005). A voxel-based morphometry study of patterns of brain atrophy in ALS and ALS/FTLD. *Neurology*, **65**, 75–80.
12. Agosta F, Pagani E, Rocca MA, *et al.* (2007). Voxel-based morphometry study of brain volumetry and diffusivity in amyotrophic lateral sclerosis patients with mild disability. *Hum Brain Mapp*, **28**(12), 1430–1438.
13. Thivard L, Pradat PF, Lehericy S, *et al.* (2007). Diffusion tensor imaging and voxel based morphometry study in amyotrophic lateral sclerosis: relationships with motor disability. *J Neurol Neurosurg Psychiatry*, **78**(8), 889–892.
14. Agosta F, Gorno-Tempini ML, Pagani E, *et al.* (2009). Longitudinal assessment of grey matter contraction in amyotrophic lateral sclerosis: A tensor based morphometry study. *Amyotroph Lateral Scler*, **10**(3), 168–174.
15. Avants B, Khan A, McCluskey L, Elman L, Grossman M. (2009). Longitudinal cortical atrophy in amyotrophic lateral sclerosis with frontotemporal dementia. *Arch Neurol*, **66**, 138–139.
16. Brambati SM, Renda NC, Rankin KP, *et al.* (2007). A tensor based morphometry study of longitudinal gray matter contraction in FTD. *Neuroimage*, **35**(3), 998–1003.
17. Knopman DS, Jack CR, Jr, Kramer JH, *et al.* (2009). Brain and ventricular volumetric changes in frontotemporal lobar degeneration over 1 year. *Neurology*, **72**(21), 1843–1849.
18. Chan D, Fox NC, Jenkins R, Scahill RI, Crum WR, Rossor MN. (2001). Rates of global and regional cerebral atrophy in AD and frontotemporal dementia. *Neurology*, **57**(10), 1756–1763.
19. Gordon E, Rohrer JD, Kim LG, *et al.* (2010). Measuring disease progression in frontotemporal lobar degeneration: a clinical and MRI study. *Neurology*, **74**(8), 666–673.
20. Whitwell JL, Jack CR, Jr, Parisi JE, *et al.* (2007). Rates of cerebral atrophy differ in different degenerative pathologies. *Brain*, **130**(Pt 4), 1148–1158.

21. Pioro EP, Antel JP, Cashman NR, Arnold DL. (1994). Detection of cortical neuron loss in motor neuron disease by proton magnetic resonance spectroscopic imaging *in vivo*. *Neurology*, **44**(10), 1933–1938.
22. Block W, Karitzky J, Traber F, *et al.* (1998). Proton magnetic resonance spectroscopy of the primary motor cortex in patients with motor neuron disease: subgroup analysis and follow-up measurements. *Arch Neurol*, **55**(7), 931–936.
23. Strong MJ, Grace GM, Orange JB, Leeper HA, Menon RS, Aere C. (1999). A prospective study of cognitive impairment in ALS. *Neurology*, **53**(8), 1665–1670.
24. Bowen BC, Pattany PM, Bradley WG, *et al.* (2000). MR imaging and localized proton spectroscopy of the precentral gyrus in amyotrophic lateral sclerosis. *AJNR Am J Neuroradiol*, **21**(4), 647–658.
25. Pohl C, Block W, Karitzky J, *et al.* (2001). Proton magnetic resonance spectroscopy of the motor cortex in 70 patients with amyotrophic lateral sclerosis. *Arch Neurol*, **58**(5), 729–735.
26. Abe K, Takanashi M, Watanabe Y, *et al.* (2001). Decrease in N-acetylaspartate/creatine ratio in the motor area and the frontal lobe in amyotrophic lateral sclerosis. *Neuroradiology*, **43**(7), 537–541.
27. Suhy J, Miller RG, Rule R, *et al.* (2002). Early detection and longitudinal changes in amyotrophic lateral sclerosis by (1)H MRSI. *Neurology*, **58**(5), 773–779.
28. Kalra S, Genge A, Arnold D. (2003). A prospective, randomized, placebo-controlled evaluation of corticoneuronal response to intrathecal BDNF therapy in ALS using magnetic resonance spectroscopy: feasibility and results. *Amyotroph Lateral Scler Other Motor Neuron Disord* **4**, 22–26.
29. Rule RR, Suhy J, Schuff N, Gelinas DF, Miller RG, Weiner MW. (2004). Reduced NAA in motor and non-motor brain regions in amyotrophic lateral sclerosis: a cross-sectional and longitudinal study. *Amyotroph Lateral Scler Other Motor Neuron Disord*, **5**(3), 141–149.
30. Mitsumoto H, Ulug AM, Pullman SL, *et al.* (2007). Quantitative objective markers for upper and lower motor neuron dysfunction in ALS. *Neurology*, **68**(17), 1402–1410.
31. Cwik VA, Hanstock CC, Allen PS, Martin WR. (1998). Estimation of brainstem neuronal loss in amyotrophic lateral sclerosis with *in vivo* proton magnetic resonance spectroscopy. *Neurology*, **50**, 72–77.
32. Pioro EP, Majors AW, Mitsumoto H, Nelson DR, Ng TC. (1999). 1H-MRS evidence of neurodegeneration and excess glutamate + glutamine in ALS medulla. *Neurology*, **53**, 71–79.
33. De SN, Filippi M, Miller D, *et al.* (2007). Guidelines for using proton MR spectroscopy in multicenter clinical MS studies. *Neurology*, **69**(20), 1942–1952.
34. Ellis CM, Simmons A, Jones DK, *et al.* (1999). Diffusion tensor MRI assesses corticospinal tract damage in ALS. *Neurology*, **53**(5), 1051–1058.
35. Sach M, Winkler G, Glauche V, *et al.* (2004). Diffusion tensor MRI of early upper motor neuron involvement in amyotrophic lateral sclerosis. *Brain*, **127**(Pt 2), 340–350.
36. Abe O, Yamada H, Masutani Y, *et al.* (2004). Amyotrophic lateral sclerosis: diffusion tensor tractography and voxel-based analysis. *NMR Biomed*, **17**(6), 411–416.
37. Graham JM, Papadakis N, Evans J, *et al.* (2004). Diffusion tensor imaging for the assessment of upper motor neuron integrity in ALS. *Neurology*, **63**(11), 2111–2119.
38. Cosottini M, Giannelli M, Siciliano G, *et al.* (2005). Diffusion-tensor MR imaging of corticospinal tract in amyotrophic lateral sclerosis and progressive muscular atrophy. *Radiology*, **237**, 258–264.
39. Wong JC, Concha L, Beaulieu C, Johnston W, Allen PS, Kalra S. (2007). Spatial profiling of the corticospinal tract in amyotrophic lateral sclerosis using diffusion tensor imaging. *J Neuroimaging*, **17**(3), 234–240.
40. Pyra T, Hui B, Hanstock C, *et al.* (2010). Combined structural and neurochemical evaluation of the corticospinal tract in amyotrophic lateral sclerosis. *Amyotroph Lateral Scler*, **11**(1–2), 157–165.
41. Sage CA, Peeters RR, Gorner A, Robberecht W, Sunaert S. (2007). Quantitative diffusion tensor imaging in amyotrophic lateral sclerosis. *Neuroimage*, **34**(2), 486–499.

42. Charil A, Corbo M, Filippi M, *et al.* (2009). Structural and metabolic changes in the brain of patients with upper motor neuron disorders: a multiparametric MRI study. *Amyotroph Lateral Scler*, **10**(5–6), 269–279.
43. Senda J, Ito M, Watanabe H, *et al.* (2009). Correlation between pyramidal tract degeneration and widespread white matter involvement in amyotrophic lateral sclerosis: a study with tractography and diffusion-tensor imaging. *Amyotroph Lateral Scler*, **10**(5–6), 288–294.
44. Blain CR, Williams VC, Johnston C, *et al.* (2007). A longitudinal study of diffusion tensor MRI in ALS. *Amyotroph Lateral Scler*, **8**(6), 348–355.
45. Agosta F, Rocca MA, Valsasina P, *et al.* (2009). A longitudinal diffusion tensor MRI study of the cervical cord and brain in amyotrophic lateral sclerosis patients. *J Neurol Neurosurg Psychiatry*, **80**, 53–55.
46. Lule D, Diekmann V, Kassubek J, *et al.* (2007). Cortical plasticity in amyotrophic lateral sclerosis: motor imagery and function. *Neurorehabil Neural Repair*, **21**(6), 518–526.
47. Lule D, Diekmann V, Anders S, *et al.* (2007). Brain responses to emotional stimuli in patients with amyotrophic lateral sclerosis (ALS). *J Neurol*, **254**(4), 519–527.
48. Kalra S, Cashman NR, Genge A, Arnold DL. (1998). Recovery of N-acetylaspartate in corticomotor neurons of patients with ALS after riluzole therapy. *Neuroreport*, **9**(8), 1757–1761.
49. Kalra S, Tai P, Genge A, Arnold DL. (2006). Rapid improvement in cortical neuronal integrity in amyotrophic lateral sclerosis detected by proton magnetic resonance spectroscopic imaging. *J Neurol*, **253**(8), 1060–1063.
50. Vielhaber S, Kaufmann J, Kanowski M, *et al.* (2001). Effect of creatine supplementation on metabolite levels in ALS motor cortices. *Exp Neurol*, **172**(2), 377–382.
51. Kalra S, Cashman NR, Caramanos Z, Genge A, Arnold DL. (2003). Gabapentin therapy for amyotrophic lateral sclerosis: lack of improvement in neuronal integrity shown by MR spectroscopy. *AJNR Am J Neuroradiol*, **24**(3), 476–480.
52. Angenstein F, Niessen HG, Goldschmidt J, Vielhaber S, Ludolph AC, Scheich H. (2004). Age-dependent changes in MRI of motor brain stem nuclei in a mouse model of ALS. *Neuroreport*, **15**(14), 2271–2274.
53. Niessen HG, Angenstein F, Sander K, Kunz WS, Teuchert M, Ludolph AC, *et al.* (2006). In vivo quantification of spinal and bulbar motor neuron degeneration in the G93A-SOD1 transgenic mouse model of ALS by T2 relaxation time and apparent diffusion coefficient. *Exp Neurol*, **201**(2), 293–300.
54. Niessen HG, Bska-Vielhaber G, Sander K, *et al.* (2007). Metabolic progression markers of neurodegeneration in the transgenic G93A-SOD1 mouse model of amyotrophic lateral sclerosis. *Eur J Neurosci*, **25**(6), 1669–1677.
55. Andreassen OA, Jenkins BG, Dedeoglu A, *et al.* (2001). Increases in cortical glutamate concentrations in transgenic amyotrophic lateral sclerosis mice are attenuated by creatine supplementation. *J Neurochem*, **77**(2), 383–390.
56. Leist TP, Marks S. (2010). Magnetic resonance imaging and treatment effects of multiple sclerosis therapeutics. *Neurology*, **74** (Suppl 1), S54–S61.
57. Jack CR, Jr, Shiung MM, Weigand SD, *et al.* (2005). Brain atrophy rates predict subsequent clinical conversion in normal elderly and amnestic MCI. *Neurology*, **65**(8), 1227–1231.

Chapter 16

Differentiating normal from pathological atrophy: when is frontotemporal atrophy normal?

Tiffany W. Chow

Although we would all prefer to believe that our brains will not atrophy with age, it has been widely observed that the frontal lobe atrophies as we age, to an extent greater than the other lobes. For example, the ratio of frontal pole to total brain volume decreases over age 20 to 40 years in normal controls (1). Raz and colleagues have shown in volumetric studies that the dorsolateral prefrontal cortex, as opposed to the anterior cingulate gyrus or the orbitofrontal cortex shows the most substantial age-related decline (2).

In a binary logistic regression analysis to determine which semiautomated volumetrics could discriminate patients with frontotemporal dementia (FTD) from healthy controls, only two regions within the frontal and temporal lobes were helpful. The left anterior cingulate and left anterior temporal regions were most consistently atrophied in patients with FTD, and this applied to behavioural variant FTD as well as cases with primary progressive aphasia (3). Three control subjects had subthreshold volumes for either the left anterior temporal or the left anterior cingulate volumes of interest, but none of these three were subthreshold for both volumes of interest.

The same investigators have pursued whether clinicians can detect these critical atrophies in the left anterior cingulate and anterior temporal lobe, to apply the volumetric findings to real-life practice. Research magnetic resonance imaging (MRI) data from the original 2008 study were converted to the MRI slices usually available from a clinical radiology practice (transaxial, sagittal, and coronal views). While there was high inter rater agreement as to whether each volume of interest was atrophied versus normal and these ratings correlated well with the actual volumes, the four neurologists still had difficulty using this information to accurately differentiate FTD from healthy elderly and patients with Alzheimer's disease (AD). The raters' accuracy for distinguishing between FTD and healthy controls averaged 59.5%, while differentiation from AD was no less difficult for the raters, reaching an average accuracy of 63.1% (4).

Kipps and colleagues reported that good inter-rater reliability exists when temporal lobe atrophy is observed on coronal slices, and that patients with semantic dementia (focal atrophy of the left temporal lobe) can be easily identified (5). However, they also noted that nearly half of patients with behavioural variant FTD had scans that appeared much closer to normal. This was not an artifact of the patients with behavioural variant FTD being scanned at an earlier stage of illness than the ones with semantic dementia.

In a more optimistic comparison between visual raters and results of voxel-based morphometry that also used only coronal MRI views (6), the anterior fusiform gyrus, anterior hippocampus, and temporal pole were identified as significantly atrophied for the semantic dementia group, and the anterior cingulate and orbitofrontal volumes of interest for behavioural variant FTD. Although the latter case series was smaller (36 subjects) and the number of regions assessed was larger (15, as opposed to just left anterior cingulate and anterior temporal lobe), this suggests that visual rating perhaps requires a less focused approach.

Volumetric analyses are difficult to translate into routine clinical practice. Structural neuroimaging, in conjunction with a complete history from a reliable informant and neuropsychological testing, can help distinguish FTD from normal ageing. If the history equivocates between the prominence of memory impairment and the onset of new behavioural disturbances and the age of onset is later than 70 years, the main differential diagnostic debate is between FTD and AD. Routine clinical MRIs may appear very similar to the naked eye among subjects with FTD, AD, and controls with age-related atrophy (see Figures 16.1–16.3). At best, MRI atrophy ratings can predict poor outcome more reliably than duration of illness, cognitive testing, behavioural inventory score, and functional disability at presentation to a clinic can (7).

Future considerations should include whether it is more clinically useful to attend to the brain regions reported from volumetric studies (8–10) or instead to measures of cortical thinning (11). The importance of the fronto-opercular–insular region as a target of FTD proteinopathy is also emerging rapidly and may serve as an additional area of interest for volumetric or functional analysis (9,12).

Refining a diagnosis of amyotrophic lateral sclerosis to FTD/amyotrophic lateral sclerosis or FTD/motor neurone disease should definitely include the clinical history, behavioural inventories, and neuropsychological assessment (13,14). In the search for the most appropriate biomarker, there is a distinct possibility that functional imaging may be more useful in this context than cortical atrophy.

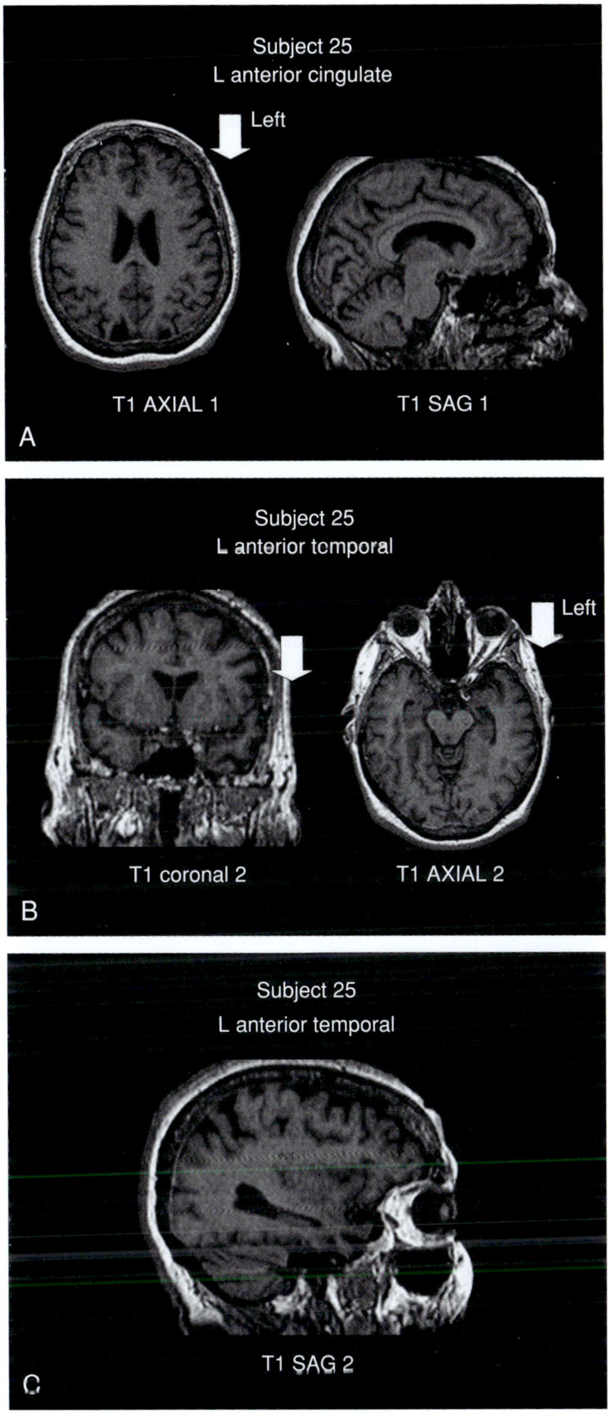

Fig. 16.1 (A–C) Subject 25, a woman aged 75 years, had a 10-year course of Alzheimer's disease determined by NINCDS-ADRDA criteria and MMSE score of 24 at the time of this scan. Note the moderate extent of atrophy in both the left anterior cingulate gyrus and the left anterior temporal lobe.

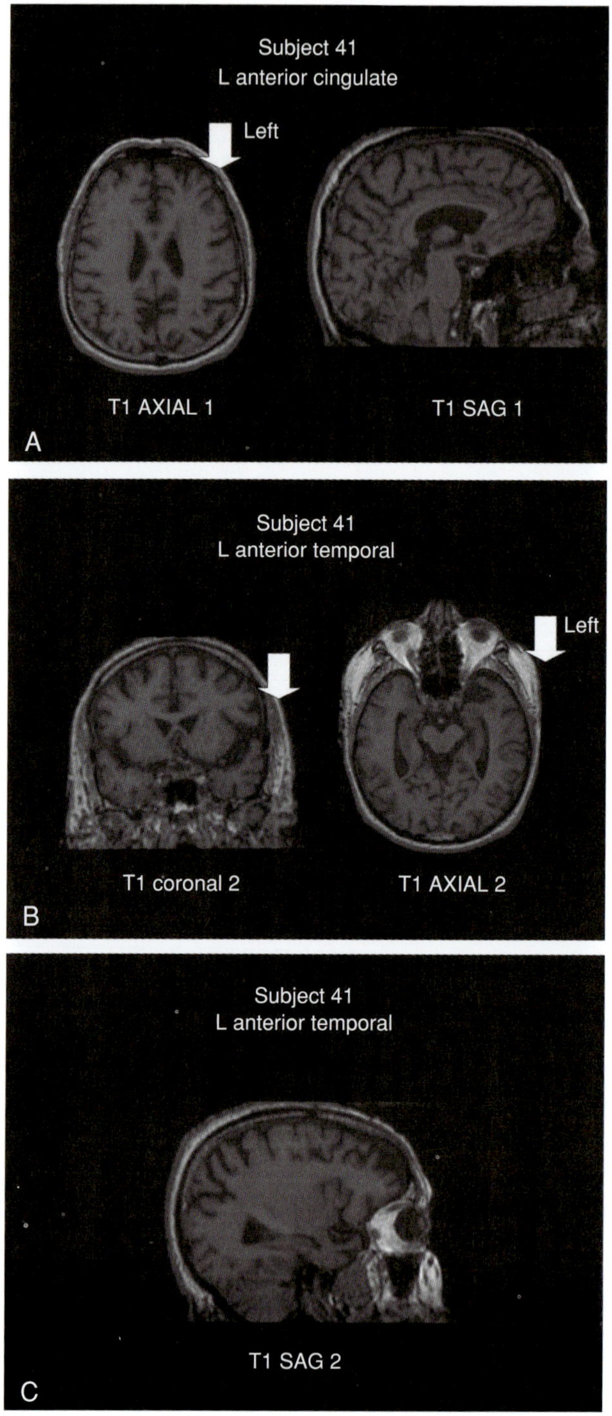

Fig. 16.2 (A–C): Subject 41, a man aged 71 years, had behavioural variant FTD by clinical consensus criteria for 5 years and MMSE score of 30 at the time of this scan. The degree of atrophy in left anterior cingulate and left anterior temporal lobe is similar to that of the Alzheimer's case in Fig. 16.1.

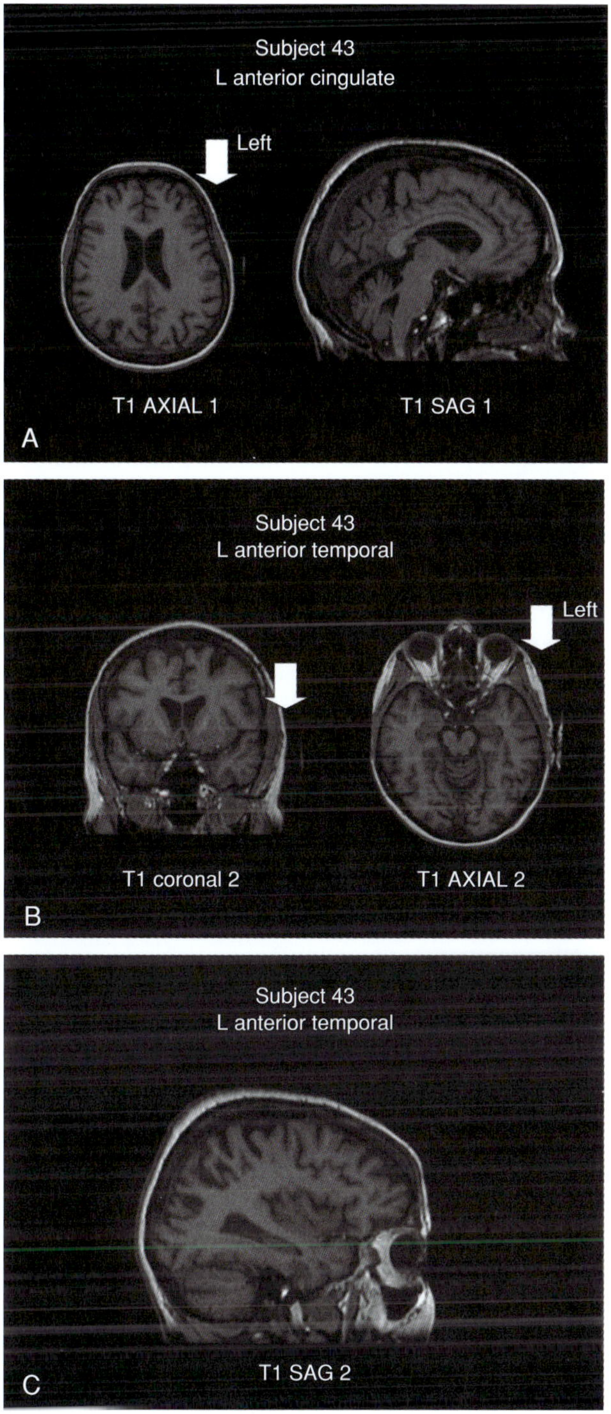

Fig. 16.3 (A–C) Subject 43, a woman aged 69 years, was a control subject with no cognitive complaints and MMSE score of 27. This subject does have cortical atrophy in right more so than left dorsoparietal brain regions, which could easily distract a clinician into suspecting cognitive impairment due to a neurodegenerative process, unless the range of age-associated atrophy was taken into consideration. Given that her MMSE score was 27, cognitive re-evaluation in a year might be warranted, with no repeat imaging unless a clear decline in mental status or neuropsychological testing scores was noted.

References

1. John JP, Burgess PW, Yashavantha BS, *et al.* (2009). Differential relationship of frontal pole and whole brain volumetric measures with age in neuroleptic-naive schizophrenia and healthy subjects. *Schizophr Res*, **109**, 148–158.
2. Raz N, Gunning FM, Head D, *et al.* (1997). Selective aging of the human cerebral cortex observed *in vivo*: differential vulnerability of the prefrontal gray matter. *Cereb Cortex*, **7**, 268–282.
3. Chow TW, Binns MA, Freedman M, *et al.* (2008). Overlap in frontotemporal atrophy between normal aging and patients with frontotemporal dementias. *Alzheimer Dis Assoc Disord*, **22**, 327–335.
4. Chow TW, Gao F, Links KA, *et al.* (2011). Visual rating versus volumetry to detect frontotemporal dementia. *Dement Geriatr Cogn Disord*, **31**, 371–378.
5. Kipps CM, Davies RR, Mitchell J, *et al.* (2007). Clinical significance of lobar atrophy in frontotemporal dementia: application of an MRI visual rating scale. *Dement Geriatr Cogn Disord*, **23**, 334–342.
6. Davies RR, Scahill VL, Graham A, *et al.* (2009). Development of an MRI rating scale for multiple brain regions: comparison with volumetrics and with voxel-based morphometry. *Neuroradiology*, **51**, 491–503.
7. Davies RR, Kipps CM, Mitchell J, *et al.* (2006). Progression in frontotemporal dementia: identifying a benign behavioral variant by magnetic resonance imaging. *Arch Neurol*, **63**, 1627–1631.
8. Perry RJ, Hodges JR, (2000). Differentiating frontal and temporal variant frontotemporal dementia from Alzheimer's disease. *Neurology*, **54**, 2277–2284.
9. Rabinovici GD, Seeley WW, Kim EJ, *et al.* (2007). Distinct MRI atrophy patterns in autopsy-proven Alzheimer's disease and frontotemporal lobar degeneration. *Am J Alzheimers Dis Other Demen*, **22**, 474–488.
10. Rosen HJ, Gorno-Tempini ML, Goldman WP, *et al.* (2002). Patterns of brain atrophy in frontotemporal dementia and semantic dementia. *Neurology*, **58**, 198–208.
11. Gordon E, Rohrer JD, Kim LG, *et al.* (2010). Measuring disease progression in frontotemporal lobar degeneration: a clinical and MRI study. *Neurology*, **74**, 666–673.
12. Zhou J, Greicius MD, Gennatas ED, *et al.* (2010). Divergent network connectivity changes in behavioural variant frontotemporal dementia and Alzheimer's disease. *Brain*, **133**, 1352–1367.
13. Strong MJ. (2008). The syndromes of frontotemporal dysfunction in amyotrophic lateral sclerosis. *Amyotroph Lateral Scler*, **9**, 323–338.
14. Strong MJ, Grace GM, Freedman M, *et al.* (2009). Consensus criteria for the diagnosis of frontotemporal cognitive and behavioural syndromes in amyotrophic lateral sclerosis. *Amyotroph Lateral Scler*, **10**, 131–146.

Chapter 17

Cerebrospinal fluid-based biomarkers for amyotrophic lateral sclerosis

Robert Bowser, James Connor, and Martin Turner

A biomarker is defined by both the US Food & Drug Administration and the UK Medical Research Council as an objective measurement that acts as an indicator of normal biological processes, pathogenic processes, or pharmacological responses to therapeutic intervention. It is nearly half a century since the first published putative biomarker for amyotrophic lateral sclerosis (ALS)—namely the observation of altered serum levels in response to oral arginine compared with controls (1). Many and varied biomarker candidates have subsequently emerged as a result of advances in molecular biological and other techniques (2,3). These studies have led to a greater understanding of underlying molecular mechanisms (4), but also to improved clinical recognition and characterization of the heterogeneous syndrome of ALS. The concept of the 'ALS signature' is attractive, with the corollary of earlier perhaps ultimately preventative intervention. However, the inherent clinical heterogeneity in ALS, the lack of understanding of the 'at-risk' population and where the 'clinical horizon' lies in relation to the earliest pathogenic events, present major challenges to translation of such candidates into meaningful biomarkers.

Ideal biomarkers for amyotrophic lateral sclerosis

In ALS, the ideal biomarker characteristics can be summarized (Table 17.1). Biomarkers in ALS have potential value on several levels, but the benchmarks are already high for some of these and the challenges significant (Table 17.2). An important question is the biofluid or tissue source that will be assessed for the biomarker. Although the *sine qua non* of ALS is anterior horn cell degeneration resulting in the lower motor neurone (LMN) clinical features of fasciculation and wasting, there is undoubtedly also a parallel upper motor neurone (UMN) in all forms of the wider syndrome of ALS (including those with so-called progressive muscular atrophy (5)), as well as an extramotor cerebral process involving clinicopathological overlap with frontotemporal dementia (6). How these processes interrelate is not yet certain (7), but raises the issue that biofluids or tissue sources may be remote from one or more of the three disease compartments, so that ultimately a multimodal biomarker approach will be required.

Table 17.1 The ideal biomarker

1. Sensitive and specific for the heterogeneous syndrome of ALS
2. Detectable before onset of significant wasting/weakness
3. Discriminate between clinical phenotypes based on:
   - (a) Upper and lower motor neurone involvement (e.g. progressive muscular atrophy and primary lateral sclerosis)
   - (b) Patterns of regional involvement (e.g. flail arm/leg, progressive bulbar palsy)
   - (c) Cognitive involvement (i.e. ALS/mild cognitive impairment versus ALS/FTD)
   - (d) Extremes of survival (i.e. 'aggressive'; 1–2-year survival from symptom onset versus 'slow' 5–10 year) course
4. Able to predict regional involvement and the pattern of spread in advance:
   - (a) Bulbar dysfunction for early percutaneous endoscopic gastrostomy
   - (b) Respiratory dysfunction for early non-invasive ventilation (possibly diaphragm pacing)
   - (c) Cognitive impairment
5. Change in a predictable way with disease progression
6. Sensitivity to confidently judge therapeutic response within weeks of challenge
7. Easily accessible and affordable technology
8. Practical to measure in the physically disabled patient

Non-destructive biopsy of central nervous system tissue is currently unrealistic, and though muscle biopsies are a potential tissue source in which one could develop biomarker assays (8), they may only reflect end-organ involvement remote from a large proportion of the pathology and possibly the very earliest steps in the pathogenic cascade. Furthermore, the particularly invasive nature of the collection procedure coupled with the challenge of performing longitudinal biopsies further limit this tissue source as a viable option for biomarker discovery or validation.

There are a number of biofluids that have been used to measure biomarkers, including blood, urine, cerebrospinal fluid (CSF), and saliva (9). Each has advantages and disadvantages, and for the purpose of this discussion, we will focus on CSF, which intuitively appears to offer most overlap between the cerebral, corticospinal tract, and anterior horn cell pathology, notwithstanding significant accompanying challenges.

Why cerebrospinal fluid?

Although urine and saliva also have potential as biomarker sources, blood (serum) and CSF are currently viewed as the richest potential source for biomarkers across a range of neurological disorders; the relative advantages of each are summarized in Table 17.3. CSF is compartmentalized with respect to other organ systems and biofluids and therefore in

Table 17.2 Categories of biomarker

Category	Purpose	Current benchmark	Challenges
Diagnostic	To reduce diagnostic delay (current mean ~1 year from symptom onset) To distinguish ALS from mimic disorders; Permit earlier therapeutic intervention	Clinical acumen ALS neurologists in tertiary referral centres >95% sensitive and specific, but possibly inflated as a result of current referral delay	Who are the 'at-risk' population? Where is the 'clinical horizon' in relation to pathogenesis? The true mimics are not healthy controls, but pure LMN and pure UMN syndromes
Prognostic	To identify those with poor prognosis who may require earlier intervention or care planning Identify the minority for whom cognitive involvement likely to be significant and intrusive	Prognostic modelling of survival with clinical parameters probably >90% accurate, e.g. (65,66)	Prognostic modelling based on tertiary referral centre data Need to establish how earlier intervention in 'aggressive' ALS might actually be beneficial Those with ALS/FTD often present with early dementia before motor features are apparent
Monitoring	To provide a marker of early therapeutic benefit in clinical trials Reduce size and duration of studies Reduce need for placebo arms	Survival as main endpoint, which requires trials of >200 patients over 12–24 months Amyotrophic Lateral Sclerosis Functional Rating Scale-Revised and forced vital capacity are alternative surrogate endpoints	Heterogeneous syndrome of ALS may distort all trial outcome measures due to different efficacy across phenotypes
Mechanistic	Biomarkers may provide clues to pathogenesis via pathway analysis and thence provide new candidates	Cellular inclusions (e.g. TDP-43 and FUS) indicate abnormal RNA processing may be important in pathogenesis	Distinguishing pathogenic pathways from epiphenomena

proximity to the ongoing disease process. However, this necessitates an invasive procedure to collect the fluid and therefore impedes its diagnostic evaluation and clinical utility (Figure 17.1). CSF likely harbours proteins released from injured or dying cells that may represent biomarkers, in addition to proteins or molecules released from neurones and glia throughout the disease pathogenesis. These proteins may be at higher concentrations in the CSF than in blood, urine, or saliva. Thus, CSF may be well suited for unbiased biomarker discovery efforts, and biomarker discovery efforts in the CSF may identify proteins that can subsequently be measured in other biofluids within focused biomarker discovery and validation studies.

Table 17.3 Relative advantages of different biofluids for biomarker discovery

Characteristic	Blood	CSF	Urine	Saliva
Proximity to CNS pathology	++	+++	+	+
Lack of molecular complexity	+	+	++	+++
Less invasive	++	+	+++	+++
Practicality of sampling	+++	++	+++	++
Handling and storage	++	+*	++	+
Resistance to exogenous drug contamination	+	+++	+	++
Candidate molecules to date	++	+++	+	+

*Bloody tap contamination potential and need for rapid centrifugation.

While CSF has advantages, there are also significant disadvantages that must be considered for all biomarker-related studies. Similar to blood, there is a wide concentration range of proteins in the CSF (10). Therefore, investigators may first have to enrich proteins within specific concentration ranges (e.g. abundant versus low abundant proteins). The protein complexity of the CSF is much less than blood, but hundreds to thousands of proteins can be detected in the human CSF proteome (10,11). CSF collection and preprocessing steps have been varied across different laboratories, which may add to disparate results between study results. The spinal tap procedure can also introduce a number of artefacts, including introduction of blood during the procedure and varied time from sample collection to storage. Diurnal rhythms and CSF flow rate also influence protein concentrations. Therefore, the time of the day for the sample collection affects protein concentration within the CSF. CSF proteome stability over time has been the subject of investigation, and results demonstrate that proteome alterations can be detected as early as 1–2 hours after CSF withdraw, even when stored at 4°C (12). Figure 17.2 shows results of CSF stability over 24 hours at two different temperatures. Similar findings were reported

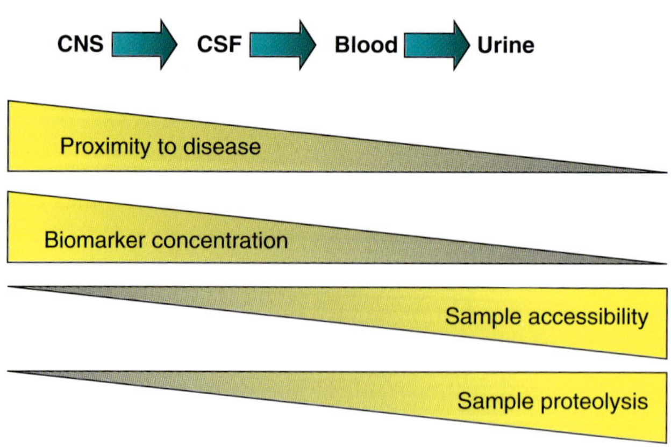

Fig. 17.1 CSF protein stability over time. Relative biomarker concentration, proximity to disease, ease of access and degree of protein degradation within the various body biofluids commonly used for biomarker discovery efforts for amyotrophic lateral sclerosis.

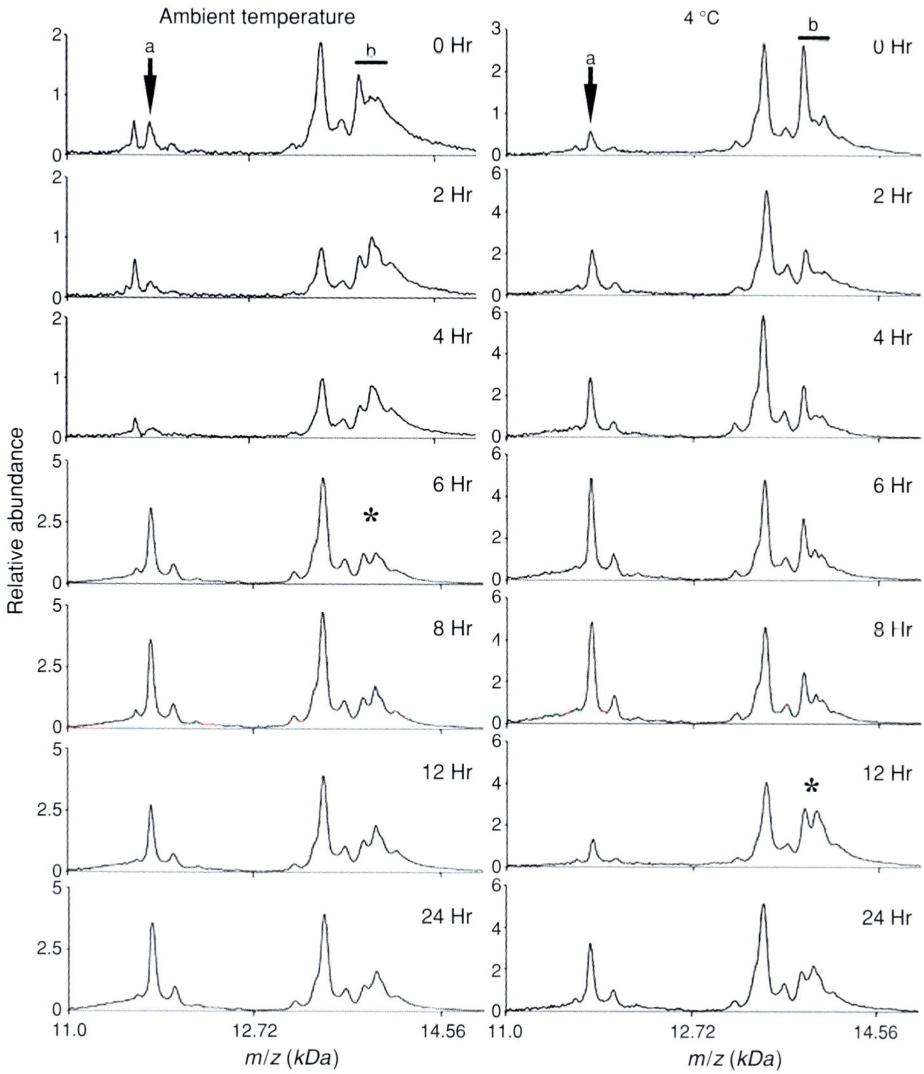

Fig. 17.2 Surface enhanced laser-desorption/ionization time-of-flight mass spectrometry of CSF maintained at either ambient temperature (left panel) or at 4°C (right panel) and assayed by mass spectrometry over the course of 24 hours. The m/z profiles between 11 and 15 kDa are shown for 0, 2, 4, 6, 8, 12, and 24 hours. The arrow denoted by 'a' and the line denoted by 'b' mark specific peaks that rapidly exhibit alterations over time.

for collection, processing, and storage of CSF for metabolomic biomarker studies (13). Repeated sample thawing can also introduce protein alterations that would introduce variability and artefacts into biomarker discovery and validation efforts.

Finally, recent studies have suggested early defects in the blood–brain barrier (BBB) in both rodent models of ALS and in patients with ALS (14–16). The most common biochemical methods to determine BBB integrity include counting red blood cells in the CSF, determining the albumin quotient, or measurements of blood-borne proteins in the CSF such as haemoglobin, apolipoprotein B (17). It is currently uncertain if BBB compromise is a primary or secondary event in ALS. Therefore elimination of CSF samples that contain evidence of BBB breakdown may eliminate early disease events and compromise the ability to identify early biomarkers of disease. In addition, therapeutics that target the BBB may be most effective in patients the exhibit BBB alterations. Clearly, more investigations are required to examine the role of BBB in ALS pathogenesis and progression.

Subject populations used for biomarker studies

ALS biomarker discovery efforts are typically performed using a group of clinically defined ALS patients and control groups that may contain a combination of non-neurological disease controls and neurological disease controls. Ultimately, the sensitivity and specificity of any putative biomarker is defined during large validation studies in relation to the control population. However, the latter has been quite variable in its definition to date. A diagnostic biomarker is likely to be most helpful in the context of phenotypic mimics, which are relatively rare in ALS. While the pre-symptomatic 'at-risk' population remains uncharacterized, healthy controls may be less useful as a comparative population for diagnostic biomarkers, with neurological disease groups (e.g. other motor neuropathies versus progressive muscular atrophy, and primary progressive multiple sclerosis for primary lateral sclerosis) being more pertinent.

The implication of transactive response DNA-binding protein of 43 kDa (TDP-43) across a range of disorders (18), suggests that inclusion of other neurodegenerative diseases may be useful to determine the specificity of candidate biomarkers to ALS. Some forms of frontotemporal dementia (FTD) are clearly relevant to ALS, and a significant percentage of patients with ALS will develop detectable cognitive impairment within the FTD spectrum (19). However, this generates additional challenges, as patients with ALS may have subclinical FTD reflected in early biomarker changes exhibiting equivalent biomarker alterations to 'pure' FTD subjects. The relative merits of several control populations are considered in Table 17.4.

Biomarker discovery methods

An agnostic ('fishing') approach to biomarkers is entirely reasonable in the face of so much uncertainty about the pathogenic process in ALS, including when and where the first events in the cascade occur. However, there are consistent themes of research into disease pathogenesis over many years, including excitotoxicity, axonal transport, and the role of inflammatory pathways (4), as well as the growing interest in RNA processing (20), that make focused hypothesis-led screening for candidate molecules equally useful. A recent study identified specific proteins derived from neurones, astrocytes, or inflammatory molecules that were elevated or decreased in ALS or specific motor neurone disease subtypes, with glial CSF markers correlating to patient survival (21).

The agnostic approaches have often used mass spectrometry, two-dimensional gel electrophoresis, antibody microarray analysis, or cytokine profiling techniques for

Table 17.4 Advantages and disadvantages of different control populations

Category of control	Advantage	Disadvantage
Healthy	'Pure' sample Maximize sensitivity	Ethical approval for invasive procedures especially spinal tap, although research is reassuring (67) Age-matching additionally challenging Reduced specificity
'Ward traffic': CSF as part of investigation with additional sampling volume	Availability Ethical approval and consent easier as it is part of routine care	Diagnosis may be idiopathic (e.g. 'headache', 'paraesthesiae') with a need for follow-up to categorize later as further information comes to light (with the need for ethical approval in this respect) Experience from routine lumbar drainage suggests multiple confounds (68)
Other NDs	Explore disease specificity of putative markers, especially neuronal FTLD particularly relevant to ALS	Disparate collection procedures across diseases Relevance of other NDs to ALS? Poor clinical diagnostic accuracy in other NDs (69,70)
Other motor neuropathies (e.g. MFMN)	Clinical 'mimic'	Scarcity Only serve as mimic for PMA MFMN is immune-based pathology, not degenerative
Neuroinflammatory diseases	Relatively common Explore specificity of putative markers, especially glial May be some 'mimic' potential (e.g. primary progressive multiple sclerosis versus PLS)	Relevance of primary immune-based conditions to ALS, including age, natural history, and treatments?

MFMN, multifocal motor neuropathy with conduction block; ND, neurodegenerative disorders.

biomarker discovery (22). More hypothesis-driven studies have used enzyme-linked immunosorbent assay or immunoblot for detection methods of specific proteins.

Probing the origin of candidate biomarkers

Once a biomarker has been identified, the cell type origin of the protein can provide insight into disease mechanisms. There have been a number of reviews listing the protein candidate biomarkers for ALS within the CSF, that include broad categories such as hormones, growth factors, inflammatory markers and markers of oxidative stress (2,3,23,24). A recent review also highlighted the cell type origin for a number of candidate biomarkers useful in neurological diseases (25). Further insight into mechanisms of disease may be obtained by examining the subcellular origin of biomarker candidates detected in the CSF. We will highlight cell-type-specific ALS biomarkers with respect to their potential significance in disease pathogenesis.

Neuronal markers

Numerous biomarker candidates originate from neurones, a logical cell-type origin given that injured or dying neurones release proteins into the brain and spinal cord parenchyma, which then accumulate within the CSF before elimination into the blood. Notwithstanding the fact that release of such proteins through cell death may be a long way from the earliest pathogenic steps, and the pattern of proteins secreted may reflect those of neuronal cell death and not necessarily processes specific to ALS, valuable insights into disease mechanisms may still be obtained by subsequent in-depth examination of where these proteins reside within the living neurone.

Multiple studies have identified increased levels of neurofilament light chain (NF_L) or neurofilament heavy chain (NF_H) in the CSF of patients with ALS (26–28). In addition, increased NF_L levels have been reported for ALS versus progressive muscular atrophy (28), and in more rapid progressors (29). Increased NF_H has been observed in upper motor neurone dominant ALS and rapid progressors (27). Disruption to these proteins fits with the long-established concept that axonal transport may be critical in ALS pathology (30,31), though the presence of neurofilaments per se is unlikely to be disease specific (32).

The microtubule-associated protein tau has also been shown to be increased in the CSF of patients with ALS (21,33). CSF tau levels are also increased in upper motor neurone diseases when compared with lower motor neurone diseases (21). Both neurofilament and tau are located predominately in axons. This can be interpreted as evidence of white matter axonal injury during ALS.

Altered levels and/or function of neuroendocrine proteins, including neuroendocrine protein 7B2 and chromogranin A have been observed in ALS CSF and linked to disease (34,35). These proteins further highlight subcellular trafficking deficiencies during ALS. Altered levels of numerous growth factors have also been observed in the CSF (2,24). These changes may occur due to combined effects from inhibition of proper secretion, injury/death of cells that produce and secrete the trophic factors, or increased proteolysis of trophic factors. However, these findings indicate that axonal trafficking, release of synaptic vesicles and subsequent signalling via trophic factors is altered during ALS and contributes to the disease pathogenesis.

Intracellular protein aggregation has been well documented in ALS, though questions remain about the degree to which this is an epiphenomenon to more remote and currently obscure pathogenic events. Superoxide dismutase-1 (*SOD1*) containing aggregates accumulate in neuronal cell bodies and the outer membrane of mitochondria in patients with familial *SOD1* mutations and transgenic animal models of disease (36,37). However there are no changes in SOD1 protein level or enzymatic activity within the CSF of patients with ALS (38). RNA-binding proteins, including TDP-43 and FUS (fused in sarcoma) develop cytoplasmic aggregates and skeins in neurones in ALS (reviewed in references (20,39)). The recent generation of antibodies to TDP-43 has enabled the search for this protein in the CSF. Increased CSF levels of TDP-43 have been detected in patients with ALS by enzyme-linked immunosorbent assay or immunoblot analysis (40,41). CSF levels of TDP-43 were similar between patients with ALS and FTLD, though lower in patients with ALS/FTD (40). The significance of this finding is unclear and further studies using a much larger number of subjects and a more quantitative method are required to verify this result. The CSF levels of TDP-43 are higher in patients when monitored closest to onset of symptoms, suggesting that highest levels of TDP-43 within the CSF occur early in the disease process (41). Mass spectrometric detection of these proteins is hindered by limited protease digestion of the aggregates, resulting in few peptides that are detectable by the mass spectrometer. These studies continue to reinforce the importance of RNA metabolism to the pathogenesis of ALS.

Decreased CSF levels of cystatin C have been reported in patients with ALS (34,42,43). Cystatin C is produced and secreted into the CSF via choroid plexus cells, but neurones also express cystatin C and it is located in Bunina bodies in spinal cord motor neurones during ALS (44). While extracellular protein aggregates have not been observed in spinal cord tissues of patients with ALS, decreased levels of amyloid-beta 1–42 and transthyretin have been observed in the CSF of patients with ALS (34,45). As both of these proteins can act as the fundamental subunit of the aggregates found in some forms of familial cerebral amyloid angiopathy, further exploration of potential extracellular protein deposits within the parenchyma are warranted.

From these studies, neuronal-derived candidate biomarkers in the CSF include proteins for axonal (within white matter) and somal (grey matter) injury. It appears thus far that markers of white matter damage are more commonly detected though they may reflect previous pathological events at the cell body.

Glial/inflammatory markers

The exposure of glial cells in culture to CSF from patients with ALS results in their activation (46,47). This bioassay approach was among the early indicators for the presence of glial-activating factors in the CSF. Although a number of trophic factors can be present in the CSF, there are also inflammatory cytokines known to activate glial cells. Some of these cytokines are secreted by astrocytes and microglial cells and may be used as indices of glial activation. A number of studies have examined inflammatory markers in the CSF in patients with ALS and not all have found consistent results. Some of the reasons for lack of consistency are technical and others have to do with the types of control groups that have been discussed elsewhere in this chapter. One of the limitations in evaluation of cytokines in CSF has been the approach to consider one cytokine at a time rather than evaluate the cytokines as representing a pattern of expression using multifactorial analyses that determine patterns of profile expression similar to what is used for gene array analyses. For example, in a recent study using a multiplex system, 14 cytokines were found that differed between ALS and controls, but by using a 'leave one out' strategy for analysing the protein patterns, five inflammatory cytokines (interleukin (IL)-10, IL-6, granulocyte-macrophage colony-stimulating factor, IL-2, and IL-15) could be identified that would distinguish patients with ALS from neurological disease controls with greater than 89% accuracy (48). Rentzos and colleagues reported that IL-12 and IL-15 were elevated in CSF of patients with ALS (49), suggesting an emerging cytokine profile for ALS. However, the disease specificity of these cytokine alterations is unclear.

In the study by Mitchell *et al.*, expression of IL-8 correlated negatively with Amyotrophic Lateral Sclerosis Functional Rating Scale-Revised suggesting that specific cytokine levels may correlate to rate of disease progression. Monocyte chemoattractant protein (MCP-1) has also been reported as a potential predictor of disease course. MCP-1 was found elevated in CSF of patients with ALS compared with controls in a number of studies (48,50–54) and higher levels of MCP-1 might predict more rapid disease progression (51). CCL2 and CXCL8 levels have been negatively correlated with Amyotrophic Lateral Sclerosis Functional Rating Scale-Revised whereas CCL4 was positively correlated but the latter along with CXCL10 showed negative correlations with disease progression (55). Changes in protein levels may also be dependent upon the individual genotype and potential genetic risk factors for ALS, as elevated CSF levels of MCP-1 has been correlated to patients with ALS that carry a variant of the HFE gene, a reported risk factor for ALS (56). We also suggest that one should consider evaluation of relationships and patterns of protein expression instead of individual protein differences, as the ratio of MCP-1 to vascular endothelial growth factor in the CSF has been suggested to be a diagnostic indicator (52).

In addition to predictive value, the ideal biomarker(s) will also provide targets for therapeutic interventions. An example may be that of prostaglandin E_2 (PGE_2). Almer *et al.* report that 82% of the patients with ALS studied had two to 10 times higher PGE_2 levels in CSF compared with normal control subjects (57). The levels of PGE_2 were also elevated in post-mortem spinal cords from patients with ALS. Inhibition of a key PGE_2-synthesizing enzyme, cyclooxygenase-2, is neuroprotective in an *in vitro* model of ALS and thus provides a therapeutic target (57).

The type of inflammatory agents appearing in the CSF of patients with ALS is consistent with the overall concept that microglia activation and recruitment are important contributors of ALS pathogenesis. As such, the degree of activation at any given time is, of course, going to impact the profile of cytokines collected at a single time point. Longitudinal lumbar taps are necessary to evaluate changes in the cytokine profile during disease progression, though a reliable serum-based marker for neuroinflammation would supplant the collection of CSF. Recent studies have suggested that serum ferritin is elevated in ALS (58–60); though additional larger studies are necessary to validate these findings.

Next steps to advance candidate biomarkers

There have been many CSF-based biomarker discovery studies, using a multitude of methodologies, and a list of individual substances rapidly becomes overwhelming, with replication of findings being the exception not the rule. While the next steps include much larger validation studies, there remain important issues to resolve before initiation of these validation studies that will require a concerted effort to collect sufficient numbers of samples from ALS and appropriate control subjects.

A consensus across the numerous participants in biomarker studies is required with respect to how to collect, process, and store CSF samples, similar to that proposed for other neurological disorders (61). This will facilitate the ability to share samples, to generate reproducible results, and to define the parameters so that candidate biomarkers can be translated to the 'real world' situation where routine assays would be carried out within hospital-based laboratories.

Longitudinal samples collected from patients with ALS are not only needed to identify biomarkers of disease progression, but will help determine the timing of biomarker alterations within the ALS population. They will be critical to identify and validate biomarkers for disease progression, or to correlate specific biomarkers to disease phenotype, patient survival or response to drug therapy. Such studies are in the early stages for ALS, whereas similar studies in other neurodegenerative diseases such as Alzheimer's disease have already yielded biomarkers for each of these important questions (62). Two studies have identified cystatin C, S100beta, and soluble CD14 as biomarker candidates for survival of patients with ALS (21,63). Incorporation of standardized CSF collection procedures into all ALS clinical trials will facilitate the discovery and validation of prognostic biomarkers for survival, progression, and response to drug treatment.

As ALS is a heterogeneous disease, standardized collection and storage procedures are critical and may also help identify patient subpopulations from a biochemical rather than simply clinicogenetic perspective. Standardized protocols also help stimulate collaboration among those in the field, though international shipping barriers still exist that must be addressed in order to facilitate world-wide collaborative studies. Alternatively, experimental methods could be standardized and qualified such that a small number of experimental sites in different continents could generate data that are shared by investigators around the globe.

The methodology used for biomarker measurement will help determine the types of bioinformatics approaches used to properly interpret the data and avoid type I errors that commonly occur in diseases with a high level of complexity. Highly complex data sets generated by mass spectrometry or microarray technologies often require computer-based learning algorithms to generate biomarker panels (64). However, this can easily lead to false positive or negative results due to the large number of data points collected per individual sample.

In conclusion, the last decade has seen tremendous advancements in biomarker discovery and validation in neurological disorders. While hypothesis-driven biomarker discovery efforts based on presumed mechanisms relevant to ALS have continued to make important contributions, the use of unbiased biomarker discovery efforts has led to new candidate biomarkers and opportunities. To date, the CSF-based biomarkers best verified in ALS include those related to axonal injury and inflammation. It is likely that for a heterogeneous disease such as ALS a multiprotein panel will be required to classify ALS from control groups and to monitor disease progression. We look forward to translation of validated biomarkers into the clinic to aid physicians in early diagnosis and improved methods to monitor disease progression and drug response.

References

1. Poser CM, Johnson M, Bunch LD. (1965). Serum amino acid studies in amyotrophic lateral sclerosis I. Results of arginine tolerance tests. *Arch Neurol*, **12**, 604–609.
2. Ryberg H, Bowser R. (2008). Protein biomarkers for amyotrophic lateral sclerosis. *Expert Rev Proteomics*, **5**, 249–262.
3. Turner MR, Kiernan MC, Leigh NP, Talbot K. (2009). Biomarkers in amyotrophic lateral sclerosis. *Lancet Neurol*, **8**, 94–109.
4. Rothstein JD. (2009). Current hypotheses for the underlying biology of amyotrophic lateral sclerosis. *Ann Neurol*, **65**, S3–S9.
5. Ince PG, Evans J, Knopp M, *et al.* (2003). Corticospinal tract degeneration in the progressive muscular atrophy variant of ALS. *Neurology*, **60**, 1252–1258.
6. Phukan J, Pender NP, Hardiman O. (2007). Cognitive impairment in amyotrophic lateral sclerosis. *Lancet Neurol*, **6**, 994–1003.
7. Ravits JM, La Spada AR. (2009). ALS motor phenotype heterogeneity, focality, and spread: deconstructing motor neuron degeneration. *Neurology*, **73**, 805–811.
8. Pradat PF, Bruneteau G, Gonzalez de Aguilar JL, *et al.* (2007). Muscle Nogo-A expression is a prognostic marker in lower motor neuron syndromes. *Ann Neurol*, **62**, 15–20.
9. Hu S, Loo JA, Wong DT. (2006). Human body fluid proteome analysis. *Proteomics*, **6**, 6326–6353.
10. Huhmer AF, Biringer RG, Amato H, Fonteh AN, Harrington MG. (2006). Protein analysis in human cerebrospinal fluid: Physiological aspects, current progress and future challenges. *Dis Markers*, **22**, 3–26.
11. Pan S, Zhu D, Quinn JF, *et al.* (2007). A combined dataset of human cerebrospinal fluid proteins identified by multi-dimensional chromatography and tandem mass spectrometry. *Proteomics*, **7**, 469–473.
12. Ranganathan S, Polshyna A, Nicholl G, Lyons-Weiler J, Bowser R. (2006). Assessment of protein stability in cerebrospinal fluid using surface-enhanced laser desorption/ionization time-of-flight mass spectrometry protein profiling. *Clin Proteomics*, **2**, 91–102.
13. Wuolikainen A, Hedenstrom M, Moritz T, Marklund SL, Antti H, Andersen PM. (2009). Optimization of procedures for collecting and storing of CSF for studying the metabolome in ALS. *Amyotroph Lateral Scler*, **10**, 229–236.
14. Garbuzova-Davis S, Haller E, Saporta S, Kolomey I, Nicosia SV, Sanberg PR. (2007). Ultrastructure of blood-brain barrier and blood-spinal cord barrier in SOD1 mice modeling ALS. *Brain Res*, **1157**, 126–137.
15. Garbuzova-Davis S, Saporta S, Haller E, *et al.* (2007). Evidence of compromised blood-spinal cord barrier in early and late symptomatic SOD1 mice modeling ALS. *PLoS ONE*, **2**, e1205.
16. Zlokovic BV. (2008). The blood-brain barrier in health and chronic neurodegenerative disorders. *Neuron*, **57**, 178–201.
17. Roheim PS, Carey M, Forte T, Vega GL. (1979). Apolipoproteins in human cerebrospinal fluid. *Proc Natl Acad Sci USA*, **76**, 4646–4649.
18. Geser F, Martinez-Lage M, Kwong LK, Lee VM, Trojanowski JQ. (2009). Amyotrophic lateral sclerosis, frontotemporal dementia and beyond: the TDP-43 diseases. *J Neurol*, **256**, 1205–1214.
19. Lomen-Hoerth C, Murphy J, Langmore S, Kramer JH, Olney RK, Miller B. (2003). Are amyotrophic lateral sclerosis patients cognitively normal? *Neurology*, **60**, 1094–1097.
20. Bäumer D, Ansorge O, Almeida M, Talbot K. (2010). The role of defects in RNA processing in the pathogenesis of motor neuron degeneration. *Expert Rev Mol Med*, **12**, e21.
21. Sussmuth SD, Sperfeld AD, Hinz A, *et al.* (2010). CSF glial markers correlate with survival in amyotrophic lateral sclerosis. *Neurology*, **74**, 982–987.

22. Romeo MJ, Espina V, Lowenthal M, Espina BH, Petricoin EF, Liotta LA. (2005). CSF proteome: a protein repository for potential biomarker identification. *Exp Rev Proteomics*, **2**, 57–70.
23. Kolarcik C, Bowser R. (2006). Plasma and cerebrospinal fluid-based protein biomarkers for motor neuron disease. *Mol Diagn Ther*, **10**, 281–292.
24. Sussmuth SD, Brettschneider J, Ludolph AC, Tumani H. (2008). Biochemical markers in CSF of ALS patients. *Curr Med Chem*, **15**, 1788–1801.
25. Deisenhammer F, Egg R, Giovannoni G, *et al.* (2009). EFNS guidelines on disease-specific CSF investigations. *Eur J Neurol*, **16**, 760–770.
26. Boylan K, Yang C, Crook J, *et al.* (2009). Immunoreactivity of the phosphorylated axonal neurofilament H subunit (pNF-H) in blood of ALS model rodents and ALS patients: evaluation of blood pNF-H as a potential ALS biomarker. *J Neurochem*, **111**, 1182–1191.
27. Brettschneider J, Petzold A, Submuth SD, Ludolph AC, Tumani H. (2006). Axonal damage markers in cerebrospinal fluid are increased in ALS. *Neurology*, **66**, 852–856.
28. Rosengren LE, Karlsson JE, Karlsson JO, Persson LI, Wikkelso C. (1996). Patients with amyotrophic lateral sclerosis and other neurodegenerative diseases have increased levels of neurofilament protein in CSF. *J Neurochem*, **67**, 2013–2018.
29. Zetterberg H, Jacobsson J, Rosengren L, Blennow K, Andersen PM. (2007). Cerebrospinal fluid neurofilament light levels in amyotrophic lateral sclerosis: impact of *SOD1* genotype. *Eur J Neurol*, **14**, 1329–1333.
30. Figlewicz DA, Krizus A, Martinoli MG, *et al.* (1994). Variants of the heavy neurofilament subunit are associated with the development of amyotrophic lateral sclerosis. *Hum Mol Genet*, **3**, 1757–1761.
31. Williamson TL, Cleveland DW. (1999). Slowing of axonal transport is a very early event in the toxicity of ALS-linked SOD1 mutants to motor neurons. *Nat Neurosci*, **2**, 50–56.
32. Norgren N, Rosengren L, Stigbrand T. (2003). Elevated neurofilament levels in neurological diseases. *Brain Res*, **987**, 25–31.
33. Sussmuth SD, Tumani H, Ecker D, Ludolph AC. (2003). Amyotrophic lateral sclerosis: disease stage related changes of tau protein and S100 beta in cerebrospinal fluid and creatine kinase in serum. *Neurosci Lett*, **353**, 57–60.
34. Ranganathan S, Williams E, Ganchev P, *et al.* (2005). Proteomic profiling of cerebrospinal fluid identifies biomarkers for amyotrophic lateral sclerosis. *J Neurochem*, **95**, 1461–1471.
35. Urushitani M, Sik A, Sakurai T, Nukina N, Takahashi R, Julien J-P. (2006). Chromogranin-mediated secretion of mutant superoxide dismutase proteins linked to amyotrophic lateral sclerosis. *Nat Neurosci*, **9**, 108–118.
36. Watanabe M, Dykes-Hoberg M, Culotta VC, Price DL, Wong PC, Rothstein JD. (2001). Histological evidence of protein aggregation in mutant SOD1 transgenic mice and in amyotrophic lateral sclerosis neural tissues. *Neurobiol Dis*, **8**, 933–941.
37. Higgins CMJ, Jung C, Ding H, Xu Z. (2002). Mutant Cu, Zn superoxide dismutase that causes motoneuron degeneration is present in mitochondria in the CNS. *J Neurosci*, **22**, RC215, 1–6.
38. Jacobsson J, Jonsson PA, Andersen PM, Forsgren L, Marklund SL. (2001). Superoxide dismutase in CSF from amyotrophic lateral sclerosis patients with and without CuZn-superoxide dismutase mutations. *Brain*, **124**, 1461–1466.
39. Lagier-Tourenne C, Cleveland DW. (2009). Rethinking ALS: the FUS about TDP-43. *Cell* **136**, 1001–1004.
40. Steinacker P, Hendrich C, Sperfeld AD, *et al.* (2008). TDP-43 in cerebrospinal fluid of patients with frontotemporal lobar degeneration and amyotrophic lateral sclerosis. *Arch Neurol*, **65**, 1481–1487.
41. Kasai T, Tokuda T, Ishigami N, *et al.* (2009). Increased TDP-43 protein in cerebrospinal fluid of patients with amyotrophic lateral sclerosis. *Acta Neuropathol*, **117**, 55–62.

42. Pasinetti GM, Ungar LH, Lange DJ, *et al.* (2006). Identification of potential CSF biomarkers in ALS. *Neurology*, **66**, 1218–1222.
43. Tsuji-Akimoto S, Yabe I, Niino M, Kikuchi S, Sasaki H. (2009). Cystatin C in cerebrospinal fluid as a biomarker of ALS. *Neurosci Lett*, **452**, 52–55.
44. Okamoto K. (1993). Bunina bodies in amyotrophic lateral sclerosis immunostained with rabbit anti-cystatin C serum. *Neurosci Lett*, **162**, 125–128.
45. Sjogren M, Davidsson P, Wallin A, *et al.* (2002). Decreased CSF-beta-amyloid 42 in Alzheimer's disease and amyotrophic lateral sclerosis may reflect mismetabolism of beta-amyloid induced by disparate mechanisms. *Dement Geriatr Cogn Disord*, **13**, 112–118.
46. Shahani N, Nalini A, Gourie-Devi M, Raju TR. (1998). Reactive astrogliosis in neonatal rat spinal cord after exposure to cerebrospinal fluid from patients with amyotrophic lateral sclerosis. *Exp Neurol*, **149**, 295–298.
47. Shobha K, Alladi PA, Nalini A, Sathyaprabha TN, Raju TR. (2010). Exposure to CSF from sporadic amyotrophic lateral sclerosis patients induces morphological transformation of astroglia and enhances GFAP and S100beta expression. *Neurosci Lett*, **473**, 56–61.
48. Mitchell RM, Freeman WM, Randazzo WT, *et al.* (2009). A CSF biomarker panel for identification of patients with amyotrophic lateral sclerosis. *Neurology*, **72**, 14–19.
49. Rentzos M, Rombos A, Nikolaou C, *et al.* (2010). Interleukin-15 and interleukin-12 are elevated in serum and cerebrospinal fluid of patients with amyotrophic lateral sclerosis. *Eur Neurol*, **63**, 285–290.
50. Baron P, Bussini S, Cardin V, *et al.* (2005). Production of monocyte chemoattractant protein-1 in amyotrophic lateral sclerosis. *Muscle Nerve*, **32**, 541–544.
51. Kuhle J, Lindberg RL, Regeniter A, *et al.* (2009). Increased levels of inflammatory chemokines in amyotrophic lateral sclerosis. *Eur J Neurol*, **16**, 771–774.
52. Nagata T, Nagano I, Shiote M, *et al.* (2007). Elevation of MCP-1 and MCP-1/VEGF ratio in cerebrospinal fluid of amyotrophic lateral sclerosis patients. *Neurol Res*, **29**, 772–776.
53. Tanaka M, Kikuchi H, Ishizu T, *et al.* (2006). Intrathecal upregulation of granulocyte colony stimulating factor and its neuroprotective actions on motor neurons in amyotrophic lateral sclerosis. *J Neuropathol Exp Neurol*, **65**, 816–825.
54. Wilms H, Sievers J, Dengler R, Bufler J, Deuschl G, Lucius R. (2003). Intrathecal synthesis of monocyte chemoattractant protein-1 (MCP-1) in amyotrophic lateral sclerosis: further evidence for microglial activation in neurodegeneration. *J Neuroimmunology*, **144**, 139–142.
55. Tateishi T, Yamasaki R, Tanaka M, *et al.* (2010). CSF chemokine alterations related to the clinical course of amyotrophic lateral sclerosis. *J Neuroimmunol*, **222**, 76–81.
56. Mitchell R. (2009). Influence of HFE variants and cellular iron on monocyte chemoattractant protein-1. *J Neuroinflammation*, **6**, 1–12.
57. Almer G, Teismann P, Stevic Z, *et al.* (2002). Increased levels of the pro-inflammatory prostaglandin PGE2 in CSF from ALS patients. *Neurology*, **58**, 1277–1279.
58. Goodall EF, Haque MS, Morrison KE. (2008). Increased serum ferritin levels in amyotrophic lateral sclerosis (ALS) patients. *J Neurol*, **255**, 1652–1656.
59. Mitchell RM, Simmons Z, Beard JL, Stephens HE, Connor JR. (2010). Plasma biomarkers associated with ALS and their relationship to iron homeostasis. *Muscle Nerve*, **42**, 95–103.
60. Qureshi M, Brown RHJ, Rogers JT, Cudkowicz ME. (2008). Serum ferritin and metal levels as risk factors for amyotrophic lateral sclerosis. *Open Neurol J*, **12**, 51–54.
61. Teunissen CE, Petzold A, Bennet CL, *et al.* (2009). A consensus protocol for the standardization of cerebrospinal fluid collection and biobanking. *Neurology*, **73**, 1914–1922.
62. Shaw LM, Vanderstichele H, Knapik-Czajka M, *et al.* (2009). Cerebrospinal fluid biomarker signature in Alzheimer's disease neuroimaging initiative subjects. *Ann Neurol*, **65**, 403–413.

63. Ryberg H, An J, Darko S, *et al.* (2010). Discovery and verification of amyotrophic lateral sclerosis biomarkers by mass spectrometry based proteomics. *Muscle Nerve*, **42**, 104–111.
64. Lustgarten JL, Visweswaran S, Bowser RP, Hogan WR, Gopalakrishnan V. (2009). Knowledge-based variable selection for learning rules from proteomic data. *BMC Bioinformatics*, **10**, S16.
65. Haverkamp LJ, Appel V, Appel SH. (1995). Natural history of amyotrophic lateral sclerosis in a database population. Validation of a scoring system and a model for survival prediction. *Brain*, **118** (Pt 3), 707–719.
66. Turner MR, Bakker M, Sham P, Shaw CE, Leigh PN, Al-Chalabi A. (2002). Prognostic modelling of therapeutic interventions in amyotrophic lateral sclerosis. *Amyotroph Lateral Scler Other Motor Neuron Disord*, **3**, 15–21.
67. Peskind ER, Riekse R, Quinn JF, *et al.* (2005). Safety and acceptability of the research lumbar puncture. *Alzheimer Dis Assoc Disord*, **19**, 220–225.
68. Tarnaris A, Toma AK, Chapman MD, *et al.* (2009). The longitudinal profile of CSF markers during external lumbar drainage. *J Neurol Neurosurg Psychiatry*, **80**, 1130–1133.
69. Homer AC, Honavar M, Lantos PL, Hastie IR, Kellett JM, Millard PH. (1988). Diagnosing dementia: do we get it right? *BMJ*, **297**, 894–896.
70. Hughes AJ, Daniel SE, Kilford L, Lees AJ. (1992). Accuracy of clinical diagnosis of idiopathic Parkinson's disease: a clinico-pathological study of 100 cases. *J Neurol Neurosurg Psychiatry*, **55**, 181–184.

Chapter 18

Neuropathology of frontotemporal lobar degeneration

Nigel J. Cairns

Frontotemporal dementia (FTD) is a clinical syndrome associated with several neurodegenerative diseases that are characterized by frontotemporal lobar degeneration (FTLD) (1–5). After Alzheimer's disease (AD) and dementia with Lewy bodies (DLB), FTLD is the most common neurodegenerative disorder, affecting between 5 and 20% of pre-senile patients. It has a worldwide distribution and affects both men and women. As many as one-half of all cases of FTD have a family history of a similar dementing disorder (6,7). Within the last few years, there has been rapid progress in delineating the molecular pathology of most cases and several genes have been identified that make FTLD clinically, neuropathologically, and genetically heterogeneous (Figure 18.1). For practising neuropathologists, most of these diseases are characterized by the pathological aggregation of misfolded proteins, either in neurones or glial cells, or both. The most frequent FTLD molecular pathology, accounting for more than half of all cases in most autopsy series, is characterized by abnormal intracellular accumulations of the transactive response (TAR) DNA-binding protein of 43 kDa (TDP-43), collectively called TDP-43 proteinopathies or FTLD-TDP (3,8,9). A number of genes have been associated with TDP-43 proteinopathy, including: progranulin (*GRN*) (10–15), the most frequent gene defect causing FTLD; the gene encoding TDP-43 (*TARDBP*) (16,17); valosin-containing protein (*VCP*) (18); and, in cases with combined familial FTLD and motor neurone disease (FTLD/MND), there is linkage to chromosome 9 (19,20) and a mutation in the chromosome 9 open reading frame 72 (*C9ORF72*) gene has been reported (161,162). Recently, a multicentre genome-wide scan identified common variants at 7p21 that are also associated with FTLD-TDP (21), further adding to the genetic heterogeneity of TDP-43 proteinopathy.

The second most frequent molecular pathology has neuronal or glial inclusions containing the microtubule-associated protein tau encoded by the *MAPT* gene. The term *tauopathy* has been applied to this group of diseases, which includes: Pick's disease (PiD), corticobasal degeneration (CBD), progressive supranuclear palsy (PSP), tangle predominant form of senile dementia or 'tangle-only' dementia (TOD), multiple system tauopathy with dementia (MSTD), a recently described tauopathy called white matter tauopathy with globular glial inclusions, and FTLD with *MAPT* mutation, previously called FTD with parkinsonism linked to chromosome 17 (FTDP-17) (2–5).

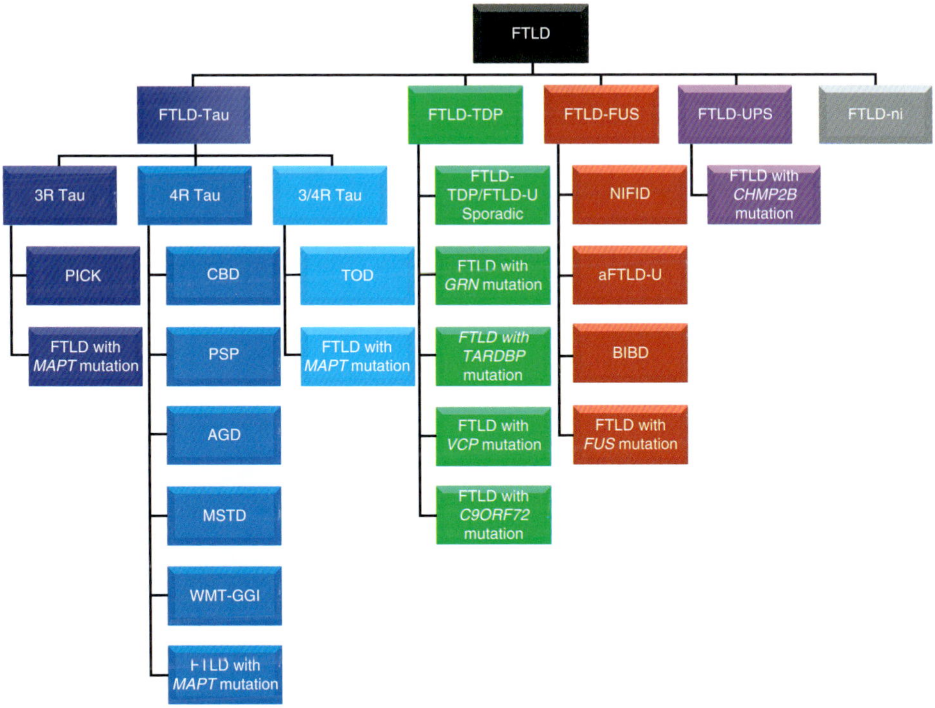

Fig. 18.1 Molecular classification of FTLD. Three distinct neuropathological categories may be identified based on the molecular pathology of the misfolded protein within the inclusion: FTLD-Tau, FTLD-TDP, and FTLD-FUS; the molecular pathology of a fourth category, FTLD with epitopes of the ubiquitin–proteasome system (FTLD-UPS), and a fifth category with no inclusions (FTLD-ni), remain indeterminate. 3R, 4R, 3R/4R; the predominant tau isoform within the inclusion; PICK, Pick's disease; FTLD with microtubule-associated protein tau (*MAPT*) mutation with inclusions of 3R, 4R, or 3R and 4R tau protein; CBD, corticobasal degeneration; PSP, progressive supranuclear palsy; MSTD, multiple system tauopathy with dementia; white matter tauopathy with globular glial inclusions (WMT-GGI); AGD, argyrophilic grain disease; TOD, tangle-only dementia; FTLD-U, FTLD with ubiquitin inclusions, now called FTLD-TDP; FTLD with progranulin (*GRN*) mutation; FTLD with transactive response DNA-binding protein of 43 kDa (*TARDBP*) mutation; FTLD with valosin-containing protein (*VCP*) mutation; FTLD with chromosome 9 open reading frame 72 (*C9ORF72*) gene mutation. NIFID, neuronal intermediate filament inclusion disease; BIBD, basophilic inclusion body disease; aFTLD-U, atypical FTLD with ubiquitin inclusions; FTLD with fused in sarcoma (*FUS*) mutation; FTLD with charged multivesicular body protein 2B (*CHMP2B*) mutation. Within each molecular pathology, there may be unclassified entities. Adapted from references (3–5).

Some rare FTLD entities have been characterized by neuronal and glial inclusions containing the *fused in sarcoma* (FUS) protein called FTLD-FUS in the new nosology (5) and include: neuronal intermediate filament inclusion disease (NIFID) (22), basophilic inclusion body disease (BIBD) (23), and atypical FTLD with ubiquitin-immunoreactive inclusions (aFTLD-U) (24).

A fourth group of patients with FTLD lacks TDP-43, tau, and FUS inclusions. This unique entity, limited to a single Danish pedigree, has mutations in the charged multivesicular body protein 2B (*CHMB2B*) gene (25). To date, ubiquitin and P62, components of the ubiquitin–proteasome system (UPS), are the only proteins that have been reported in the inclusions associated with this gene defect (25). As the pathological protein of the inclusions has yet to be identified, this entity has been called, tentatively, FTLD-UPS. The molecular pathology of most FTLD entities has now been defined and most cases of FTLD without inclusions (26,27), also called dementia lacking distinctive histopathology (6) or frontal lobe degeneration of non-Alzheimer type (28), have been reassigned to one of the FTLD entities with known molecular pathology. In very rare cases of FTLD, where no inclusions have been detected, an entity called FTLD with no inclusions in the revised nomenclature (5) may be present. Sporadic and familial cases of FTLD may be found alone or in combination with AD, DLB, or, rarely, other neurodegenerative diseases and vascular disease.

Frontotemporal lobar degeneration with TDP-43 proteinopathy

Among the neurodegenerative diseases, FTLD is neuropathologically very heterogeneous (3,5,9). This pathological heterogeneity may be explained, in part, by different genetic loci in familial FTLD (Table 18.1). Recently, the pathological protein in the ubiquitin-immunoreactive inclusions of most cases of FTLD with ubiquitin-positive inclusions (FTLD-U), FTLD-MND, and amyotrophic lateral sclerosis (ALS) was identified as the TDP-43 (29,30) (Figures 18.2–18.6). The discovery of mutations in the gene encoding TDP-43, *TARDBP*, demonstrated that abnormal TDP-43 is sufficient to cause neurodegenerative disease (16,31–33). TDP-43 is a 414 amino acid protein that is located, predominantly, in the nucleus, but in pathological states the protein is translocated to the

Table 18.1 Genes involved in FTLD

Chromosome	Gene name (*symbol*)	Molecular pathology (common name)	Mutations
1p	Transactive response (TAR) DNA-binding protein of 43 kDa (*TARDBP*)	FTLD/TDP	34
17q	Progranulin (*GRN*)	FTLD/TDP	69
9p	Valosin-containing protein (*VCP*)	FTLD/TDP (FTLD with inclusion body myopathy and Paget's disease of bone)	17
9p	Chromosome 9 open reading frame 72 (*C9ORF72*)	FTLD/TDP (FTLD/MND)	GGGGCC repeat expansion
17q	Microtubule-associated protein tau (*MAPT*)	FTLD-tau	44
16p	Fused in sarcoma (*FUS*)	FTLD/FUS	23
3p	Chromatin modifying protein 2B (*CHMP2B*)	FTLD/UPS	4

Alzheimer Disease & Frontotemporal Dementia Mutation Database. Available at: http://www.molgen.ua.ac.be/FTDMutations/(accessed on 1 January 2012).

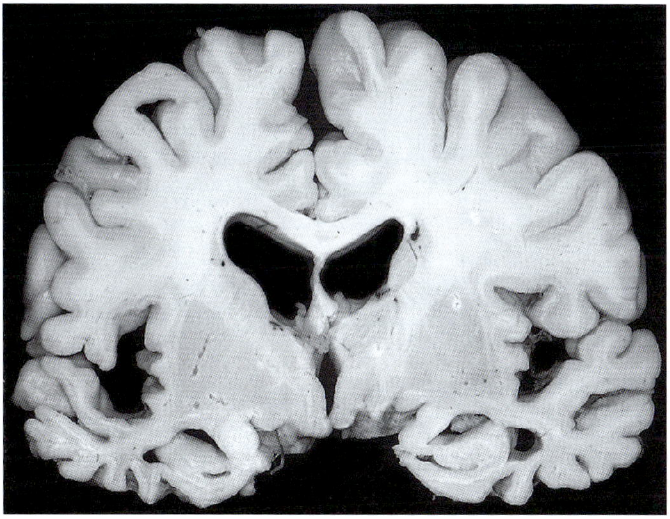

Fig. 18.2 FTLD-TDP. There is dilatation of the lateral ventricles, increased space in the lateral fissure, and pronounced atrophy of the temporal lobes. With permission from Cairns, N.J., Lee, V.M.-Y., Trojanowski, J.Q. pp. 382–407. In The Human Frontal Lobes: Functions and Disorders. Second Edition. Edited by Bruce L. Miller and Jeffrey L. Cummings. The Guilford Press, New York, 2007.

cytoplasm in most affected neurones and glial cells (9,30,34). TDP-43 has multiple functions, including RNA and DNA splicing and transcription, and neuronal plasticity; for a review see (35). It is likely, therefore, that different genes causing FTLD-TDP cause inclusion formation and neurodegeneration by different cellular pathways. In pathological conditions, TDP-43 forms a relatively insoluble aggregate, which is ubiquitinated and

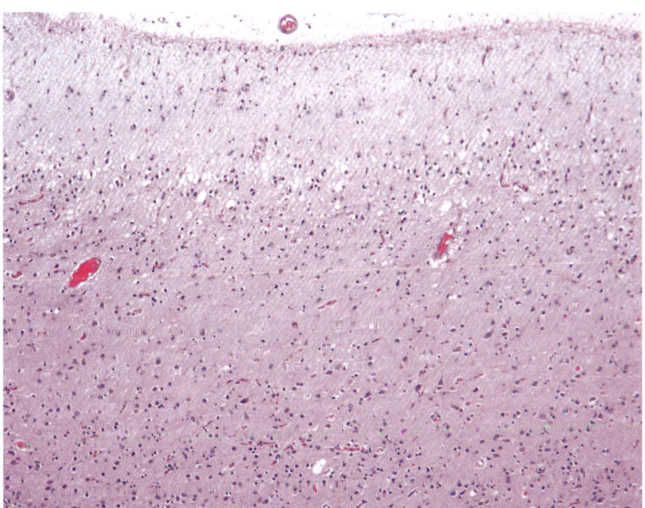

Fig. 18.3 FTLD-TDP. There is neuronal loss and microvacuolation in the superficial cortical layers. In the most severely affected areas, neuronal loss and vacuolation may extend to the full thickness of the cortex. Haematoxylin and eosin. With permission from Cairns, N.J., Lee, V.M.-Y., Trojanowski, J.Q. pp. 382–407. In The Human Frontal Lobes: Functions and Disorders. Second Edition. Edited by Bruce L. Miller and Jeffrey L. Cummings. The Guilford Press, New York, 2007.

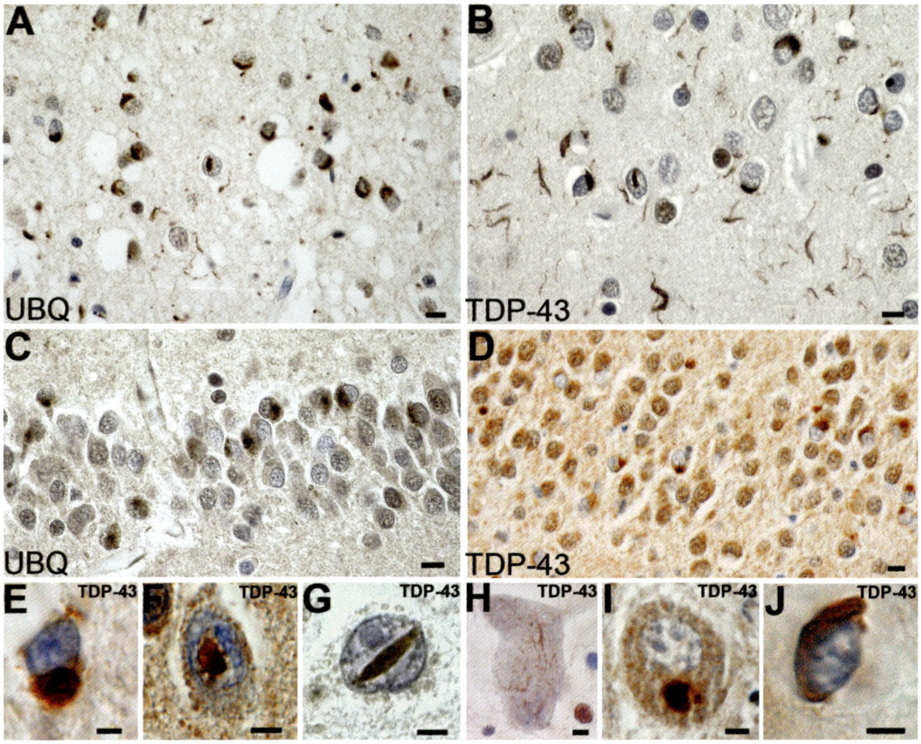

Fig. 18.4 FTLD-TDP. Adjacent sections of superficial frontal neocortex showing NCI, DN, and isolated NII, stained for both ubiquitin (A) and TDP-43 (B). NCI in the dentate granule cells stained for ubiquitin (C) and TDP-43 (D). Neuronal and glial inclusions include NCI (E), round and lentiform NII (F,G); skein-like (H) and compact round (I) NCI in lower motor neurones; and a glial cytoplasmic inclusion (J). (A,C) Ubiquitin immunohistochemistry. (B,D,E–J) TDP-43 immunohistochemistry. Bars: 10 μm (A–D); 5 μm (E–J). Adapted from (9). This figure was published in *Am J Pathol*, **171**, Cairns NJ, Neumann M, Bigio EH, et al., TDP-43 in familial and sporadic frontotemporal lobar degeneration with ubiquitin inclusions, 227–40, Copyright Elsevier 2007.

hyperphosphorylated to generate a 45 kDa species and cleaved to form a 25 kDa band, which may be detected by immunoblotting (9,30,36).

Early reports described four subtypes of FTLD-TDP, which were based on the morphology and distribution of inclusions and appeared to relate to the causative gene defects (Figure 18.7). Three types of neuronal inclusions are recognized: neuronal cytoplasmic inclusions (NCI), neuronal intranuclear inclusions (NII), and dystrophic neurites (DN) (3,9,37). In addition, glial inclusions may be seen in some cases (30,38). In one classification scheme (3,9,37), FTLD-TDP type 1 is characterized by long DNs in superficial laminae. Type 2 has mainly NCI in superficial and deep cortical laminae and has been reported in both sporadic cases and familial cases of FTLD/MND with *C9ORF72* mutation. . The most frequent pattern is type 3, which has NCI, DN, and NII; this type is seen in sporadic cases and in many, but not all, cases of FTLD with *GRN* mutation (15,39–41). Type 4 shows a predominance of NII, with fewer DN, and is characteristic of FTLD with *VCP* mutation. Quantitative studies that are more recent indicate that FTLD-TDP is composed of a spectrum

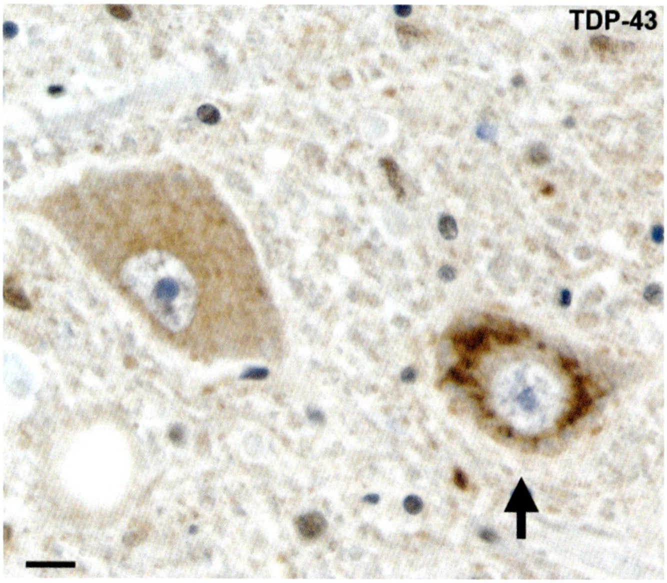

Fig. 18.5 FTLD-TDP with MND. Granular TDP-43 perinuclear staining in a motor neurone (arrow). TDP-43 immunohistochemistry. Bar: 10 μm. Adapted from (3)

of TDP-immunoreactive inclusions with overlapping features of each subtype (42). Different genes may contribute some of the variance in the patterns of inclusion types but additional studies of large cohorts are needed to corroborate these findings.

Atrophy in FTLD-TDP, like all FTLD entities, is variable. It may be limited to the frontal lobe or may be more pronounced in the anterior temporal lobe. The parietal lobes are typically relatively well preserved and most cases show symmetrical cerebral atrophy, although a few cases show asymmetrical atrophy. In addition to neocortical thinning, there may also be atrophy of nuclei of the limbic system, particularly the amygdala and hippocampus. The striatum is often affected and there may be pallor of the pigmented nuclei of the brainstem. These cases often show extrapyramidal signs. Microscopy typically reveals neuronal loss in superficial cortical laminae (II and III), which is often associated with microvacuolation and in the most severe cases this extends to the full thickness of the cortex. As status spongiosus is often the only dramatic feature of the histology, the possibility of prion disease arises. However, prion protein immunohistochemistry (43) and Western blotting (44) exclude prion disease from the differential diagnosis. The distribution of neuronal loss is accompanied by gliosis and swollen achromatic neurones are seen in most cases. The complete absence of argyrophilic inclusions by silver impregnation methods, the presence of ubiquitin- and TDP-43-immunoreactive inclusions and the absence of tau, α-synuclein, prion, polyglutamine, and FUS lead to FTLD-TDP being a distinct neuropathological entity.

Frontotemporal lobar degeneration with motor neurone disease-type inclusions

The association between MND and dementia has been recognized in several studies (45,46) and in a number of patients, dementia may be present without the pathological changes

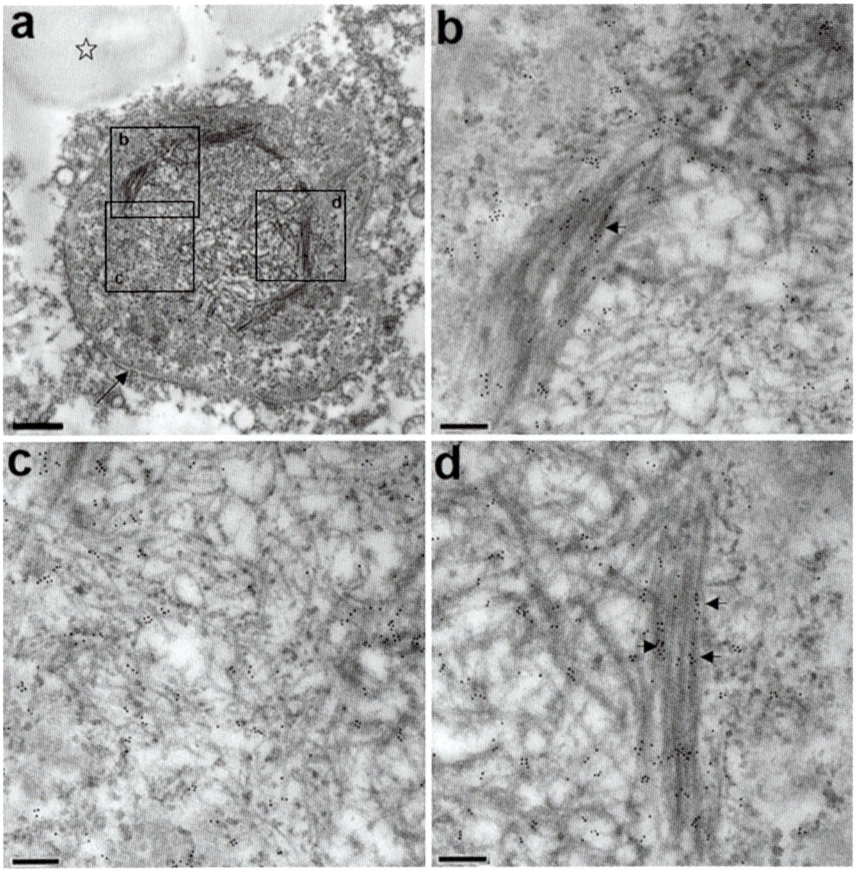

Fig. 18.6 FTLD-TDP. Fine structure of a neuronal intranuclear inclusion in the superficial laminae of the frontal neocortex of a case of FTLD-TDP. (a) Low-power electron micrograph of NII (the arrow indicates the nuclear envelope and the asterisk identifies a lipofuscin granule). (b–d) High-power electron micrographs of the corresponding boxed areas in (a). (b,d) Arrows indicate TDP-43 labelling along the fibrils of the inclusion. TDP-43 transmission immunogold electron microscopy. Bars: 1 µm (a) and 0.2 µm (b–d). Adapted from (158).

seen in the spinal cord in MND (47). Among patients with FTD, FTLD-MND, previously called 'MND-inclusion dementia', is one of the more common neuropathological diagnoses. FTLD-MND, with or without the clinical and pathological features of classical MND, presents with cognitive impairment and in some, but not all patients, an amyotrophic picture develops (weakness and wasting of limb muscles and bulbar palsy leading to dysarthria, dysphagia, and wasting of the tongue). The disease often starts in the sixth decade of life and has an average duration of 2–3 years, considerably shorter than that of AD. More men are affected than women with a ratio of 2:1. Although mainly a sporadic disorder, familial occurrence accounts for 15–20% of cases. The sex ratio, age at onset, and disease duration do not vary between familial and sporadic forms (48). A number of families with FTLD-MND have been linked to *TARDBP, FUS and C9ORF72* gene defects (49–51,161,162).

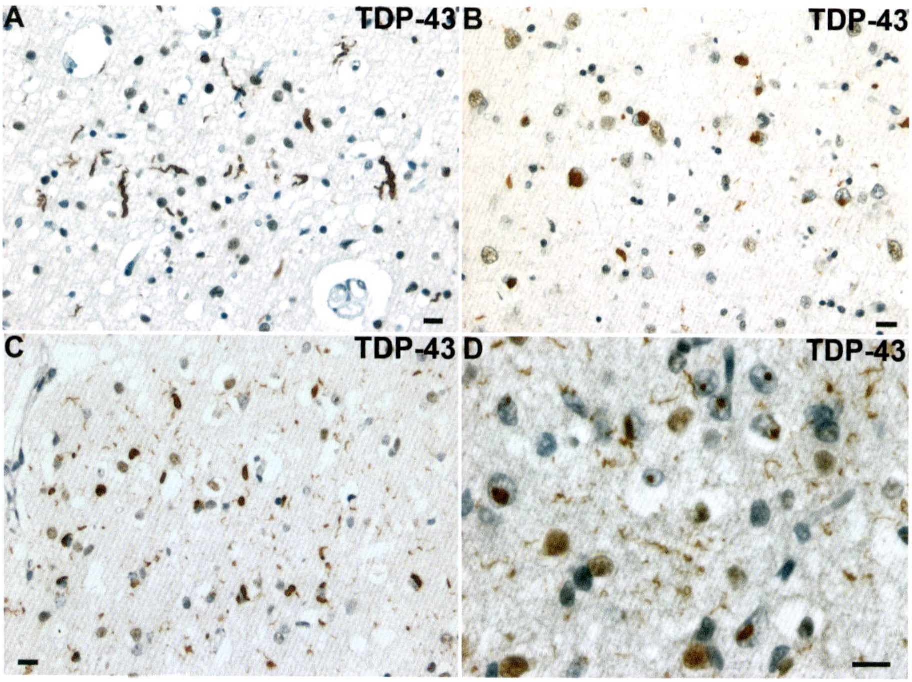

Fig. 18.7 FTLD-TDP subtypes 1–4. (A) Type 1 is characterized by long and tortuous DN in laminae II/III with relatively few NCI and no NII. (B) Type 2, frequently seen in FTLD with *C9ORF72* mutation, has numerous NCI, relatively few DN, and no NII. (C) Type 3, often seen in FTLD with *GRN* mutation, has numerous NCI and DN and an occasional NII in lamina II. (D) Type 4 pathology, most often seen in FTLD with *VCP* mutation, is characterized by numerous NII and DN but few NCI. TDP-43 immunohistochemistry. Bars: 10 µm. Adapted from (9).

Typically, there is mild to moderate atrophy of the frontal, anterior temporal, and parietal lobes (Figure 18.2). The atrophy is often less dramatic than that seen in PiD. Coronal slices often have dilated lateral ventricles with rounding of the angles and the corpus callosum is thin. There may be loss of pigment from the substantia nigra. Microscopy shows neuronal loss, microvacuolation, and astrocytosis in the superficial layers of the cortex, and intraneuronal non-argyrophilic, TDP-43- and ubiquitin-positive, tau-negative inclusions both in the cortex and in the granule cells of the dentate gyrus (Figures 18.3–18.5). Neuronal inclusions are also seen in the amygdala (52), but the highest densities are observed in the dentate fascia. Ubiquitin-positive neuronal inclusions have been reported in both familial cases of FTLD-MND (53,54) and in sporadic cases (8). In the most severely affected areas, there may be neuronal loss extending across all cortical laminae with widespread astrocytosis and microglial activation. There is usually severe neuronal loss in the substantia nigra. The pathological changes found in MND may also be present in FTLD-MND with clinical and pathological MND, including neurone loss in the anterior horns of the spinal cord, motor nuclei of the brainstem, and motor cortex. Surviving neurones contain both TDP-43- and ubiquitin-positive, skein-like, and other inclusions of MND. In addition to the clinical phenotypes of FTD and MND, the pathological changes of FTLD-MND may also be present in cases of semantic dementia (55). The occurrence of clinically distinct behavioural variant FTD (bvFTD), progressive nonfluent aphasia (PNFA), semantic dementia (SD), MND, and PSP with similar pathological changes may relate to spatial variation in neuronal loss, vacuolation, dendritic, and synaptic loss in neocortex, limbic, and subcortical nuclei.

Frontotemporal lobar degeneration with *GRN* mutation

Progranulin, encoded by the *GRN* gene, is a ubiquitously expressed secreted precursor protein that contains tandem repeats of a 10- or 12-cysteine motif, which are proteolytically cleaved to form seven granulin (grn) peptides (10,56,57). Progranulin and granulin peptides have been implicated in several biological processes, including cell cycle regulation, wound repair, tumour growth, and inflammation. Elevated progranulin levels have been described in some tumours (56–58). It is also expressed in cortical and hippocampal neurones of the central nervous system, Pathogenic *GRN* mutations in FTLD are dominant loss-of-function mutations, including whole gene deletions and non-sense and frameshift mutations leading to premature termination codons with subsequent non-sense-mediated mRNA decay of the mutant transcript, mutations in the signal peptide leading to protein mislocalization and degradation, and mutations in the initiation codon preventing translation (10,11,13).

The dominant null allele mutations in *GRN* result in progranulin haploinsufficiency (loss of 50% of progranulin), implying that progranulin behaves like a growth factor and is critical for neurone survival. The loss of progranulin in FTLD with *GRN* mutation is consistent with the absence of progranulin in the ubiquitinated inclusions (13). In most cases of FTLD with *GRN* mutation the pattern of TDP-43 inclusions is most consistent with type 3, that is NCI, NII, and DN are all present but in varying numbers often reflecting the stage of disease (3,13) (Figures 18.8 and 18.9). Biochemically, both sporadic and familial FTLD/TDP (*GRN, VCP* and *C9ORF72* mutations) have a similar signature (Figure 18.10). As progranulin enhances axonal outgrowth and granulin promotes survival of cultured neurones its diminution may contribute to neurodegeneration (59). Although FTD is the most common clinical phenotype associated with *GRN* mutations, *GRN* mutations have also been reported in some cases of AD and Parkinson's disease (60–63). Interestingly, *GRN* null mutations have not been reported in ALS/MND where there is also TDP-43 proteinopathy, indicating that motor neurones may be less sensitive to a reduction in progranulin. In FTLD with *GRN* mutation, it is not clear how progranulin is linked with the pathological accumulation of TDP-43. Mutant *TARDBP* is clearly sufficient to cause TDP-43 pathology in ALS and some cases of FTLD-MND and FTLD, but mutations and variants in FTLD with *TARDBP* mutation are rare (16,17).

Frontotemporal lobar degeneration with *VCP* mutation

FTLD with *VCP* mutation or hereditary inclusion body myopathy (IBM) associated with Paget's disease of bone (PDB) and early-onset FTD (IBMPFD) is a rare, lethal, autosomal dominant progressive disease linked to chromosome 9p13.3–p12 (64). The disease

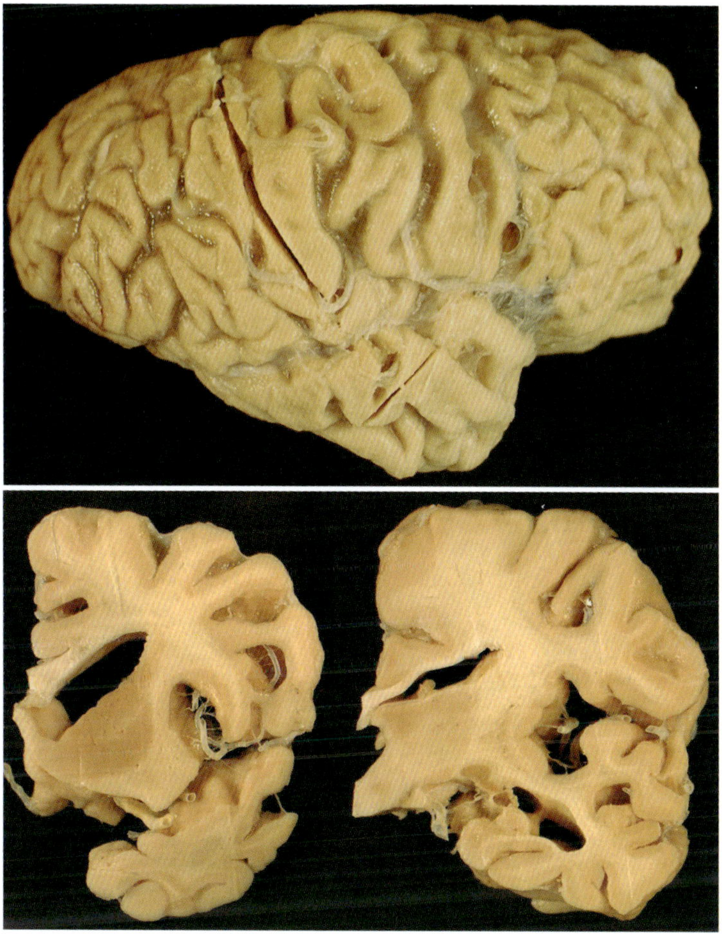

Fig. 18.8 FTLD-TDP: FTLD with *GRN* mutation. The right cerebral hemisphere of FTLD with GRN A9T mutation (top). There is pronounced atrophy of the frontal, temporal, and parietal lobes. Coronal slices (bottom) demonstrate marked dilatation of the lateral ventricle and narrowing of gyri (bottom left) and thinned corpus callosum, increased space in the Sylvian fissure and inferior horn of the lateral ventricle, but the hippocampus is relatively well preserved (bottom right). With permission from Mukherjee O, Pastor P, Cairns NJ, et al. (2006). *Ann Neurol*, **60**(3), 314–22, Wiley.

features adult-onset proximal and distal muscle weakness, early-onset PDB in many and, in cases, FTD. The phenotypic variation in this disease is remarkable and death may precede overt clinical symptoms in one or more of the affected tissues. In one study, 13 families in which mutations in the *VCP* gene were reported, 82% had myopathy, 49% had PDB, and 30% had early-onset FTD (65). The mean age at presentation was 42 years for both IBM and PDB, whereas FTD typically developed somewhat later at age 53 years, possibly indicating greater functional reserve in brain tissue. In IBMPFD myopathic muscle and PDB osteoclasts, similar inclusions are seen indicating common pathogenetic mechanisms. Seventeen missense mutations in *VCP* have been reported (Table 18.1). Human VCP (also called p97, ter94, or CDC48) is a 644 amino acid protein encoded by a gene

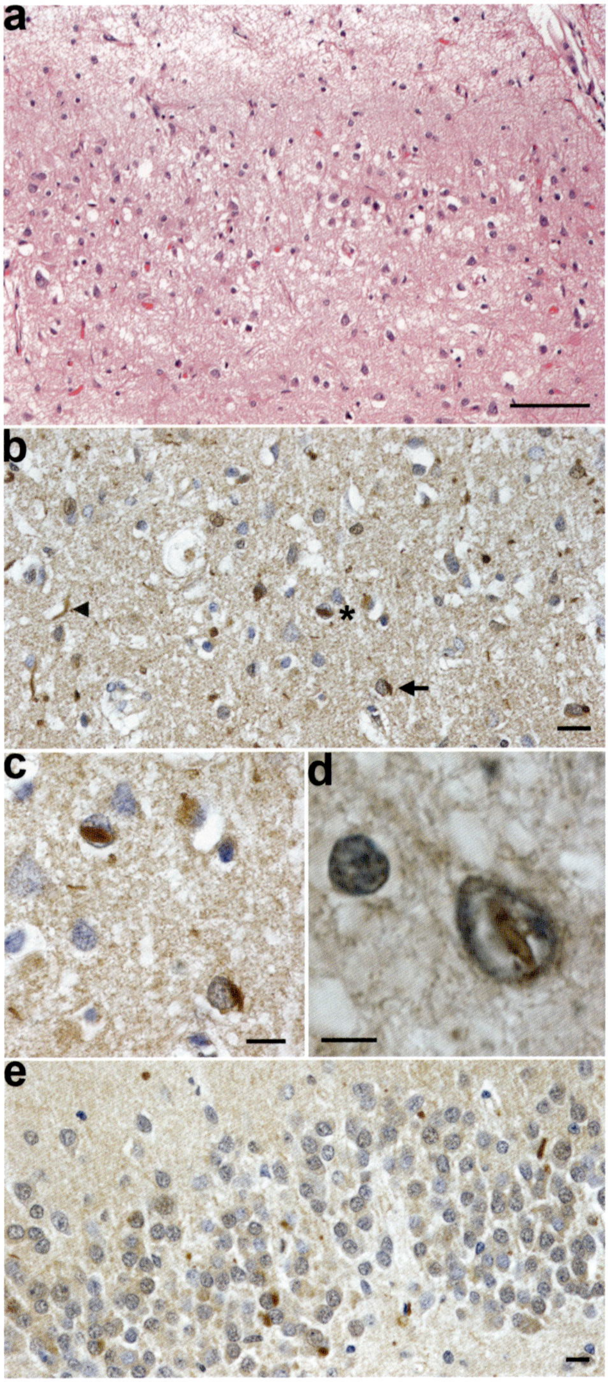

Fig. 18.9 FTLD-TDP: FTLD with *GRN* mutation. Microscopy of chromosome FTLD with *GRN* A9T mutation. (A) Neuronal loss, microvacuolation, and astrocytosis in laminae II and III of the anterior cingulate gyrus. Haematoxylin and eosin. (B) Ubiquitin-positive neuronal inclusions: a neuronal cytoplasmic inclusion (arrow), a neuronal intranuclear inclusion (asterisk), and a dystrophic neurite (arrowhead) in lamina III of the middle frontal gyrus. (C) High-power photomicrograph of the neuronal cytoplasmic and intranuclear inclusions in (B). (D) Fusiform ubiquitin-positive neuronal intranuclear inclusion in lamina III of the parietal lobe. (E) Neuronal cytoplasmic inclusions in the dentate fascia. (B–E) Ubiquitin immunohistochemistry. Scale bars: 100 µm (A); 10 µm (B,C,E); 5 µm (D). With permission from Mukherjee O, Pastor P, Cairns NJ, et al. (2006). *Ann Neurol*, **60**(3), 314–22, Wiley (13).

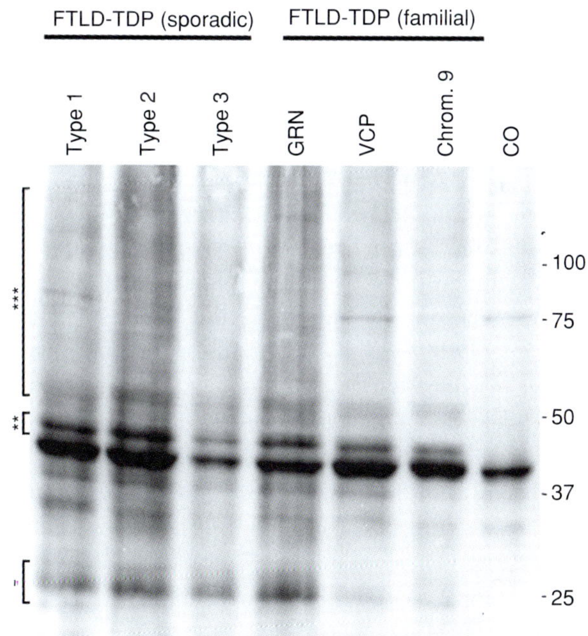

Fig. 18.10 FTLD/TDP: biochemical analysis. Immunoblot of insoluble frozen brain tissue fractions probed with anti-TDP-43 antibodies demonstrate a distinct pathological profile of TDP-43 with variable presence of pathological ≈25-kDa bands (*), 45-kDA bands (**), and a high molecular smear (***) in all sporadic and familial FTLD-TDP brains (FTLD-TDP types 1–3), including those with progranulin ((*GRN*), *VCP*, and *C9ORF72* mutations linked to chromosome 9p) and VCP (Chapter 9). Pathological TDP-43 bands were not detected in control brain (CO). Adapted from (9).

with 17 exons, which maps to chromosome 9. It is a member of the ATPases associated with diverse cellular activities (AAA-ATPase) superfamily involved in vesicle transport and fusion, 26S proteasome function, and assembly of peroxisomes. VCP is a structural protein and is associated with the assembly of clathrin, and the heat-shock protein HSP70. VCP has been implicated in a number of cellular events regulated during mitosis, including homotypic membrane fusion, spindle pole body function, and ubiquitin-dependent protein degradation. Most of the families with IBMPFD have an amino acid substitution at codon 155 in VCP and all are present within the N-terminal CDC48 domain, which is involved in ubiquitin binding (66) indicating that mutations in this region may compromise the normal ubiquitin protein degradation pathway.

To date, few brains of patients with IBMPFD have been examined. Of those patients with FTD, the characteristic features of FTLD have been observed: atrophy of the frontal lobe, neuronal loss, status spongiosus, and reactive astrocytosis (67). The atrophy is less pronounced than in other FTLD entities. The neuropathological hallmark lesion is the neuronal ubiquitin- and TDP-43-immunoreactive NII; type 4 in the classification of FTLD/TDP (9,18) (Figure 18.7). Large focal inclusions and smaller foci containing VCP are present in muscle fibres of patients with IBMPFD (68). This pattern of staining is not specific to IBMPFD as VCP aggregates are also seen in muscle fibres in sporadic IBM. The mechanism by which mutant *VCP* causes FTLD/TDP is unknown.

Frontotemporal lobar degeneration with *C9ORF72* mutation

Familial FTD-MND is a rare neurodegenerative disorder inherited in an autosomal dominant manner. A locus was mapped to chromosome 9 (9p21.3–p13.3) (19,20) and recently the gene defect causing chromosome 9-linked MND, FTLD-MND, and FTLD was identified (161,162). The gene defect is a GGGCC hexanucleotide repeat expansion in the first intron of the *C9ORF72* gene. The repeat expansion was present in one-third of familial ALS cases of outbred European descent, making it the most common genetic cause of these fatal neurodegenerative diseases identified to date. Additionally, in patients of Finnish descent, the mutation was found in 22 of 75 (29.3%) cases (161). Typically, patients present with either FTD, or MND, or both disorders. Neuropathologically, TDP-43-immunoreactive NCIs, with few DNs, are found in the frontal and temporal cortex, hippocampus, and spinal cord. In the typology of FTLD-TDP, the predominance of NCI makes this entity a TDP-43 proteinopathy type 2 (9) (Figure 18.7). Granular, so-called 'pre-inclusions', may be present that are not detected by ubiquitin immunohistochemistry may also be seen. The majority of chromosome 9p-linked cases also have evidence of ubiquitin- and TDP-positive inclusions in upper and lower motor neurones, identical to those encountered in sporadic MND. A recent neuropathological study of FTLD with *C9ORF72* mutation revealed, in addition to TDP-43 proteinopathy previously reported, unusual TDP-43 synaptic-like pathology was observed in the hippocampus of some cases (163). Biochemistry shows that full-length TDP-43 is present in soluble and insoluble fractions of affected and unaffected brain regions of FTLD linked to chromosome 9p cases, similar to sporadic FTLD-TDP and control brains (9). Additional protein bands of 25 and 45 kDa are detected in detergent-insoluble urea fractions from affected regions of cases of FTLD-TDP linked to chromosome 9p and other sporadic and familial forms of FTLD-TDP, but not in normal control subjects. The quantity of these modified TDP-43 species is variable but correlates with the amount of pathology detected by immunohistochemistry. Biochemical methods show that the abnormal 45 kDa species shifts into the 43 kDa band on dephosphorylation with alkaline phosphatase, indicating that TDP-43 is abnormally phosphorylated. Thus, these data suggest that, despite the distinct genetic differences between FTLD with *GRN* and *VCP* mutations, the biochemical signature of TDP-43 proteinopathy in FTLD linked chromosome 9p with *C9ORF72* mutation is similar.

Transgenic models of TDP-43 proteinopathies

TDP-43 proteinopathy is found in both sporadic and familial cases. Several genes have been associated with this molecular pathology, including *TARDBP*, *GRN*, and *VCP*, and defects in these genes have been used recently in various transgenic (TG) model systems, including *Caenorhabditis elegans*, *Drosophila melanogaster*, zebrafish, mouse, and rat (69–75). As with all models, some features of the human disease are variably recapitulated. The development of these early model systems holds promise of facilitating the dissection of molecular pathways leading to neurodegeneration, which may translate into therapeutic strategies.

Frontotemporal lobar degeneration with tauopathy

Several sporadic and familial neurodegenerative diseases are characterized by the formation of argyrophilic, filamentous deposits of abnormal brain proteins. Thus, a heterogeneous group of FTLD entities is linked by the presence of pathological intracellular glial and neuronal inclusions of tau. Despite the diverse phenotypic expression, brain dysfunction and neurodegeneration are linked to the progressive accumulation of abnormal filamentous protein, and this, together with the absence of other disease-specific neuropathological abnormalities, provides evidence implicating tau in disease onset and progression in up to one-half of all cases of FTLD. The discovery of multiple mutations in the *MAPT* gene in FTLD with *MAPT* mutation, also called FTD with parkinsonism linked to chromosome 17 (FTDP-17), has led to the unequivocal evidence that tau abnormalities alone are sufficient to cause neurodegenerative disease. These discoveries have opened up new avenues of research into the role of tau in mechanisms of brain dysfunction and neurodegeneration.

Tau proteins are low-molecular-weight microtubule (MT)-associated proteins that are abundant in the CNS where they are expressed predominantly in axons, and at low levels in astrocytes and oligodendrocytes. Human tau proteins are encoded by a single gene on chromosome 17q21 of 16 exons with CNS isoforms generated by alternative mRNA splicing (Figure 18.11). In the adult human brain, alternative splicing of exons 2, 3, and 10 generates six tau isoforms ranging from 352 to 441 amino acids in length, which differ by the presence of either three or four MT binding repeats (3R tau or 4R tau, respectively) consisting of repeat sequences of 31 or 32 amino acids each encoded by exons 9–12. Additionally, alternative splicing of exons 2 and 3 leads to the absence (0N) or presence of inserted sequences of 29 (1N) or 58 (2N) amino acids in the amino-terminal third of the molecule. In the adult human brain, the ratio of 3R/4R tau isoforms is approximately 1:1.

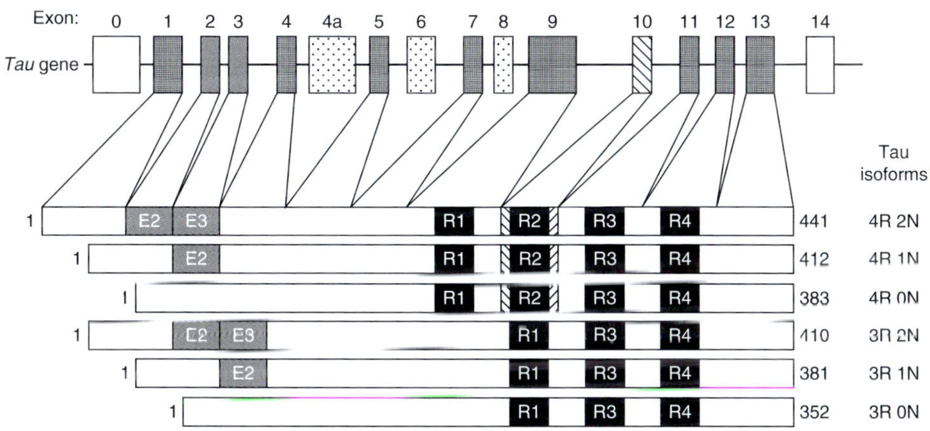

Fig. 18.11 FTLD-Tau. Schematic representation of the human MAPT gene and six human CNS tau isoforms generated by alternative splicing. Exons 1, 4, 5, 7, 9, and 11–13 are constitutively expressed. Alternative splicing of exons 2 (E2), 3 (E3), and 10 produces the six alternative tau isoforms. The black bars depict the 18 amino acid microtubule binding repeats and are designated R1–R4. The relative sizes of the exons and introns are not drawn to scale. With permission from Cairns NJ, Lee VM, Trojanowski JQ (2004). *J Pathol* **204**(4), 438–449, Wiley (157,160).

Tau binds to, and stabilizes, MTs and promotes MT polymerization. The MT binding domains of tau are localized within the four MT binding motifs. These motifs are composed of highly conserved binding elements. The function of tau as an MT binding protein is regulated by phosphorylation. Several protein kinases and protein phosphatases have been implicated in regulating the phosphorylation state and thus the function of tau. The phosphorylation sites are clustered in regions flanking the MT binding repeats, and increasing tau phosphorylation at multiple sites regulates MT binding. However, in both sporadic and familial tauopathies tau is hyperphosphorylated, and it is this 'abnormal' tau that is the principal component of the filamentous aggregates in neurones and glia that are the pathological hallmarks of these disorders. The tauopathies may be broadly grouped according to the pattern of tau immunostaining and tau isoform ratios as demonstrated by Western blotting (Figure 18.12).

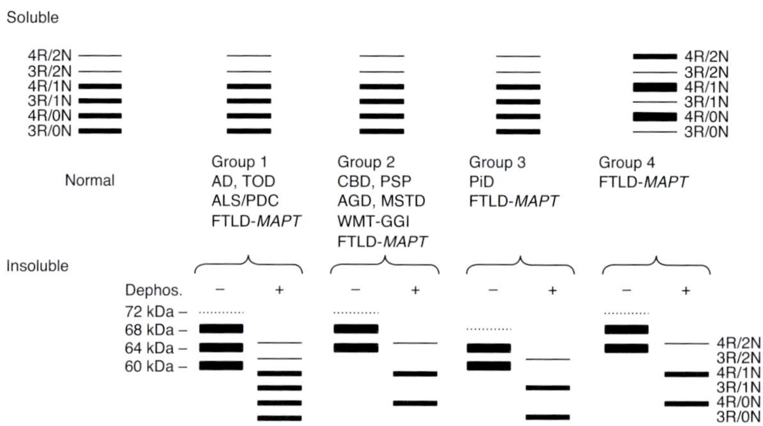

Fig. 18.12 FTLD-Tau. Cartoon representing immunoblot banding patterns of soluble and insoluble tau from different tauopathies. The figure depicts the typical banding pattern of soluble tau (top panels) and insoluble and filamentous tau (bottom panels) from the brains of patients with FTLD with *MAPT* mutation as well as sporadic tauopathies resolved by electrophoresis and demonstrated by immunoblotting with anti-tau antibodies. The FTLD with *MAPT* mutations show several different immunoblot banding patterns of soluble and insoluble tau protein that are depicted as groups 1–4. The soluble fraction from the brains of unaffected (normal) individuals, sporadic tauopathies, and FTLD with *MAPT* mutation that does not affect tau splicing show expression of all six tau isoforms (group 1). Insoluble tau from the brain of patients with AD, TOD, amyotrophic lateral sclerosis/parkinsonism–dementia complex (ALS/PDC), and FTLD with *MAPT* mutation, group 1, resolve as three major proteins of 68-, 64- and 60-kDa; and a minor band of 72 kDa. When dephosphorylated, they resolve into six proteins that correspond to all six tau isoforms similar to the soluble fraction. In CBD, PSP, AGD, MSTD, WMT-GGI, and FTLD with *MAPT* mutation (group 2), two prominent 68- and 64-kDa protein bands are detected (the 72 kDa minor band is variably detected) that align with 4R tau following dephosphorylation, indicating selective aggregation of 4R tau. In PiD and FTLD with *MAPT* mutation (group 3) the 64 and 60 kDa insoluble tau protein isoforms predominate and align with 3R tau isoforms following dephosphorylation indicating selective aggregation of 3R tau. In FTLD with *MAPT* mutations that affect mRNA splicing, there is expression of predominantly 4R tau. With permission from Cairns NJ, Lee VM, Trojanowski JQ (2004). *J Pathol* **204**(4), 438–449, Wiley (160).

Pick's disease

Arnold Pick first reported a form of presenile dementia with circumscribed lobar atrophy in 1892 (76). However, it was Alois Alzheimer, in 1911, who first described the histological lesions characteristic of the disease (i.e. intraneuronal, argyrophilic, globular inclusions) (77). Classical cases of PiD may be readily distinguished from AD on clinical grounds but many patients with PiD have symptoms which are indistinguishable from those found in AD. In contrast, it is easier to distinguish PiD from AD pathologically. PiD is an uncommon cause of dementia and accounts for less than 5% of cases (78). The age at onset varies between 45 and 65 years and rarely beyond 75 years. Thus, unlike most patients with AD, patients with PiD have, typically, an early-onset dementia. The duration of the disease is on average 5–10 years. Women appear to be slightly more affected than men and the disease has a worldwide distribution. It is largely a sporadic disease and as familial cases have come under greater scrutiny the original diagnosis in some has been revised to take account of advances in immunohistochemistry and molecular genetics. Most familial cases have now been reassigned to FTLD with *MAPT* mutation. However, in one family with tau-positive inclusions, a novel presenilin 1 (*PSEN1*) mutation was reported (79) demonstrating that PiD, like AD, is genetically heterogeneous. Two extended haplotypes cover the human *MAPT* gene and there is complete disequilibrium between polymorphisms that span the gene (which covers approximately 100 kb of DNA). This suggests that the establishment of the two haplotypes was an ancient event and either that recombination is suppressed in this region, or that recombinant genes are selected against. The more common haplotype (H1) is significantly over-represented in patients with PSP (80), but there is no difference between the tau H2 haplotype or H2/H2 genotype frequency in PiD cases when compared with control subjects, and no tau mutations have been found in pathologically typical cases of PiD (81).

Macroscopically, the PiD brain may have striking atrophy localized to the frontal or temporal lobe or both and, less commonly, to the parietal lobe (Figure 18.13). In classical cases, the temporal pole may be particularly affected with relative sparing of the posterior part of the superior temporal gyrus. In the frontal lobes, the inferior aspect, including the orbitofrontal region, is often severely shrunken. The loss of brain substance may lead to a brain weight below 1000 g. Coronal slicing of the cerebral hemispheres reveals narrowing of the gyri and widening of sulci in the frontal and temporal lobes. The amygdala and hippocampus are often severely affected and the caudate nucleus may be so atrophied as to give the appearance of that seen in advanced Huntington's disease. Associated with this devastation, the lateral ventricles may be grossly dilated. These changes can be contrasted with the relatively well-preserved remainder of the brain. Although these changes are typical of PiD, they may not be present in all cases. The patient may die at an early stage of the disease and atrophy may not be particularly extensive. In those patients who have the longest clinical history the brain may be the most atrophied.

The diagnostic histological feature of PiD is the Pick body. Pick bodies are well-circumscribed, spherical, argyrophilic, and tau-immunoreactive neuronal intracytoplasmic inclusions. In addition, there are swollen achromatic so-called 'ballooned' neurones or Pick cells, neuronal loss, and astrocytosis (Figures 18.14 and 18.15). Granulovacuolar

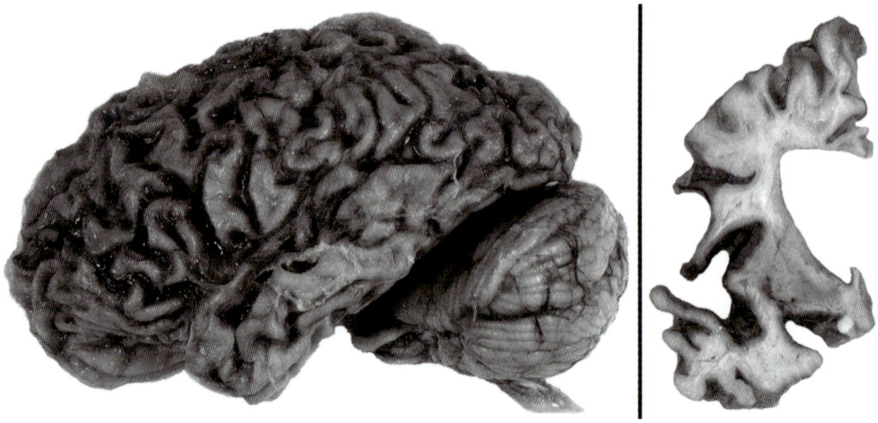

Fig. 18.13 FTLD-Tau: Pick's disease. (*Left panel*) There is striking atrophy of the frontal and temporal lobes and the parietal lobe is also affected. The gyri are markedly thinned and the sulci widened. (*Right panel*) A coronal slice of the hemi-brain in the left panel. The lateral ventricle is severely dilated, lateral fissure is enlarged, gyri are narrowed, and cortical ribbon is thinned. Adapted and with permission from Cairns, N.J., Lee, V.M.-Y., Trojanowski, J.Q. pp. 382–407. In The Human Frontal Lobes: Functions and Disorders. Second Edition. Edited by Bruce L. Miller and Jeffrey L. Cummings. The Guilford Press, New York, 2007.

degeneration may be seen in the hippocampus. These additional changes are not specific to PiD because they are also found in other neurodegenerative disorders. Pick bodies are found most abundantly in the granule cells of the dentate gyrus. The predilection for the cells of the dentate gyrus distinguishes PiD from AD where neurofibrillary tangles (NFT) are rarely found in the granule cells. Pick bodies are found at lower densities in

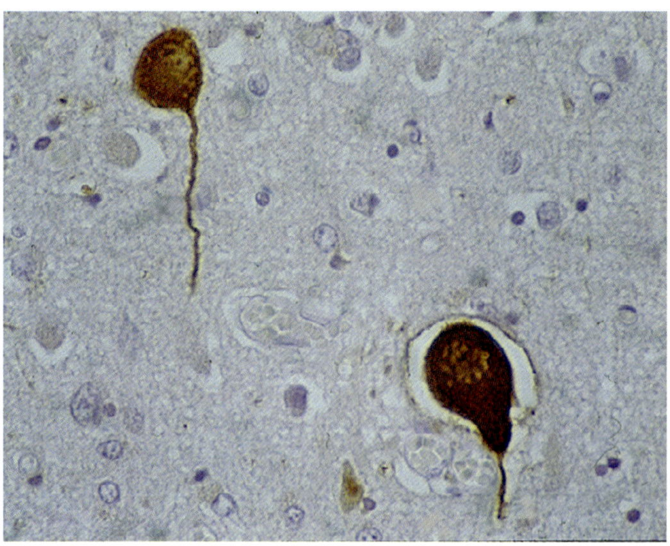

Fig. 18.14 FTLD-Tau. Swollen achromatic neurones, co-called 'ballooned' or Pick cells, in the frontal lobe in Pick's disease. αB-crystallin immunohistochemistry. Adapted and with permission from Cairns, N.J., Lee, V.M.-Y., Trojanowski, J.Q. pp. 382–407. In The Human Frontal Lobes: Functions and Disorders. Second Edition. Edited by Bruce L. Miller and Jeffrey L. Cummings. The Guilford Press, New York, 2007.

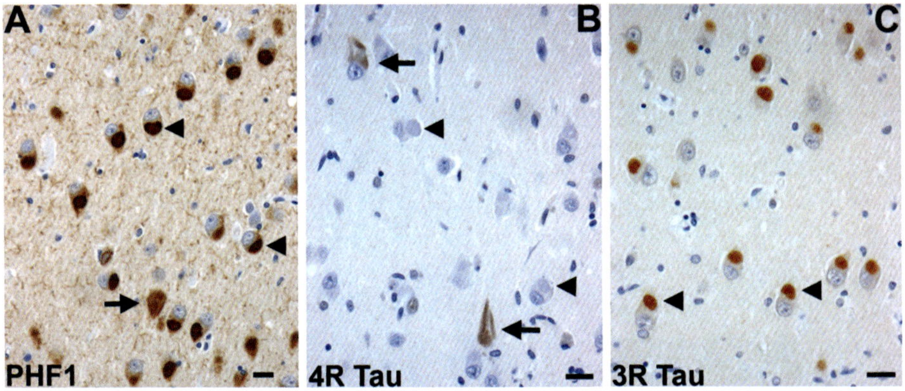

Fig. 18.15 FTLD-Tau. Pick bodies in Pick's disease. Pick bodies (arrowheads) and a neurofibrillary tangle (arrow) in the subiculum (a) are immunolabelled by antiphosphorylated tau antibodies (PHF1 immunohistochemistry). Pick bodies are not immunolabelled with anti-4R tau antibodies (arrowheads), while neurofibrillary tangles are immunolabelled (arrows) (b). Anti-3R tau antibodies clearly label Pick bodies (arrowheads) (c). (b) 4R tau (ET3) and (c) 3R tau (RD3) immunohistochemistry. Bars 10 μm. Adapted from (3).

the pyramidal neurones of the frontal and temporal neocortex. The distribution of Pick bodies may be uni- or bilaminar and this difference may reflect the stage of progression of the disease. These neurones can be contrasted with those in AD where NFT are found predominantly in the large pyramidal neurones of layers III and V, the major corticocortical projecting neurones. Spatial pattern analysis has shown that Pick bodies appear in regular clusters throughout affected cortical areas (82). The size of Pick bodies depends on the size of the neurone in which they are found: Pick bodies in the pyramidal cells of the hippocampus are larger than those found in dentate granule cells. Pick bodies may be found outside the hippocampus, temporal and frontal neocortex, including the amygdala, striatum, thalamus, hypothalamus, brainstem nuclei, and the spinal cord.

Ultrastructurally, Pick bodies consist mainly of bundles of disorganized straight fibrils, which are labelled by anti-tau antibodies. Although the Pick body is well-demarcated by light microscopy, ultrastructurally, they do not appear to have a limiting membrane. Immunohistochemically, Pick bodies are labelled most intensely by anti-ubiquitin and anti-tau antibodies. They have a similar staining pattern to NFTs, but the immunohistochemical and biochemical profile of tau in PiD is different from that in AD: in PiD, 3R tau isoforms are predominant (83–85).

Swollen achromatic neurones are readily seen in haematoxylin and eosin-stained sections. The nucleus is usually in an eccentric position in relation to the cytoplasm. They are typically present in the deep layers of the cortex. They are not present in all cases and are usually absent from the most severely affected regions of the cortex. Electron microscopic studies reveal filaments similar to those seen in Pick bodies together with granular material and some degenerate organelles. Ballooned neurones have a slightly different immunohistochemical profile to that of Pick bodies. Like Pick bodies, the swollen neurones are labelled by anti-ubiquitin and anti-tau antibodies, but the intensity of staining is usually less and variable within the cytoplasm of ballooned neurones. They are also labelled by the heat-shock protein anti-αB-crystallin antibodies. The significance of ballooned neurones in the pathogenesis of PiD is unclear.

Corticobasal degeneration

The clinicopathological description of corticodentatonigral degeneration with neuronal achromasia was first made by Rebeiz *et al.* in 1967 (86), but it was Gibb *et al.* who coined the term CBD in 1989 (87). Males and females are equally affected and the age at onset of sporadic cases is in the sixth to eighth decades. In rare familial cases that have been reported there is an earlier age at onset. Duration of illness ranges from 7 to 10 years. The neuronal and glial inclusions of CBD may be compared with those of PiD and PSP. The presence of swollen neurones, particularly when demonstrated by immunohistochemistry, is a striking feature of this disease. As with familial cases of PiD, the discovery of mutations in the *MAPT* gene in familial cases of CBD has resulted in these cases being reassigned to FTLD with *MAPT* mutation. In sporadic cases, genetic analysis of the tau gene has resulted in two major forms, or haplotypes, called H1 and H2 and the frequency of the H1 haplotype is increased in CBD and several cases are H1/H1 homozygous (81).

Characteristically, the brain is atrophied asymmetrically in the posterior frontal and parietal lobes; both the pre- and post-central gyri are affected. Cortical atrophy is not usually as pronounced as in PiD. There is dilatation of the lateral ventricles and the striatum may be shrunken. The corticospinal tracts and corpus callosum may appear thinned. The substantia nigra appears pale in the majority of cases but there is not the brainstem atrophy typically found in patients with PSP.

The loss of neurones may be more severe in the outer cortical laminae and generate status spongiosus. The white matter underlying the affected areas of cortex may be rarefied and display a reactive astrocytosis. Ballooned neurones are readily seen. They are found most frequently in the deeper cortical laminae (III, V, and VI) and occasionally in subcortical areas, but may be absent in the most severely affected cortical areas. As in PiD, swollen neurones are variably labelled by ubiquitin, neurofilament (NF), and tau antibodies, and are best demonstrated by αB-crystallin immunohistochemistry (88). Ultrastructurally, swollen neurones contain 10–15 nm filaments and a smaller number of thicker 25–30 nm filaments, granular material, and lipofuscin (89).

There is usually severe neuronal loss and accompanying astrocytosis in the substantia nigra. A characteristic feature is the intraneuronal basophilic inclusion. These 'corticobasal inclusions' are argyrophilic and fibrillar and are labelled by anti-ubiquitin and anti-tau antibodies (Figure 18.16). Histologically, they resemble the NFTs of PSP. Ultrastructurally, the filaments of the inclusions are mainly straight with a diameter of 15 nm (89). Similar inclusions may be found in the locus coeruleus and other brainstem nuclei. In addition to these corticobasal inclusions, small neuronal tau-positive inclusions and neuropil threads can be found in the superficial layers of the cortex.

A striking feature of CBD is glial pathology in the affected areas. Filamentous argyrophilic structures are seen most commonly in astrocytes and less frequently in oligodendrocytes. Clusters of astrocytic tangles may form astrocytic plaques. The inclusions

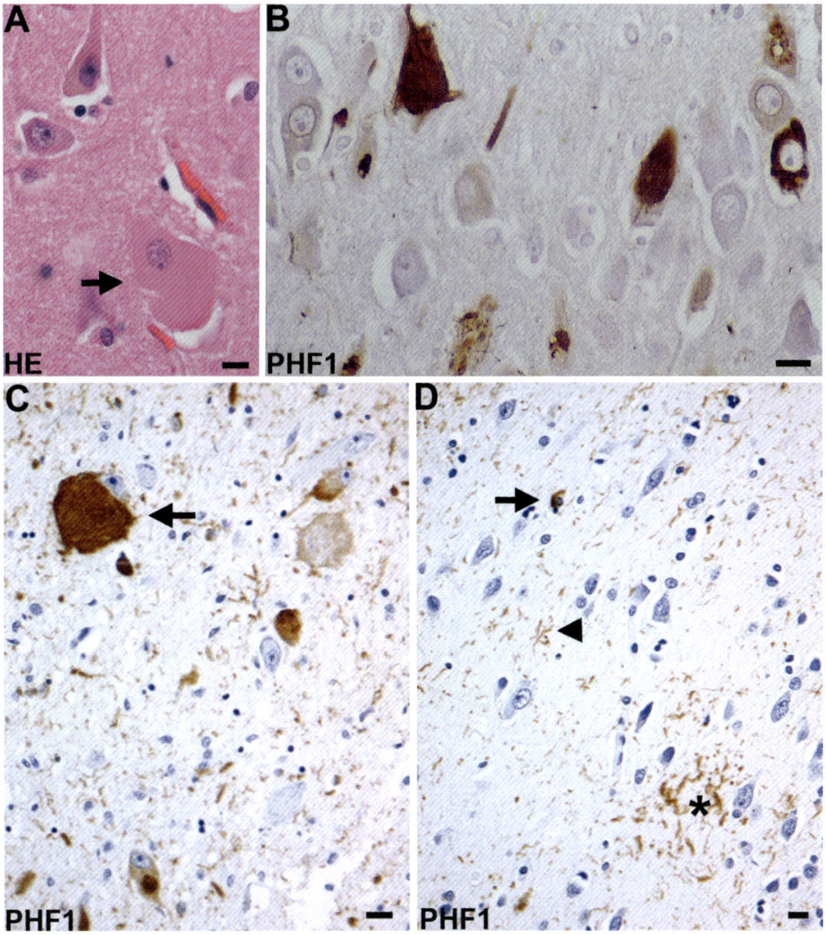

Fig. 18.16 FTLD-Tau: corticobasal degeneration. (a) A swollen achromatic neurone (arrow) in the middle frontal gyrus. Haematoxylin and eosin. (b) Tau-positive neurofibrillary tangles in the pyramidal neurones of the CA1 hippocampal subfield. (c) A globose neurofibrillary tangle (arrow) in the locus coeruleus. (d) An astrocytic plaque (asterisk), coiled body (arrow), and threads (arrowhead) in the deep cortical laminae and white matter of the parietal lobe. (b–d) Phosphorylated tau (PHF1) immunohistochemistry. Bars: 10 μm. Adapted from (3).

in oligodendrocytes are argyrophilic, fibrillary structures. Both the astrocytic and oligodendroglial inclusions in CBD are labelled by anti-ubiquitin and anti-tau antibodies. They are not recognized by α-synuclein antibodies, the major component of the glial cytoplasmic inclusions of multiple system atrophy (90). Although it has been suggested that the glial cytoplasmic inclusions are not specific to multiple system atrophy and are found in corticobasal degeneration and PSP, the oligodendroglial inclusions of corticobasal degeneration are morphologically and immunohistochemically different from the glial cytoplasmic inclusions of multiple system atrophy. The tau protein in CBD is predominantly 4R tau, which is different from that of both AD and PiD.

Progressive supranuclear palsy

PSP was first defined as a clinical and neuropathological entity in 1964 by Steele *et al.* (91). Approximately 4% of patients with Parkinson's disease have PSP or four cases per million per year. The age at onset is about 60 years, an average duration of 6 years, and a slight male preponderance; the ratio of male to female is 60%:40%. The clinical features include parkinsonism, vertical supranuclear gaze palsy, cognitive impairment consistent with FTD, dysarthria, and dysphasia. Frontal lobe signs may be prominent (92). The parkinsonian symptoms include bradykinesia, rigidity, gait disorder, masked fascies, neck dystonia, and falls, but there is no tremor and the patient does not respond to levodopa. The disease is sporadic although rare autosomal dominant familial cases have been reported. Some familial cases with a PSP phenotype have *MAPT* mutations and these have been reassigned to FTLD with *MAPT* mutation; however, some familial cases of PSP fail to show mutations in *MAPT*. Two extended haplotypes cover the human *MAPT* gene and there is complete disequilibrium between polymorphisms that span the gene. The more common haplotype (H1) is significantly over-represented in patients with PSP, extending earlier reports of an association between an intronic dinucleotide polymorphism and PSP (80).

Macroscopically, the brain may appear normal or atrophied. The atrophy may include the globus pallidus, thalamus, subthalamic nucleus, and occasionally the brainstem and cerebellum (Figure 18.17). The substantia nigra and locus coeruleus often appear pale. Histology reveals NFTs, neuropil threads, glial inclusions, neuronal loss, and astrocytosis (93). The predominant hallmark of PSP is the NFT (Figure 18.18). They are found in the substantia nigra, globus pallidus, subthalamic nucleus, nucleus basalis of Meynert, pretectal area, tegmentum of the midbrain and pons, locus coeruleus, raphé nuclei, and the nuclei of various cranial nerves. The tangles are readily seen by silver impregnation methods but are best visualized by tau immunohistochemistry. Electron microscopy demonstrates that the tangles contain straight filaments of 12–15 nm (94), which in turn are composed of six or more protofilaments of 2–5 nm (95). Paired helical filaments and intermediate forms may be seen. Many astrocytes show inclusions, so-called astrocytic tangles, and the tuft-shaped astrocyte is the most frequent lesion although thorn-shaped astrocytes have also been observed. Oligodendrocytes may also contain tau-positive inclusions called coiled bodies, which are different from the glial cytoplasmic inclusions of multiple system atrophy. Predominantly 4R tau isoforms are present in PSP (84).

The diagnosis is based on a semiquantitative assessment of the distribution of NFTs. The criteria also take into account the presence of neuropil threads and tau-positive astrocytes. Based on neuropathological criteria, three types of PSP can be distinguished: typical, atypical, and combined (96). Typical cases show the pathological features as originally described, while atypical cases are variants of the histological changes characteristic of PSP. In combined cases, in addition to PSP there is another disease process such as AD or vascular disease.

Argyrophilic grain disease

Argyrophilic grain disease (AGD), a neuropathological entity, was first described by Braak and colleagues in 1987 and 1989 (97,98). It is a neurodegenerative disease characterized by argyrophilic grains in the entorhinal cortex, hippocampus, amygdala, and neighbouring

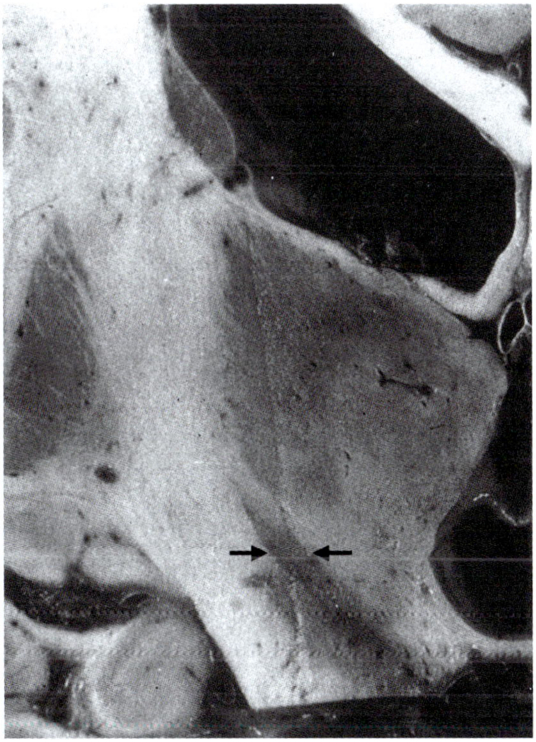

Fig. 18.17 FTLD-Tau: progressive supranuclear palsy. Atrophy of the subthalamic nucleus (between arrows). With permission from Cairns, N.J., Lee, V.M.-Y., Trojanowski, J.Q. pp. 382–407. In The Human Frontal Lobes: Functions and Disorders. Second Edition. Edited by Bruce L. Miller and Jeffrey L. Cummings. The Guilford Press, New York, 2007

temporal cortex in a subset of patients who suffer from adult-onset dementia. When they are present, clinical symptoms of AGD include cognitive decline and dementia. Behavioural abnormalities, personality changes and emotional and mood disorder have been noted in some cases (99,100). Episodic memory is a common finding in most subjects (100). Although the early descriptions described the relative absence of Alzheimer changes, subsequent studies have shown association of AGD with other neurodegenerative diseases, including AD, PiD, PSP, TOD, and rarely other neurodegenerative diseases. AGD has also been reported in cognitively normal elderly subjects and the presence of this pathology raises the question about the contribution, if any, of AGD to dementia. In autopsy series, 5–10% of adults have some degree of AGD (99,101) and there is an increase in the incidence of AGD with age.

The neuropathology of AGD was characterized, initially, by the presence of 'argyrophilic grains' and visualized best by the Gallyas silver impregnation method. Grains are small, spindle shaped, rod-like, or round bodies in the neuropil and about 4–8 μm in diameter. The grains are most numerous in the transentorhinal and entorhinal cortex, CA1 area of the hippocampus, adjacent temporal cortex, orbitofrontal cortex, and amygdala. Coiled bodies in oligodendrocytes and 'tufted' astrocytes similar to those seen in PSP are often seen, as are swollen achromatic neurones and tau-immunoreactive 'pre-tangles.'

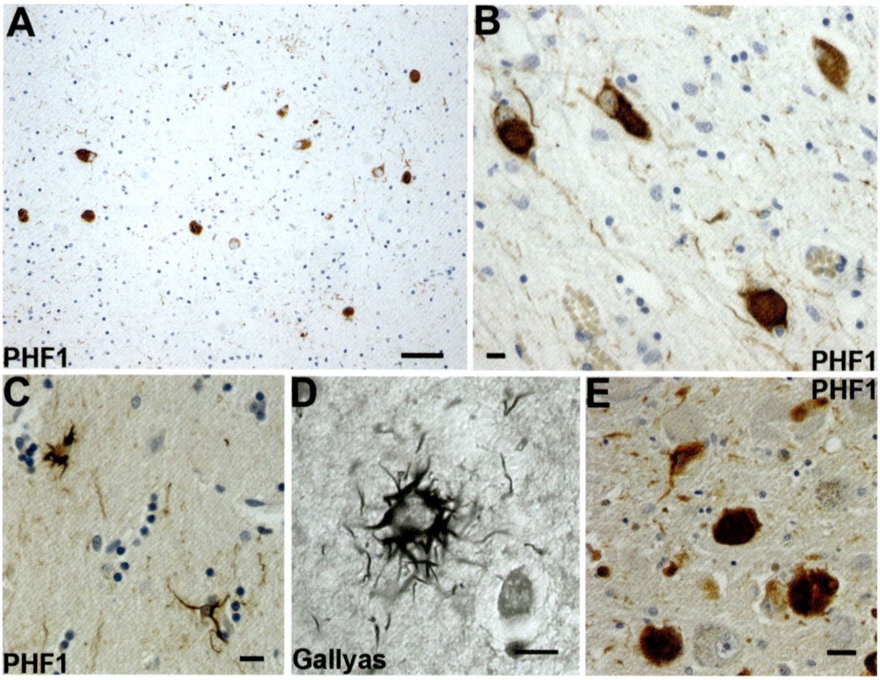

Fig. 18.18 FTLD-Tau: progressive supranuclear palsy. Neurofibrillary tangles in the subthalamic nucleus (a), occulomotor nucleus (b), and locus coeruleus (e). Tau-immunoreactive astrocytes in the putamen (c,d). (a–c,e) Phosphorylated tau (PHF1) immunohistochemistry. (d) Gallyas silver impregnation. Scale bars: (a) 50 µm, (b–e) 10 µm. Adapted from (3).

Tau immunohistochemistry typically reveals more pathology than that seen by the Gallyas silver stain and is now the method of choice for detecting neuronal and glial inclusions (Figure 18.19). The presence of 4R tau in the inclusions of AGD indicates that this disorder, like PSP and CBD may be classified as a 4R tauopathy (102). As with other neurodegenerative diseases, attempts have been made to stage the progression of AGD (103), but none has been universally accepted.

Electron microscopy of the inclusions of AGD reveals straight filaments or tubules measuring 9–25 nm (102). Coiled bodies are found in almost all cases and are morphologically and immunohistochemically similar to those observed in other 4R tauopathies and they lack specificity. Gel electrophoresis of insoluble fractions has been useful in detecting a double band of 68 and 64 kDa, similar to the 4R pattern found in PSP and CBD. The development of 3R- and 4R-specific antibodies has facilitated the detection of 3R and 4R tau by immunohistochemistry, which may be used to complement the biochemical findings obtained in the research laboratory.

Sporadic multiple system tauopathy with dementia

Rare forms of FTLD with tauopathy have been reported and it is not yet clear whether sporadic MSTD (104) represents a unique entity or is part of a spectrum of white matter

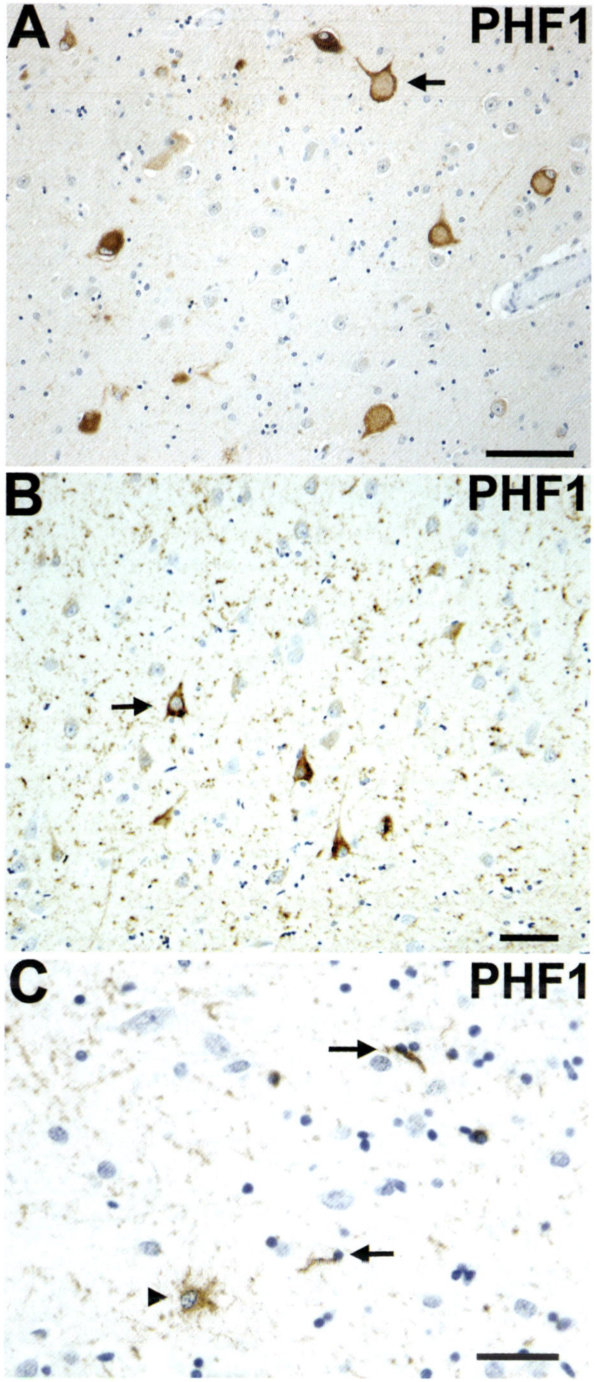

Fig. 18.19 FTLD-Tau: argyrophilic grain disease. A swollen achromatic neurone (arrow) with pale centre and more intense tau-immunoreactive periphery in the subiculum. Tau-immunoreactive grains in the neuropil and diffusely stained pyramidal neurones (arrow) indicating a pre-neurofibrillary tangle stage in the pyramidal layer of the hippocampus (b). A tau-immunoreactive astrocytic inclusion (arrowhead) and oligodendroglial cytoplasmic inclusions called coiled bodies (arrows) in the CA1 subfield of the hippocampus. (a–c) Phosphorylated tau (PHF1) immunohistochemistry. Scale bars (a) 100 μm and (b,c) 50 μm. Adapted from (3).

tauopathies, which also include white matter tauopathy with globular glial inclusions (105). In one report, where neuropathology of MSTD was described, there was a late age at onset of 75 years, consistent with the non-familial nature of the disease (104). There were frontal lobe symptoms (including abnormalities in behaviour, personality, and executive functions). Parkinsonism and eye movement disorders were not present.

Macroscopy revealed mild atrophy of the frontal and parietal lobes and severe atrophy of the temporal lobes. Microscopically, there were sparse filamentous tau-positive inclusions and more numerous globular neuronal and glial tau-positive inclusions in both grey and white matter (Figure 18.20). Inclusions were also seen in subcortical regions, including the substantia nigra, globus pallidus, subthalamic nucleus, and dentate nucleus. Fine structural studies revealed predominantly straight filaments, while other inclusions resembled 'fingerprint' bodies. The filamentous inclusions were composed of tau. Immunoblotting of sarkosyl-insoluble tau revealed two major bands of 64 and 68 kDa, predominantly 4R tau. Sequence analysis of *MAPT* revealed that there were no mutations in either exons 9–13 or the adjacent intronic sequences. Thus, sporadic multiple system tauopathy with dementia represents a distinct phenotype in the spectrum of tauopathies.

White matter tauopathy with globular glial inclusions

A disease with predominant white matter tauopathy with globular glial inclusions was described in seven individuals with a 4R tauopathy (105). Clinically, the patients presented with frontal lobe signs consistent with the behavioural variant of FTD (bvFTD) and included pyramidal signs in some cases. Neuropathologically, there was marked

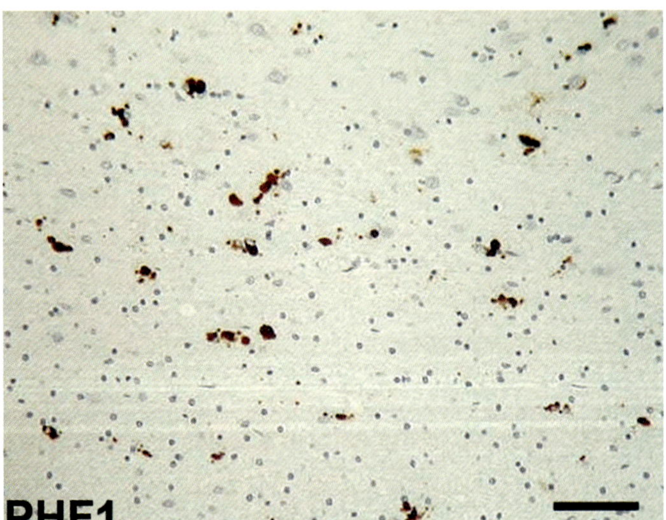

Fig. 18.20 FTLD-Tau: Sporadic multiple system tauopathy with dementia. Neuronal and glial globular inclusions at the grey/white junction. Phosphorylated tau (PHF1) immunohistochemistry. Scale bar 100 μm. Adapted from (3).

neuronal loss in the frontal and temporal cortex, subiculum, and amygdala. Adjacent white matter had numerous globular glial inclusions composed of abnormal filaments present mostly in oligodendrocytes (Figure 18.21). Immunoblotting of sarkosyl-insoluble tau demonstrated the presence of two major tau bands of 64 and 68 kDa and consistent with the pattern seen in other 4R tauopathies. No mutations in the *MAPT* gene were detected. The presence of 4R tau-immunoreactive globular glial inclusions in these cases represents a novel FTLD-Tau. The presence of glial tau-immunoreactive inclusions appears to overlap with another 4R tauopathy, MSTD, but future studies will be required to determine whether these two entities are distinct or are part of the spectrum of 4R tauopathies with variable clinical and pathological phenotypes.

Tangle-only dementia

NFT predominant form of senile dementia of Alzheimer type, also called senile dementia of the NFT type, or TOD is characterized clinically by late onset (106–108). In one study, the mean age at onset was 83.8 ± 6.8 (mean ± standard deviation) years and the mean age at death was 88.1 ± 7.6 years (108). Memory loss is the usual presenting symptom followed by deficits in activities in daily living; this phenotype overlaps clinically with the early features of AD. In one study, the prevalence of TOD was eight of 207 (3.9%) (108). As in AD, there may be mild to moderate diffuse atrophy with or without atrophy of the hippocampus. Microscopy reveals numerous NFT in the medial temporal lobe with few or no neocortical tangles, and there is an absence of Aβ and neuritic plaques (Figure 18.22). There is considerable overlap between the numbers of NFT in the hippocampus in TOD, AD, and cognitively normal aged subjects (108). As in AD, the tau isoform pattern is 3R and 4R. In some cases, but not all, sparse additional glial pathology (coiled bodies, tufted and thorny astrocytes) may be present, similar to that seen in CBD, PSP, and AGD (106).

Frontotemporal lobar degeneration with *MAPT* mutation

Several families with FTD with and without movement disorder have been identified with mutations in the *MAPT* gene. Although this group of disorders has been referred to as FTD and parkinsonism linked to chromosome 17 (FTDP-17) not all cases have parkinsonism (109,110). *MAPT* gene mutations cause tau dysfunction by several mechanisms. Intronic and some exonic mutations affect the alternative splicing of exon 10 and, consequently, alter the relative proportions of 3R and 4R tau. Other exonic mutations impair the ability of tau to bind MTs and to promote MT assembly. Some mutations also promote the assembly of tau into pathological amyloid filaments. Intronic mutations clustered around the 5′ splice site of exon 10, as well as several mutations within exon 10, increase the ratio of 4R/3R tau by altering exon splicing (111–114). As a result of these mutations there is a relative increase in mRNA containing exon 10. Biochemical analysis of insoluble tau extracted from FTLD with *MAPT* mutation brain tissue reveals predominantly 4R tau isoforms. Furthermore, 4R tau protein levels are increased in both affected and unaffected regions of FTLD with *MAPT* mutation brains (115–117).

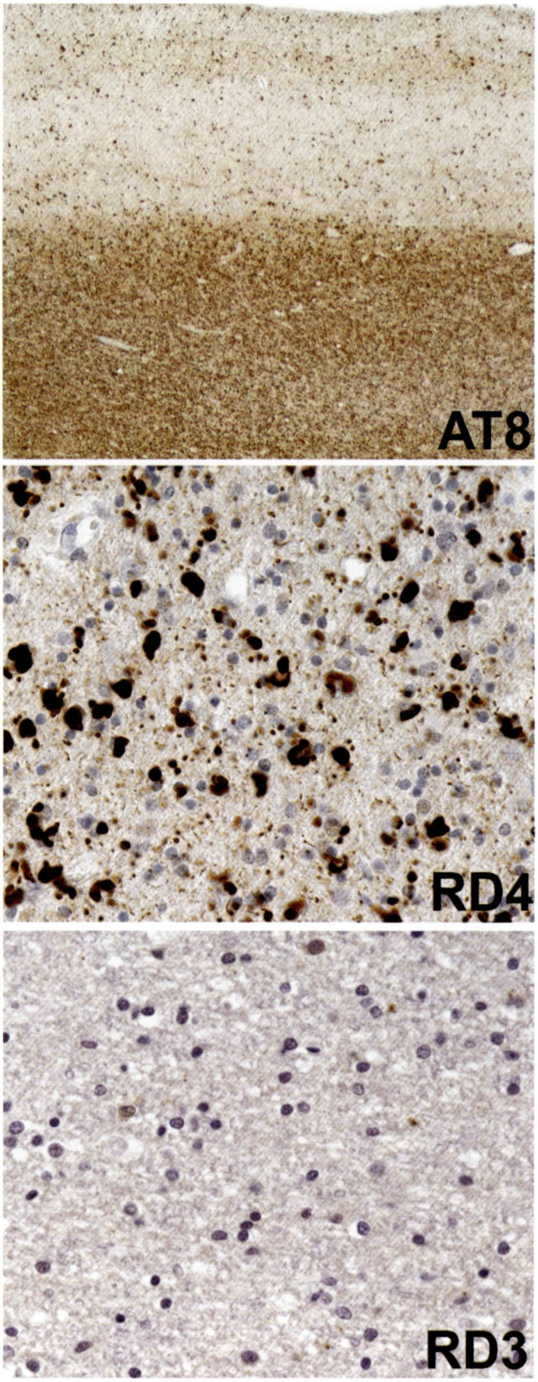

Fig. 18.21 FTLD-Tau: white matter tauopathy with globular glial inclusions. (*Upper panel*) Globular glial inclusions are prominent at the border between the cortex and white matter of the frontal lobe. Phosphorylated tau (AT8) immunohistochemistry. (*Centre panel*) Abundant globular glial inclusions in the underlying white matter contain 4R tau (RD4 immunohistochemistry). The white matter inclusions (of the *lower panel*) do not contain 3R tau (RD3 immunohistochemistry). Kindly provided by Dr Gabor Kovacs, Medical University of Vienna, Austria.

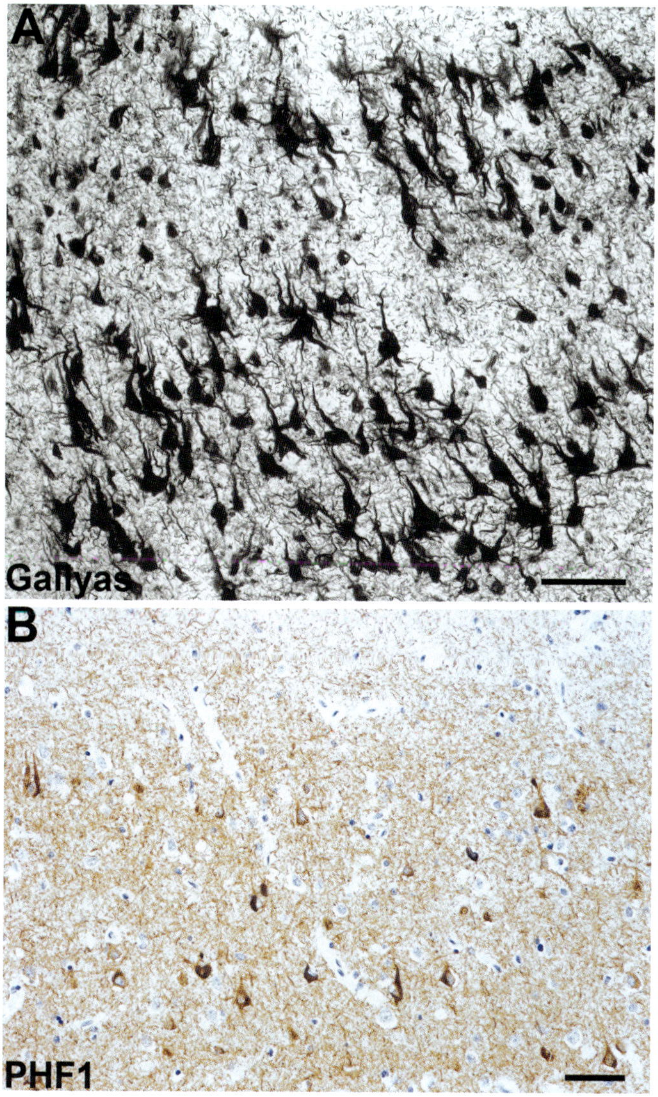

Fig. 18.22 FTLD-Tau: tangle-only dementia. (a,b) Numerous neurofibrillary tangles in the upper and lower pyramidal neurones of the occipitotemporal cortex; no neuritic plaques or amyloid deposits are present. (a) Gallyas silver impregnation. (b) Phosphorylated tau (PHF1) immunohistochemistry. Scale bars: 50 μm. Adapted from (3).

Mutations alter exon 10 splicing of *MAPT* by affecting several of the regulatory elements described above. The mechanisms by which changes in the ratio of 3R/4R tau lead to neuronal and glial dysfunction and cell death remain unclear. However, 3R and 4R tau may bind to distinct sites on MT (118), and it is possible that a specific ratio of tau isoforms is necessary for normal MT function (119). Thus, the altered ratio of 3R/4R tau may directly affect MT function. In addition, overproduction of 4R tau isoforms may lead to an excess of free tau in the cytoplasm that is prone to aggregate and polymerize into filaments over time. Conversely, overproduction of 3R tau may have the opposite effect: an absence of tau inclusions and the phenotype of FTLD (120).

Another subset of the mutations has no effect on splicing, but instead alters the ability of tau to interact with MT, reduces the binding of tau to MT, and decrease its ability to promote MT stability and assembly *in vitro* (121–123). In contrast to mutations that affect the splicing of *MAPT*, these mutations do not alter the expression pattern of 3R and 4R tau (116). A moderate decrease in soluble 4R tau with the P301L mutation is caused by the selective aggregation of mutant 4R tau isoforms (116,124,125). These mutations generate a variety of biochemical patterns of insoluble tau extracted from brain tissue of patients.

Tau aggregation in FTLD with *MAPT* mutation may be caused, in part, by a subset of missense *MAPT* mutations. *In vitro* studies demonstrate that mutations, including K257T and R406W, promote heparin- or arachidonic acid-induced tau filament formation relative to wild-type tau (125–127). Tau function may also be altered by *MAPT* mutations by altering its phosphorylation state and several mutations decrease the binding affinity of tau for phosphatase 2A, a phosphatase implicated in the regulation of the MT-binding activity of tau (128).

These familial cases typically have atrophy of the frontal and temporal lobes (Figure 18.23). Microscopically, neuronal loss, astrocytosis, microvacuolation, and swollen neurones are found in affected areas together with a spectrum of tau pathology, including intraneuronal NFT-like inclusions, neuronal globose tangle-like inclusions, intraneuronal Pick body-like inclusions, astrocytic tangle-like inclusions, and oligodendroglial inclusions resembling coiled bodies and DNs (Figure 18.24). In a subset of cases with *MAPT* mutations, there may be sufficient NFT and β-amyloid plaques to fulfil the neuropathological criteria for AD, but these cases, in addition to the *MAPT* mutation, may also have an apolipoprotein E ε4 allele, a risk factor for AD. (129). Mutations in the *MAPT* gene generate a heterogeneous biochemical phenotype: mutations may generate predominantly either 3R or 4R tau or a

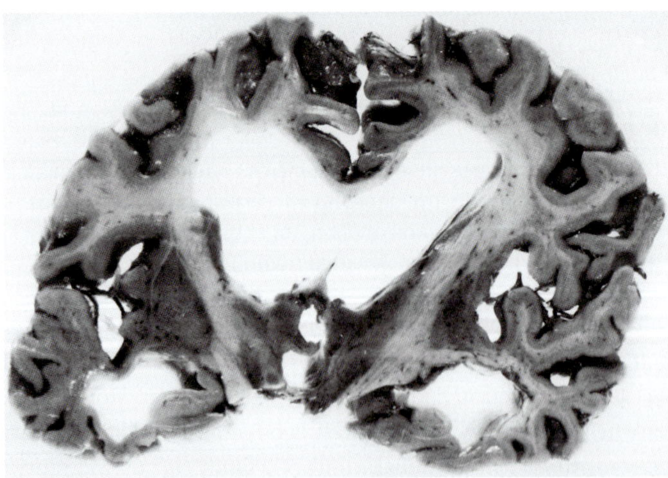

Fig. 18.23 FTLD-Tau: FTLD with *MAPT* mutation. Atrophy of the frontal and temporal lobes at the level of the red nucleus in a case with FTLD with *MAPT* intron 10+16. Adapted from Lantos PL, Cairns NJ, Khan MN, et al. (2002). Neuropathologic variation in frontotemporal dementia due to the intronic tau 10 (+16) mutation. *Neurology*, **58**(8), 1169–1175.

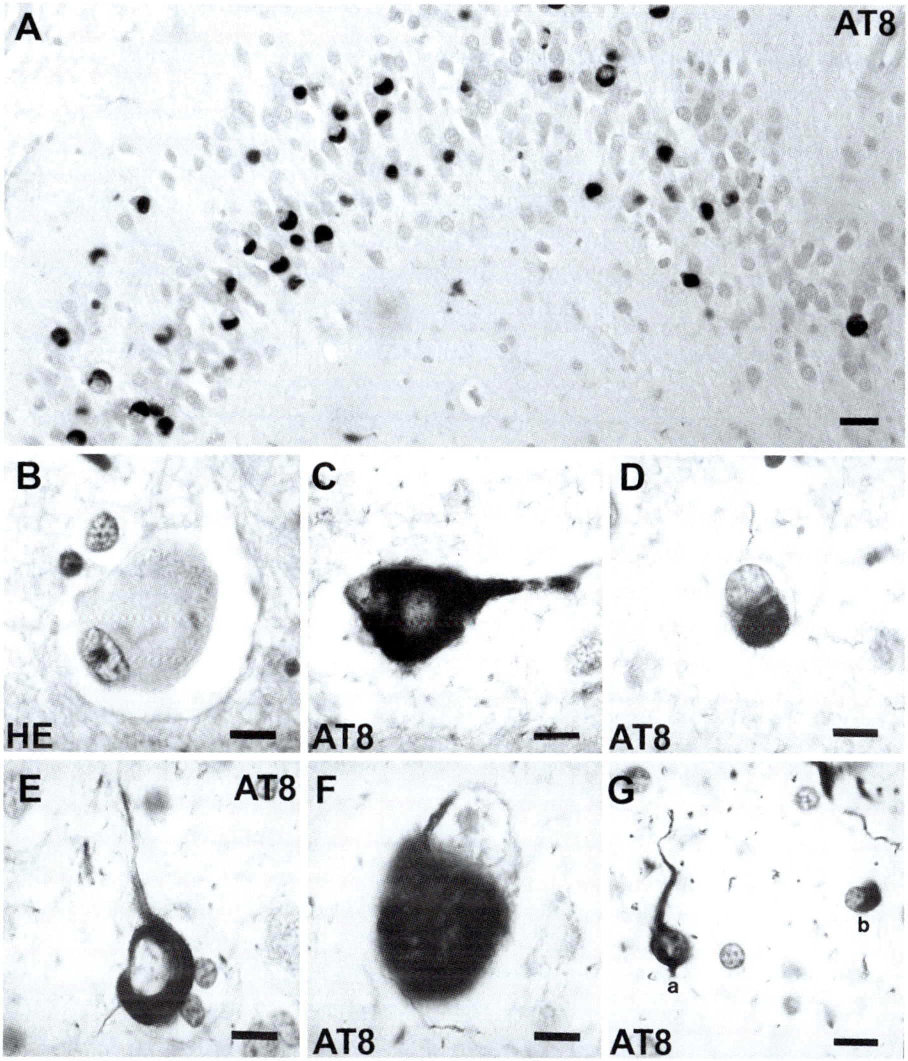

Fig. 18.24 FTLD-Tau: FTLD with *MAPT* mutation. Spectrum of neuronal and glial tau inclusions in FTLD with *MAPT* mutation. Inclusions in FTLD with *MAPT* G389R mutation (A) and *MAPT* intron 10+16 mutation (B–G). (A) Numerous Pick body-like inclusions in the granule neurones of the dentate fascia. (B) A swollen achromatic neurone (haematoxylin and eosin). (C) A swollen neurone with a central area of pale tau immunoreactivity surrounded by more intense staining. (D) An intraneuronal inclusion resembling a Pick body in the frontal lobe. (E) A neurofibrillary tangle-like inclusion in a pyramidal neurone of the frontal lobe. (F) A globose neurofibrillary tangle-like inclusion in the dorsal raphé nucleus. (G) An astrocytic fibrillary inclusion (a) and a coiled body (b) in an oligodendrocyte in the white matter of the frontal lobe. (B–F) Tau immunohistochemistry. Scale bars: 10 μm. Adapted from Lantos PL, Cairns NJ, Khan MN, et al. (2002) Neuropathologic variation in frontotemporal dementia due to the intronic tau 10 (+16) mutation. *Neurology*, **58**(8), 1169–1175.

combination of the two. Thus, an extraordinarily wide range of tau pathology has been observed in these familial cases.

Although there is clinical and neuropathological overlap between the neurodegenerative tauopathies, each can be distinguished with variable probability by the distribution, severity, and morphology of tau-positive inclusions. In cases with a *MAPT* gene mutation, in addition to extensive neuronal loss and astrocytosis, tau-positive neuronal and glial inclusions may resemble those seen in AD, PSP, CBD, and PiD. This neuropathological heterogeneity is a striking feature of FTLD with *MAPT* mutation and it is complemented by biochemical heterogeneity where there is variation in the proportions of tau isoforms, not only with different mutations, but also within the same brain. Nevertheless, cases with *MAPT* gene mutations may be broadly grouped according to the pattern of tau immunostaining and tau isoform ratios as demonstrated by Western blotting (Figure 18.12).

Transgenic models of tauopathies

To simulate the pathogenesis of tau inclusion bodies, TG models have been generated by overexpressing human tau proteins in mice (130,131). However, these mice are either asymptomatic or develop pathology that is localized to the spinal cord or lacks many of the pathological changes of tau-based disorders. In contrast, the introduction of the P301L mutation led to the development of TG mice that develop age- and gene dose-dependent accumulation of tau tangles in the brain and spinal cord with associated nerve cell loss and gliosis as well as behavioural abnormalities (130). The tau inclusions were composed of only mutant human tau thus implicating the P301L mutation in the aggregation of mutant tau. Various aspects of human tauopathies have been modelled, including a TG mouse overexpressing the shortest human tau isoform, which acquired age-dependent tau pathology similar to that seen in FTLD with *MAPT* mutation and ALS/Parkinsonism-dementia complex of Guam (132). The fruit fly, *Drosophila melanogaster*, has been used to overexpress either wild-type or mutant tau (R406W and V337M) and shows features of tauopathy, including adult-onset progressive neurodegeneration with accumulation of abnormal tau (133), but the neurodegeneration occurs in the absence of NFT formation. NFT-like pathology has been generated in another fly model when tau was coexpressed with shaggy, a homologue of glycogen synthase 3-kinase, an enzyme implicated in tau phosphorylation (134). A tau TG *Caenorhabditis elegans* model has been used to demonstrate neurodegeneration and defective neurotransmission. In this model, pan-neuronal expression of normal and mutant tau resulted in altered behaviour, accumulation of insoluble phosphorylated tau, age-dependent loss of axons and neurones, and structural damage to axonal tracts (159). Thus, a spectrum of models is being developed that recapitulates various features of tau pathology and these models will facilitate understanding of the molecular mechanisms underlying neurodegeneration in the tauopathies.

Frontotemporal lobar degeneration with FUS inclusions

Following the discovery of pathogenic mutations in *TARDBP* in familial ALS, investigators identified a related gene on chromosome 16 in some autosomal dominant ALS families.

Mutations in the *FUS* (fusion in sarcoma) gene cause one form of familial ALS (135,136). Like TDP-43, FUS is an RNA/DNA processing protein. Like TDP-43, FUS is associated with heterogeneous ribonucleoprotein, and its functions include: DNA repair, transcription, RNA splicing, transport of mRNA to and RNA translation at the synapse, and microRNA processing (for review, see Lagier-Tourenne and Cleveland (137)). Most mutations identified in *FUS* have been found in the C-terminus (135,136), resembling the C-terminal clustering of pathogenic mutations in *TARDBP*.

In spinal cord and brain tissue of *FUS* mutation carriers, NCIs containing mutant FUS protein have been observed. These inclusions do not contain TDP-43 indicating that different metabolic pathways are involved in neurodegeneration caused by mutant FUS (135,136). Mutations may result in a loss of normal function or a gain of toxic function of FUS in the nucleus, resulting in impaired RNA processing and cell death. Three FTLD/FUS entities have been identified: NIFID, BIBD, and aFTLD-U.

Neuronal intermediate filament inclusion disease

NIFID is a rare neurological disease with a clinically heterogeneous phenotype, including atypical dementia, and pyramidal and extrapyramidal signs presenting at a young age (138–140). In a series of 10 cases, the mean age at onset was 40 (range 23–56) years, the mean duration of disease was 4.5 (range 2.7–13) years, and the mean age at death was 45 (range 28–61) years (140). Both sexes are affected, the ratio of men to women being 2:3. NIFID is largely a sporadic disorder and only one case has been reported where the father had parkinsonism and dementia indicating evidence of hereditability (141). The presenting symptoms included personality change, apathy, blunted affect, and disinhibition. There may also be memory loss, cognitive impairment, and language deficits in half of the cases. Motor weakness may be evident at presentation in a minority of patients. Extrapyramidal features are present in most cases, and less frequently buccofacial apraxia and supranuclear ophthalmoplegia. Personality and behavioural changes, and memory and language deficits are seen in the majority of patients. Hyper-reflexia is a common finding and most patients became mute with advanced disease. Structural brain imaging typically shows atrophy of the frontal and temporal lobes and the caudate nucleus may be atrophied. Atrophy of the caudate may raise the possibility of Huntington's disease, but no expansion in the huntingtin *(HTT)* gene has been reported.

The brain often shows severe atrophy of the frontal and temporal lobes with mild parietal atrophy. The loss of brain substance may lead to a brain weight below 1000 g. The caudate nucleus is markedly atrophied in most cases. While the severity and pattern of atrophy varies from case to case, the frontal and temporal poles and caudate nucleus are often the most severely affected. In all cases, there is variable atrophy of subcortical nuclei, including the basal ganglia, amygdala, and thalamus. The brainstem, cerebellum, and spinal cord appear unremarkable. Coronal slices further confirm frontotemporal atrophy: the gyri are narrowed and the intervening sulci widened with enlargement of the lateral ventricles. In the more severely affected cases the cortical ribbon is thinned. In some cases, there is striking atrophy of the amygdala and hippocampus. The histological changes include the stereotypic lesions of FTLD: neuronal loss, status spongiosus, and astrocytosis in temporal and frontal isocortex. Swollen achromatic neurones are also seen. However, the most striking feature is the presence of inclusions containing FUS protein, a proportion of which also contains neuronal IF proteins (i.e. the NF triplet proteins and α-internexin) (Figures 18.25 and 18.26). The severity of each of these histological abnormalities varies from case to case.

Microscopy reveals extensive neuronal loss and reactive astrocytosis in the frontal, medial temporal, and parietal lobes, and varying degrees of loss in subcortical nuclei, including the caudate nucleus, putamen, globus pallidus, amygdala, substantia nigra, and locus coeruleus. A variable degree of neuronal loss and axonal swellings may be present in the cerebellum. Occasional swollen achromatic neurones are observed in affected areas. In areas of neuronal loss, faintly eosinophilic, intraneuronal, cytoplasmic inclusions are present. In haematoxylin and eosin and cresyl violet-stained sections, hyaline aggregates of neuronal IFs are observed. The inclusions are variably argyrophilic with modified Bielschowsky and Bodian silver impregnations and superficially resemble the Pick bodies of PiD. Immunohistochemistry demonstrates the presence within the inclusions of FUS (22). Many NCI are ubiquitinated and contain class IV IF proteins (NF-L, NF-M, NF-L, and α-internexin). FUS immunohistochemistry reveals pathology that is more extensive: NII and glial inclusions contain FUS but not neuronal IF. The morphology of the inclusions is extremely variable throughout the neuraxis. Axonal swellings, similar to those found in ALS and in normal ageing, but which are not specific to any neurodegenerative disease, are also seen in affected areas and in underlying white matter, corticospinal tracts, and other white matter tracts. In cases with pyramidal signs, there may be evidence of corticospinal tract degeneration in the spinal cord. However, motor neurones in the anterior horns are relatively spared and the number of pyknotic neurones is much lower than that typically seen in classical MND.

The cytoplasmic inclusions of NIFID are variably ubiquitinated as demonstrated by immunohistochemistry. FUS-, ubiquitin-, and neuronal IF-positive inclusions are most numerous in the youngest cases (140). Ubiquitinated inclusions are found in the neocortex and subcortical nuclei and in the neurones of the dentate gyrus in all cases where they resemble those seen in FTLD/MND. Single and multiple round and elongated intranuclear inclusions may also be observed in neurones containing cytoplasmic inclusions. The intranuclear inclusions in NIFID contain FUS and ubiquitin, but they are not labelled by antineuronal IF antibodies.

Ultrastructural study of the NCIs in NIFID reveals aggregates of granular filamentous material with no apparent limiting membrane (142). The granular material resembles the morphology of ribosomes and the filaments have an apparent diameter of 10–25 nm. Immunoelectron microscopy demonstrates that the filaments of the inclusions contain epitopes of neuronal IF proteins (140).

Basophilic inclusion body disease

Rare cases of BIBD may present as juvenile (143,144) or adult-onset MND (145,146), FTD (147), or a combination of both (148). Typically, patients are younger when symptoms

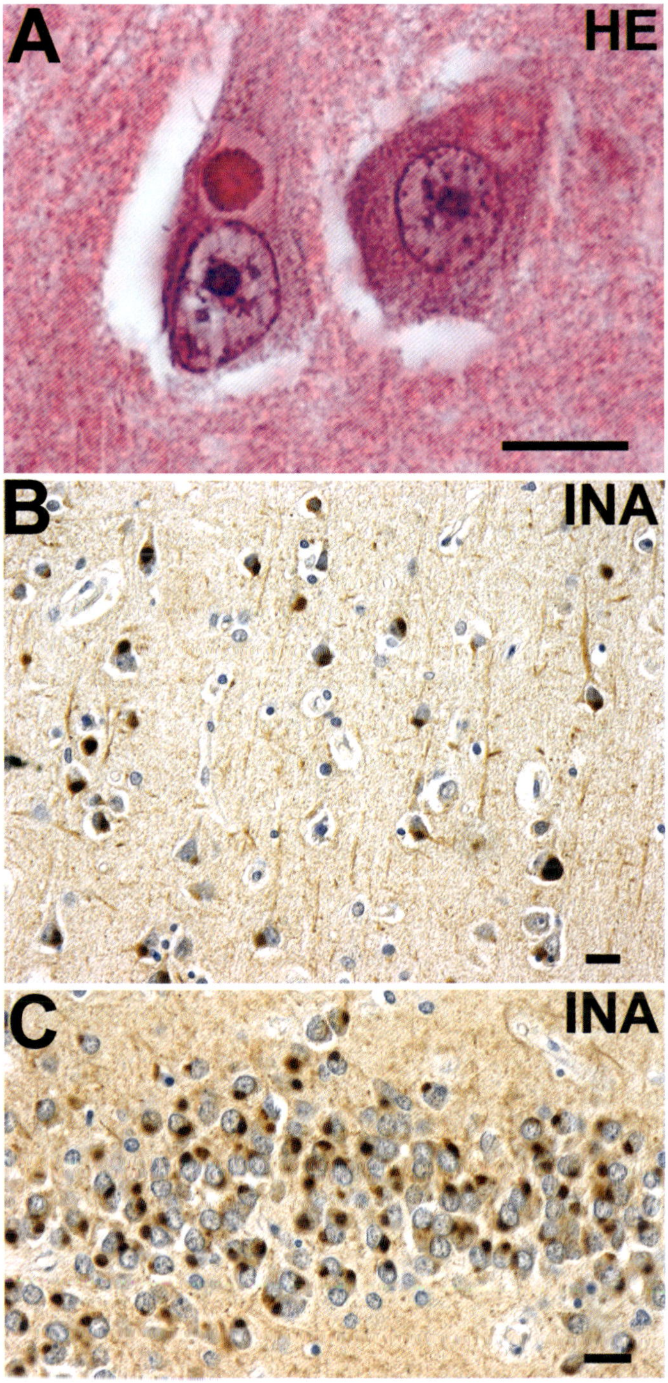

Fig. 18.25 FTLD-FUS: neuronal intermediate filament inclusion disease. (a) Eosinophilic Lewy body-like NCI in a pyramidal neurone of the CA1 subfield of the hippocampus. (b) α-Internexin immunoreactive NCI in layer III of the superior temporal gyrus. (c) Numerous α-internexin immunoreactive NCI in the granule neurones of the dentate fascia. (a) Haematoxylin and eosin; (b,c) α-internexin (INA) immunohistochemistry. Scale bars: 10 μm. Adapted from (3).

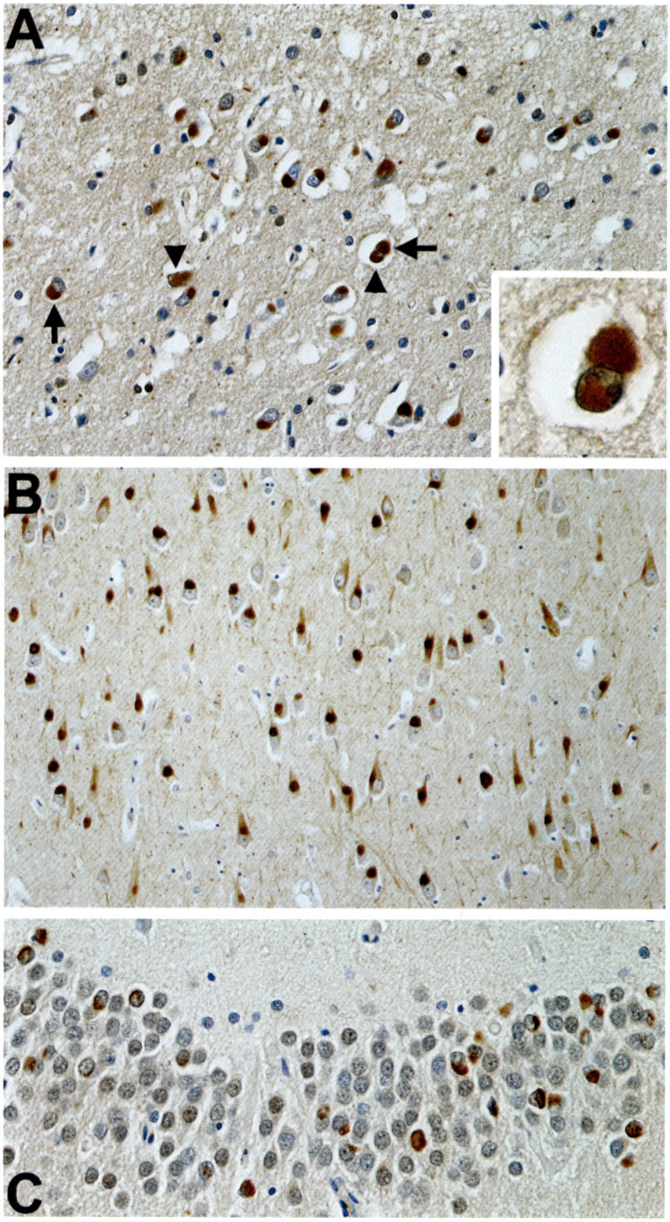

Fig. 18.26 FTLD/FUS: neuronal intermediate filament inclusion disease. (A) FUS-immunoreactive NCI (arrow) and NII (arrowhead) in the superficial laminae of the frontal lobe. Insert, a neurone containing both an NCI and an NII. FUS-immunoreactive NCI in the CA1 subfield of the hippocampus (B) and dentate fascia (C). FUS immunohistochemistry. With kind permission from Springer Science+Business Media: Acta Neuropathol. The spectrum and severity of FUS-immunoreactive inclusions in the frontal and temporal lobes of ten cases of neuronal intermediate filament inclusion disease. **121**, 2011, 219–28, Armstrong RA, Gearing M, Bigio EH, Cruz-Sanchez FF, Duyckaerts C, Mackenzie IR, Perry RH, Skullerud K, Yokoo H, Cairns NJ.

develop (29–30 years (147) and 52–58 years (149)) than those with PiD. Features of MND and FTD are comparable with the heterogeneous phenotype of NIFID. The early age at onset of this widespread, but rare, disease hints at a genetic cause, but none has been identified.

Cases typically show pronounced atrophy of the frontal and temporal lobes with less involvement of the parietal lobe. Coronal slices reveal marked atrophy of the striatum, often with a thinned caudate nucleus, thalamus, and amygdala. The substantia nigra is also depigmented. Microscopy shows the stereotypic features of FTLD: severe neuronal loss, superficial microvacuolation, reactive astrocytosis, and swollen achromatic neurones. The histological hallmark of this disease is the basophilic inclusion body (147) (Figure 18.27), which contain epitopes of FUS (23), but neither tau, nor α-synuclein, nor neuronal IF proteins are present. Basophilic inclusion bodies are found in affected neocortex preferentially affecting the superficial laminae similar to the distribution in PiD (150). Unlike Pick bodies in PiD, basophilic inclusion bodies are not usually found in the hippocampus and dentate gyrus. However, inclusions are found in subcortical nuclei, including the putamen, caudate nucleus, globus pallidus, nucleus basalis of Meynert, red

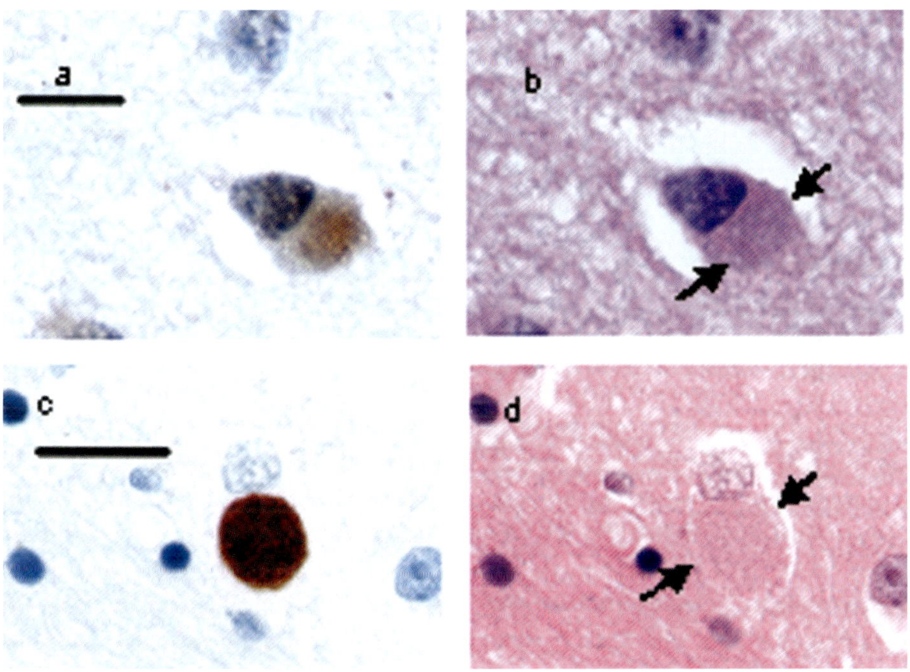

Fig. 18.27 FTLD/FUS: basophilic inclusion body disease. (a) FUS antibodies label a basophilic inclusion. Following FUS immunohistochemistry using 3-amino-9-ethylcarbazole (AEC), a water-soluble dye, the same neurones were photographed before (a,c) and after (b,d) destaining in water and haematoxylin and eosin staining. (a,b) cerebral cortex, (c,d) putamen. (b,d) Haematoxylin and eosin; (a,c) FUS immunohistochemistry. Scale bars: 20 mm. Adapted from (23).

nucleus, subthalamic nucleus, periaqueductal gray and in the anterior horns of the spinal cord. Unlike in MND, Bunina bodies and ubiquitin-positive, skein-like inclusions are not seen in cases of BIBD. The inclusions are variably basophilic, and occasionally eosinophilic, in haematoxylin and eosin-stained sections. The inclusions are variably ubiquitinated and contain variable amounts of RNA as shown by acridine orange staining. Misfolded proteins seen in tauopathies and synucleinopathies, and neuronal IF proteins are absent from these inclusions. Electron microscopy shows that the inclusions are not membrane bound and contain fibrils with a diameter between 13 and 25 nm and variably granular in appearance (147). Swollen axons and axonal spheroids are also present, but these are not specific to BIBD as they are commonly seen in other neurodegenerative diseases and normal ageing.

Atypical frontotemporal lobar degeneration with ubiquitin-immunoreactive inclusions

A third FTLD/FUS entity has been described. Initially, cases of this subgroup of FTLD were reported with ubiquitin-positive, tau- and TDP-43-negative inclusions (i.e. aFTLD-U) (151). Clinically, most of these cases have an early-onset bvFTD but a variable proportion has psychotic symptoms, including eating disorder. Memory is only affected late in the disease course. Mild parkinsonism is present in some, but none shows pyramidal signs. No cases with a family history of similar disease have been identified.

The clinical and pathological overlap between FTLD and ALS led investigators to explore the inclusions of aFTLD-U and found that FUS was a component of both neuronal and glial inclusions (152). Biochemistry has revealed an increase in the amount of insoluble FUS in aFTLD-U. Although no FUS mutations have been found in NIFID, BIBD, or aFTLD-U, a mutation has been reported in a case presenting with FTD and later developing MND. Thus, the contribution of FUS to pathogenesis in these disorders is uncertain. The presence of FUS in both ALS and FTLD reinforces the concept that FTLD and ALS are closely related disorders.

Macroscopic findings include symmetric atrophy of the frontal and temporal lobes and caudate nucleus. Microscopically, there is evidence of neuronal loss and gliosis in the frontal and temporal neocortex, hippocampus, striatum, globus pallidus, and substantia nigra. No pathological changes are seen with silver impregnation methods and immunohistochemical studies fail to show epitopes of Aβ, phosphorylated tau, α-synuclein, neuronal intermediate filament proteins, TDP-43, or expanded polyglutamine repeats.

The inclusions of aFTLD-U are ubiquitinated and contain FUS (Figure 18.28) and have variable morphology, including round and crescentic NCI, and vermiform or rod-like NII. The NII are most numerous in the dentate granule cells but they are also found in pyramidal neurones of the neocortex and hippocampus and some subcortical nuclei. Unlike NCI and DN, NII of aFTLD-U contain epitopes of ubiquitin, but not P62, the latter being a marker of the UPS. In cases of aFTLD-U, immunohistochemistry reveals FUS-immunoreactive NCI, DN, and NII of similar shape, number, and distribution as are demonstrated with ubiquitin antibodies.

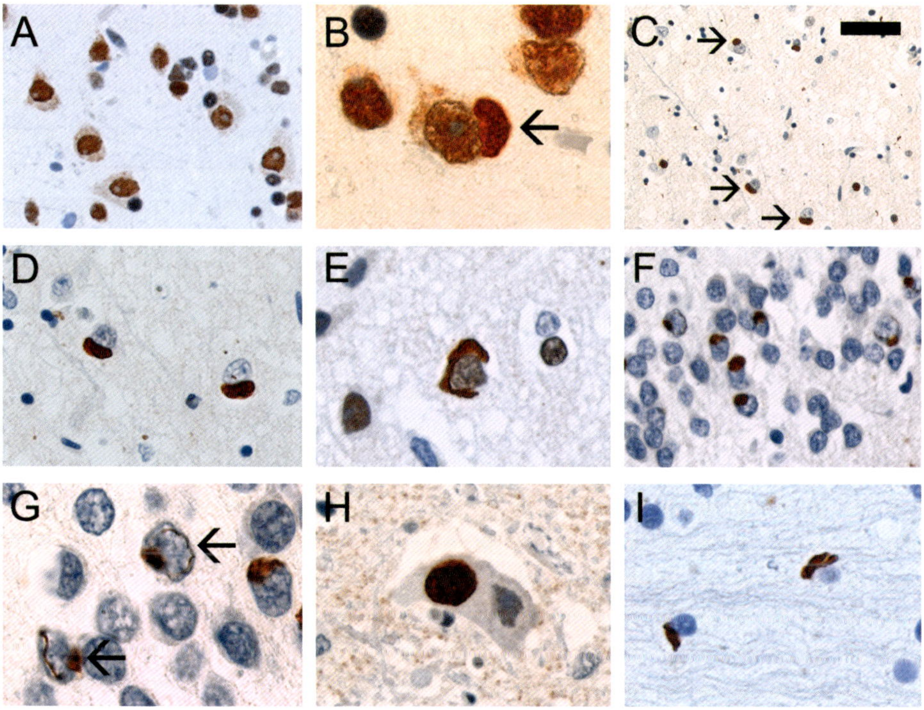

Fig. 18.28 FTLD/FUS: atypical FTLD with ubiquitin-immunoreactive inclusions (aFTLD-U). FUS immunohistochemistry performed on sections of post-mortem brain tissue from normal control (A) and aFTLD-U subjects (B–I). The normal physiological staining pattern, consisting of strong immunoreactivity of neuronal nuclei, weaker but consistent staining of neuronal cytoplasm and more variable reactivity of glial nuclei was demonstrated in all cases, including normal controls (A), neurological controls and aFTLD-U subjects (B). In patients with aFTLD-U, neurones with inclusions (arrow) retained at least some of the normal nuclear and cytoplasmic staining (B). Neuronal cytoplasmic inclusions (NCI) were most numerous in the middle and deeper layers of neocortex (C–E) and dentate granule cells of the hippocampus (F) and ranged in morphology from round or oval (D,F) to crescentic (E). Dentate granule cells with vermiform neuronal intranuclear inclusions (arrows) often also had NCI (G). Globular NCI were present in lower motor neurones (H). Flame-shaped glial cytoplasmic inclusions were present in white matter (I). FUS IHC with concentration of primary antibody adjusted to demonstrate normal physiological staining (A,B) or optimize visualization of pathological inclusions. (C–I). Scale bars: (A,H) 20 μm; (B,E,G,I) 10 μm; (C) 50 μm; (D) 15 μm; (F) 30 μm. Figure kindly provided by Dr Ian Mackenzie, Vancouver General Hospital, Vancouver, Canada. Adapted from (151).

Frontotemporal lobar degeneration with ubiquitin-immunoreactive inclusions

In the molecular classification of FTLD (Figure 18.1) there is a fourth group of patients who have inclusions that do not contain TDP-43, tau, or FUS proteins. This unique entity, limited to a single Danish pedigree, has mutations in the charged multivesicular body protein 2B (*CHMB2B*) gene (153). To date, ubiquitin and P62, a component of the

UPS, are the only proteins that have been reported in the inclusions associated with this gene defect (25) (Figure 18.29). As the pathological protein of the inclusions has yet to be identified, this entity has been called, tentatively, FTLD/UPS (4,5).

Frontotemporal lobar degeneration with no inclusions

FTLD is characterized by stereotypic features: atrophy of the frontal and temporal lobes, neuronal loss, microvacuolation, and astrocytosis (2,27). This disease is distinguished by the absence of any hallmark inclusion. Previously, this nosological entity combined clinical syndromes with pathological substrates and was referred to variously as: PiD Group C in the classification scheme of Constantinidis *et al.* (154), frontal lobe degeneration of non-Alzheimer type (155), dementia of frontal type, FTD, and dementia lacking distinctive histopathology (6,156). As new molecular pathologies have been described, immunohistochemistry has revealed inclusions not previously seen and this has resulted in this diagnostic entity being assigned to a dwindling number of cases.

Conclusions

The accumulation of misfolded proteins in inclusion bodies is a common feature of a wide variety of sporadic and familial neurodegenerative disorders that present clinically with FTD. These diseases are distinguished by the distinct topographic and cell type-specific distribution of inclusions. The biochemical and ultrastructurally characteristics of the inclusions also reveal a significant phenotypic overlap. The discovery of multiple mutations in the *MAPT*, *GRN*, *C9ORF72*, *TARDBP*, *VCP*, and *FUS* genes leading to abnormal filamentous inclusions demonstrates that neuronal and glial dysfunction is sufficient to produce neurodegenerative disease. Experimental evidence indicates that mutations lead to specific alterations in expression, function, and biochemistry of tau, progranulin, TDP-43, VCP, and FUS proteins. Similarly, mutations in *CHMP2B* result in misfolding, protein aggregation, ubiquitination of inclusions, and neurodegeneration in FTLD with *CHMP2B* mutation. The identification of gene mutations in FTLD or polymorphisms at distinct genetic loci that either cause or are risk factors for disease will provide additional insights into disease pathogenesis as well as in the development of new models and novel strategies for treatment and prevention.

Acknowledgements

Support for this work was provided by grants from the National Institute on Aging of the National Institutes of Health, USA (P01-AG03991 and P50-AG05681). We would also like to thank the members of the Alzheimer's Disease Research Center, Washington University School of Medicine, St Louis, Missouri, USA, and the many patients studied and their families, for making the research reviewed here possible.

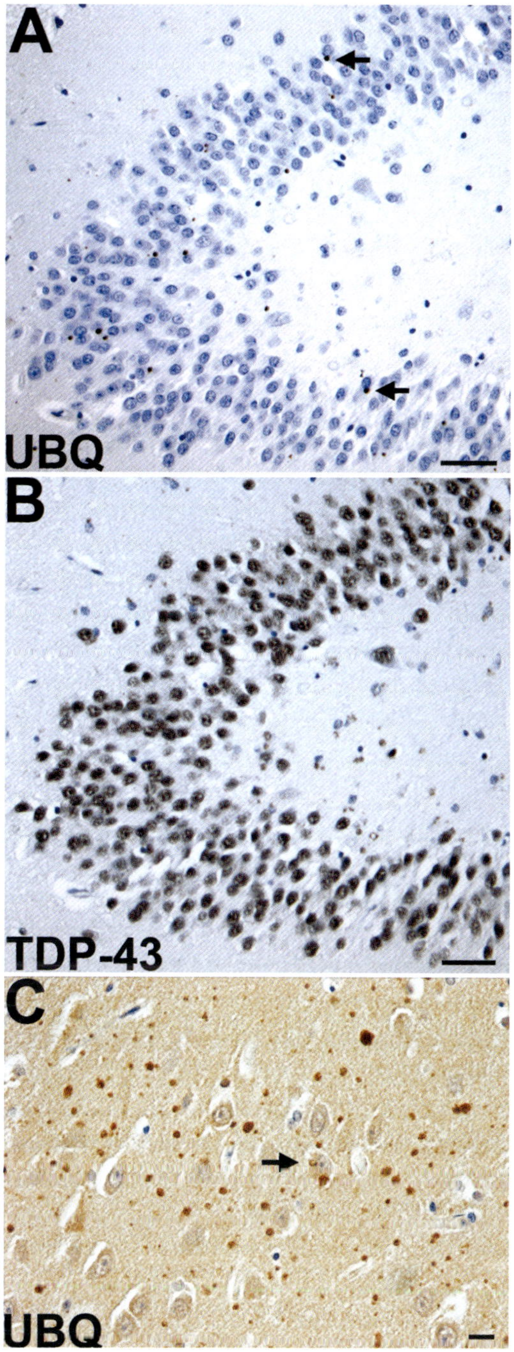

Fig. 18.29 FTLD/UPS: FTLD with CHMP2B mutation. (a) Sparse ubiquitin-immunoreactive NCI (arrows) in the granule neurones of the dentate fascia. The NCIs are not labelled with anti-TDP-43 antibodies (b). Ubiquitin-positive neuropil aggregates and a sparse NCI (arrow) in the frontal lobe of an affected 61-year-old woman (c). Scale bars: (a,b) 50 μm, (c) 10 μm. Adapted from (3).

References

1. Brun A, Englund B, Gustafson L, *et al.* (1994). Clinical and neuropathological criteria for frontotemporal dementia. *J Neurol Neurosurg Psychiatry*, **57**(4), 416–418.
2. McKhann GM, Albert MS, Grossman M, Miller B, Dickson D, Trojanowski JQ. (2001). Clinical and pathological diagnosis of frontotemporal dementia: report of the Work Group on Frontotemporal Dementia and Pick's Disease. *Arch Neurol*, **58**(11), 1803–1809.
3. Cairns NJ, Bigio EH, Mackenzie IR, *et al.* (2007). Neuropathologic diagnostic and nosologic criteria for frontotemporal lobar degeneration: consensus of the Consortium for Frontotemporal Lobar Degeneration. *Acta Neuropathol*, **114**, 5–22.
4. Mackenzie IR, Neumann M, Bigio EH, *et al.* (2009). Nomenclature for neuropathologic subtypes of frontotemporal lobar degeneration: consensus recommendations. *Acta Neuropathol*, **117**, 15–18.
5. Mackenzie IR, Neumann M, Bigio EH, *et al.* (2010). Nomenclature and nosology for neuropathologic subtypes of frontotemporal lobar degeneration: an update. *Acta Neuropathol*, **119**, 1–4.
6. Knopman DS, Mastri AR, Frey WH, Sung JH, Rustan T. (1990). Dementia lacking distinctive histologic features: a common non-Alzheimer degenerative dementia. *Neurology*, **40**(2), 251–256.
7. Chow TW, Miller BL, Hayashi VN, Geschwind DH. (1999). Inheritance of frontotemporal dementia. *Arch Neurol*, **56**(7), 817–822.
8. Bigio EH, Johnson NA, Rademaker AW, *et al.* (2004). Neuronal ubiquitinated intranuclear inclusions in familial and non-familial frontotemporal dementia of the motor neuron disease type associated with amyotrophic lateral sclerosis. *J Neuropathol Exp Neurol*, **63**(8), 801–811.
9. Cairns NJ, Neumann M, Bigio EH, *et al.* (2007). TDP-43 in familial and sporadic frontotemporal lobar degeneration with ubiquitin inclusions. *Am J Pathol*, **171**, 227–240.
10. Baker M, Mackenzie IR, Pickering-Brown SM, *et al.* (2006). Mutations in progranulin cause tau-negative frontotemporal dementia linked to chromosome 17. *Nature*, **442**(7105), 916–919.
11. Cruts M, Gijselinck I, van der ZJ, *et al.* (2006). Null mutations in progranulin cause ubiquitin-positive frontotemporal dementia linked to chromosome 17q21. *Nature*, **442**(7105), 920–924.
12. Gass J, Cannon A, Mackenzie IR, *et al.* (2006). Mutations in progranulin are a major cause of ubiquitin-positive frontotemporal lobar degeneration. *Hum Mol Genet*, **15**(20), 2988–3001.
13. Mukherjee O, Pastor P, Cairns NJ, *et al.* (2006). HDDD2 is a familial frontotemporal lobar degeneration with ubiquitin-positive, tau-negative inclusions caused by a missense mutation in the signal peptide of progranulin. *Ann Neurol*, **60**(3), 314–322.
14. Behrens MI, Mukherjee O, Tu PH, *et al.* (2007). Neuropathologic heterogeneity in HDDD1: a familial frontotemporal lobar degeneration with ubiquitin-positive inclusions and progranulin mutation. *Alzheimer Dis Assoc Disord*, **21**, 1–7.
15. Mackenzie IR. (2007). The neuropathology and clinical phenotype of FTD with progranulin mutations. *Acta Neuropathol*, **114**, 49–54.
16. Benajiba L, Le Ber I, Camuzat A, *et al.* (2009). TARDBP mutations in motoneuron disease with frontotemporal lobar degeneration. *Ann Neurol*, **65**(4), 470–473.
17. Gitcho MA, Bigio EH, Mishra M, *et al.* (2009). TARDBP 3 -UTR variant in autopsy-confirmed frontotemporal lobar degeneration with TDP-43 proteinopathy. *Acta Neuropathol*, **118**(5), 633–645.
18. Neumann M, Mackenzie IR, Cairns NJ, *et al.* (2007). TDP-43 in the ubiquitin pathology of frontotemporal dementia with VCP gene mutations. *J Neuropathol Exp Neurol*, **66**(2), 152–157.
19. Morita M, Al Chalabi A, Andersen PM, *et al.* (2006). A locus on chromosome 9p confers susceptibility to ALS and frontotemporal dementia. *Neurology*, **66**(6), 839–844.
20. Vance C, Al Chalabi A, Ruddy D, *et al.* (2006). Familial amyotrophic lateral sclerosis with frontotemporal dementia is linked to a locus on chromosome 9p13.2–21.3. *Brain*, **129**(Pt 4), 868–876.

21. Holzer M, Craxton M, Jakes R, Arendt T, Goedert M. (2004). Tau gene (MAPT) sequence variation among primates. *Gene*, **341**, 313–322.
22. Neumann M, Roeber S, Kretzschmar HA, Rademakers R, Baker M, Mackenzie IR. (2009). Abundant FUS-immunoreactive pathology in neuronal intermediate filament inclusion disease. *Acta Neuropathol*, **118**(5), 605–616.
23. Munoz DG, Neumann M, Kusaka H, *et al.* (2009). FUS pathology in basophilic inclusion body disease. *Acta Neuropathol*, **118**(5), 629–631.
24. Neumann M, Rademakers R, Roeber S, Baker M, Kretzschmar HA, Mackenzie IR. (2009). A new subtype of frontotemporal lobar degeneration with FUS pathology. *Brain*, **132**(Pt 11), 2922–2931.
25. Holm IE, Isaacs AM, Mackenzie IR. (2009). Absence of FUS-immunoreactive pathology in frontotemporal dementia linked to chromosome 3 (FTD-3) caused by mutation in the CHMP2B gene. *Acta Neuropathol*, **118**, 719–720.
26. Neary D, Snowden JS, Gustafson L, *et al.* (1998). Frontotemporal lobar degeneration: a consensus on clinical diagnostic criteria. *Neurology*, **51**(6), 1546–1554.
27. Trojanowski JQ, Dickson D. (2001). Update on the neuropathological diagnosis of frontotemporal dementias. *J Neuropathol Exp Neurol*, **60**(12), 1123–1126.
28. Brun A, Passant U. (1996). Frontal lobe degeneration of non-Alzheimer type. Structural characteristics, diagnostic criteria and relation to other frontotemporal dementias. *Acta Neurol Scand Suppl*, **168**, 28–30.
29. Arai T, Hasegawa M, Akiyama H, *et al.* (2006). TDP-43 is a component of ubiquitin-positive tau-negative inclusions in frontotemporal lobar degeneration and amyotrophic lateral sclerosis. *Biochem Biophys Res Commun*, **351**(3), 602–611.
30. Neumann M, Sampathu DM, Kwong LK, *et al.* (2006). Ubiquitinated TDP-43 in frontotemporal lobar degeneration and amyotrophic lateral sclerosis. *Science*, **314**(5796), 130–133.
31. Gitcho MA, Baloh RH, Chakraverty S, *et al.* (2008). TDP-43 A315T mutation in familial motor neuron disease. *Ann Neurol*, **63**(4), 535–538.
32. Kabashi E, Valdmanis PN, Dion P, *et al.* (2008). TARDBP mutations in individuals with sporadic and familial amyotrophic lateral sclerosis. *Nat Genet*, **40**(5), 572–574.
33. Mackenzie IR, Bigio EH, Ince PG, *et al.* (2007). Pathological TDP-43 distinguishes sporadic amyotrophic lateral sclerosis from amyotrophic lateral sclerosis with SOD1 mutations. *Ann Neurol*, **61**(5), 427–434.
34. Ayala YM, Zago P, D'Ambrogio A, *et al.* (2008). Structural determinants of the cellular localization and shuttling of TDP-43. *J Cell Sci*, **121**(Pt 22), 3778–3785.
35. Buratti E, Baralle FE. (2008). Multiple roles of TDP-43 in gene expression, splicing regulation, and human disease. *Front Biosci*, **13**, 867–878.
36. Hasegawa M, Arai T, Nonaka T, *et al.* (2008). Phosphorylated TDP-43 in frontotemporal lobar degeneration and amyotrophic lateral sclerosis. *Ann Neurol*, **64**, 60–70.
37. Sampathu DM, Neumann M, Kwong LK, *et al.* (2006). Pathological heterogeneity of frontotemporal lobar degeneration with ubiquitin-positive inclusions delineated by ubiquitin immunohistochemistry and novel monoclonal antibodies. *Am J Pathol*, **169**(4), 1343–1352.
38. Neumann M, Kwong LK, Truax AC, *et al.* (2007). TDP-43-positive white matter pathology in frontotemporal lobar degeneration with ubiquitin-positive inclusions. *J Neuropathol Exp Neurol*, **66**(3), 177–183.
39. Mackenzie IR, Baker M, Pickering-Brown S, *et al.* (2006). The neuropathology of frontotemporal lobar degeneration caused by mutations in the progranulin gene. *Brain*, **129**(Pt 11), 3081–3090.
40. Josephs KA, Ahmed Z, Katsuse O, *et al.* (2007). Neuropathologic features of frontotemporal lobar degeneration with ubiquitin-positive inclusions with progranulin gene (PGRN) mutations. *J Neuropathol Exp Neurol*, **66**(2), 142–151.

41. Seelaar H, Schelhaas HJ, Azmani A, *et al.* (2007). TDP-43 pathology in familial frontotemporal dementia and motor neuron disease without progranulin mutations. *Brain*, **130**(Pt 5), 1375–1385.
42. Armstrong RA, Ellis W, Hamilton RL, *et al.* (2010). Neuropathological heterogeneity in frontotemporal lobar degeneration with TDP-43 proteinopathy: a quantitative study of 94 cases using principal components analysis. *J Neural Transm*, **117**(2), 227–239.
43. Caselli RJ, Windebank AJ, Petersen RC, *et al.* (1993). Rapidly progressive aphasic dementia and motor neuron disease. *Ann Neurol*, **33**(2), 200–207.
44. Pollanen MS, Bergeron C, Weyer L. (1993). Absence of protease-resistant prion protein in dementia characterized by neuronal loss and status spongiosus. *Acta Neuropathol*, **86**(5), 515–517.
45. Mitsuyama Y, Takamiya S. (1979). Presenile dementia with motor neuron disease in Japan. A new entity? *Arch Neurol*, **36**(9), 592–593.
46. Neary D, Snowden JS, Mann DM, Northen B, Goulding PJ, Macdermott N. (1990). Frontal lobe dementia and motor neuron disease. *J Neurol Neurosurg Psychiatry*, **53**, 23–32.
47. Jackson M, Lennox G, Lowe J. (1996). Motor neurone disease-inclusion dementia. *Neurodegeneration*, **5**(4), 339–350.
48. Mann DM. (1998). Dementia of frontal type and dementias with subcortical gliosis. *Brain Pathol*, **8**(2), 325–338.
49. Hosler BA, Siddique T, Sapp PC, *et al.* (2000). Linkage of familial amyotrophic lateral sclerosis with frontotemporal dementia to chromosome 9q21–q22. *JAMA*, **284**(13), 1664–1669.
50. Savioz A, Kovari E, Anastasiu R, *et al.* (2000). Search for a mutation in the tau gene in a Swiss family with frontotemporal dementia. *Exp Neurol*, **161**, 330–335.
51. Savioz A, Riederer BM, Heutink P, *et al.* (2003). Tau and neurofilaments in a family with frontotemporal dementia unlinked to chromosome 17q21–22. *Neurobiol Dis*, **12**, 46–55.
52. Anderson VE, Cairns NJ, Leigh PN. (1995). Involvement of the amygdala, dentate and hippocampus in motor neuron disease. *J Neurol Sci*, **129** Suppl, 75–78.
53. Mackenzie IR, Feldman H. (2003). Neuronal intranuclear inclusions distinguish familial FTD-MND type from sporadic cases. *Acta Neuropathol*, **105**(6), 543–548.
54. Cairns NJ, Brännström T, Khan MN, Rossor MN, Lantos PL. (2003). Neuronal loss in familial frontotemporal dementia with ubiquitin-positive, tau-negative inclusions. *Exp Neurol*, **181**(2), 319–326.
55. Rossor MN, Revesz T, Lantos PL, Warrington EK. (2000). Semantic dementia with ubiquitin-positive tau-negative inclusion bodies. *Brain*, **123** (Pt 2), 267–276.
56. He Z, Bateman A. (2003). Progranulin (granulin-epithelin precursor, PC-cell-derived growth factor, acrogranin) mediates tissue repair and tumorigenesis. *J Mol Med*, **81**(10), 600–612.
57. Daniel R, He Z, Carmichael KP, Halper J, Bateman A. (2000). Cellular localization of gene expression for progranulin. *J Histochem Cytochem*, **48**(7), 999–1009.
58. He Z, Bateman A. (1999). Progranulin gene expression regulates epithelial cell growth and promotes tumor growth *in vivo*. *Cancer Res*, **59**(13), 3222–3229.
59. Van Damme P, Van Hoecke A, Lambrechts D, *et al.* (2008). Progranulin functions as a neurotrophic factor to regulate neurite outgrowth and enhance neuronal survival. *J Cell Biol*, **181**, 37–41.
60. Benussi L, Binetti G, Sina E, *et al.* (2008). A novel deletion in progranulin gene is associated with FTDP-17 and CBS. *Neurobiol Aging*, **29**(3), 427–435.
61. Brouwers N, Nuytemans K, van der ZJ, *et al.* (2007). Alzheimer and Parkinson diagnoses in progranulin null mutation carriers in an extended founder family. *Arch Neurol*, **64**(10), 1436–1446.
62. Le Ber I, Camuzat A, Hannequin D, *et al.* (2008). Phenotype variability in progranulin mutation carriers: a clinical, neuropsychological, imaging and genetic study. *Brain*, **131**(Pt 3), 732–46.

63. Wider C, Wszolek ZK. (2007). Clinical genetics of Parkinson's disease and related disorders. *Parkinsonism Relat Disorder*, **13** Suppl 3, S229–232.
64. Kovach MJ, Waggoner B, Leal SM, *et al.* (2001). Clinical delineation and localization to chromosome 9p13.3–p12 of a unique dominant disorder in four families: hereditary inclusion body myopathy, Paget disease of bone, and frontotemporal dementia. *Mol Genet Metab*, **74**(4), 458–475.
65. Watts GD, Wymer J, Kovach MJ, *et al.* (2004). Inclusion body myopathy associated with Paget disease of bone and frontotemporal dementia is caused by mutant valosin-containing protein. *Nat Genet*, **36**(4), 377–381.
66. Dai RM, Li CC. (2001). Valosin-containing protein is a multi-ubiquitin chain-targeting factor required in ubiquitin-proteasome degradation. *Nat Cell Biol*, **3**(8), 740–744.
67. Forman MS, Mackenzie IR, Cairns NJ, *et al.* (2006). Novel ubiquitin neuropathology in frontotemporal dementia with valosin-containing protein gene mutations. *J Neuropathol Exp Neurol*, **65**(6), 571–581.
68. Weihl CC, Temiz P, Miller SE, *et al.* (2008). TDP-43 accumulation in inclusion body myopathy muscle suggests a common pathogenic mechanism with frontotemporal dementia. *J Neurol Neurosurg Psychiatry*, **79**(10), 1186–1189.
69. Ayala YM, Pantano S, D'Ambrogio A, *et al.* (2005). Human, Drosophila, and C.elegans TDP43: nucleic acid binding properties and splicing regulatory function. *J Mol Biol*, **348**(3), 575–588.
70. Li Y, Ray P, Rao EJ, *et al.* (2010). A Drosophila model for TDP-43 proteinopathy. *Proc Natl Acad Sci USA*, **107**(7), 3169–3174.
71. Kabashi E, Lin L, Tradewell ML, *et al.* (2010). Gain and loss of function of ALS-related mutations of TARDBP (TDP-43) cause motor deficits *in vivo*. *Hum Mol Genet*, **19**(4), 671–683.
72. Wegorzewska I, Bell S, Cairns NJ, Miller TM, Baloh RH. (2009). TDP-43 mutant transgenic mice develop features of ALS and frontotemporal lobar degeneration. *Proc Natl Acad Sci USA*, **106**(44), 18809–18814.
73. Braun RJ, Buttner S, Ring J, Kroemer G, Madeo F. (2010). Nervous yeast: modeling neurotoxic cell death. *Trends Biochem Sci*, **35**(3), 135–144.
74. Johnson BS, McCaffery JM, Lindquist S, Gitler AD. (2008). A yeast TDP-43 proteinopathy model: exploring the molecular determinants of TDP-43 aggregation and cellular toxicity. *Proc Natl Acad Sci USA*, **105**(17), 6439–6444.
75. Zhou H, Huang C, Chen H, *et al.* (2010). Transgenic rat model of neurodegeneration caused by mutation in the TDP gene. *PLoS Genet*, 6(3): e1000887.
76. Pick A (1892). Über die Beziehungen der senilen Hirnatrophie zur Aphasie. *Prag Med Wochenschr*, **17**, 165–167.
77. Alzheimer A. (1911) Über eigenartige Krankheitsfälle des späteren Alters. *Z Gesamte Neurol Psychiatr*, **4**, 356–385.
78. Boller F, Lopez OL, Moossy J. (1989). Diagnosis of dementia: clinicopathologic correlations. *Neurology*, **39**, 76–79.
79. Dermaut B, Kumar-Singh S, Engelborghs S, *et al.* (2004). A novel presenilin 1 mutation associated with Pick's disease but not beta-amyloid plaques. *Ann Neurol*, **55**(5), 617–926.
80. Baker M, Litvan I, Houlden H, *et al.* (1999). Association of an extended haplotype in the tau gene with progressive supranuclear palsy. *Hum Mol Genet*, **8**(4), 711–715.
81. Morris HR, Baker M, Yasojima K, *et al.* (2002). Analysis of tau haplotypes in Pick's disease. *Neurology*, **59**(3), 443–445.
82. Armstrong RA, Cairns NJ, Lantos PL. (1998). Clustering of Pick bodies in patients with Pick's disease. *Neurosci Lett*, **242**(2), 81–84.
83. Delacourte A, Robitaille Y, Sergeant N, *et al.* (1996). Specific pathological Tau protein variants characterize Pick's disease. *J Neuropathol Exp Neurol*, **55**(2), 159–168.

84. Delacourte A. (1999). Biochemical and molecular characterization of neurofibrillary degeneration in frontotemporal dementias. *Dement Geriatr Cogn Disord*, **10** (Suppl 1), 75–79.
85. Bell K, Cairns NJ, Lantos PL, Rossor MN. (2000). Immunohistochemistry distinguishes: between Pick's disease and corticobasal degeneration. *J Neurol Neurosurg Psychiatry*, **69**(6), 835–836.
86. Rebeiz JJ, Kolodny EH, Richardson EP, Jr. (1967). Corticodentatonigral degeneration with neuronal achromasia: a progressive disorder of late adult life. *Trans Am Neurol Assoc*, **92**, 23–26.
87. Gibb WR, Luthert PJ, Marsden CD. (1989). Corticobasal degeneration. *Brain*, **112** (Pt 5), 1171–1192.
88. Lowe J, Errington DR, Lennox G, *et al.* (1992). Ballooned neurons in several neurodegenerative diseases and stroke contain alpha B crystallin. *Neuropathol Appl Neurobiol*, **18**(4), 341–350.
89. Wakabayashi K, Oyanagi K, Makifuchi T, *et al.* (1994). Corticobasal degeneration: etiopathological significance of the cytoskeletal alterations. *Acta Neuropathol*, **87**(6), 545–553.
90. Spillantini MG, Crowther RA, Jakes R, Cairns NJ, Lantos PL, Goedert M. (1998). Filamentous alpha-synuclein inclusions link multiple system atrophy with Parkinson's disease and dementia with Lewy bodies. *Neurosci Lett*, **251**(3), 205–208.
91. Steele JC, Richardson JC, Olszewski J. (1964). Progressive supranuclear palsy. A heterogeneous degneration involving the brain stem, basal ganglia and cerebellum with vertical gaze and pseudobulbar palsy, nuchal dystonia and dementia. *Arch Neurol*, **10**, 333–359.
92. Golbe LI, Davis PH, Schoenberg BS, Duvoisin RC. (1988). Prevalence and natural history of progressive supranuclear palsy. *Neurology*, **38**(7), 1031–1034.
93. Bergeron C, Davis A, Lang AE. (1998). Corticobasal ganglionic degeneration and progressive supranuclear palsy presenting with cognitive decline. *Brain Pathol*, **8**(2), 355–365.
94. Tellez-Nagel I, Wisniewski HM. (1973). Ultrastructure of neurofibrillary tangles in Steele-Richardson-Olszewski syndrome. *Arch Neurol*, **29**(5), 324–327.
95. Montpetit V, Clapin DF, Guberman A. (1985). Substructure of 20 nm filaments of progressive supranuclear palsy. *Acta Neuropathol*, **68**(4), 311–318.
96. Hauw JJ, Daniel SE, Dickson D, *et al.* (1994). Preliminary NINDS neuropathologic criteria for Steele-Richardson-Olszewski syndrome (progressive supranuclear palsy). *Neurology*, **44**(11), 2015–2019.
97. Braak H, Braak E. (1987). Argyrophilic grains: characteristic pathology of cerebral cortex in cases of adult onset dementia without Alzheimer changes. *Neurosci Lett*, **76**, 124–127.
98. Braak H, Braak E. (1989). Cortical and subcortical argyrophilic grains characterize a disease associated with adult onset dementia. *Neuropathol Appl Neurobiol*, **15**, 13–26.
99. Braak H, Braak E. (1998). Argyrophilic grain disease: frequency of occurrence in different age categories and neuropathological diagnostic criteria. *J Neural Transm*, **105**(8–9), 801–819.
100. Ikeda K, Akiyama H, Arai T, Matsushita M, Tsuchiya K, Miyazaki H. (2000). Clinical aspects of argyrophilic grain disease. *Clin Neuropathol*, **19**(6), 278–284.
101. Tolnay M, Clavaguera F. (2004). Argyrophilic grain disease: a late-onset dementia with distinctive features among tauopathies. *Neuropathology*, **24**(4), 269–283.
102. Togo T, Sahara N, Yen SH, *et al.* (2002). Argyrophilic grain disease is a sporadic 4-repeat tauopathy. *J Neuropathol Exp Neurol*, **61**(6), 547–556.
103. Saito Y, Ruberu NN, Sawabe M, *et al.* (2004). Staging of argyrophilic grains: an age-associated tauopathy. *J Neuropathol Exp Neurol*, **63**(9), 911–918.
104. Bigio EH, Lipton AM, Yen SH, *et al.* (2001). Frontal lobe dementia with novel tauopathy: sporadic multiple system tauopathy with dementia. *J Neuropathol Exp Neurol*, **60**(4), 328–341.
105. Kovacs GG, Majtenyi K, Spina S, *et al.* (2008). White matter tauopathy with globular glial inclusions: a distinct sporadic frontotemporal lobar degeneration. *J Neuropathol Exp Neurol*, **67**(10), 963–975.

106. Bancher C, Jellinger KA. (1994). Neurofibrillary tangle form of senile dementia of Alzheimer type: a rare subtype in very old subjects. *Acta Neuropathol*, **88**, 565–570.

107. Jellinger KA, Bancher C. (1998). Senile dementia with tangles (tangle predominant form of senile dementia. *Brain Pathol*, **8**(2), 367–376.

108. Noda K, Sasaki K, Fujimi K, *et al.* (2006). Quantitative analysis of neurofibrillary pathology in a general population to reappraise neuropathological criteria for senile dementia of the neurofibrillary tangle type (tangle-only dementia): the Hisayama study. *Neuropathology*, **26**, 508–518.

109. Spillantini MG, van Swieten JC, Goedert M. (2000). Tau gene mutations in frontotemporal dementia and parkinsonism linked to chromosome 17 (FTDP-17). *Neurogenetics*, **2**(4), 193–205.

110. Spillantini MG, Goedert M. (2001). Tau gene mutations and tau pathology in frontotemporal dementia and parkinsonism linked to chromosome 17. *Adv Exp Med Biol*, **487**, 21–37.

111. Hutton M, Lendon CL, Rizzu P, *et al.* (1998). Association of missense and 5′-splice-site mutations in tau with the inherited dementia FTDP-17. *Nature*, **393**(6686), 702–705.

112. D'Souza I, Poorkaj P, Hong M, *et al.* (1999). Missense and silent tau gene mutations cause frontotemporal dementia with parkinsonism-chromosome 17 type, by affecting multiple alternative RNA splicing regulatory elements. *Proc Natl Acad Sci USA*, **96**(10), 5598–5603.

113. Grover A, Houlden H, Baker M, *et al.* (1999). 5′ splice site mutations in tau associated with the inherited dementia FTDP-17 affect a stem-loop structure that regulates alternative splicing of exon 10. *J Biol Chem*, **274**(21), 15134–15143.

114. D'Souza I, Schellenberg GD. (2000). Determinants of 4-repeat tau expression. Coordination between enhancing and inhibitory splicing sequences for exon 10 inclusion. *J Biol Chem*, **275**(23), 17700–17709.

115. Spillantini MG, Murrell JR, Goedert M, Farlow MR, Klug A, Ghetti B. (1998). Mutation in the tau gene in familial multiple system tauopathy with presenile dementia. *Proc Natl Acad Sci USA*, **95**(13), 7737–7741.

116. Hong M, Zhukareva V, Vogelsberg-Ragaglia V, *et al.* (1998). Mutation-specific functional impairments in distinct tau isoforms of hereditary FTDP-17. *Science*, **282**(5395), 1914–1917.

117. Goedert M, Spillantini MG, Crowther RA, *et al.* (1999). Tau gene mutation in familial progressive subcortical gliosis. *Nat Med*, **5**(4), 454–457.

118. Goode BL, Feinstein SC. (1994). Identification of a novel microtubule binding and assembly domain in the developmentally regulated inter-repeat region of tau. *J Cell Biol*, **124**(5), 769–782.

119. Goode BL, Denis PE, Panda D, *et al.* (1997). Functional interactions between the proline-rich and repeat regions of tau enhance microtubule binding and assembly. *Mol Biol Cell*, **8**(2), 353–365.

120. Stanford PM, Shepherd CE, Halliday GM, *et al.* (2003). Mutations in the tau gene that cause an increase in three repeat tau and frontotemporal dementia. *Brain*, **126** (Pt 4), 814–826.

121. Rizzini C, Goedert M, Hodges JR, *et al.* (2000). Tau gene mutation K257T causes a tauopathy similar to Pick's disease. *J Neuropathol Exp Neurol*, **59**(11), 990–1001.

122. Rizzu P, van Swieten JC, Joosse M, *et al.* (1999). High prevalence of mutations in the microtubule-associated protein tau in a population study of frontotemporal dementia in the Netherlands. *Am J Hum Genet*, **64**(2), 414–421.

123. Hasegawa M, Smith MJ, Goedert M. (1998). Tau proteins with FTDP-17 mutations have a reduced ability to promote microtubule assembly. *FEBS Lett*, **437**(3), 207–210.

124. Rizzu P, Joosse M, Ravid R, *et al.* (2000). Mutation-dependent aggregation of tau protein and its selective depletion from the soluble fraction in brain of P301L FTDP-17 patients. *Hum Mol Genet*, **9**(20), 3075–3082.

125. Miyasaka T, Morishima-Kawashima M, Ravid R, Kamphorst W, Nagashima K, Ihara Y. (2001). Selective deposition of mutant tau in the FTDP-17 brain affected by the P301L mutation. *J Neuropathol Exp Neurol*, **60**(9), 872–884.
126. Goedert M, Jakes R, Crowther RA. (1999). Effects of frontotemporal dementia FTDP-17 mutations on heparin-induced assembly of tau filaments. *FEBS Lett*, **450**(3), 306–311.
127. Gamblin TC, King ME, Dawson H, *et al.* (2000). In vitro polymerization of tau protein monitored by laser light scattering: method and application to the study of FTDP-17 mutants. *Biochemistry*, **39**(20), 6136–6144.
128. Goedert M, Satumtira S, Jakes R, *et al.* (2000). Reduced binding of protein phosphatase 2A to tau protein with frontotemporal dementia and parkinsonism linked to chromosome 17 mutations. *J Neurochem*, **75**(5), 2155–2162.
129. Lantos PL, Cairns NJ, Khan MN, *et al.* (2002). Neuropathologic variation in frontotemporal dementia due to the intronic tau 10(+16) mutation. *Neurology*, **58**(8), 1169–1175.
130. Götz J, Chen F, Barmettler R, Nitsch RM. (2001). Tau filament formation in transgenic mice expressing P301L tau. *J Biol Chem*, **276**, 529–34.
131. Götz J. (2001). Tau and transgenic animal models. *Brain Res Rev*, **35**(3), 266–286.
132. Ishihara T, Hong M, Zhang B, *et al.* (1999). Age-dependent emergence and progression of a tauopathy in transgenic mice overexpressing the shortest human tau isoform. *Neuron*, **24**(3), 751–762.
133. Wittmann CW, Wszolek MF, Shulman JM, *et al.* (2001). Tauopathy in Drosophila: neurodegeneration without neurofibrillary tangles. *Science*, **293**(5530), 711–714.
134. Jackson GR, Wiedau-Pazos M, Sang TK, *et al.* (2002). Human wild-type tau interacts with wingless pathway components and produces neurofibrillary pathology in Drosophila. *Neuron*, **34**(4), 509–519.
135. Kwiatkowski TJ, Jr, Bosco DA, Leclerc AL, *et al.* (2009). Mutations in the FUS/TLS gene on chromosome 16 cause familial amyotrophic lateral sclerosis. *Science*, **323**(5918), 1205–1208.
136. Vance C, Rogelj B, Hortobagyi T, *et al.* (2009). Mutations in FUS, an RNA processing protein, cause familial amyotrophic lateral sclerosis type 6. *Science*, **323**(5918), 1208–1211.
137. Lagier-Tourenne C, Cleveland DW. (2009). Rethinking ALS: the FUS about TDP-43. *Cell*, **136**(6), 1001–1004.
138. Bigio EH, Lipton AM, White CL, III, Dickson DW, Hirano A. (2003). Frontotemporal and motor neurone degeneration with neurofilament inclusion bodies: additional evidence for overlap between FTD and ALS. *Neuropathol Appl Neurobiol*, **29**(3), 239–253.
139. Josephs KA, Holton JL, Rossor MN, *et al.* (2003). Neurofilament inclusion body disease: a new proteinopathy? *Brain*, **126** (Pt 10), 2291–3303.
140. Cairns NJ, Grossman M, Arnold SE, *et al.* (2004). Clinical and neuropathologic variation in neuronal intermediate filament inclusion disease. *Neurology*, **63**(8), 1376–1384.
141. Josephs KA, Tsuboi Y, Cookson N, Watt H, Dickson DW. (2004). Apolipoprotein E epsilon 4 is a determinant for Alzheimer-type pathologic features in tauopathies, synucleinopathies, and frontotemporal degeneration. *Arch Neurol*, **61**(10), 1579–1584.
142. Mosaheb S, Thorpe JR, Hashemzadeh-Bonehi L, Bigio EH, Gearing M, Cairns NJ. (2005). Neuronal intranuclear inclusions are ultrastructurally and immunologically distinct from cytoplasmic inclusions of neuronal intermediate filament inclusion disease. *Acta Neuropathol*, **110**, 360–368.
143. Nelson JS, Prensky AL. (1972). Sporadic juvenile amyotrophic lateral sclerosis. A clinicopathological study of a case with neuronal cytoplasmic inclusions containing RNA. *Arch Neurol*, **27**(4), 300–306.
144. Matsumoto S, Kusaka H, Murakami N, Hashizume Y, Okazaki H, Hirano A. (1992). Basophilic inclusions in sporadic juvenile amyotrophic lateral sclerosis: an immunocytochemical and ultrastructural study. *Acta Neuropathol*, **83**(6), 579–583.

145. Kusaka H, Matsumoto S, Imai T. (1990). An adult-onset case of sporadic motor neuron disease with basophilic inclusions. *Acta Neuropathol*, **80**(6), 660–665.
146. Kusaka H, Matsumoto S, Imai T. (1993). Adult-onset motor neuron disease with basophilic intraneuronal inclusion bodies. *Clin Neuropathol*, **12**(4), 215–218.
147. Munoz-Garcia D, Ludwin SK. (1984). Classic and generalized variants of Pick's disease: a clinicopathological, ultrastructural, and immunocytochemical comparative study. *Ann Neurol*, **16**(4), 467–480.
148. Hamada K, Fukazawa T, Yanagihara T, *et al.* (1995). Dementia with ALS features and diffuse Pick body-like inclusions (atypical Pick's disease?). *Clin Neuropathol*, **14**, 1–6.
149. Ito H, Kusaka H, Matsumoto S, Imai T. (1995). Topographic involvement of the striatal efferents in basal ganglia of patients with adult-onset motor neuron disease with basophilic inclusions. *Acta Neuropathol*, **89**(6), 513–518.
150. Armstrong RA, Cairns NJ, Lantos PL. (1999). Laminar distribution of Pick bodies, Pick cells and Alzheimer disease pathology in the frontal and temporal cortex in Pick's disease. *Neuropathol Appl Neurobiol*, **25**(4), 266–271.
151. Mackenzie IR, Foti D, Woulfe J, Hurwitz TA. (2008). Atypical frontotemporal lobar degeneration with ubiquitin-positive, TDP-43-negative neuronal inclusions. *Brain*, **131** (Pt 5), 1282–1293.
152. Neumann M, Rademakers R, Roeber S, Baker M, Kretzschmar HA, Mackenzie IR. (2009). Frontotemporal lobar degeneration with FUS pathology. *Brain*, **132** (Pt 11), 2922–2931.
153. Skibinski G, Parkinson NJ, Brown JM, *et al.* (2005). Mutations in the endosomal ESCRTIII-complex subunit CHMP2B in frontotemporal dementia. *Nat Genet*, **37**(8), 806–808.
154. Constantinidis J, Richard J, Tissot R. (1974). Pick's disease. Histological and clinical correlations. *Eur Neurol*, **11**(4), 208–217.
155. Brun A. (1987). Frontal lobe degeneration of non-Alzheimer type. I. Neuropathology. *Arch Gerontol Geriatr*, **6**(3), 193–208.
156. Mackenzie IR, Shi J, Shaw CL, *et al.* (2006). Dementia lacking distinctive histology (DLDH) revisited. *Acta Neuropathol*, **112**(5), 551–559.
157. Cairns NJ. (2006). Neuropathology of frontotemporal lobar degenerations. In: Strong MJ (ed.), *Dementia and Motor Neuron Disease*, pp. 147–166. Informa UK Ltd, London.
158. Thorpe JR, Tang H, Atherton J, Cairns NJ. (2008). Fine structural analysis of the neuronal inclusionsof frontotemporal lobar degeneration with TDP-43 proteinopathy. *J Neural Transm*, **115**, 1661–1671.
159. Kraemer BC, Zhang B, Leverenz JB, *et al.* (2003). Neurodegeneration and defective neurotransmission in Caenorhabditis elegans model of tauopathy. *PNAS USA*, **100**, 9980–9985.
160. Cairns NJ, Lee VM, Trojanowski JQ. (2004). The cytoskeleton in neurodegenerative diseases. *J Pathol*, **204**(4), 438–449.
161. Renton AE, Majounie E, Waite A, *et al.* (2011). A hexanucleotide repeat in C9ORF72 is the cause of chromosome 9p21-linked ALS-FTD. *Neuron*, **72**(2), 257–268.
162. De Jesus-Hernandez M, Mackenzie IR, Boeve BF, *et al.* (2011). Expanded GGGCC hexanucleotide repeat in noncoding region of C9ORF72 causes chromosome 9p-linked FTD and ALS. *Neuron*, **72**(2), 245–256.
163. Stewart H, Rutherford NJ, Briemberg H, *et al.* (2012). Clinical and Pathological features of amyotrophic lateral sclerosis caused by mutation in the C9ORF72 gene on chromosome 9p. *Acta Neuropathol.*, **122**, 673–690.

Chapter 19

The neuropathology of the motor neurone diseases

J. Robin Highley and Paul G. Ince

This chapter describes the neuropathology of a core group of motor neurone diseases (MNDs), including amyotrophic lateral sclerosis (ALS), progressive muscular atrophy (PMA), and primary lateral sclerosis (PLS). Other motor neurone disorders are not discussed, and the reader is directed elsewhere (1).

Pathological and clinical investigation of MND have proceeded hand in hand ever since its first description by Charcot (2). The last two decades have seen an exponential growth in our neuropathological understanding of MND, shifting the emphasis from an exclusively motor system disease to a disease that affects multiple brain systems as part of a spectrum of disorders. The existence of this book attests to considerable pathological overlap between MND and frontotemporal lobar degeneration (FTLD), covered in Chapter 18 by Cairns.

Classical motor neurone disease pathology

Classical MND is characterized by degeneration of the pyramidal motor system at all levels. This is characterized by neuronal loss with concomitant gliosis. The neuropathological hallmark of MND is the ubiquitylated, transactive response DNA-binding protein of 43 kDa (TDP-43)-immunoreactive neuronal cytoplasmic inclusion (NCI), one of a number of inclusions that characterize the disease.

Inclusions

The neuropathological literature pertaining to MND contains reference to a bewildering array of inclusion bodies, including Bunina bodies, hyaline conglomerate inclusions, eosinophilic, basophilic, or amphophilic round inclusion bodies. Some eosinophilic inclusions have a halo earning themselves the appellation 'Lewy-like' or 'Lewy-like hyaline' inclusion (3,4). There has been little attempt to systematize terminology such that definitions can be variable from report to report. However, the arrival of immunohistochemistry has brought clarification. In the current understanding, the most important inclusion for the diagnosis of MND is the ubiquitylated, TDP-43-positive, neuronal cytoplasmic inclusion.

The authors believe the inclusion literature should be viewed in the light of immunohistochemistry so that studies can be divided into those that did and did not use this.

Thus, basophilic inclusions in one study appear to correspond to ubiquitylated cytoplasmic inclusions (5). The term 'Lewy-like' appears to correspond variously to compact, ubiquitylated, TDP-43-immunoreactive cytoplasmic inclusions (see below) (5), hyaline conglomerate inclusions (6) or in studies that pre-date ubiquitin immunohistochemistry (7). The term 'Lewy-like' confuses those unacquainted with the minutiae of neuropathological cytoplasmic inclusions and its use is discouraged, particularly given that these inclusions are α-synuclein negative in contrast to true Lewy bodies (8).

Ubiquitylated, transactive response DNA-binding protein of 43 kDa-immunoreactive neuronal cytoplasmic inclusions

The ubiquitylated neuronal cytoplasmic inclusion, first described in the late 1980s (9,10), are a near universal finding in MND (11). However, they may also be absent or nearly absent in severe, end-stage disease characterized by a near total loss motor neurones, in cases associated with mutations of *FUS* (see below) or atypical cases (12). Greater numbers of NCI relate to a more rapid decline from disease onset to death (13,14).

Polyubiquitylation is a process whereby a protein is targeted for proteasomal degradation, implying the protein is abnormal, denatured, or misfolded. It was not until 2006 that two groups independently demonstrated that the predominant protein in the ubiquitylated cytoplasmic inclusions of both FTLD and MND was TDP-43 (15,16). TDP-43 is a ubiquitously expressed nuclear protein that binds the transactive response (TAR) region of DNA of HIV-1 and regulates gene transcription and mRNA splicing as well as stabilizing neurofilament light mRNA (17) (see also Buratti, Chapter 24, and Volkening and Strong, Chapter 22).

NCI tend to take one of three forms using TDP-43, ubiquitin, and p62 immunohistochemistry (18,19): 'Skeins' are loosely aggregated thread-like structures (Figure 19.1c). Compact inclusions are more dense filamentous structures of a similar size, or larger than, the nucleus (Figure 19.1d). Dot-like inclusions are smaller, round, usually perinuclear and approximately 1–3 μm diameter (Figure 19.1e). Skeins and compact inclusions are largely seen in lower motor neurones with dot-like inclusions seen elsewhere. Intermediate forms are frequent. In general, skeins are more common. In addition, TDP-43 immunohistochemistry reveals neurones with more diffuse, sometimes granular labelling of the cytoplasm, a loss of nuclear TDP-43, but no well-defined solid inclusion (Figure 19.1b) (18). These have been referred to as pre-inclusions and are not ubiquitylated (15,19).

At the ultrastructural level, pre-inclusions appear as linear wisps of TDP-43-immunoreactive matter. Skeins, compact, and dot-like inclusions appear to be formed from loose, randomly arranged filaments with associated granular material. Skeins additionally contain filaments arranged into cord-like bundles (18).

In addition to ubiquitylation, the pathological TDP-43 of inclusions is phosphorylated and fragmented (15,16). Antibodies specific for phosphorylated TDP-43 label only pathological deposits, leaving the non-pathological nuclear TDP-43 unlabelled (20).

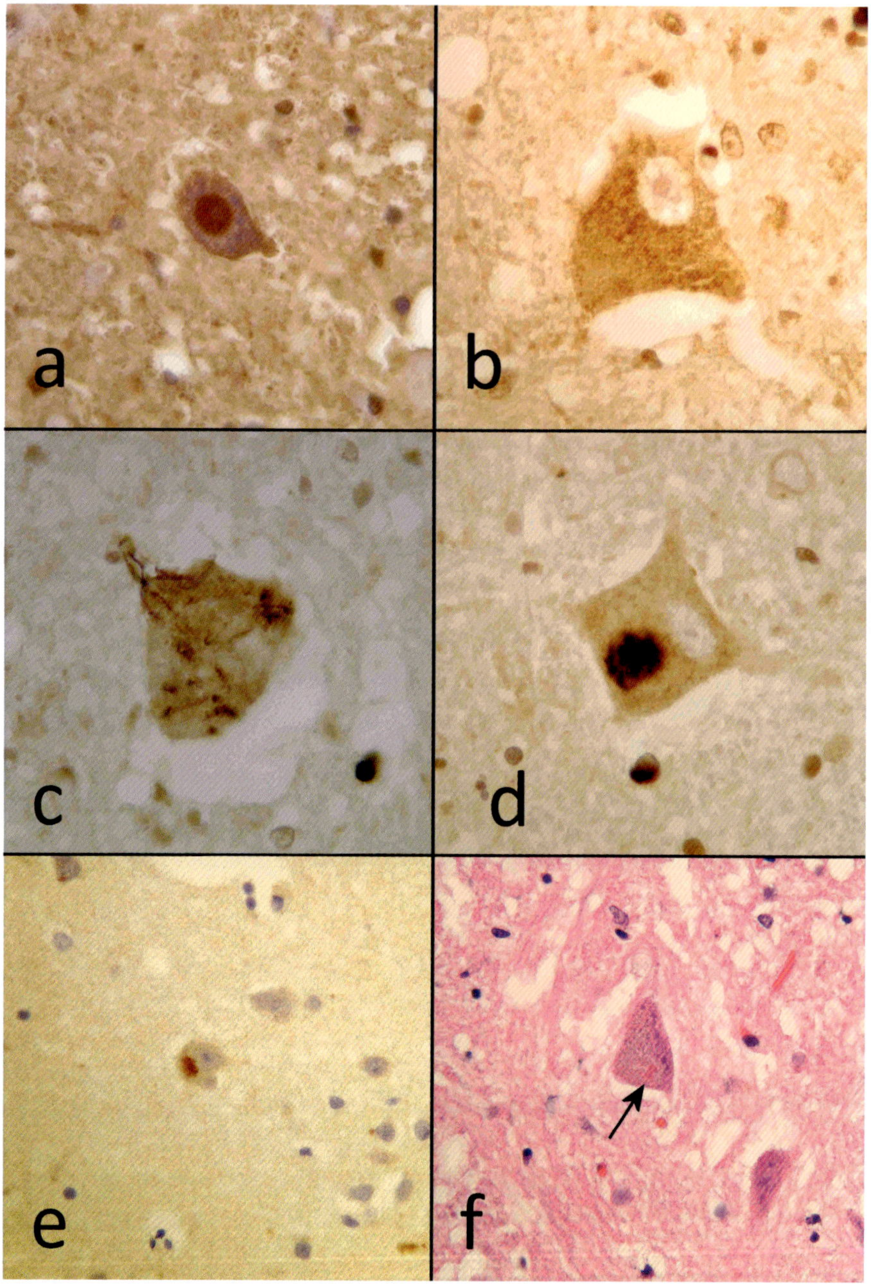

Fig. 19.1 (a) TDP-43 immunohistochemistry in a normal motor neurone showing strong nuclear labelling with only a small amount of cytoplasmic expression. The nucleolus is unstained. (b) A neurone with a so-called pre-inclusion with loss of nuclear TDP-43, diffuse cytoplasmic labelling, but no well-formed cytoplasmic inclusion. (c) A skein-like neuronal cytoplasmic inclusion is a loose aggregate of thread-like TDP-43-positive material. (d) A compact neuronal cytoplasmic inclusion is more dense than a skein. (e) A dot-like inclusion is a small perinuclear aggregate of TDP-43. (f) A Bunina body is a small, intracytoplasmic, intensely eosinophilic inclusion in an haematoxylin and eosin preparation.

Bunina bodies

Bunina bodies are 3–4 μm refractile eosinophilic, cytoplasmic inclusions (Figure 19.1f) seen in surviving lower motor neurones in approximately 86% of MND cases (11). They are specific to MND and tend to co-occur in the same neurones as TDP-43 NCI (21). They are immunopositive for cystatin C (22) and transferrin (23), but negative for p62 (5) and TDP-43 (24), with only a small proportion positive for ubiquitin (25). The relationship between Bunina bodies and TDP-43-immunoreactive inclusions is unresolved.

Hyaline conglomerate inclusions

Hyaline conglomerate inclusions are large, multifocal patches of material that occupy 50–70% of the cell body, displacing normal cellular constituents, including the nucleus (see Figure 19.2) (26). They are rare, but are particularly associated with mutations of *SOD1* (see below).

Hyaline conglomerate inclusions do not stain for antisera to TDP-43 (24) or ubiquitin (26), but are strongly argyrophilic. They label with antibodies to neurofilament, predominantly medium and heavy chain (27–29), both phosphorylated and unphosphorylated, suggesting a generalized defect in neurofilament distribution and biology in affected cells (26).

Axonal spheroids

Axonal spheroids are seen in the spinal cord anterior horns of both normal and diseased individuals (30). Like hyaline conglomerate inclusions they label with neurofilament on immunohistochemistry and their numbers may be increased in MND (31).

Lower motor neurone disease

MND is almost universally characterized by lower motor neurone pathology. Neuronal loss in the spinal cord ventral horn is in the region of 50% but varies by case and anatomical factors in individuals (32). Not all populations of lower motor neurones are equally affected; in the spinal cord, the ventral horns are affected and in brainstem, the facial nerve, motor trigeminal, ambiguus, and hypoglossal nuclei are predominantly affected. However, there is relative sparing of the oculomotor cranial nerve nuclei (33) and the nucleus of Onufrowicz that innervates the voluntary muscle of the pelvic floor and regulates urinary bladder and bowel function (34). The reason for sparing of these lower motor neurone groups is unresolved.

Upper motor neurone disease

The degree of upper motor neurone pathology and symptomatology shows considerable variability. It is manifest in the motor cortex by neuronal and glial cytoplasmic inclusions as well as gliosis, microvacuolation, and neuronal loss. To a variable degree and secondary to upper motor neurone disease, degeneration of the white matter pathways of the corticospinal tracts can be observed in the spinal cord.

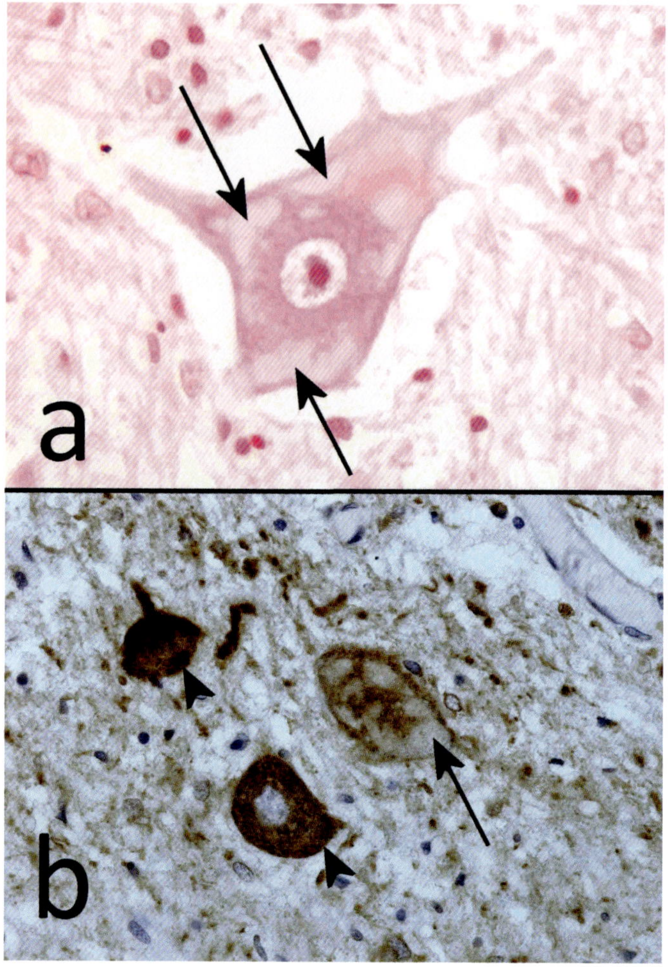

Fig. 19.2 (a) Haematoxylin and eosin staining of a lower motor neurone from a patient with ALS due to a mutation of SOD1 showing hyaline conglomerate inclusions (arrows) in the cytoplasm. These are large, glassy pale areas occupying a large proportion of the cytoplasm. (b) Two normal motor neurones (arrowheads) and a motor neurone bearing a hyaline conglomerate inclusion (arrow). Immunohistochemistry for SOD1 protein reveals staining of the cytoplasm of the normal motor neurones and the residual cytoplasm around the hyaline conglomerate inclusion, but not the inclusion itself.

Early studies of the primary motor cortex in MND suggest there may be a reduction in the number of neurones (35,36). However, stereological studies have revealed no difference in the total number (37) or size (38) of upper motor neurones. In many cases, upper motor neurone pathology is only reflected by distal axonal loss in the corticospinal tracts with normal motor cortex histology.

Descending tracts

In the descending corticospinal tracts, upper motor neurone pathology may be manifest by axonal loss with concomitant myelin loss and a glial reaction. This process is easily demonstrated as pale staining with tinctorial preparations for myelin. However, the most sensitive method is CD68 immunohistochemistry to demonstrate a microglial reaction (39).

Gliosis and glial pathology

Astrogliosis is said to be present in both upper and lower motor neurone-containing regions (40). Certainly, some cases of MND do show astrocytic hyperplasia and hypertrophy in deeper cortical layers as well as the grey–white matter junction. However, it is the authors' experience that this is a common feature of neurodegenerative disease and not a disease-specific feature (32).

Importantly, recent research has demonstrated that NCI in MND are accompanied by glial cytoplasmic inclusions readily demonstrated by both p62 and TDP-43 immunohistochemistry (16,41).

Immunohistochemistry in neuropathological investigation of motor neurone disease

Traditionally, immunohistochemical demonstration of NCI has been used to map the extent of MND pathology. Initially, this used antisera to ubiquitin, but these label a large amount of non-specific, extracellular features, including so-called 'ubiquitin dot profiles', which occur outside cell bodies in the neuropil and are not pathological (42).

Antibodies to p62 (also known as sequestosome 1) provided a better tool for characterizing MND neuropathology (43). p62 binds polyubiquitylated proteins and shuttles them to the proteasome (44). Antibodies to p62 label pathological, ubiquitylated protein aggregates, including TDP-43 (45) with greater specificity than ubiquitin antibodies, leaving non-pathological features largely unlabelled. Further, p62 antibodies label neuronal inclusions more intensely than ubiquitin and label more inclusions, more clearly than either TDP-43 or ubiquitin antibodies (5,45,46).

Both ubiquitin and p62 immunohistochemistry, however, label most ubiquitylated protein aggregates. In lower motor neurones, the NCI of MND are easily identified by their unique morphology and location. However, elsewhere in the nervous system, ubiquitin or p62 immunopositivity is not specific for TDP-43, and thus the MND/FTLD spectrum disorders. Thus confirmatory staining, in limited blocks, with a TDP-43 antibody is always recommended.

TDP-43 raised against non-phosphorylated protein stain cell nuclei with great intensity, making microscopy problematic, as slides have to be examined at high power to distinguish pathological inclusions from cell nuclei. The development of antisera to phosphorylated TDP-43 offers a more specific tool for immunohistochemical studies (20).

Extramotor pathology

It has long been known that the pathology of ALS is not always restricted to the motor system (35). Extramotor pathology is variable in its severity and extent within the nervous system, but is often considerable. In a survey of TDP-43 pathology in 31 brains from patients with MND, all of the 27 extramotor regions examined were involved in at least one case (47).

Sensory system pathology

A few studies have considered the issue of peripheral nervous system pathology in MND, with reports of sensory nerve degeneration (48) and cell loss in the dorsal root ganglia (49). In the brain, the thalamus shows gliosis (35) and TDP-43 pathology (47). However, most central nervous system studies have focused on the ascending white matter pathways.

Spinocerebellar tracts

The dorsal spinocerebellar tract arises from neurones in Clarke's column in the spinal cord. Early reports that suggested a significant reduction in neuronal number in Clarke's column (50) were not replicated, although there was evidence of Bunina body formation (51). Immunohistochemical studies of NCI have reported an inclusion in one of five cases in one study (52), no inclusions in a total of 28 cases in another (53). Case reports of familial MND have recorded NCI in Clarke's column in association with mutations of *SOD1* (27) and *FUS* (54).

The dorsal column–medial lemniscus pathway

The dorsal columns are located posteriorly between the two spinal cord dorsal horns. They relay proprioception with vibration and fine tactile sensation. There is a long literature describing dorsal column pathology in MND (35,55). Pallor of myelin staining in the dorsal columns can be seen in up to 50% of sporadic MND cases (39).

Substantia nigra and basal ganglia

The substantia nigra in MND may show neuronal loss and gliosis (35,56), as well as TDP-43-immunoreactive neuronal or glial cytoplasmic inclusions (57–59). Many studies have additionally detailed pallidoluysian pathology (57,58), striatal pathology (53), or both (11,35,47,58).

Many reports of nigral and basal ganglia pathology in MND stress an association with dementia (11,47,53,59), although only a handful of cases show parkinsonian clinical features (58–60). This may be due to the latter features being masked by more classical MND motor features.

In this context, it should be recalled that the ALS/parkinsonism–dementia complex of Guam is characterized by tau and α-synuclein pathology as well as TDP-43-positive, neuronal, and glial cytoplasmic inclusions of the type seen in classical MND (61). Sporadic reports of associated Parkinson's disease and MND are infrequent (62).

Hippocampal and neocortical pathology

Shortly after the first descriptions of ubiquitylated NCI in motor neurones in MND similar lesions were described in the hippocampus (63,64) and frontal and temporal neocortices of demented patients with MND (11,53,63,65–69). The majority of these reports suggest that the granule cell layer of the dentate gyrus is the most consistently affected region, followed by the entorhinal cortex. The association with dementia is not absolute.

The pathological relationship between motor neurone disease and frontotemporal lobar degeneration

While extramotor pathology is common in MND, studies of FTLD also reveal motor pathology identical to that seen in patients with MND (70,71). The pathological labels assigned to these cases has varied over the years, but the consensus is now to refer to them as FTLD with ubiquitylated or TDP-43 inclusions, with or without MND (72) (see Cairns, Chapter 18).

There is thus a pathological continuum with considerable overlap between syndromes ranging across 'pure' MND to FTLD/MND and 'pure' FTLD. Immunohistochemical studies with p62 and TDP-43 that pool MND and FTLD cases reveal a correlation between the pattern of motor versus extramotor pathological involvement and the clinical manifestation of MND or frontotemporal dementia. These studies show a considerable overlap with clinically 'pure' MND cases showing considerable extramotor pathology and clinically 'pure' dementia cases all showing some form of motor pathology (73,74). The hypothesis that MND and FTLD and cases with mixed pathology are all manifestations of the same disease process (75) is confirmed by this continuum of TDP-43 pathology. Mutations of *TARDBP*, the gene that encodes TDP-43 can cause either MND or FTLD or both (see Traynor, Chapter 20).

This pathological continuum raises the question of what factors dictate where disease in the nervous system is anatomically expressed. Underlying genetic and environmental factors remain to be determined. However, at a molecular level, there is evidence that the aberrant processing of TDP-43 may differ between the brain and spinal cord (76).

The neuropathology of familial motor neurone disease

A number of genes responsible for familial forms of MND have been described. Regrettably, autopsy data are available only for a small number of genes and specific mutations and many autopsy reports are limited in the data provided or the genetic characterization.

SOD1-related motor neurone disease

Mutations of *SOD1* are responsible for approximately 15–20% of cases of familial MND with about 130 mutations described. Some of these (26,77) are associated with NCI that are evident on ubiquitin in many forms of *SOD1*-related MND (24,80).

As noted above, hyaline conglomerate inclusions, composed of neurofilaments, characterize some, but not all, *SOD1* mutations (26,27,81). The reason why some mutations are associated with hyaline conglomerate inclusions while others are not is yet to be determined.

Normal human motor neurones show very strong *SOD1* immunoreactivity (see Figure 19.2b). Some light and electron microscopic studies appear to demonstrate that the hyaline conglomerate inclusions of *SOD1*-related MND label with SOD1 antibodies (3,82,83). However, in the authors' experience, hyaline conglomerate inclusions, although positive for phosphorylated neurofilament, are not positive for SOD1, although residual neuronal cytoplasm may label for this. The G127insTGGG *SOD1* mutation results in the formation of a truncated protein with a nonsense terminal sequence (84). Antibodies against the resultant epitope show marked cytoplasmic accumulation of the mutant enzyme that does not co-localize with either hyaline conglomerate or NCI.

TARDBP-related motor neurone disease

Some individuals with MND/FTLD spectrum disorders have associated mutations of *TARDBP*, the gene that encodes TDP-43. Eight cases have been published with neuropathological examination by four research groups (85–89). The clinical and pathological diagnoses of these cases range from FTLD with MND to pure MND with classical pathological features, but no distinguishing features peculiar to *TARDBP* mutations.

FUS/TLS-related motor neurone disease

The FUS/TLS protein (henceforth FUS) is expressed by most body tissues, being largely present in the nucleus, but with some cytoplasmic expression (90). In common with TDP-43, FUS binds nucleic acids and has a role in alternative splicing of mRNA (91). Mutations of *FUS* account for approximately 3–5% of cases of familial MND (92,93). The neuropathological features of a number of cases of MND due to *FUS* mutations have been described (54,92,94–98). FUS-positive NCI appear to be universally present, a feature not seen in controls or MND cases, which are not due to *FUS* mutations. In contrast, TDP-43-immunoreactive inclusions are absent (54,93,94,96) and ubiquitylated NCI are either absent or very few in many (93,95,96) but not all (54,94) cases.

Angiogenin

One case of MND due to a mutation of *angiogenin* (*ANG*), an angiogenic compound that additionally has a role in nucleic acid metabolism has been described at autopsy (99,100). There was a loss of α-actinin-2 in skeletal muscle. Eosinophilic neuronal intranuclear inclusions in the pyramidal neurones of the hippocampus and frontal cortex were immunoreactive for ubiquitin, p62, and α-smooth muscle actin but negative for *ANG* (99,100). In common with classical MND, there were neuronal and glial TDP-43-immunoreactive cytoplasmic inclusions in residual motor neurones.

CHMP2B

Mutations of the gene encoding charged multivesicular body protein 2B (*CHMP2B*), a protein that is believed to be involved in endosomal function, has been linked to both FTLD and MND. The neuropathology of four ALS cases due to mutations in *CHMP2B* has been described (101,102). These generally show lower motor neurone-predominant disease with widespread glial cytoplasmic inclusions on p62 and TDP-43 immunohistochemistry. Ubiquitylated, TDP-43-immunoreactive NCI are evident in residual lower motor neurones.

References

1. Ince PG, Wharton SB. (2007). Cytopathology of the motor neuron. In: Eisen AA, Shaw PJ (eds.), *Motor Neuron Disorders and Related Diseases*, pp. 89–119. Elsevier, Amsterdam.

2. Goetz CG. (2000). Amyotrophic lateral sclerosis: early contributions of Jean-Martin Charcot. *Muscle Nerve*, **23**, 336–343.
3. Sasaki S, Ohsawa Y, Yamane K, *et al.* (1998). Familial amyotrophic lateral sclerosis with widespread vacuolation and hyaline inclusions. *Neurology*, **51**, 871–873.
4. Murayama S, Ookawa Y, Mori H, *et al.* (1989). Immunocytochemical and ultrastructural study of Lewy body-like hyaline inclusions in familial amyotrophic lateral sclerosis. *Acta Neuropathol*, **78**, 143–152.
5. Mizuno Y, Amari M, Takatama M, *et al.* (2006). Immunoreactivities of p62, an ubiqutin-binding protein, in the spinal anterior horn cells of patients with amyotrophic lateral sclerosis. *J Neurol Sci*, **249**, 13–18.
6. Ohi T, Nabeshima K, Kato S, *et al.* (2004). Familial amyotrophic lateral sclerosis with His46Arg mutation in Cu/Zn superoxide dismutase presenting characteristic clinical features and Lewy body-like hyaline inclusions. *J Neurol Sci*, **225**, 19–25.
7. Kato T, Katagiri T, Hirano A, *et al.* (1988). Sporadic lower motor neuron disease with Lewy body-like inclusions: a new subgroup? *Acta Neuropathol*, **76**, 208–211.
8. Sasaki S, Komori T, Iwata M. (2006). Neuronal inclusions in sporadic motor neuron disease are negative for alpha-synuclein. *Neurosci Lett*, **397**, 15–19.
9. Leigh PN, Anderton BH, Dodson A, *et al.* (1988). Ubiquitin deposits in anterior horn cells of motor neuron disease. *Neurosci Lett*, **93**, 197–203.
10. Lowe J, Lennox G, Jefferson D, *et al.* (1988). A filamentous inclusion body within anterior horn neurones in motor neurone disease defined by immunocytochemical localisation of ubiquitin. *Neurosci Lett*, **94**, 203–210.
11. Piao YS, Wakabayashi K, Kakita A, *et al.* (2003). Neuropathology with clinical correlations of sporadic amyotrophic lateral sclerosis: 102 autopsy cases examined between 1962 and 2000. *Brain Pathol*, **13**, 10–22.
12. Borthwick GM, Taylor RW, Walls TJ, *et al.* (2006). Motor neuron disease in a patient with a mitochondrial tRNAIle mutation. *Ann Neurol*, **59**, 570–574.
13. Sumi H, Kato S, Mochimaru Y, *et al.* (2009). Nuclear TAR DNA binding protein 43 expression in spinal cord neurons correlates with the clinical course in amyotrophic lateral sclerosis. *J Neuropathol Exp Neurol*, **68**, 37–47.
14. Nishihira Y, Tan CF, Hoshi Y, *et al.* (2009). Sporadic amyotrophic lateral sclerosis of long duration is associated with relatively mild TDP-43 pathology. *Acta Neuropathol*, **117**, 45–53.
15. Neumann M, Sampathu DM, Kwong LK, *et al.* (2006). Ubiquitinated TDP-43 in frontotemporal lobar degeneration and amyotrophic lateral sclerosis. *Science*, **314**, 130–133.
16. Arai T, Hasegawa M, Akiyama H, *et al.* (2006). TDP-43 is a component of ubiquitin-positive tau-negative inclusions in frontotemporal lobar degeneration and amyotrophic lateral sclerosis. *Biochem Biophys Res Commun*, **351**, 602–611.
17. Buratti E and Baralle FE. (2008). Multiple roles of TDP-43 in gene expression, splicing regulation, and human disease. *Front Biosci*, **13**, 867–878.
18. Mori F, Tanji K, Zhang H-X, *et al.* (2008). Maturation process of TDP-43-positive neuronal cytoplasmic inclusions in amyotrophic lateral sclerosis with and without dementia. *Acta Neuropathol*, **116**, 193–203.
19. Dickson DW, Josephs KA, Amador-Ortiz C. (2007). TDP-43 in differential diagnosis of motor neuron disorders. *Acta Neuropathol*, **114**, 71–79.
20. Arai T, Hasegawa M, Nonoka T, *et al.* (2010). Phosphorylated and cleaved TDP-43 in ALS, FTLD and other neurodegenerative disorders and in cellular models of TDP-43 proteinopathy. *Neuropathology*, **30**, 170–181.
21. Mori F, Tanji K, Miki Y, *et al.* (2010). Relationship between Bunina bodies and TDP-43 inclusions in spinal anterior horn in amyotrophic lateral sclerosis, *Neuropathol Appl Neurobiol*, **36**, 345–352.
22. Okamoto K, Hirai S, Amari M, *et al.* (1993). Bunina bodies in amyotrophic lateral sclerosis immunostained with rabbit anti-cystatin C serum. *Neurosci Lett*, **162**, 125–128.

23. Mizuno Y, Amari M, Takatama M, *et al.* (2006). Transferrin localizes in Bunina bodies in amyotrophic lateral sclerosis. *Acta Neuropathol*, **112**, 597–603.
24. Tan C-F, Eguchi H, Tagawa A, *et al.* (2007). TDP-43 immunoreactivity in neuronal inclusions in familial amyotrophic lateral sclerosis with or without SOD1 gene mutation. *Acta Neuropathol*, **113**, 535–542.
25. Murayama S, Mori H, Ihara Y, *et al.* (1990). Immunocytochemical and ultrastructural studies of lower motor neurons in amyotrophic lateral sclerosis. *Ann Neurol*, **27**, 137–148.
26. Ince PG, Tomkins J, Slade JY, *et al.* (1998). Amyotrophic lateral sclerosis associated with genetic abnormalities in the gene encoding Cu/Zn superoxide dismutase: molecular pathology of five new cases, and comparison with previous reports and 73 sporadic cases of ALS. *J Neuropathol Exp Neurol*, **57**, 895–904.
27. Kokubo Y, Kuzuhara S, Narita Y, *et al.* (1999). Accumulation of neurofilaments and SOD1-immunoreactive products in a patient with familial amyotrophic lateral sclerosis with I113T SOD1 mutation. *Arch Neurol*, **56**, 1506–1508.
28. Kondo A, Iwaki T, Tateishi J, *et al.* (1986). Accumulation of neurofilaments in a sporadic case of amyotrophic lateral sclerosis. *Jpn J Psychiatry Neurol*, **40**, 677–684.
29. Munoz DG, Greene C, Perl DP, *et al.* (1988). Accumulation of phosphorylated neurofilaments in anterior horn motoneurons of amyotrophic lateral sclerosis patients. *J Neuropathol Exp Neurol*, **47**, 9–18.
30. Carpenter S. (1968). Proximal axonal enlargement in motor neuron disease. *Neurology*, **18**, 841–851.
31. Sobue G, Hashizume Y, Yasuda T, *et al.* (1990). Phosphorylated high molecular weight neurofilament protein in lower motor neurons in amyotrophic lateral sclerosis and in other neurodegenerative diseases involving ventral horn cells. *Acta Neuropathol*, **79**, 402–408.
32. Ince, P. 2000. Neuropathology. In: Brown, Jr RH, Meininger V, Swash M (eds.), *Amyotrophic Lateral Sclerosis*, pp. 83–112. Martin Dunitz, London.
33. Okamoto K, Hirai S, Amari M, *et al.* (1993). Oculomotor nuclear pathology in amyotrophic lateral sclerosis. *Acta Neuropathol*, **85**, 458–462.
34. Kihira T, Yoshida S, Yoshimasu F, *et al.* (1997). Involvement of Onuf's nucleus in amyotrophic lateral sclerosis. *J Neurol Sci*, **147**, 81–88.
35. Brownell B, Oppenheimer DR, Hughes JT. (1970). The central nervous system in motor neurone disease. *J Neurol Neurosurg Psychiatry*, **33**, 338–357.
36. Nihei K, McKee AC, Kowall NW. (1993). Patterns of neuronal degeneration in the motor cortex of amyotrophic lateral sclerosis patients. *Acta Neuropathol*, **86**, 55–64.
37. Gredal O, Pakkenberg H, Karlsborg M, *et al.* (2000). Unchanged total number of neurons in motor cortex and neocortex in amyotrophic lateral sclerosis: a stereological study. *J Neurosci Methods*, **95**, 171–176.
38. Toft MH, Gredal O, Pakkenberg B. (2005). The size distribution of neurons in the motor cortex in amyotrophic lateral sclerosis. *J Anat*, **207**, 399–407.
39. Ince PG, Evans J, Knopp M, *et al.* (2003). Corticospinal tract degeneration in the progressive muscular atrophy variant of ALS. *Neurology*, **60**, 1252–1258.
40. Barbeito LH, Pehar M, Cassina P, *et al.* (2004). A role for astrocytes in motor neuron loss in amyotrophic lateral sclerosis. *Brain Res Brain Res Rev*, **47**, 263–274.
41. Hiji M, Takahashi T, Fukuba H, *et al.* (2008). White matter lesions in the brain with frontotemporal lobar degeneration with motor neuron disease: TDP-43-immunopositive inclusion co-localize with p62, but not ubiquitin. *Acta Neuropathol*, **116**, 183–191.
42. Dickson DW, Wertkin A, Kress Y, *et al.* (1990). Ubiquitin immunoreactive structures in normal human brains. Distribution and developmental aspects. *Lab Invest*, **63**, 87–99.
43. Zatloukal K, Stumptner C, Fuchsbichler A, *et al.* (2002). p62 is a common component of cytoplasmic inclusion in protein aggregation diseases. *Am J Pathol*, **160**, 255–263.

44. Wooten MW, Hu X, Babu JR, *et al.* (2006). Signaling, polyubiquitination, trafficking, and inclusions: sequestosome 1/p62's role in neurodegenerative disease. *J Biomed Biotechnol*, **2006**, 62079.
45. Kuusisto E, Kauppinen T, Alafuzoff I. (2008). Use of p62/SQSTM1 antibodies for neuropathological diagnosis. *Neuropathol Appl Neurobiol*, **34**, 169–180.
46. Pikkarainen M, Hartikainen P, Alafuzoff I. (2008). Neuropathologic features of frontotemporal lobar degeneration with ubiquitin-positive inclusions visualized with ubiquitin-binding protein p62 immunohistochemistry. *J Neuropathol Exp Neurol*, **67**, 280–298.
47. Geser F, Brandmeir NJ, Kwong LK, *et al.* (2008). Evidence of multisystem disorder in whole-brain map of pathological TDP-43 in amyotrophic lateral sclerosis. *Arch Neurol*, **65**, 636–641.
48. Isaacs JD, Dean AF, Shaw CE, *et al.* (2007). Amyotrophic lateral sclerosis with sensory neuropathy: part of a multisystem disorder? *J Neurol Neurosurg Psychiatry*, **78**, 750–753.
49. Kawamura Y, Dyck PJ, Shimono M, *et al.* (1981). Morphometric comparison of the vulnerability of peripheral motor and sensory neurons in amyotrophic lateral sclerosis. *J Neuropathol Exp Neurol*, **40**, 667–675.
50. Averback P and Crocker P. (1982). Regular involvement of Clarke's nucleus in sporadic amyotrophic lateral sclerosis. *Arch Neurol*, **39**, 155–156.
51. Takahashi H, Oyanagi K, Ohama E, *et al.* (1992). Clarke's column in sporadic amyotrophic lateral sclerosis. *Acta Neuropathol*, **84**, 465–470.
52. Nakano T, Nakaso K, Nakashima K, *et al.* (2004). Expression of ubiquitin-binding protein p62 in ubiquitin-immunoreactive intraneuronal inclusions in amyotrophic lateral sclerosis with dementia: analysis of five autopsy cases with broad clinicopathological spectrum. *Acta Neuropathol*, **107**, 359–364.
53. Nishihira Y, Tan CF, Onodera O, *et al.* (2008). Sporadic amyotrophic lateral sclerosis: two pathological patterns shown by analysis of distribution of TDP-43-immunoreactive neuronal and glial cytoplasmic inclusions. *Acta Neuropathol*, **116**, 169–182.
54. Tateishi T, Hokonohara T, Yamasaki R, *et al.* (2010). Multiple system degeneration with basophilic inclusions in Japanese ALS patients with FUS mutation. *Acta Neuropathol*, **119**, 355–364.
55. Hudson AJ. (1981). Amyotrophic lateral sclerosis and its association with dementia, parkinsonism and other neurological disorders: A review. *Brain*, **194**, 217–247.
56. Kato S, Oda M, Tanabe H. (1993). Diminution of dopaminergic neurons in the substantia nigra of sporadic amyotrophic lateral sclerosis. *Neuropathol Appl Neurobiol*, **19**, 300–304.
57. Miki Y, Mori F, Nunomura J, *et al.* (2010). Sporadic amyotrophic lateral sclerosis with pallido-nigro-luysian degeneration: a TDP-43 immunohistochemical study. *Neuropathology*, **30**, 149–153.
58. Sudo S, Fukutani Y, Matsubara R, *et al.* (2002). Motor neuron disease with dementia combined with degeneration of striatonigral and pallidoluysian systems. *Acta Neuropathol*, **103**, 521–525.
59. Zhang H, Tan C-F, Mori F, *et al.* (2008). TDP-43-immunoreactive neuronal and glial inclusions in the neostriatum in amyotrophic lateral sclerosis with and without dementia. *Acta Neuropathol*, **115**, 115–122.
60. Mochizuki A, Komatsuzaki Y, Iwamoto H, *et al.* (2004). Frontotemporal dementia with ubiquitinated neuronal inclusions presenting with primary lateral sclerosis and parkinsonism: clinicopathological report of an autopsy case. *Acta Neuropathol*, **107**, 377–380.
61. Miklossy J, Steele JC, Yu S, *et al.* (2008). Enduring involvement of tau, beta-amyloid, alpha-synuclein, ubiquitin and TDP-43 pathology in the amyotrophic lateral sclerosis/parkinsonism-dementia complex of Guam (ALS/PDC). *Acta Neuropathol*, **116**, 625–637.
62. Williams TL, Shaw PJ, Lowe J, *et al.* (1995). Parkinsonism in motor neuron disease: case report and literature review. *Acta Neuropathol*, **89**, 275–283.
63. Okamoto K, Hirai S, Yamazaki T, *et al.* (1991). New ubiquitin-positive intraneuronal inclusions in the extra-motor cortices in patients with amyotrophic lateral sclerosis. *Neurosci Lett*, **129**, 233–236.
64. Wightman G, Anderson VER, Martin J, *et al.* (1992). Hippocampal and neocortical ubiquitin-immunoreactive inclusions in amyotrophic lateral sclerosis with dementia. *Neurosci Lett*, **139**, 269–274.

65. Leigh PN, Whitwell H, Garofalo O, *et al.* (1991). Ubiquitin-immunoreactive intraneuronal inclusions in amyotrophic lateral sclerosis. Morphology, distribution, and specificity. *Brain*, **114** (Pt 2), 775–788.
66. Kato S, Oda M, Hayashi H, *et al.* (1994). Participation of the limbic system and its associated areas in the dementia of amyotrophic lateral sclerosis. *J Neurol Sci*, **126**, 62–69.
67. Kawashima T, Doh-ura K, Kikuchi H, *et al.* (2001). Cognitive dysfunction in patients with amyotrophic lateral sclerosis is associated with spherical or crescent-shaped ubiquitinated intraneuronal inclusions in the parahippocampal gyrus and amygdala, but not in the neostriatum. *Acta Neuropathol*, **102**, 467–472.
68. Mackenzie IR and Feldman H. (2003). The relationship between extramotor ubiquitin-immunoreactive neuronal inclusions and dementia in motor neuron disease. *Acta Neuropathol*, **105**, 98–102.
69. Wilson CM, Grace GM, Munoz DG, *et al.* (2001). Cognitive impairment in sporadic ALS. A pathological continuum underlying a multisystem disorder. *Neurology*, **57**, 651–657.
70. Holton JL, Revesz T, Crooks R, *et al.* (2002). Evidence for pathological involvement of the spinal cord in motor neuron disease-inclusion dementia. *Acta Neuropathol*, **103**, 221–227.
71. Okamoto K, Murakami N, Kusaka H, *et al.* (1992). Ubiquitin-positive intraneuronal inclusions in the motor cortices of presenile dementia patients with motor neuron disease. *J Neurol*, **239**, 426–430.
72. Cairns NJ, Bigio EH, Mackenzie IRA, *et al.* (2007). Neuropathological diagnostic and nosologic criteria for frontotemporal lobar degeneration: consensus of the Consortium for Frontotemporal Lobar Degeneration. *Acta Neuropathol*, **114**, 5–22.
73. Geser F, Martinez-Lage M, Robinson J, *et al.* (2009). Clinical and pathological continuum of multisystem TDP-43 proteinopathies. *Arch Neurol*, **66**, 180–189.
74. Mackenzie IR, Feldman HH. (2005). Ubiquitin immunohistochemistry suggests classic motor neuron disease, motor neuron disease with dementia, and frontotemporal dementia of the motor neuron disease type represent a clinicopathologic spectrum. *J Neuropathol Exp Neurol*, **64**, 730–739.
75. Ince PG, Lowe J, Shaw PJ. (1998). Amyotrophic lateral sclerosis: curent issues in classification, pathogenesis and molecular pathology. *Neuropathol Appl Neurobiol*, **24**, 104–117.
76. Igaz LM, Kwong LK, Xu Y, *et al.* (2008). Enrichment of C-terminal fragments in TAR DNA-binding protein-43 cytoplasmic inclusions in brain but not in spinal cord of frontotemporal lobar degeneration and amyotrophic lateral sclerosis. *Am J Pathol*, **173**, 182–194.
77. Tan CF, Piao YS, Hayashi S, *et al.* (2004). Familial amyotrophic lateral sclerosis with bulbar onset and a novel Asp101Tyr Cu/Zn superoxide dismutase gene mutation. *Acta Neuropathol*, **108**, 332–336.
78. Shimizu T, Kawata A, Kato S, *et al.* (2000). Autonomic failure in ALS with a novel SOD1 gene mutation. *Neurology*, **54**, 1534–1537.
79. Suzuki M, Irie T, Watanabe T, *et al.* (2008). Familial amyotrophic lateral sclerosis with Gly93Ser mutation in Cu/Zn superoxide dismutase: a clinical and neuropathological study. *J Neurol Sci*, **268**, 140–144.
80. Mackenzie IRA, Bigio EH, Ince PG, *et al.* (2007). Pathological TDP-43 distinguishes sporadic amyotrophic lateral sclerosis from amyotrophic lateral sclerosis with *SOD1* mutations. *Ann Neurol*, **61**, 427–434.
81. Rouleau GA, Clark AW, Rooke K, *et al.* (1996). SOD1 mutation is associated with accumulation of neurofilaments in amyotrophic lateral sclerosis. *Ann Neurol*, **39**, 128–131.
82. Shibata N, Hirano A, Kobayashi M, *et al.* (1996). Intense superoxide dismutase-1 immunoreactivity in intracytoplasmic hyaline inclusions of familial amyotrophic lateral sclerosis with posterior column involvement. *J Neuropathol Exp Neurol*, **55**, 481–490.
83. Chou SM, Wang HS, Taniguchi A. (1996). Role of SOD-1 and nitric oxide/cyclic GMP cascade on neurofilament aggregation in ALS/MND. *J Neurol Sci*, **139**, 16–26.
84. Jonsson PA, Ernhill K, Andersen PM, *et al.* (2004). Minute quantities of misfolded mutant superoxide dismutase-1 cause amyotrophic lateral sclerosis. *Brain*, **127**, 73–88.

85. Gitcho MA, Bigio EH, Mishra M, *et al.* (2009). TARDBP 3'-UTR variant in autopsy-confirmed frontotemporal lobar degeneration with TDP-43 proteinopathy. *Acta Neuropathol*, **118**, 633–645.
86. Kovacs GG, Murrell JR, Horvath S, *et al.* (2009). TARDBP variation associated with frontotemporal dementia, supranuclear gaze palsy, and chorea. *Mov Disord*, **24**, 1843–1847.
87. Tamaoka A, Arai M, Itokawa M, *et al.* (2010). TDP-43 M337V mutation in familial amyotrophic lateral sclerosis in Japan. *Intern Med*, **49**, 331–334.
88. Van Deerlin VM, Leverenz JB, Bekris LM. *et al.* (2008). TARDBP mutations in amyotrophic lateral sclerosis with TDP-43 neuropathology: a genetic and histological analysis. *Lancet Neurol*, **7**, 416.
89. Yokoseki A, Shiga A, Tan C-F, *et al.* (2008). TDP-43 mutation in familial amyotrophic lateral sclerosis. *Ann Neurol*, **63**, 538–542.
90. Andersson MK, Stahlberg A, Arvidsson Y, *et al.* (2008). The multifunctional FUS, EWS and TAF15 proto-oncoproteins show cell type-specific expression patterns and involvement in cell spreading and stress response. *BMC Cell Biol*, **9**, 37.
91. Strong MJ. (2010). The evidence for altered RNA metabolism in amyotrophic lateral sclerosis (ALS). *J Neurol Sci*, **288**, 1–12.
92. Kwiatkowski TJ, Jr, Bosco DA, Leclerc AL, *et al.* (2009). Mutations in the FUS/TLS gene on chromosome 16 cause familial amyotrophic lateral sclerosis. *Science*, **323**, 1205–1208.
93. Vance C, Rogelj B, Hortobágyi T, *et al.* (2009). Mutations in FUS, an RNA processing protein, cause familial amyotrophic lateral sclerosis type 6. *Science*, **323**, 1208–1211.
94. Blair IP, Williams KL, Warraich ST, *et al.* (2010). FUS mutations in amyotrophic lateral sclerosis: clinical, pathological, neurophysiological and genetic analysis. *J Neurol Neurosurg Psychiatry*, **81**, 639–645.
95. Groen EJ, van Es MA, van Vught PW, *et al.* (2010). FUS mutations in familial amyotrophic lateral sclerosis in the Netherlands. *Arch Neurol*, **67**, 224–230.
96. Hewitt C, Kirby J, Highley JR, *et al.* (2010). Novel FUS/TLS mutations and pathology in familial and sporadic amyotrophic lateral sclerosis. *Arch Neurol*, **67**, 455–461.
97. Suzuki N, Aoki M, Warita H, *et al.* (2010). FALS with FUS mutation in Japan, with early onset, rapid progress and basophilic inclusion. *J Hum Genet*, **55**, 252–254.
98. Van den Berg-Vos RM, Van den Berg LH, Jansen GH, *et al.* (2001). Hereditary pure lower motor neuron disease with adult onset and rapid progression. *J Neurol*, **248**, 290–296.
99. Seilhean D, Takahashi J, El Hachimi KH, *et al.* (2004). Amyotrophic lateral sclerosis with neuronal intranuclear protein inclusions. *Acta Neuropathol*, **108**, 81–87.
100. Seilhean D, Cazeneuve C, Thuriès V, *et al.* (2009). Accumulation of TDP-43 and α-actin in an amyotrophic lateral sclerosis patient with the K171 ANG mutation. *Acta Neuropathol*, **118**, 561–573.
101. Parkinson N, Ince PG, Smith MO, *et al.* (2006). ALS phenotypes with mutations in CHMP2B (charges multivesicular body protein 2B). *Neurology*, **67**, 1074–1077.
102. Cox LE, Ferraiuolo L, Goodall EF, *et al.* (2010). Mutations in CHMP2B in lower motor neuron predominant amyotrophic lateral sclerosis (ALS). *PLoS One*, **5**, e9872.

Chapter 20

Genetics of frontotemporal dementia*

Bryan J. Traynor and Stuart Pickering-Brown

Frontotemporal dementia (FTD) is the second or third most common cause of dementia, accounting for approximately 10% of all cases and an even higher proportion of cases under the age of 65 years (1,2). In contrast to Alzheimer's disease, which increases in prevalence after the age of 65, the median age of onset of FTD is 52.8 years of age, albeit with a relatively wide range (3). Clinically, the disease is characterized by abnormalities in personality, behaviour, and language with relatively preserved memory. About 10% of FTD cases manifest motor neurone dysfunction at some stage during the course of disease (4,5). Median survival is typically 7 years (2), though it tends to be significantly less in the presence of concomitant motor neurone disease (6). Importantly from the perspective of genetics, a significant portion of FTD has a family history; as high as 40% in some studies (2,7).

To date, mutations in six genes have been described as causes of familial FTD, namely *MAPT*, *PRGN*, *CHMP2B*, *VCP*, *TYROBP*, and *TREM2*. In addition, a 120 kb locus on chromosome 9p21 appears to account for a significant proportion of familial FTD and FTD/amyotrophic lateral sclerosis (ALS), though the precise genetic defect underlying this locus has not yet been determined. Cumulatively, these genes account for well less than half of all familial cases suggesting that additional pathogenic genes remain to be found. Regardless of the absolute number of cases caused by mutations in each gene, each one has provided fundamental insights into the biology of the disease. Indeed many of the molecular biology work, including animal models, biomarker studies, and therapeutic development, that is ongoing in the field at present is driven by identification of one of these genes.

Most of the genes known for FTD were discovered by linkage analysis of large families followed by positional cloning of the genes in the linked region. More recently, genomic techniques (i.e. testing the entire genome agnostic of biological function) have been applied to FTD with interesting results (see below). In addition to detection of the previously identified chromosome 9p21 region, genetic variation on chromosome 7p21 was associated with altered risk for developing this fatal neurodegenerative disease (8).

In this review, we will describe each of these six genes in terms of their initial discovery, the phenotype associated with them, and proposed mechanisms of action. We will then describe the results of genome-wide association studies (GWAS) that have been performed in this fatal neurodegenerative disease. We will conclude with a discussion about what future of FTD genetics holds in store.

Microtubule-associated protein tau (OMIM 157140)

Linkage to the chromosome 17 was first described in a FTD family in 1994 (9,10), and was followed relatively shortly afterwards by the finding of missense and splice-site mutations in the microtubule-associated protein tau (*MAPT*) gene within this region (11–13). There was particular excitement surrounding this finding, as *MAPT* was the first gene described as a cause of FTD. Furthermore, *MAPT* had been described as the major component of the neurofibrillary tangles and Pick bodies, which are the pathological hallmark of the disease (14).

The genetic mechanism by which *MAPT* mutations lead to disease was particularly illuminating in terms of understanding the pathogenesis of FTD. The biological function of MAPT is mediated through its interaction with microtubules, which regulates the assembly and organization of neuronal microtubular network that acts as the scaffold for axonal transport (15–17). *MAPT* within the central nervous system exits in six alternatively spliced isoforms, three of them containing three repeat domains in the C-terminal end of the protein and three of them containing four repeat domains (18,19). These repeat domains are encoded by exons 9–12 of the *MAPT* gene, where inclusion of exon 10 leads to four repeat tau domains and exclusion yields three repeat tau. The importance of these imperfect repeat domains is that they are responsible for the binding of MAPT to microtubules with four repeat isoforms binding more strongly than isoforms with just three repeats (20). In normal brain, the balance between three repeat and four repeat tau is maintained in near equilibrium. In contrast, mutations in the splice region of exon 10 disrupt a stem–loop motif that prevents skipping of this exon leading to altered production of four repeat tau (11,13,19,21,22). Indeed, other diseases associated with tau neuropathology are characterized by shifts in this balance between three and four repeat tau.

To date, over 30 different mutations have been described in 80 families (http://www.molgen.ua.ac.be/ADMutations/) (21,23,24). Cumulatively, *MAPT* mutations account for about 5–10% of familial FTD cases (25–27) with the vast majority of these mutations concentrated in exons 9–13 that encode the microtubule binding repeats (17). Aside from those mutations affecting exon 10 splicing, these other mutations disrupt the repeat domains and thus the interaction between tau and the microtubule (28–31). However, while the splicing mutations demonstrate the importance of the 4R:3R tau isoform ratio, it remains unclear exactly how disruption of this ratio (in either direction) results in neurodegeneration (17). Despite this, it looks as though mutations in *MAPT* may result in a toxic gain of function. Genetic screening of this gene is available, and most clinical centres routinely sequence this gene in patients with FTD, particularly those with a family history of disease.

A correlation has been observed between the type of *MAPT* mutation and the observed tau neuropathology. In patients with mutations affecting exon 10 splicing or affecting the repeat domain encoded by exon 10, the neurofibrillary inclusions consist almost entirely of 4R tau. Furthermore, these inclusions are typically seen in both neurones and glia. Patients with mutations involving exons 9, 11, 12, and 13 typically have neuronal lesions resembling Pick-like bodies or neurofibrillary tangles similar to those observed in Alzheimer's disease (13,32–34).

Progranulin (OMIM 138945)

Progranulin (*PGRN*) is a 68.5 kDa secreted growth factor that regulates a variety of cellular processes, including development, wound repair, and inflammation (see Gass and Petrucelli, Chapter 25). This gene is located on the long arm of chromosome 17, less than 2 Mb away from the *MAPT* gene. Indeed, the close proximity of these two genes delayed the cloning of PGRN as an FTD gene. Since its initial discovery in 2006 (35,36), over 60 truncating and non-sense mutations of *PGRN* have been found in FTD (http://www.molgen.ua.ac.be/ADMutations/). Importantly, the neuropathological features of these cases distinguish them from patients with *MAPT* mutations, in that it is characterized by ubiquitin and TAR-DNA binding protein 43 (TDP-43)-positive, tau-negative inclusions (35). Primary progressive aphasia and corticobasal syndrome have also been described as being caused by mutations in *PGRN* (37–40). To date, it would appear that *PGRN* mutations are a rare cause of isolated ALS syndrome, if at all (41,42). Overall, *PGRN* mutations account for about 10% of familial FTD cases, which is similar to the occurrence of *MAPT* mutations in this particular population (43).

PGRN mutations appear to cause disease through loss of protein function, either through truncation or frameshift mutations that lead to non-sense-mediated decay of mRNA, or by disruption of the nuclear export signal leading to nuclear degradation of the protein (35,36,44). Mutations of the start methionine of *PGRN* have also been described (36). These observations point to haploinsufficiency as the mechanism underlying disease, and suggest that therapeutic interventions aimed at boosting the amount of *PGRN* may ameliorate disease.

Valosin-containing protein (OMIM 601023)

Valosin-containing protein (*VCP*) was initially identified in 2004 as the cause of an unusual syndrome characterized by the clinical triad of inclusion body myopathy, early-onset Paget's disease of the bone and FTD (45). The unifying pathological substrate between these diverse tissue types is the presence of ubiquitin inclusions (46). Furthermore, at least in the case of muscle and frontal cortex, there is aberrant TDP-43 staining (47), and it has been shown that mutant *VCP* is associated with redistribution of this protein within the cell (48–50). A striking feature of *VCP*-associated disease is the marked clinical heterogeneity associated with disease (51). Even within the same family carrying the same mutant allele, different generations manifest distinct features of the disease either in isolation or in combination with other. Of the three cardinal features, FTD is the least common, being present in only a third of cases (45). Neuropathologically, these cases manifest ubiquitin-positive, VCP-positive neuronal intranuclear inclusions. Surprisingly, there are no published studies examining the role of this gene in uncomplicated FTD.

The exact mechanism by which *VCP* mutations gives rise to disease is not clear. VCP is a member of the AAA-ATPase family of proteins and appears to have a number of cellular processes, including vesicle transport and fusion, 26S proteasome function, assembly of peroxisomes, spindle pole body function, and, importantly, ubiquitin-dependent protein degradation. The protein exists as a hexamer, surrounding a central pore (47). The majority of the 17 mutations that have been described in VCP to date occur in exons 3, 5, and 6, which encode the cleft that interacts between VCP monomers (46). This has given rise to the hypothesis that these mutations disrupt the conformational change of the VCP protein that occurs with activation, thereby interfering with the process. Furthermore, assuming that a wild-type and a mutant allele are expressed in equimolar concentrations, then only 1.5% of VCP hexamers would be composed of just wild-type VCP monomers. This suggests that heterozygous mutations of this gene could reduce the effective function of this protein by more than 50%. Based on these observations, it is likely that mutations in VCP result in a complex loss of function involving disruption of the hexamer.

Chromatin modifying protein 2B (OMIM 609512)

Chromatin modifying protein 2B (*CHMP2b*) is thought to be involved in endosomal trafficking, which is increasingly recognized as being important in neurodegeneration (52). The gene was first identified in a large Danish family with behavioural variant FTD with motor neurone dysfunction appearing later in the disease (53). The region on chromosome 3p had been previously identified based on linkage analysis of the same family (54–56). The mutation in this family was located within the acceptor splice site of exon 6. Since then, two additional mutations have been described, supporting the pathogenic nature of mutations in this gene (57). However, *CHMP2B* mutations are a relatively rare cause of FTD accounting for less than 1% of cases (58,59). Interestingly, the neuropathological picture observed within this family is distinct from that in other families with FTD in that there was a notable lack of tau-positive, synuclein-positive pathology (54,60), though ubiquitin-positive inclusions have been observed. In terms of effect of the mutations on function, the precise mechanism has not been elucidated, but evidence points in the direction of a complex misfunction of the CHMP2b protein.

TYRO protein tyrosine kinase-binding protein (OMIM 604142) and triggering receptor expressed on myeloid cells 2 (OMIM 605086)

TYRO protein tyrosine kinase binding protein (TYROBP) on chromosome 19q and triggering receptor expressed on myeloid cells 2 (TREM2) on chromosome 6p encode different subunits of the same signalling complex. Recessive mutations with these two genes are responsible for a rare syndrome clinically characterized by a combination of bone cysts, often presenting as fractures, and early-onset FTD (61–63). Mutations in these genes have only been described in Japanese and Scandinavian families, and it appears to be very rare outside of these regions.

Genome-wide association studies of frontotemporal dementia

In this section, we will discuss the results of GWAS that have been completed in FTD and in ALS/FTD.

Van Deerlin and colleagues published the first (and to date only) GWAS for FTD (8). Based on 515 cases, they detected significant risk loci on chromosome 17 corresponding to the *PGRN* locus, and on chromosome 7p21. Within this locus, *TMEM106B* has been nominated as the causative gene based on its proximity of the peak associated single nucleotide polymorphism (SNP). To a certain extent, these results may reflect the manner in which the cases were selected for inclusion in the study: about 20% of the cases carried a known *PGRN* mutation. Interestingly, the chromosome 7 locus continued to have an effect on disease risk when the analysis was confined to those patients with *PGRN* mutations, suggesting that the locus may important in influencing the clinical expression and phenotype in these cases.

Recently, we published that a locus on chromosome 9p21 increased the risk of familial ALS, and accounted for a large proportion of cases seen in Finland (64). Finland was an ideal location for a study of this nature as it is has one of the highest rates of ALS reported in the world (65), and because of the remarkably genetically homogeneous nature of the Finnish population arising from the population history of small founder population and multiple bottlenecks. Importantly, the clinical phenotype associated with this locus is ALS with FTD, and the haplotype identified in the Finnish population overlapped with that identified in the FTD GWAS (8), suggesting that this locus may be also relevant in the pathogenesis of frontal lobe degeneration. Furthermore, the families in which this locus was originally described manifested both ALS and FTD (66,67) At present the precise genetic defect underlying this locus is unknown, but it is a subject of much study in laboratories around the world.

Ubiquitin-associated protein 1 (UBAP1), also located on the short arm of chromosome 9, has been identified as a potential risk for developing FTD based on a number of cohorts. Expression analysis demonstrated a significant reduction of expression from the disease-associated haplotype. Interestingly, UBAP1 and TDP-43 colocalized in the neuronal cytoplasmic inclusions in the brain of an affected individual, suggesting a mechanistic relationship between this protein and TDP-43 (68).

Interpreting the results of genome-wide association studies

Since the publication of the first GWAS in 2005, there has been a flood of such studies. Indeed, the catalogue of GWAS maintained by the National Human Genome Research Institute now lists 702 publications with 3406 associated SNPs involving 420 diseases and traits, and this number is increasing on a nearly daily basis (http://www.genome.gov/gwastudies/, accessed 17 October 2010) (69).

Despite the evident success of this technique, a number of caveats are worth highlighting, so that the causal reader can critically evaluate the results of such a study. First, the technique of genome-wide association is best applied to diseases that conform to the common disease–common variant hypothesis (70). This is because the SNPs on a genotyping chip were specifically chosen by their manufacturers to have a minor allele frequency in the general population greater than 5%. Rare variants are, by and large, missed in this paradigm. Despite this, it is possible to apply, albeit with diminishing returns, the technique of GWAS to rare diseases, but in that instance the sample size must be dramatically increased. Furthermore, more recent versions of Illumina genotyping arrays aim to include SNPs with a minor allele frequency down as low as 1%. An alternative strategy is to specifically target homogeneous populations where the genetic heterogeneity (i.e. the number of genes in a population causing disease) and the allelic heterogeneity (i.e. the number of pathogenic alleles of a particular gene existing within a population) is reduced, thereby decreasing the signal to noise ratio (71).

The advent of GWAS and the need to genotype several thousand well-phenotyped samples has placed much greater emphasis on sample availability and interlaboratory collaboration (72). The NINDS Coriell Repository is an example of attempts to overcome this bottleneck. This repository was funded to collect and distribute DNA from several thousand ALS, Parkinson's disease, stroke cases, and controls. The success of Coriell is in large part to the fact that the samples are made publicly available to all, rather than having limited access.

Second, false positive associations remain a significant problem in the field, and are driven largely by the sheer number of tests (sometimes in the region of millions) performed on any GWAS data set. Such spurious associations can mislead a field for many years resulting in wasted time and resources (73). To overcome this, most scientific journals now require that SNPs achieve genome-wide significance after application of the Bonferroni correction for multiple testing (74). Even such stringent thresholds are associated with a 5% chance of false positive findings. Consequently, most top tier journals require that the results be replicated in an independent cohort of samples before publication. This replication cohort must be suitably sized to detect what can often be a locus with small effects, and ideally would be drawn from separate populations/regions to discount the possibility of population stratification.

Third, population stratification remains a major issue in GWA studies. Simply put, this is where a positive association arises because of differences in the population from which cases and controls are drawn, rather than being due to a genetic risk factor that distinguishes the cases from the controls as it alters risk of disease. This is a particular problem within outbred heterogeneous populations such as the United States, where historical immigration patterns have yielded considerable genetic heterogeneity. Although statistical techniques can be employed to minimize this problem, large-scale epidemiological studies probably provide the ideal solution by providing the infrastructure to collect large, well-phenotyped samples from affected and unaffected individuals drawn from similar ethnic backgrounds (75).

Fourth, understanding the biological relevance of associated SNPs detected by GWAS remains a priority. Indeed, it should be remembered that GWAS identify loci, not genes, and determining which of the multiple genes in a block of linkage disequilibrium is responsible for disease can be challenging. Significant inroads are being made into this issue to understand the effect of genetic variation on neighbouring gene expression (76,77). Several online data sets now exist that allow researchers to evaluate quickly the effect of such variation (http://eqtl.uchicago.edu), and the National Institutes of Health is currently undertaking a large-scale project to map expression quantitative trait loci across multiple tissues (the GTEx (Genotype–Tissue Expression) project, http://nihroadmap.nih.gov/GTEx/). It is also worth noting that the odds ratio associated with an associated allele represents only the allele that is most common in the case population. Other risk alleles may be present in the same locus that either individually or cumulatively explain a far higher proportion of disease than suggested by the original report. Deep re-sequencing of the region by next generation sequencing is likely to elucidate these rarer variants further (78).

Finally, GWAS are often criticized as not yet having yielded any new therapies for diseases. To our mind, this is an unfair criticism, especially when one considers the timeline involved. At best, it takes a decade of pre-clinical, animal screening, and clinical trials before a therapeutic agent is licensed for the market. Given that the first GWAS was published in 2005, it is premature to say that this technique has failed to yield clinically useful results. True, translating genetic discoveries into clinical practice is a long, tedious process, but the chances of success for such endeavours is increased when the therapeutic target is well defined.

In conclusion, the last decade has seen considerable progress in unravelling the genetic aetiology of FTD. These advances have provided fundamental insight into neurodegeneration, and underpin much of the molecular biology currently ongoing in laboratories around the world. The advent of next generation sequencing and our ability to perform exome sequencing will likely lead to an improved understanding of Mendelian form of FTD, perhaps identifying common pathways between the various causes.

References

1. Knopman DS, Petersen RC, Edland SD, *et al.* (2004). The incidence of frontotemporal lobar degeneration in Rochester, Minnesota, 1990 through 1994. *Neurology*, **62**, 506–508.
2. Rosso SM, Donker Kaat L, Baks T, *et al.* (2003). Frontotemporal dementia in The Netherlands: patient characteristics and prevalence estimates from a population-based study. *Brain*, **126**, 2016–2022.
3. Ratnavalli E, Brayne C, Dawson K, Hodges JR. (2002). The prevalence of frontotemporal dementia. *Neurology*, **58**, 1615–1621.
4. Neary D, Snowden JS, Mann DM. (2000). Classification and description of frontotemporal dementias. *Ann N Y Acad Sci*, **920**, 46–51.
5. Neary D, Snowden JS, Mann DM. (2000). Cognitive change in motor neurone disease/amyotrophic lateral sclerosis (MND/ALS). *J Neurol Sci*, **180**, 15–20.
6. Chio A, Logroscino G, Hardiman O, *et al.* (2009). Prognostic factors in ALS: a critical review. *Amyotroph Lateral Scler*, **10**, 310–323.

7. Chow TW, Miller BL, Hayashi VN, Geschwind DH. (1999). Inheritance of frontotemporal dementia. *Arch Neurol*, **56**, 817–822.
8. Van Deerlin VM, Sleiman PM, Martinez-Lage M, *et al.* (2010). Common variants at 7p21 are associated with frontotemporal lobar degeneration with TDP-43 inclusions. *Nat Genet*, **42**, 234–239.
9. Wilhelmsen K.C, Lynch T, Pavlou E, *et al.* (1994). Localization of disinhibition-dementia-parkinsonism-amyotrophy complex to 17q21–22. *Am J Hum Genet*, **55**, 1159–1165.
10. Lynch T, Sano M, Marder KS, *et al.* (1994). Clinical characteristics of a family with chromosome 17-linked disinhibition-dementia-parkinsonism-amyotrophy complex. *Neurology*, **44**, 1878–1884.
11. Hutton M, Lendon CL, Rizzu P, *et al.* (1998). Association of missense and 5'-splice-site mutations in tau with the inherited dementia FTDP-17. *Nature*, **393**, 702–705.
12. Poorkaj P, Bird TD, Wijsman E, *et al.* (1998). Tau is a candidate gene for chromosome 17 frontotemporal dementia. *Ann Neurol*, **43**, 815–825.
13. Spillantini MG, Murrell JR, Goedert M, *et al.* (1998). Mutation in the tau gene in familial multiple system tauopathy with presenile dementia. *Proc Natl Acad Sci USA*, **95**, 7737–7741.
14. Dickson DW. (1997). Neurodegenerative diseases with cytoskeletal pathology: a biochemical classification. *Ann Neurol*, **42**, 541–544.
15. Lopresti P, Szuchet S, Papasozomenos SC, *et al.* (1995). Functional implications for the microtubule-associated protein tau: localization in oligodendrocytes. *Proc Natl Acad Sci USA*, **92**, 10369–10373.
16. Ebneth A, Godemann R, Stamer K, *et al.* (1998). Overexpression of tau protein inhibits kinesin-dependent trafficking of vesicles, mitochondria, and endoplasmic reticulum: implications for Alzheimer's disease. *J Cell Biol*, **143**, 777–794.
17. Pickering-Brown S, Hutton M. (2008). The genetics of frontotemporal dementia. *Handb Clin Neurol*, **89**, 383–392.
18. Goedert M, Spillantini MG, Jakes R, *et al.* (1989). Multiple isoforms of human microtubule-associated protein tau: sequences and localization in neurofibrillary tangles of Alzheimer's disease. *Neuron*, **3**, 519–526.
19. Goedert M, Spillantini MG, Potier MC, *et al.* (1989). Cloning and sequencing of the cDNA encoding an isoform of microtubule-associated protein tau containing four tandem repeats: differential expression of tau protein mRNAs in human brain. *EMBO J*, **8**, 393–399.
20. Lee G, Neve RL, Kosik KS. (1989). The microtubule binding domain of tau protein. *Neuron*, **2**, 1615–1624.
21. Rademakers R, Cruts M, Van Broeckhoven C. (2004). The role of tau (MAPT). in frontotemporal dementia and related tauopathies. *Hum Mutat*, **24**, 277–295.
22. Stanford PM, Shepherd CE, Halliday GM, *et al.* (2003). Mutations in the tau gene that cause an increase in three repeat tau and frontotemporal dementia. *Brain*, **126**, 814–826.
23. Gijselinck I, Van Broeckhoven C, Cruts M. (2008). Granulin mutations associated with frontotemporal lobar degeneration and related disorders: an update. *Hum Mutat*, **29**, 1373–1386.
24. Cruts M, Van Broeckhoven C. (1998). Presenilin mutations in Alzheimer's disease. *Hum Mutat*, **11**, 183–190.
25. Houlden H, Baker M, Adamson J, *et al.* (1999). Frequency of tau mutations in three series of non-Alzheimer's degenerative dementia. *Ann Neurol*, **46**, 243–248.
26. Morris HR, Khan MN, Janssen JC, *et al.* (2001). The genetic and pathological classification of familial frontotemporal dementia. *Arch Neurol*, **58**, 1813–1816.
27. Poorkaj P, Grossman M, Steinbart E, *et al.* (2001). Frequency of tau gene mutations in familial and sporadic cases of non-Alzheimer dementia. *Arch Neurol*, **58**, 383–387.

28. Dayanandan R, Van Slegtenhorst M, Mack TG, *et al.* (1999). Mutations in tau reduce its microtubule binding properties in intact cells and affect its phosphorylation. *FEBS Lett*, **446**, 228–232.
29. Hasegawa M, Smith MJ, Goedert M. (1998). Tau proteins with FTDP-17 mutations have a reduced ability to promote microtubule assembly. *FEBS Lett*, **437**, 207–210.
30. Hong M, Zhukareva V, Vogelsberg-Ragaglia V, *et al.* (1998). Mutation-specific functional impairments in distinct tau isoforms of hereditary FTDP-17. *Science*, **282**, 1914–1917.
31. Pickering-Brown SM, Baker M, Nonaka T, *et al.* (2004). Frontotemporal dementia with Pick-type histology associated with Q336R mutation in the tau gene. *Brain*, **127**, 1415–1426.
32. Neumann M, Schulz-Schaeffer W, Crowther RA, *et al.* (2001). Pick's disease associated with the novel Tau gene mutation K369I. *Ann Neurol*, **50**, 503–513.
33. Ghetti B, Murrell JR, Zolo P, *et al.* (2000). Progress in hereditary tauopathies: a mutation in the Tau gene (G389R). causes a Pick disease-like syndrome. *Ann N Y Acad Sci*, **920**, 52–62.
34. Pickering-Brown S, Baker M, Yen SH, *et al.* (2000). Pick's disease is associated with mutations in the tau gene. *Ann Neurol*, **48**, 859–867.
35. Baker M, Mackenzie IR, Pickering-Brown SM, *et al.* (2006). Mutations in progranulin cause tau-negative frontotemporal dementia linked to chromosome 17. *Nature*, **442**, 916–919.
36. Cruts M, Gijselinck I, Van Der Zee J, *et al.* (2006). Null mutations in progranulin cause ubiquitin-positive frontotemporal dementia linked to chromosome 17q21. *Nature*, **442**, 920–924.
37. Davion S, Johnson N, Weintraub S, *et al.* (2007). Clinicopathologic correlation in PGRN mutations. *Neurology*, **69**, 1113–1121.
38. Borroni B, Archetti S, Alberici A, *et al.* (2008). Progranulin genetic variations in frontotemporal lobar degeneration: evidence for low mutation frequency in an Italian clinical series. *Neurogenetics*, **9**, 197–205.
39. Spina S, Murrell JR, Huey ED, *et al.* (2007). Corticobasal syndrome associated with the A9D Progranulin mutation. *J Neuropathol Exp Neurol*, **66**, 892–900.
40. Masellis M, Momeni P, Meschino W, *et al.* (2006). Novel splicing mutation in the progranulin gene causing familial corticobasal syndrome. *Brain*, **129**, 3115–3123.
41. Schymick JC, Yang Y, Andersen PM, *et al.* (2007). Progranulin mutations and amyotrophic lateral sclerosis or amyotrophic lateral sclerosis-frontotemporal dementia phenotypes. *J Neurol Neurosurg Psychiatry*, **78**, 754–756.
42. Del Bo R, Corti S, Santoro D, *et al.* (2011). No major progranulin genetic variability contribution to disease etiopathogenesis in an ALS Italian cohort. *Neurobiol Aging*, **32**, 1157–1158.
43. Yu CE, Bird TD, Bekris LM, *et al.* (2010). The spectrum of mutations in progranulin: a collaborative study screening 545 cases of neurodegeneration. *Arch Neurol*, **67**, 161–170.
44. Van Der Zee J, Rademakers R, Engelborghs S, *et al.* (2006). A Belgian ancestral haplotype harbours a highly prevalent mutation for 17q21-linked tau-negative FTLD. *Brain*, **129**, 841–852.
45. Watts GD, Wymer J, Kovach MJ, *et al.* (2004). Inclusion body myopathy associated with Paget disease of bone and frontotemporal dementia is caused by mutant valosin-containing protein. *Nat Genet*, **36**, 377–381.
46. Ju JS, Weihl CC. (2010). Inclusion body myopathy, Paget's disease of the bone and fronto-temporal dementia: a disorder of autophagy. *Hum Mol Genet*, **19**, R38–45.
47. Weihl CC, Pestronk A, Kimonis VE. (2009). Valosin-containing protein disease: inclusion body myopathy with Paget's disease of the bone and fronto-temporal dementia. *Neuromuscul Disord*, **19**, 308–315.
48. Ritson GP, Custer SK, Freibaum BD, *et al.* (2010). TDP-43 mediates degeneration in a novel Drosophila model of disease caused by mutations in VCP/p97. *J Neurosci*, **30**, 7729–7739.

49. Custer SK, Neumann M, Lu H, Wright AC, Taylor JP. (2010). Transgenic mice expressing mutant forms VCP/p97 recapitulate the full spectrum of IBMPFD including degeneration in muscle, brain and bone. *Hum Mol Genet*, **19**, 1741–1755.
50. Gitcho MA, Strider J, Carter D, *et al.* (2009). VCP mutations causing frontotemporal lobar degeneration disrupt localization of TDP-43 and induce cell death. *J Biol Chem*, **284**, 12384–12398.
51. Van Der Zee J, Pirici D, Van Langenhove T, *et al.* (2009). Clinical heterogeneity in 3 unrelated families linked to VCP p. Arg159His. *Neurology*, **73**, 626–632.
52. Nixon RA. (2005). Endosome function and dysfunction in Alzheimer's disease and other neurodegenerative diseases. *Neurobiol Aging*, **26**, 373–382.
53. Skibinski G, Parkinson NJ, Brown JM, *et al.* (2005). Mutations in the endosomal ESCRTIII-complex subunit CHMP2B in frontotemporal dementia. *Nat Genet*, **37**, 806–808.
54. Gydesen S, Hagen S, Klinken L, *et al.* (1987). Neuropsychiatric studies in a family with presenile dementia different from Alzheimer and Pick disease. *Acta Psychiatr Scand*, **76**, 276–284.
55. Brown J, Ashworth A, Gydesen S, *et al.* (1995). Familial non-specific dementia maps to chromosome 3. *Hum Mol Genet*, **4**, 1625–1628.
56. Yancopoulou D, Crowther RA, Chakrabarti L, *et al.* (2003). Tau protein in frontotemporal dementia linked to chromosome 3 (FTD-3). *J Neuropathol Exp Neurol*, **62**, 878–882.
57. Van Der Zee J, Urwin H, Engelborghs S, *et al.* (2008). CHMP2B C-truncating mutations in frontotemporal lobar degeneration are associated with an aberrant endosomal phenotype *in vitro*. *Hum Mol Genet*, **17**, 313–322.
58. Cannon A, Baker M, Boeve B, *et al.* (2006). CHMP2B mutations are not a common cause of frontotemporal lobar degeneration. *Neurosci Lett*, **398**, 83–84.
59. Momeni P, Rogaeva E, Van Deerlin V, *et al.* (2006). Genetic variability in CHMP2B and frontotemporal dementia. *Neurodegener Dis*, **3**, 129–133.
60. Mackenzie IR, Feldman H. (2003). The relationship between extramotor ubiquitin-immunoreactive neuronal inclusions and dementia in motor neuron disease. *Acta Neuropathol*, **105**, 98–102.
61. Kondo T, Takahashi K, Kohara N, *et al.* (2002). Heterogeneity of presenile dementia with bone cysts (Nasu-Hakola disease): three genetic forms. *Neurology*, **59**, 1105–1107.
62. Paloneva J, Kestila M, Wu J, *et al.* (2000). Loss-of-function mutations in TYROBP (DAP12). result in a presenile dementia with bone cysts. *Nat Genet*, **25**, 357–361.
63. Paloneva J, Manninen T, Christman G, *et al.* (2002). Mutations in two genes encoding different subunits of a receptor signaling complex result in an identical disease phenotype. *Am J Hum Genet*, **71**, 656–662.
64. Laaksovirta H, Peuralinna T, Schymick JC, *et al.* (2010). Chromosome 9p21 in amyotrophic lateral sclerosis in Finland: a genome-wide association study. *Lancet Neurol*, **9**, 978–985.
65. Cronin S, Hardiman O, Traynor BJ. (2007). Ethnic variation in the incidence of ALS: a systematic review. *Neurology*, **68**, 1002–1007.
66. Morita M, Al-Chalabi A, Andersen PM, *et al.* (2006). A locus on chromosome 9p confers susceptibility to ALS and frontotemporal dementia. *Neurology*, **66**, 839–844.
67. Vance C, Al-Chalabi A, Ruddy D, *et al.* (2006). Familial amyotrophic lateral sclerosis with frontotemporal dementia is linked to a locus on chromosome 9p13.2–21.3. *Brain*, **129**, 868–876.
68. Rollinson S, Rizzu P, Sikkink S, *et al.* (2009). Ubiquitin associated protein 1 is a risk factor for frontotemporal lobar degeneration. *Neurobiol Aging* 2009; **30**, 656–665.
69. Hindorff LA, Sethupathy P, Junkins HA, *et al.* (2009). Potential etiologic and functional implications of genome wide association loci for human diseases and traits. *Proc Natl Acad Sci USA*, **106**, 9362–9367.
70. Pritchard JK, Cox NJ. (2002). The allelic architecture of human disease genes: common disease-common variant . . . or not? *Hum Mol Genet*, **11**, 2417–2423.

71. Shifman S, Darvasi A. (2001). The value of isolated populations. *Nat Genet*, **28**, 309–310.
72. Gwinn K, Corriveau RA, Mitsumoto H, *et al.* (2007). Amyotrophic lateral sclerosis: an emerging era of collaborative gene discovery. *PLoS One*, **2**, e1254.
73. Hardy J, Singleton A. (2007). Reporting and interpretation of genetic variants in cases and controls. *Neurology*, **69**, 111–112.
74. Chanock SJ, Manolio T, Boehnke M, *et al.* (2007). Replicating genotype-phenotype associations. *Nature*, **447**, 655–660.
75. Traynor BJ. (2009). The era of genomic epidemiology. *Neuroepidemiology*, **33**, 276–279.
76. Myers AJ, Gibbs JR, Webster JA, *et al.* (2007). A survey of genetic human cortical gene expression. *Nat Genet*, **39**, 1494–1499.
77. Gibbs JR, Van Der Brug MP, Hernandez DG, *et al.* (2010). Abundant quantitative trait loci exist for DNA methylation and gene expression in human brain. *PLoS Genet*, **6**, e1000952.
78. Singleton AB, Hardy J, Traynor BJ, Houlden H. (2010). Towards a complete resolution of the genetic architecture of disease. *Trends Genet*, **26**, 438–442.

Chapter 21

Genetics of the MNDs

Ashley Jones and Ammar Al-Chalabi

Amyotrophic lateral sclerosis (ALS) is commonly considered a condition that is inherited in 5% and otherwise sporadic (1–3). Although there are families in which transmission is clearly autosomal dominant with almost complete penetrance, in many cases, the situation is less clear-cut, with second- or third-degree relatives affected (4). Because many do not know their relatives beyond such relationships, it is not clear whether a more distant family history is common or even relevant in ALS, but it is likely that at least some cases of sporadic ALS represent examples of familial clustering on a coarse scale that is not apparent to patients or medical staff. The risk to relatives in such families would therefore be greater than the background lifetime risk of 1 in 400 (5). Thus, the distinction between familial and sporadic ALS is to some extent artificial, although convenient for the purposes of research.

There is now considerable evidence for a genetic contribution to both familial and sporadic ALS. Several genes have been shown to be mutated in familial ALS, and these will be discussed here. Mutations of every such gene have also been identified in sporadic ALS, and while causation is more difficult to show in this situation, it seems reasonable to assume that a pathogenic mutation causing familial ALS is responsible for sporadic ALS when found in someone with no family history (6–8). The heritability of sporadic ALS has been estimated as 0.61 (0.38–0.78) (9) and there are now several robustly replicated genetic associations. Although, in common with many other diseases, much of the heritability remains to be explained, newer genetic techniques such as next-generation sequencing and epigenetics are likely to find the genetic variation responsible. Because the list of ALS genes is frequently changing (Table 21.1), a complete list is available with relevant literature and bioinformatics links at the ALS Online Genetics Database, http://alsod.iop.kcl.ac.uk (10).

Several methods exist for gene identification. Family-based methods generally rely on a statistical method known as linkage, although other techniques such as homozygosity mapping will work in specific circumstances. When family-based methods are not possible, association studies are usually the alternative, and these can either be based on study of a specific candidate gene or by an unbiased approach such as genome-wide association.

Table 21.1 Genes implicated in familial amyotrophic lateral sclerosis

Locus	Genes	Chromosome region	Initial report(s)	Analysis type
ALS1	SOD1	21q22.1	Rosen *et al.* (2003) (13)	Linkage analysis
ALS2	Alsin	2q33	Hadano *et al.* (2001) (72)	Linkage analysis
ALS3	–	18q21	Hand *et al.* (2002) (132)	Linkage analysis
ALS4	SETX	9q34	Chen *et al.* (2004) (74)	Linkage analysis
ALS5	–	15q15.1–q21.1	Hentati *et al.* (1994) (2)	Linkage analysis
ALS6	FUS	16p11.2	Kwiatkowski *et al.* (2009) (48) Vance *et al.* (2009) (47)	Linkage analysis
ALS7	–	20p13	Sapp *et al.* (2003) (133)	Linkage analysis
ALS8	VAPB	20q13.3	Nishimura *et al.* (2004) (71)	Linkage analysis
ALS9	ANG	14q11.2	Greenway *et al.* (2004) (61) Greenway *et al.* (2006) (67)	Candidate gene
ALS10	TARDBP	1p36.2	Kabashi *et al.* (2008) (42) Sreedharan *et al.* (2008) (32) Van Deerlin *et al.* (2008) (45)	Candidate gene Linkage analysis
ALS11	FIG4	6q21	Chow *et al.* (2009) (134)	Candidate gene
ALS12	OPTN	10p15–p14	Maruyama *et al.* (2010) (60)	Homozygosity Mapping
ALS13*	ATXN2	12q24	Elden *et al.* (2010) (88)	Candidate gene
ALS/FTD	C9orf92	9p13.3–21.3	De Jesus *et al.* (2011) (81) Renton *et al.* (2011) (82)	Linkage analysis Genome-wide association studies
Suspected fALS genes	DAO	12q24	Mitchell *et al.* (2010) (68)	Linkage analysis
	NFH	22q12.2	Figlewicz *et al.* (1994) (81) Tomkins *et al.* (1998) (83) Al-Chalabi *et al.* (1999) (82)	Candidate gene

*ATXN2 was reported to have a modulatory effect on TDP-43 toxicity; caution is recommended on whether it is a primary instigator of a distinct familial ALS (fALS) subtype.

Genes identified through family-based studies

SOD1

Inherited forms of adult-onset motor neuron degeneration were recognized in the 1800s (11), and ALS was one of the first conditions in which linkage to a gene was observed. Mutations in *SOD1*, responsible for about 2% of all ALS (6), were first identified in 1993 (12,13), and there are now more than 150 known mutations of *SOD1* affecting all parts of this small, five exon gene (http://alsod.iop.kcl.ac.uk) (14,15). The pathogenic mechanism remains unknown despite intensive efforts although it is clear there is a gain of some toxic function. One of the major problems to understand is how mutations occurring almost anywhere in the molecule (16) can result in the same toxic gain of function with the same mode of inheritance and the same specificity for motor neurons.

The commonest *SOD1* mutation in the USA is A4V (17), accounting for nearly 50% of those with *SOD1* mutation (18) and associated with an aggressive form of ALS with short survival (19). The alanine at codon 4 is essential for the structural integrity of the SOD1 protein (20,21), but this is not necessarily the mechanism of action as other mutations with no such role can result in ALS as well. Efforts to classify *SOD1* mutations by structural effect have not led to any obvious relationship between phenotype and mutation effect (http://alsod.iop.kcl.ac.uk).

The D90A mutation is the commonest worldwide and is interesting in several respects. First, it is the only mutation that shows a clear recessive inheritance (22). There are individuals with ALS who are heterozygous for D90A (8,23), but it is likely that in these cases it is one of several contributors to the burden of disease liability. Second, the phenotype of those who are homozygous is characteristic, with slowly ascending symmetrical paresis. Third, the phenotype of those heterozygous for D90A is often more severe and aggressive than those with homozygous genotypes (8). Fourth, because it reaches polymorphic frequency in parts of Scandinavia, the distinction between sporadic and familial disease is meaningless, as two carrier parents can occur by chance and the familiality of the disease is then a product of chance and sibship size, while in other cases, an affected homozygous individual having children with a carrier will generate an apparently dominant pattern of inheritance. Fifth, founder studies have shown a single worldwide founder based in Russia or Scandinavia about 50 generations ago (23). In contrast to A4V, the D90A mutation does not appear to have much effect on any aspect of *SOD1* function or structure (22,24).

The G93A mutation has been the subject of extensive research through transgenic animal models (25) but again, the mechanism of action is unclear but may include inducing apoptosis, mitochondrial dysfunction, and oxidative cellular damage (26–29).

TARDBP

There remained no significant familial ALS genetic breakthrough for several years until a pathological clue led to the identification of the next familial ALS gene and a shift in our understanding of ALS. A major component of ALS pathology is the presence of ubiquitinated inclusions (30,31). Although it was known that neurofilamentous aggregates comprised at least some of these, the major component was unknown until discovered to be transactive response DNA-binding protein of 43 kDa (TDP-43), a protein involved in the response to HIV infection and in RNA splicing, with a major role in cystic fibrosis (32–36) (see also Buratti, Chapter 24). Wild-type (^{WT}) TDP-43^{WT} is believed to be multifunctional, influencing RNA splicing inhibition and exon skipping, heterogeneous ribonucleoprotein binding, transcriptional regulation, mRNA genesis, apoptosis, as well as protein–protein interactions, mainly through the C-terminus (32,35,37–39). Linkage followed by sequencing of DNA from families with ALS identified segregating mutations in the *TARDBP* gene on chromosome 1p36.22, coding for TDP-43 (40), and functional studies supported a role for the protein in motor neuron death.

Subsequently many other studies have replicated the original findings, and mutations have been found in sporadic ALS (32,33,41). The mutations nearly all affect the C-terminus; of the six ALS-causing mutations, all but one (D169G) are in exon 6, and all but one (truncating mutation Y374X) are missense mutations (42,43). The mutations result in redistribution of TDP-43 from the nucleus to the cytoplasm in neurones and glia (37, 44) in the anterior horn of the spinal cord (45). *TARDBP* mutations account for about 3% of familial ALS and 1.5% of sporadic ALS (41).

Fused in sarcoma *gene*

Shortly after identification of the pivotal role of TDP-43 in ALS, linkage of other families with ALS to chromosome 16q12 resulted in the next major target for gene identification (46). Of the many genes in the target locus, one was similar to TDP-43, and screening of this candidate, *fused in sarcoma* (*FUS*) identified many mutations in two important studies, one from the UK and one from the USA (47,48). Most mutations appear to be missense and based in exons 14 and 15 (49). These exons code for the C-terminus, with the commonest being R521C, which disrupts RNA binding and transcription processing, leading to a toxic gain-of-function (6,47,50).

FUS protein is 526 amino acids long and structurally, functionally, and proteinopathically similar to TDP-43 (41). Indeed, it has been considered that they might be acting in concert in ALS pathology (51), although current evidence points towards them being mutually exclusive (Fig. 21.1). Inclusions immunoreactive for FUS have been located within nucleic and cytoplasmic regions in several studies (52,53). FUS^{WT} is multifunctional, and has been implicated in alternative splicing (54), genomic maintenance (55), and transcription factor regulation (56).

Interestingly, mutations of exons 3, 5, and 6 account for about a third of the mutations identified so far, and may be commoner in sporadic than familial ALS (57). This part of the gene codes for the glycine-rich N-terminal and may result in aberrant mRNA synthesis (58). *FUS* mutation is estimated to account for 4.4% of familial and 0.7% of sporadic ALS (47–50,57,59).

Optineurin

Using homozygosity mapping in consanguineous families, a region of chromosome 10 was implicated in ALS in a Japanese study (60). Mutation analysis of these and other samples from people with familial and sporadic ALS, revealed mutations in a gene known to cause primary open angle glaucoma, optineurin (*OPTN*). Mutations have been found in both familial and sporadic ALS, one missense autosomal dominant (E478G), and two autosomal recessive, a deletion of exon 5 and a non-sense mutation on exon 12 (Q398X) (60). In general, those with *OPTN* mutation had a slow progression of ALS. The mechanism through which the recessive and dominant mutations result in ALS may well be different, with a loss of function likely for the recessive, and a gain of function related to mislocalization of the OPTN protein possibly important for the dominant. The impact on OPTN protein of ALS and primary open angle glaucoma linked mutations is different,

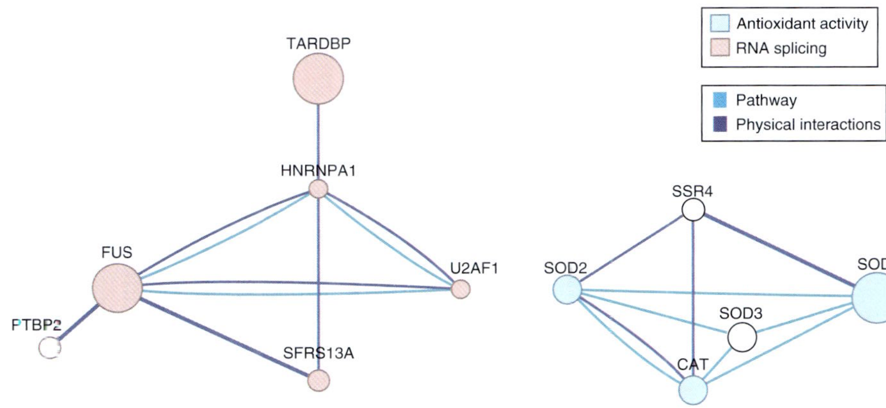

Fig. 21.1 Physical interactions and common pathways of FUS, TARDBP, and SOD1. Taken from GeneMANIA (135) (http://www.genemania.org). Query parameters were restricted to 10 genes with an automatic query-dependent weighting displaying physical interactions (96.48%) and common pathways (0.59%). Taken from The GeneMANIA prediction server: biological network integration for gene prioritization and predicting gene function Warde-Farley D, Donaldson SL, Comes O, Zuberi K, Badrawi R, Chao P, Franz M, Grouios C, Kazi F, Lopes CT, Maitland A, Mostafavi S, Montojo J, Shao Q, Wright G, Bader GD, Morris Q

with different effects on localization and different effects on nuclear factor κb signalling, and this is likely to be the reason for the difference in phenotypic expression.

Angiogenin

Angiogenin (*ANG*) on chromosome 14q11.2 was originally screened as a candidate gene in Irish and Scottish families with ALS because it shares a metabolic pathway with the vascular endothelial growth factor gene, *VEGF* (61) which is implicated in ALS (see below). Furthermore, it is in linkage disequilibrium with the apurinic endonuclease gene, *APEX1*, which was associated with ALS in other studies (62). Although *ANG* gene missense mutations have been found in affected individuals within families, linkage and segregation with disease have not been shown. *ANG* mutations have now been found in other European populations, including Italy (63), Germany (64), France (65), and Sweden (66,67). A common variant of *ANG*, rs11701, was found to be associated with sporadic ALS in Irish and Scottish populations, but has not been found in other populations (62).

D-amino oxidase gene

The D-amino oxidase gene, *DAO*, was found to be mutated in a family linked to chromosome 12q22–23. Functional studies support the pathogenic role of the mutation R199W, but other families have yet to be found harbouring mutations in this gene (68).

Valosin-containing protein gene

The valosin-containing protein gene, *VCP*, on chromosome 9 is involved in frontotemporal dementia with Paget's disease (69). A study using whole exome sequencing in Italian families with ALS has identified mutations in *VCP* with supporting functional evidence, and it seems likely that such mutations will be confirmed as a rare additional cause of ALS (70).

Genes causing atypical amyotrophic lateral sclerosis identified through family-based studies

Mutations of several genes have been found to cause atypical ALS, including the vesicle-associated membrane protein-associated protein B (*VAPB*) (71), which usually causes a lower motor neuron predominant variant of ALS, alsin (*ALS2*), which usually causes a form of young-onset hereditary spastic paraparesis (2,72,73), and senataxin (*SETX*), which causes a juvenile form of slowly progressive lower motor neuron ALS known as ALS4 (74).

Loci identified through family studies

A region on chromosome 9p21.2 has been linked to ALS with frontotemporal dementia in several studies (75–80), and also identified by association in a set of Finnish families. The genetic lesion has now been identified as a massive hexanucleotide repeat expansion (GGGGCC)n between exons 1a and 1b of the c9orf72 gene (where n is pathologically several hundred, compared with 2–8 on average in controls) and is the commonest cause of familial ALS, accounting for 30% to 50% of cases (81,82).

Genes identified through candidate gene association studies

Neurofilament heavy gene

Many genes have been proposed to be ALS susceptibility factors on the basis of association with ALS of common or rare variants within the gene (Fig. 21.2). One of the first such replicated findings was of indel mutations in the neurofilament heavy gene, *NFH* (83). Two studies found various deletions (83,84) and another study an insertion (85), all in the *NFH* tail domain, which contains a lysine-serine-proline repeat that is highly phosphorylated and involved in neurofilament assembly and spacing. All the indels were found in people with no family history of ALS, except one in someone with familial ALS (84), although segregation with disease could not be shown. Two other studies of familial ALS did not identify such variants (86,87), but this is consistent with the idea that *NFH* tail domain indels increase the general liability to ALS without being of sufficiently large effect to cause disease. A large study of familial and sporadic ALS examining all three neurofilament subunits did not identify any association of variants with ALS, but the *NFH* tail could not be amplified and was therefore excluded from the analysis (88,89).

Ataxin 2 gene

Spinocerebellar ataxia type 2, caused by triplet repeat expansion in the ataxin 2 (*ATXN2*) gene is associated with motor neuron degeneration in some case reports (90,91). ATXN2 protein expression is elevated in ALS spinal cords and it interacts with TDP-43 protein in a complex.

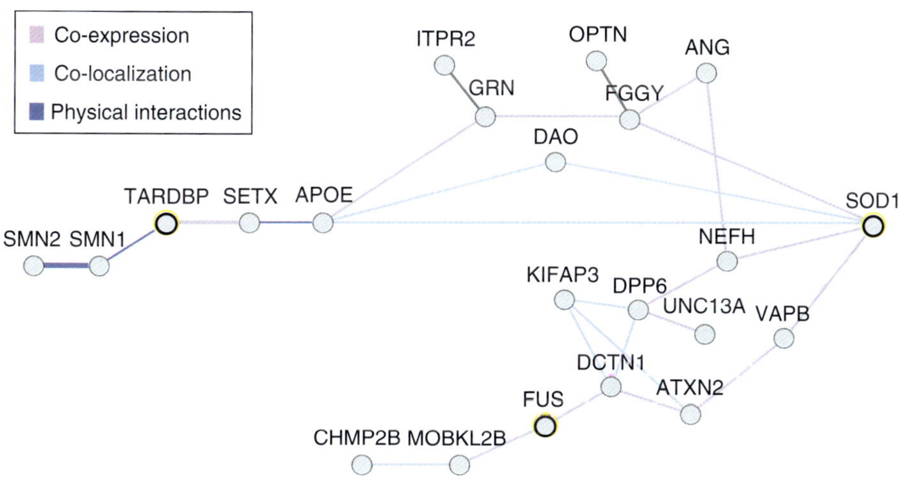

Fig. 21.2 ALS-related gene network based on co-expression, co-localization, and physical interaction. Taken from GeneMANIA (135) (http://www.genemania.org). Query parameters were restricted to 0 genes with an automatic query-dependent weighting displaying physical interactions (35.66%), co-localization (35.36%), and co-expression (28.98%). Taken from The GeneMANIA prediction server: biological network integration for gene prioritization and predicting gene function Warde-Farley D, Donaldson SL, Comes O, Zuberi K, Badrawi R, Chao P, Franz M, Grouios C, Kazi F, Lopes CT, Maitland A, Mostafavi S, Montojo J, Shao Q, Wright G, Bader GD, Morris Q

Furthermore, TDP-43 pathology is seen in spinocerebellar ataxia type 2, and ATXN2 is abnormally localized in ALS motor neurons (90). Thus, the *ATXN2* gene makes an excellent candidate for involvement in ALS. Expansions of the triplet repeat in *ATXN2* are large in spinocerebellar ataxia type 2 (more than 33 repeats), and normal in unaffected individuals (less than 27 repeats), whereas intermediate length polymorphisms increase the risk of ALS.

Survival motor neurone genes 1 and 2

The survival motor neurone genes, *SMN1* and *SMN2* are involved in the commonest childhood-onset motor neuron disease, spinal muscular atrophy (92). Homozygous deletion of *SMN1* causes spinal muscular atrophy with a phenotype that can be ameliorated by increased copies of the *SMN2* gene, which produces a less functional product (93). Copy number variation of *SMN1* appears to be a risk factor for ALS in some studies (94), although others do not find evidence for this (95), and it is not found in copy number analyses using genome-wide approaches (96–98).

Vascular endothelial growth factor gene

VEGF was identified as an ALS gene serendipitously. VEGF is involved in the vascular response to hypoxia and is therefore important in ischaemic heart disease (99–101). A mouse model of cardiovascular disease using knockout of the hypoxia response element of the *VEGF* gene had a phenotype with striking similarity to ALS (99) and a subsequent association study of the equivalent human single nucleotide polymorphisms (SNPs) found association in three of four populations studied, as well as in a joint analysis (102). These SNPs have not been associated with ALS in genome-wide association studies or replication studies and the original finding in humans may therefore have been false positive (103,104), although a second study suggested that the effect may be sex dependent (105,106). In any case, the mouse model provides evidence of the importance of VEGF to motor neurons and the rationale for generating a VEGF-based treatment.

Genes identified through genome-wide association studies of unrelated samples

Dipeptidyl peptidase 6 gene

There have been several independent genome-wide association studies in ALS, several of which have used a second cohort for replication of top hits (107–112). The first replicated gene variant implicated through such studies and achieving genome-wide significance was of the dipeptidyl peptidase 6 gene, *DPP6,* identified through a two-stage study of Dutch, Swedish, Belgian, and US samples (109). The same variant was the top hit in an Irish study but did not achieve genome-wide significance (105). Although this finding has been confirmed in an Italian study (113), subsequent joint analyses have not confirmed this association, but this may be a product of the winner's curse phenomenon (114), where an initial finding shows a higher effect size than subsequent studies.

Consistent with this idea, a weak signal not achieving genome-wide significance has been seen in association studies from samples of Italian (115,116), Polish (111), and Chinese (117) populations.

Inositol 1,4,5-triphosphate receptor type 2

Similarly, the *ITPR2* gene, coding for inositol 1,4,5-triphosphate receptor type 2, was associated with ALS in a Dutch population (108) and the finding confirmed within the same study on an independent population from Sweden, Belgium, and Holland. Again, subsequent studies have not confirmed this (116,118).

UNC13A

A large study using samples from many groups and again, with an internal replication sample, identified variation in the unc-13 homologue A (*Caenorhabditis elegans*) gene, *UNC13A* as strongly associated with ALS (110). This finding, while not confirmed in an independent study yet, still showed strong association in a joint analysis with samples from a third independent data set (112). The *UNC13A* gene is interesting because of the role of unc13 proteins in neurotransmitter release and influences on glutamatergic transmission particularly (119).

Chromosome 9p21.2

The same studies independently confirmed association with ALS of two variants on chromosome 9p21.2, rs3849942 and rs2814707, both in initial screens and on joint analysis (110,112). This region harbours three genes, Mps One Binder kinase activator-like 2B (*MOBKL2B*), interferon kappa (*IFNK*) and an open reading frame, *C9orf72*. This region had been previously implicated in familial ALS, and the genetic variant responsible is now known to be a massive hexanucleotide expansion of *c9orf72*, accounting for about 10% of apparently sporadic ALS.

Genes identified through other methods

Elongation protein 3 gene

The elongation protein 3 gene, *ELP3*, is part of a complex involved in RNA processing through elongation of messenger RNA, histone acetylation, and modification of transfer RNA wobble nucleosides (120–123). A study using microsatellites to perform genome-wide association in three populations identified variation in intron 10 of the *ELP3* gene associated with ALS (124). An independent mutagenesis study of *Drosophila* investigating the genes involved in axonal guidance and development, identified mutations of *ELP3* as a cause of defective neuronal guidance and function. Knockdown of *ELP3* in zebrafish resulted in defects of motor neuronal growth and branching. *ELP3* is a good candidate as an ALS gene because, like TDP-43, FUS, SMN, and ANG, it is involved in RNA processing, and defects of *ELP1* and *ELP4* cause familial dysautonomia and Rolandic epilepsy, two other neurodegenerative diseases (125,126).

Genes modifying phenotype

Kinesin-associated protein 3 and survival

A genome-wide study of ALS survival found variation in the kinesin-associated protein 3 (*KIFAP3*) gene was associated with a 14-month survival advantage (127). The study used clinic-based samples and a subsequent smaller study using population-based samples did not find evidence for the association (128). However, clinic populations exclude short survivors and it may be that the population-based study was therefore underpowered.

APOE *and age of onset*

There is evidence that age of onset of ALS is heritable based on a study of families with A4V and D90A *SOD1* mutations (129). The genetic basis of this is yet to be defined in detail but two studies have found an association between *APOE* genotype and age of onset of ALS (130,131).

In conclusion, genetic studies of ALS are beginning to shed light on the underlying pathways that lead to motor neuron degeneration. Axonal degeneration, synaptic signalling, and RNA processing are themes that are emerging. For example, TDP-43, FUS, ANG, SMN, and ELP3 are all RNA processing proteins. After a decade of effort at understanding ALS with models based on just one gene, *SOD1*, we now have many genes to build a picture of the pathogenic process with several more on the way. The relationship between ALS and frontotemporal dementia is becoming clearer as genes common and distinct for the two diseases become apparent, and with our greater understanding comes the hope that a new treatment will be generated.

References

1. Kurland LT, Mulder DW. (1955). Epidemiologic investigations of amyotrophic lateral sclerosis: 2. Familial aggregations indicative of dominant inheritance Part I. *Neurology*, **5**, 182–196.
2. Hentati A, Bejaoui K, Pericak-Vance MA, *et al.* (1994). Linkage of recessive familial amyotrophic lateral sclerosis to chromosome 2q33-q35. *Nat Genet*, **7**, 425–428.
3. Simpson CL, Al-Chalabi A. (2006). Amyotrophic lateral sclerosis as a complex genetic disease. *Biochim Biophys Acta*, **1762**(11–12), 973–985.
4. Fang F, Kamel F, Lichtenstein P, *et al.* (2009). Familial aggregation of amyotrophic lateral sclerosis. *Ann Neurol*, **66**(1), 94–99.
5. Johnston C, Stanton B, Turner M, *et al.* (2006). Amyotrophic lateral sclerosis in an urban setting: a population based study of inner city London. *J Neurol*, **253**, 1642–1643.
6. Pasinelli P, Brown RH. (2006). Molecular biology of amyotrophic lateral sclerosis: insights from genetics. *Nat Rev Neurosci*, **7**, 710–723.
7. Mulder DW, Kurland LT, Offord KP, Beard CM. (1986). Familial adult motor neuron disease: amyotrophic lateral sclerosis. *Neurology*, **36**, 511–517.
8. Robberecht WMDP, Aguirre TM, Van Den Bosch LP, *et al.* (1996). D90A heterozygosity in the SOD1 gene is associated with familial and apparently sporadic amyotrophic lateral sclerosis. *Neurology*, **47**, 1336–1339.
9. Al-Chalabi A, Fang F, Hanby MF, *et al.* (2010). An estimate of amyotrophic lateral sclerosis heritability using twin data. *J Neurol Neurosurg Psychiatry*, **81**, 1324–1326.
10. Wroe R, Wai-Ling Butler A, Andersen PM, *et al.* (2008). ALSOD: The Amyotrophic Lateral Sclerosis Online Database. *Amyotroph Lateral Scler*, **9**, 249–250.

11. Aran F. (1850). Recherches sur une maladie non encore decrite du systeme musculaire (atrophie musculaire progressive). *Arch Gen Med,* **14**, 5–35.
12. Siddique T, Figlewigz DA, Pericak-Vance MA, *et al.* (1991). Linkage of a gene causing familial amyotrophic lateral sclerosis to chromosome 21 and evidence of genetic-locus heterogeneity. *N Engl J Med,* **324**, 1381–1384.
13. Rosen DR, Siddique T, Patterson D, *et al.* (1993). Mutations in Cu/Zn superoxide dismutase gene are associated with familial amyotrophic lateral sclerosis. *Nature,* **362**, 59–62.
14. Turner BJ, Talbot K. (2008). Transgenics, toxicity and therapeutics in rodent models of mutant SOD1-mediated familial ALS. *Prog Neurobiol,* **85**, 94–134.
15. Shaw CE, Enayat ZE, Chioza BA, *et al.* (1998). Mutations in all five exons of SOD-1 may cause ALS. *Ann Neurol,* **43**, 390–394.
16. Valdmanis PNB, Rouleau GA. (2008). Genetics of familial amyotrophic lateral sclerosis. *Neurology,* **70**, 144–152.
17. Cudkowicz ME, McKenna-Yasek D, Sapp PE, *et al.* (1997). Epidemiology of mutations in superoxide dismutase in amyotrophic lateral sclerosis. *Ann Neurol,* **41**, 210–221.
18. Radunovíc A, Leigh PN. (1996). Cu/Zn superoxide dismutase gene mutations in amyotrophic lateral sclerosis: correlation between genotype and clinical features. *J Neurol Neurosurg Psychiatry,* **61**, 565–572.
19. Juneja T, Pericak-Vance MA, Laing NG, *et al.* (1997). Prognosis in familial amyotrophic lateral sclerosis. *Neurology,* **48**, 55–57.
20. Broom WJ, Johnson DV, Auwarter KE, *et al.* (2008). SOD1A4V-mediated ALS: absence of a closely linked modifier gene and origination in Asia. *Neurosci Lett,* **430**, 241–245.
21. DiDonato M, Craig L, Huff ME, *et al.* (2003). ALS mutants of human superoxide dismutase form fibrous aggregates via framework destabilization. *J Mol Biol,* **332**, 601–615.
22. Andersen PM, Forsgren L, Binzer M, *et al.* (1996). Autosomal recessive adult-onset amyotrophic lateral sclerosis associated with homozygosity for Asp90Ala CuZn-superoxide dismutase mutation. *Brain,* **119**, 1153–1172.
23. Al-Chalabi A, Andersen PM, Chioza B, *et al.* (1998). Recessive amyotrophic lateral sclerosis families with the D90A SOD1 mutation share a common founder: evidence for a linked protective factor. *Hum Mol Genet,* **7**, 2045–2050.
24. Själander A, Beckman G, Deng H-X, *et al.* (1995). The D90A mutation results in a polymorphism of Cu, Zn superoxide dismutase that is prevalent in northern Sweden and Finland. *Hum Mol Genet,* **4**, 1105–1108.
25. Gurney M, Pu H, Chiu A, *et al.* (1994). Motor neuron degeneration in mice that express a human Cu, Zn superoxide dismutase mutation. *Science,* **264**, 1772–1775.
26. Durham HD, Roy J, Dong L, Figlewicz DA. (1997). Aggregation of Mutant Cu/Zn Superoxide Dismutase Proteins in a Culture Model of ALS. *J Neuropathol Exp Neurol,* **56**, 523–530.
27. Higgins CMJ, Jung C, Ding H, Xu Z. (2002). Mutant Cu, Zn superoxide dismutase that causes motoneuron degeneration is present in mitochondria in the CNS. *J Neurosci,* **22**, 215.
28. Yim MB, Kang JH, Yim HS, *et al.* (1996). A gain-of-function of an amyotrophic lateral sclerosis-associated Cu, Zn-superoxide dismutase mutant: an enhancement of free radical formation due to a decrease in Km for hydrogen peroxide. *Proc Natl Acad Sci USA,* **93**, 5709–14.
29. Beckman JS, Estévez AG, Crow JP, Barbeito L. (2001). Superoxide dismutase and the death of motoneurons in ALS. *Trends Neurosci,* **24**, S15–S20.
30. Leigh P, Whitwell H, Garofalo O, *et al.* (1991). Ubiquitin-immunoreactive intraneuronal inclusions in amyotrophic lateral sclerosis. Morphology, distribution, and specificity. *Brain,* **114**, 775–788.
31. Lansbury PT, Lashuel HA. (2006). A century-old debate on protein aggregation and neurodegeneration enters the clinic. *Nature,* **443**, 774–779.

32. Sreedharan J, Blair I, Tripathi V, *et al.* (2008). TDP-43 mutations in familial and sporadic amyotrophic lateral sclerosis. *Science*, **319**, 1668–1672.
33. Gitcho MA, Baloh RH, Chakraverty S, *et al.* (2008). TDP-43 A315T mutation in familial motor neuron disease. *Ann Neurol*, **63**, 535–538.
34. Ou S, Wu F, Harrich D, Garcia-Martinez L, Gaynor R. (1995). Cloning and characterization of a novel cellular protein, TDP-43, that binds to human immunodeficiency virus type 1 TAR DNA sequence motifs. *J Virol*, **69**, 3584–3596.
35. Wang H-Y, Wang IF, Bose J, Shen CKJ. (2004). Structural diversity and functional implications of the eukaryotic TDP gene family. *Genomics*, **83**, 130–139.
36. Buratti E, Dork T, Zuccato E, *et al.* (2001). Nuclear factor TDP-43 and SR proteins promote *in vitro* and *in vivo* CFTR exon 9 skipping. *EMBO J*, **20**, 1774–1784.
37. Mackenzie I, Bigio E, Ince P, *et al.* (2007). Pathological TDP-43 distinguishes sporadic amyotrophic lateral sclerosis from amyotrophic lateral sclerosis with SOD1 mutations. *Ann Neurol*, **61**, 427–434.
38. Benajiba L, Le Ber I, Camuzat A, *et al.* (2009). TARDBP mutations in motoneuron disease with frontotemporal lobar degeneration. *Ann Neurol*, **65**, 470–473.
39. Buratti E, Brindisi A, Giombi M, *et al.* (2005). TDP-43 Binds heterogeneous nuclear ribonucleoprotein A/B through its C-terminal tail. *J Biol Chem*, **280**(45), 37572–37584.
40. Huang R, Fang D-F, Ma M-Y, *et al.* (2010). TARDBP gene mutations among Chinese patients with sporadic amyotrophic lateral sclerosis. *Neurobiol Aging*, Epub ahead of print.
41. Lagier-Tourenne C, Cleveland DW. (2009). Rethinking ALS: the FUS about TDP-43. *Cell*, **136**, 1001–1004.
42. Kabashi E, Valdmanis P, Dion P, *et al.* (2008). TARDBP mutations in individuals with sporadic and familial amyotrophic lateral sclerosis. *Nat Genet*, **40**, 572–574.
43. Daoud H, Valdmanis PN, Kabashi E, *et al.* (2009). Contribution of TARDBP mutations to sporadic amyotrophic lateral sclerosis. *J Med Genet*, **46**, 112–114.
44. Neumann M, Sampathu D, Kwong L, *et al.* (2006). Ubiquitinated TDP-43 in frontotemporal lobar degeneration and amyotrophic lateral sclerosis. *Science*, **314**, 130–133.
45. Van Deerlin VM, Leverenz JB, Bekris LM, *et al.* (2008). TARDBP mutations in amyotrophic lateral sclerosis with TDP-43 neuropathology: a genetic and histopathological analysis. *Lancet Neurol*, **7**, 409–416.
46. Ruddy DM, Parton MJ, Al-Chalabi A, *et al.* (2003). Two families with familial amyotrophic lateral sclerosis are linked to a novel locus on chromosome 16q. *Am J Hum Genet*, **73**, 390–396.
47. Vance C, Rogelj B, Hortobagyi T, *et al.* (2009). Mutations in FUS, an RNA processing protein, cause familial amyotrophic lateral sclerosis type 6. *Science*, **323**, 1208–1211.
48. Kwiatkowski TJ, Jr, Bosco DA, LeClerc AL, *et al.* Mutations in the FUS/TLS gene on chromosome 16 cause familial amyotrophic lateral sclerosis. *Science*, **323**, 1205–1208.
49. Mackenzie IRA, Rademakers R, Neumann M. (2010). TDP-43 and FUS in amyotrophic lateral sclerosis and frontotemporal dementia. *Lancet Neurol*, **9**, 995–1007.
50. Hewitt C, Kirby J, Highley JR, *et al.* (2010). Novel FUS/TLS mutations and pathology in familial and sporadic amyotrophic lateral sclerosis. *Arch Neurol*, **67**, 455–461.
51. Lagier-Tourenne C, Polymenidou M, Cleveland DW. (2010). TDP-43 and FUS/TLS: emerging roles in RNA processing and neurodegeneration. *Hum Mol Genet*, **19**(R1), R46–R64.
52. Munoz D, Neumann M, Kusaka H, *et al.* (2009). FUS pathology in basophilic inclusion body disease. *Acta Neuropathol*, **118**, 617–627.
53. Neumann M, Rademakers R, Roeber S, *et al.* (2009). A new subtype of frontotemporal lobar degeneration with FUS pathology. *Brain*, **132**, 2922–2931.

54. Yang L, Embree LJ, Tsai S, Hickstein DD. (1998). Oncoprotein TLS interacts with serine-arginine proteins involved in RNA splicing. *J Biol Chem*, **273**, 27761–4.
55. Hicks GG, Singh N, Nashabi A, *et al.* (2000). Fus deficiency in mice results in defective B-lymphocyte development and activation, high levels of chromosomal instability and perinatal death. *Nat Genet*, **24**, 175–179.
56. Uranishi H, Tetsuka T, Yamashita M, *et al.* (2001). Involvement of the pro-oncoprotein TLS (translocated in liposarcoma) in nuclear factor-κB p65-mediated transcription as a coactivator. *J Biol Chem*, **276**, 13395–13401.
57. Corrado L, Del Bo R, Castellotti B, *et al.* (2010). Mutations of FUS gene in sporadic amyotrophic lateral sclerosis. *J Med Genet*, **47**, 190–194.
58. Yang S, Warraich ST, Nicholson GA, Blair IP. (2010). Fused in sarcoma/translocated in liposarcoma: a multifunctional DNA/RNA binding protein. *Int J Biochem Cell Biol*, **42**, 1408–1411.
59. Millecamps S, Salachas F, Cazeneuve C, *et al.* (2010). SOD1, ANG, VAPB, TARDBP, and FUS mutations in familial amyotrophic lateral sclerosis: genotype–phenotype correlations. *J Med Genet*, **47**, 554–560.
60. Maruyama H, Morino H, Ito H, *et al.* (2010). Mutations of optineurin in amyotrophic lateral sclerosis. *Nature*, **465**, 223–226.
61. Greenway MJM, Alexander MDM, Ennis SP, *et al.* (2004). A novel candidate region for ALS on chromosome 14q11.2. *Neurology*, **63**, 1936–1938.
62. Hayward CP, Colville SB, Swingler RJMD, Brock DJHP. (1999). Molecular genetic analysis of the APEX nuclease gene in amyotrophic lateral sclerosis. *Neurology*, **52**, 1899–1901.
63. Gellera C, Colombrita C, Ticozzi N, *et al.* (2008). Identification of new ANG gene mutations in a large cohort of Italian patients with amyotrophic lateral sclerosis. *Neurogenetics*, **9**, 33–40.
64. Fernández-Santiago R, Hoenig S, Lichtner P, *et al.* (2009). Identification of novel Angiogenin gene missense variants in German patients with amyotrophic lateral sclerosis. *J Neurol*, **256**, 1337–1342.
65. Paubel A, Violette J, Amy M, *et al.* (2008). Mutations of the ANG gene in French patients with sporadic amyotrophic lateral sclerosis. *Arch Neurol*, **65**, 1333–1336.
66. McLaughlin RL, Phukan J, McCormack W, *et al.* (2010). Angiogenin levels and ANG genotypes: dysregulation in amyotrophic lateral sclerosis. *PLoS ONE*, **5**, e15402.
67. Greenway M, Andersen P, Russ C, *et al.* (2006). ANG mutations segregate with familial and 'sporadic' amyotrophic lateral sclerosis. *Nat Genet*, **38**, 411–413.
68. Mitchell J, Paul P, Chen H-J, *et al.* (2010). Familial amyotrophic lateral sclerosis is associated with a mutation in D-amino acid oxidase. *Proc Natl Acad Sci USA*, **107**, 7556–7561.
69. Watts GDJ, Wymer J, Kovach MJ, *et al.* (2004). Inclusion body myopathy associated with Paget disease of bone and frontotemporal dementia is caused by mutant valosin-containing protein. *Nat Genet*, **36**, 377–3781.
70. Johnson JO, Mandrioli J, Benatar M, *et al.* (2010). Exome sequencing reveals VCP mutations as a cause of familial ALS. *Neuron*, **68**, 857–864.
71. Nishimura A, Mitne-Neto M, Silva H, *et al.* (2004). A mutation in the vesicle-trafficking protein VAPB causes late-onset spinal muscular atrophy and amyotrophic lateral sclerosis. *Am J Hum Gene*, **75**, 822–831.
72. Hadano S, Hand C, Osuga H, *et al.* (2001). A gene encoding a putative GTPase regulator is mutated in familial amyotrophic lateral sclerosis 2. *Nat Genet*, **29**, 166–173.
73. Yang Y, Hentati A, Deng H, *et al.* (2001). The gene encoding alsin, a protein with three guanine nucleotide exchange factor domains, is mutated in a form of recessive amyotrophic lateral sclerosis. *Nat Genet*, **29**, 160–165.
74. Chen Y, Bennett C, Huynh H, *et al.* (2004). DNA/RNA helicase gene mutations in a form of juvenile amyotrophic lateral sclerosis (ALS4). *Am J Hum Genet*, **74**, 1128–1135.

75. Vance C, Al-Chalabi A, Ruddy D, *et al.* (2006). Familial amyotrophic lateral sclerosis with frontotemporal dementia is linked to a locus on chromosome 9p13.2–21.3. *Brain*, **129**, 868–876.
76. Morita M, Al-Chalabi A, Andersen PM, *et al.* (2006). A locus on chromosome 9p confers susceptibility to ALS and frontotemporal dementia. *Neurology*, **66**, 839–844.
77. Valdmanis PN, Dupre N, Bouchard J-P, *et al.* (2007). Three families with amyotrophic lateral sclerosis and frontotemporal dementia with evidence of linkage to chromosome 9p. *Arch Neurol*, **64**, 240–245.
78. Boxer AL, Mackenzie IR, Boeve BF, *et al.* (2011). Clinical, neuroimaging and neuropathological features of a new chromosome 9p-linked FTD-ALS family. *J Neurol Neurosurg Psychiatry*, **82**, 196–203.
79. Le Ber I, Camuzat A, Berger E, *et al.* (2009). Chromosome 9p-linked families with frontotemporal dementia associated with motor neuron disease. *Neurology*, **72**, 1669–1676.
80. Luty A, Kwok J, Thompson E, *et al.* (2008). Pedigree with frontotemporal lobar degeneration - motor neuron disease and Tar DNA binding protein-43 positive neuropathology: genetic linkage to chromosome 9. *BMC Neurol*, **8**, 32.
81. DeJesus-Hernandez M, Ian R, Mackenzie, *et al.* (2011). Expanded GGGGCC Hexanucleotide Repeat in Noncoding Region of C9ORF72 Causes Chromosome 9p-Linked FTD and ALS. *Neuron*, **72**(2), 245–256.
82. Renton, Alan E, Majounie E, *et al.* (2011). A Hexanucleotide Repeat Expansion in C9ORF72 Is the Cause of Chromosome 9p21-Linked ALS-FTD. *Neuron*, **72**(2), 257–268.
83. Figlewicz DA, Krizus A, Martinoli MG, *et al.* (1994). Variants of the heavy neurofilament subunit are associated with the development of amyotrophic lateral sclerosis. *Hum Mol Genet*, **3**, 1757–1761.
84. Al-Chalabi A, Andersen PM, Nilsson P, *et al.* (1999). Deletions of the heavy neurofilament subunit tail in amyotrophic lateral sclerosis. *Hum Mol Genet*, **8**, 157–164.
85. Tomkins J, Usher P, Slade J, *et al.* (1998). Novel insertion in the KSP region of the neurofilament heavy gene in amyotrophic lateral sclerosis (ALS). *Neuroreport*, **9**, 3967–3970.
86. Vechio JD, Bruijn LI, Xu Z, *et al.* (1996). Sequence variants in human neurofilament proteins: absence of linkage to familial amyotrophic lateral sclerosis. *Ann Neurol*, **40**, 603–610.
87. Rooke K, Figlewicz DA, Han F-Y, Rouleau GA. (1996). Analysis of the KSP repeat of the neurofilament heavy subunit in familial amyotrophic lateral sclerosis. *Neurology*, **46**, 789–790.
88. Garcia ML, Singleton AB, Hernandez D, *et al.* (2006). Mutations in neurofilament genes are not a significant primary cause of non-SOD1-mediated amyotrophic lateral sclerosis. *Neurobiol Dis*, **21**, 102–109.
89. Wong N, He B, Strong MJ. (2000). Characterization of neuronal intermediate filament protein expression in cervical spinal motor neurons in sporadic amyotrophic lateral sclerosis (ALS). *J Neuropathol Exp Neurol*, **59**, 972–982.
90. Elden AC, Kim H-J, Hart MP, *et al.* (2010). Ataxin-2 intermediate-length polyglutamine expansions are associated with increased risk for ALS. *Nature*, **466**, 1069–1075.
91. Nanetti L, Fancellu R, Tomasello C, *et al.* (2009). Rare association of motor neuron disease and spinocerebellar ataxia type 2 (SCA2): a new case and review of the literature. *J Neurol*, **256**, 1926–1928.
92. Lefebvre S, Bürglen L, Reboullet S, *et al.* (1995). Identification and characterization of a spinal muscular atrophy-determining gene. *Cell*, **80**, 155–165.
93. Parsons DW, McAndrew PE, Iannaccone ST, *et al.* (1998). Intragenic telSMN mutations: frequency, distribution, evidence of a founder effect, and modification of the spinal muscular atrophy phenotype by cenSMN copy number. *Am J Hum Genet*, **63**, 1712–1723.
94. Corcia P, Mayeux-Portas V, Khoris J, *et al.* (2002). Abnormal SMN1 gene copy number is a susceptibility factor for amyotrophic lateral sclerosis. *Ann Neurol*, **51**, 243–246.
95. Corcia P, Camu W, Halimi JM, *et al.* (2006). SMN1 gene, but not SMN2, is a risk factor for sporadic ALS. *Neurology*, **67**, 1147–1150.

96. Blauw HM, Al-Chalabi A, Andersen PM, *et al.* (2010). A large genome scan for rare CNVs in amyotrophic lateral sclerosis. *Hum Mol Genet,* **19**, 4091–4099.
97. Cronin S, Blauw HM, Veldink JH, *et al.* (2008). Analysis of genome-wide copy number variation in Irish and Dutch ALS populations. *Hum Mol Genet,* **17**, 3392–3398.
98. Wain LV, Pedroso I, Landers JE, *et al.* (2009). The role of copy number variation in susceptibility to amyotrophic lateral sclerosis: genome-wide association study and comparison with published loci. *PLoS ONE*, **4**, e8175.
99. Oosthuyse B, Moons L, Storkebaum E, *et al.* (2001). Deletion of the hypoxia-response element in the vascular endothelial growth factor promoter causes motor neuron degeneration. *Nat Genet,* **28**, 131–138.
100. Subramanian V, Crabtree B, Acharya KR. (2008). Human angiogenin is a neuroprotective factor and amyotrophic lateral sclerosis associated angiogenin variants affect neurite extension/pathfinding and survival of motor neurons. *Hum Mol Genet,* **17**, 130–149.
101. Kieran D, Sebastia J, Greenway MJ, *et al.* (2008). Control of motoneuron survival by angiogenin. *J Neurosci*, **28**, 14056–14061.
102. Lambrechts D, Storkebaum E, Morimoto M, *et al.* (2003). VEGF is a modifier of amyotrophic lateral sclerosis in mice and humans and protects motoneurons against ischemic death. *Nat Genet*, **34**, 383–394.
103. Van Vught PWJ, Sutedja NA, Veldink JH, *et al.* (2005). Lack of association between VEGF polymorphisms and ALS in a Dutch population. *Neurology*, **65**, 1643–1645.
104. Chen WM, Saeed MM, Mao HMM, *et al.* (2006). Lack of association of VEGF promoter polymorphisms with sporadic ALS. *Neurology*, **67**, 508–510.
105. Fernández-Santiago R, Sharma M, Mueller JC, *et al.* (2006). Possible gender-dependent association of vascular endothelial growth factor (VEGF) gene and ALS. *Neurology*, **66**, 1929–1931.
106. Lambrechts D, Poesen K, Fernández-Santiago R, *et al.* (2009). Meta-analysis of vascular endothelial growth factor variations in amyotrophic lateral sclerosis: increased susceptibility in male carriers of the −2578AA genotype. *J Med Genet*, **46**, 840–846.
107. Cronin S, Berger S, Ding J, *et al.* (2008). A genome-wide association study of sporadic ALS in a homogenous Irish population. *Hum Mol Genet,* **17**, 768–774.
108. van Es MA, Van Vught PW, Blauw HM, *et al.* (2007). ITPR2 as a susceptibility gene in sporadic amyotrophic lateral sclerosis: a genome-wide association study. *Lancet Neurol*, **6**, 869–877.
109. van Es MA, van Vught PWJ, Blauw HM, *et al.* (2008). Genetic variation in DPP6 is associated with susceptibility to amyotrophic lateral sclerosis. *Nat Genet,* **40**, 29–31.
110. van Es MA, Veldink JH, Saris CGJ, *et al.* (2009). Genome-wide association study identifies 19p13.3 (UNC13A) and 9p21.2 as susceptibility loci for sporadic amyotrophic lateral sclerosis. *Nat Genet*, **41**, 1083–1087.
111. Cronin S, Tomik B, Bradley DG, *et al.* (2008). Screening for replication of genome-wide SNP associations in sporadic ALS. *Eur J Hum Genet*, **17**, 213–218.
112. Shatunov A, Mok K, Newhouse S, *et al.* (2010). Chromosome 9p21 in sporadic amyotrophic lateral sclerosis in the UK and seven other countries: a genome-wide association study. *Lancet Neurol,* **9**, 986–994.
113. Bo RD, Ghezzi S, Corti S, *et al.* (2008). DPP6 gene variability confers increased risk of developing sporadic amyotrophic lateral sclerosis in Italian patients. *J Neurol Neurosurg Psychiatry,* **79**, 1085.
114. Zhong H, Prentice RL. (2010). Correcting 'winner's curse' in odds ratios from genomewide association findings for major complex human diseases. *Genet Epidemiol*, **34**, 78–91.
115. Fogh I, D'Alfonso S, Gellera C, *et al.* (2011). No association of DPP6 with amyotrophic lateral sclerosis in an Italian population. *Neurobiol Aging*, **32**(5), 966–967.
116. Chiò A, Schymick JC, Restagno G, *et al.* (2009). A two-stage genome-wide association study of sporadic amyotrophic lateral sclerosis. *Hum Mol Genet,* **18**, 1524–1532.

117. Xiao-guang L, Jiang-hu Z, Man-qing X, *et al.* (2009). Association between DPP6 polymorphism and the risk of sporadic amyotrophic lateral sclerosis in Chinese patients. *Chin Med J*, **122**, 2989–2992.
118. Fernández-Santiago R, Sharma M, *et al.* (2011). No evidence of association of FLJ10986 and ITPR2 with ALS in a large German cohort. *Neurobiol Aging*, **32**(3), 551.e1–4.
119. Varoqueaux F, Sons MS, Plomp JJ, Brose N. (2005). Aberrant morphology and residual transmitter release at the Munc13-deficient mouse neuromuscular synapse. *Mol Cell Biol*, **25**, 5973–5984.
120. Hawkes NA, Otero G, Winkler GS, *et al.* (2002). Purification and characterization of the human elongator complex. *J Biol Chem*, **277**, 3047–3052.
121. Winkler GS, Petrakis TG, Ethelberg S, *et al.* (2001). RNA polymerase II elongator holoenzyme is composed of two discrete subcomplexes. *J Biol Chem*, **276**, 32743–32749.
122. Winkler GS, Kristjuhan A, Erdjument-Bromage H, *et al.* (2002). Elongator is a histone H3 and H4 acetyltransferase important for normal histone acetylation levels *in vivo*. *Proc Natl Acad Sci USA*, **99**, 3517–3522.
123. Huang B, Johansson MJO, Bystrom AS. (2005). An early step in wobble uridine tRNA modification requires the Elongator complex. *RNA*, **11**, 424–436.
124. Simpson CL, Lemmens R, Miskiewicz K, *et al.* (2009). Variants of the elongator protein 3 (ELP3). gene are associated with motor neuron degeneration. *Hum Mol Genet*, **18**, 472–481.
125. Anderson SL, Coli R, Daly IW, *et al.* (2001). Familial dysautonomia is caused by mutations of the IKAP gene. *Am J Hum Genet*, **68**, 753–758.
126. Barton D, Braet F, Marc J, *et al.* (2009). ELP3 localises to mitochondria and actin-rich domains at edges of HeLa cells. *Neurosci Lett*, **455**, 60–64.
127. Landers JE, Melki J, Meininger V, *et al.* (2009). Reduced expression of the Kinesin-Associated Protein 3 (KIFAP3) gene increases survival in sporadic amyotrophic lateral sclerosis. *Proc Natl Acad Sci USA*, **106**, 9004–9009.
128. Traynor BJ, Nalls M, Lai S-L, *et al.* (2010). Kinesin-associated protein 3 (KIFAP3) has no effect on survival in a population-based cohort of ALS patients. *Proc Natl Acad Sci USA*, **107**, 12335–12338.
129. Fogh I, Rijsdijk F, Andersen P, *et al.* (2007). Age at onset in sod1-mediated amyotrophic lateral sclerosis shows familiality. *Neurogenetics*, **8**, 235–236.
130. Moulard B, Sefiani A, Laamri A, *et al.* (1996). Apolipoprotein E genotyping in sporadic amyotrophic lateral sclerosis: evidence for a major influence on the clinical presentation and prognosis. *J Neurol Sci*, **139**(Suppl. 1), 34–7.
131. Zetterberg H, Jacobsson J, Rosengren L, *et al.* (2008). Association of APOE with age at onset of sporadic amyotrophic lateral sclerosis. *J Neurol Sci*, **273**, 67–69.
132. Hand CK, Khoris J, Salachas F, *et al.* (2002). A novel locus for familial amyotrophic lateral sclerosis, on chromosome 18q. *Am J Hum Genet*, **70**, 251–256.
133. Sapp PC, Hosler BA, McKenna-Yasek D, *et al.* (2003). Identification of two novel loci for dominantly inherited familial amyotrophic lateral sclerosis. *Am J Hum Genet*, **73**, 397–403.
134. Chow CY, Landers JE, Bergren SK, *et al.* (2009). Deleterious variants of FIG4, a phosphoinositide phosphatase, in patients with ALS. *Am J Hum Genet*, **84**, 85–88.
135. Laaksovirta H, Peuralinna T, Schymick JC, *et al.* (2010). Chromosome 9p21 in amyotrophic lateral sclerosis in Finland: a genome-wide association study. *Lancet Neurol*, **9**, 978–985.
136. Warde-Farley D, Donaldson SL, Comes O, *et al.* (2010). The GeneMANIA prediction server: biological network integration for gene prioritization and predicting gene function. *Nucleic Acids Res*, **38**(Suppl 2), W214–W20.

Chapter 22

Perturbed RNA metabolism in amyotrophic lateral sclerosis

Kathryn Volkening and Michael J. Strong

The discovery of the involvement of the RNA-binding proteins transactive response DNA-binding protein of 43 kDa (TDP-43) and *FUS/TLS* in ALS (1–4) has given rise to the possibility that ALS is a disorder of RNA metabolism (5). Before these discoveries, it was known that ALS affected motor neurones have a selective decrease in polyadenylated mRNA and low molecular weight neurofilament (NFL) mRNA levels while sparing those of medium molecular weight neurofilament (NFM) and high molecular weight neurofilament (NFH) (6,7). That this selective NF stoichiometry alteration is of pathological relevance to ALS is supported by murine models in which NF stoichiometry was disrupted by either overexpressing NFH or knocking out or disrupting NFL expression and produce neuronal NF aggregates similar to those found in ALS (8–10). The presence of NF aggregates predisposes neurones to risk of oxidative stress, excitotoxicity, and cell death (11–15). To understand the isolated reductions of NFL mRNA in ALS, we have focused on defining the complex of proteins that regulate NFL mRNA stability and how these differ between ALS and healthy control tissues (16–20).

RNA metabolism

Messenger (m)RNA was once thought to be a simple, transient, expendable intermediate between the genetic coding of DNA and mature protein; however, it is now clear that RNA metabolism is a tightly controlled, complex cellular process. This process incorporates a highly regulated balance between transcription and degradation, via the activity of RNA polymerases, the presence or absence of enhancers and repressors of transcription, and expression of the machinery required to stabilize, transport, sequester, translate, and degrade mRNA. Changes in any of these may produce a marked change in both RNA and protein expression. In neurones, recent data have suggested that many neuronal gene expression levels are controlled mainly through the rate of RNA degradation (21).

A multitude of proteins and small non-coding (nc)RNA are associated with mRNA throughout its life cycle. The resulting protein/mRNA/ncRNA complexes form the RNA binding protein complex (RNA granule or RNP complex). Although the proteins found in RNPs are extremely varied in their nature, they usually fall into one of several groups. One group interacts with the 5′ 7-methylguanosine cap of mRNA (for example, the eIF family members, gemin5 (22,23)). Another group targets the 3′-poly(A) tail found on most mRNA (poly(A) binding protein (PABP) family, deadenylating proteins). Other proteins associate in a manner dependent on transcript sequences (*cis* elements) most commonly found in the 3′- and 5′-untranslated regions (UTRs), but occasionally in intronic or coding regions. Depending on the function of the *cis* and *trans* elements (protein or microRNA (miRNA) that interacts with the *cis* element), mRNA stabilization or destabilization may occur. For example, the embryonic lethal and abnormal vision (ELAV)-like proteins, PABP and Hu proteins all tend to stabilize (21,24–26) while tristetraproline (27,28), AU-rich RNA binding protein (RBP), also known as heterogeneous nuclear ribonucleoprotein D (29) and K-homology splicing regulatory protein (30) tend to destabilize transcripts. The final set of proteins function as adapters between proteins and/or cellular machinery required for mRNA processing. The vast majority of RNPs require some level of specificity for interaction—either a specific structure or sequence of the mRNA, or specific recruitment to another protein within the complex. Post-translational modifications, including phosphorylation and competing interactions with other proteins or mRNA, can greatly influence these interactions.

A simplified schematic of mRNA metabolism is shown in Figure 22.1. Pre-mRNA is transcribed from DNA by RNA polymerase II, then intronic regions removed by the spliceosome and the resultant mRNA bundled into a RNP complex. The RNP complex is exported and modified into specific granules targeted for transport, storage, translation, or degradation.

Transport granules are translationally quiescent RNA granules that contain the kinesin family of molecular motors, allowing for anterograde transport (31). RNPs may also be retrogradely transported using the dynein family of molecular motors (32). Stress granules store mRNA in a translationally quiescent state until such time as the protein product is required, or they may transition to P-bodies and target mRNA for degradation. Although stress granules may contain ribosomes, stalled initiation prevents translation (33). It also appears that P-bodies may transition to translationally active ribosomal complexes (34).

While mRNA degradation can occur by 3′–5′ and 5′–3′ mechanisms, these processes are distinct from each other and occur in either the exosome (3′–5′) (35) or in P-bodies (5′–3′) (36). Some mRNA destabilizing proteins act to recruit the exosome to transcripts, allowing helicases to unwind the transcript and 3′–5′ exonucleases to degrade the predominantly AU-rich RNA that appear to be preferentially degraded in the exosome (37,38). This method is widely used in RNA quality control (35). P-bodies are granules in which mRNA 5′–3′ degradation occurs (39), and are characterized by the presence of XRN1 exonuclease, GW182 RBP and decapping-associated enzymes and proteins (36,40). P-bodies are translationally quiescent and do not contain ribosomes (41).

miRNA (Figure 22.2) are increasingly recognized as being key to regulating mRNA stability. They are transcribed from non-coding regions of DNA (or rarely intronic regions) as pri-miRNA (42), cleaved by Drosha/DGCR8 into smaller 70–85 nt fragments

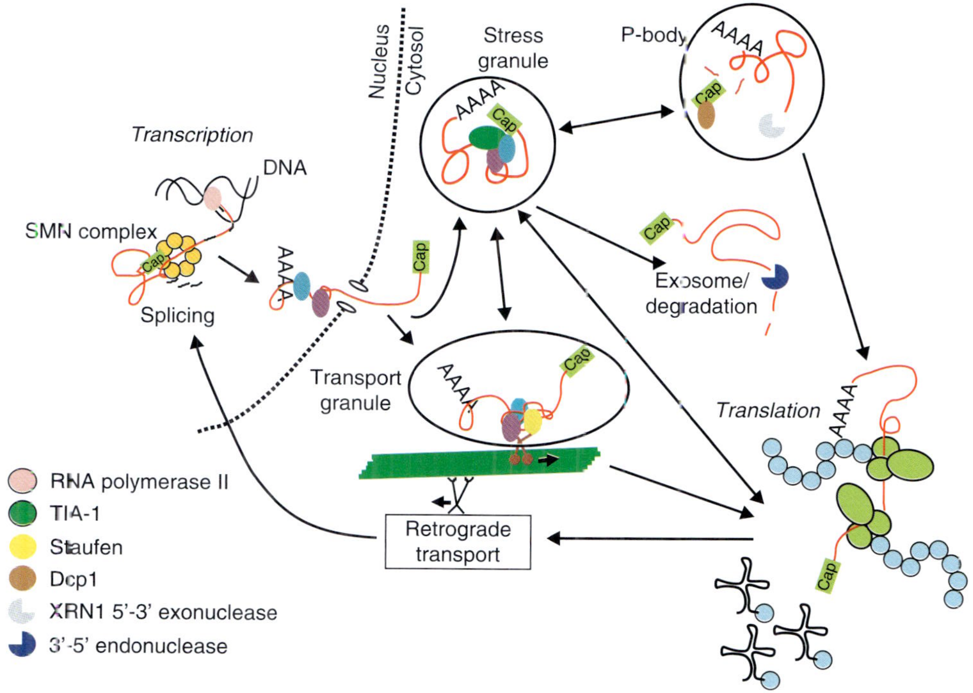

Fig. 22.1 Schematic of the mRNA metabolism pathway. RNA is transcribed, spliced in the spliceosome, exported, and the RNP formed depending on the function and requirements for the mRNA. Transport followed by translation in polysomal complexes is usual if the protein is required, while inclusion into translationally quiescent stress granules occurs if the protein is not required immediately. In the event that the mRNA is not required and must be degraded, as in cases of mRNA surveillance or extreme cellular stress, mRNA may be sent to the exosome for degradation, or degraded in P-bodies.

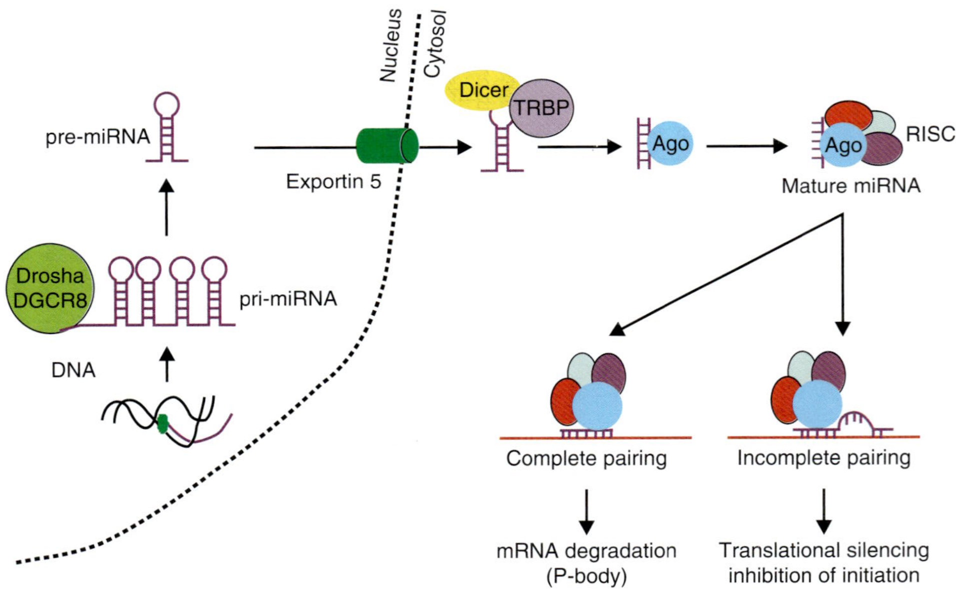

Fig. 22.2 Schematic of the microRNA pathway. MiRNA is transcribed as pri-mRNA, which are processed by cleavage by Drosha/DGCR8 to pre-miRNA. These are exported via Exportin5 to the cytosol, where Dicer/TRBP further process the miRNA. The RISC complex is formed with final maturation to a single-stranded miRNA, which then pairs with the mRNA target determining its degradation or translational silencing.

(pre-miRNA), exported by Exportin 5, and then cleaved by Dicer/TAR RBP (TRBP) (43,44). Ago is recruited to the resulting double-stranded structure, RISC (RNA-induced silencing complex) is assembled, the complementary strand degraded to leave the mature miRNA, and this complex is incorporated into the RNP (45,46). The miRNA base pairs with its *cis* mRNA recognition element (MRE) through the 5′ six to seven nucleotides of the miRNA. If complete complementarity exists the mRNA is targeted for degradation while incomplete complementarity leads to translational silencing through the inhibition of translation initiation (47). Rarely, miRNA interactions lead to enhanced translational (48). The presence of a poly(A) tail, PABP, and mRNA capping can decrease miRNA activity (49). Because miRNA recognition elements are common across mRNA, multiple miRNAs can affect the overall stability of any given mRNA and one class of miRNA may regulate many unrelated mRNA.

Linking amyotrophic lateral sclerosis with RNA metabolism

To date, several gene products have been linked to ALS or frontotemporal dementia–ALS. Of specific note, many of these proteins have a direct role in the regulation of RNA metabolism (Figure 22.3). In this next section, we will briefly describe each of these and their putative site of activity.

Transactive response DNA-binding protein of 43 kDa

TDP-43 is found in RNA and nuclear granules (50,51), can interact with DNA and RNA, is found in the spliceosome, and appears to be associated with miRNA processing (52–56). We have shown that the expression of TDP-43 is significantly upregulated and is associated with stress granules following either sciatic nerve axotomy or crush, suggesting that TDP-43 is an injury responsive factor (57,58). As reviewed elsewhere, in ALS TDP-43 expression is both upregulated and forms pathological skein-like structures in degenerating motor neurones where it is also preferentially associated with translationally quiescent granules (20). ALS-associated mutations have been identified in the glycine-rich region and C-terminal region, as well as one in the RRM1 domain (59–64). Three of these mutations have been shown to contribute to motor neurone deficits in zebrafish (65). The RRM1 mutation would be predicted to affect mRNA interaction, while other mutations would be predicted to have effects on protein–protein interaction, or overall protein structure.

FUS/TLS

FUS/TLS is a dual DNA/RBP, with similar RNA recognition motifs to those of TDP-43 (66). *FUS/TLS* is part of the heterogeneous nuclear ribonucleoprotein D complex responsible for pre-mRNA splicing and RNA export from the nucleus (66), interacts with Drosha, and participates in miRNA processing (43). ALS-associated mutations are predominantly clustered to the C-terminal region of the protein (3,4) and may disrupt RNP structure/function.

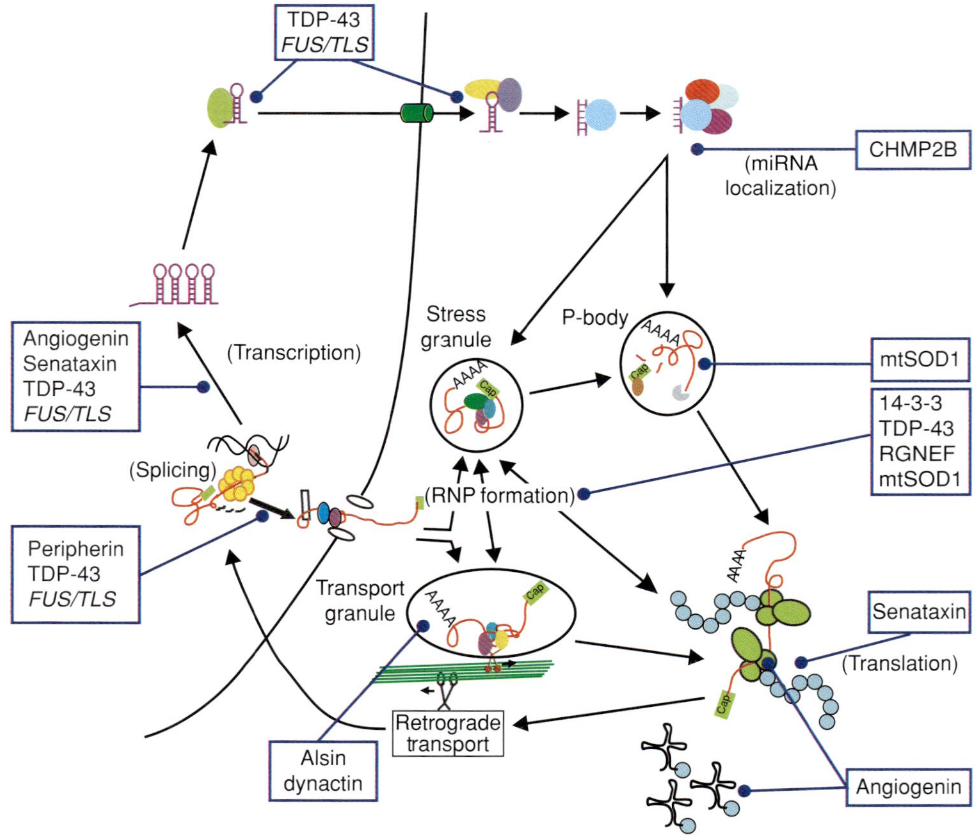

Fig.22.3 Compilation of Figures 22.1 and 22.2 showing the impact of ALS associated gene products on the mRNA metabolism pathway. Note that one protein may interfere with the mRNA metabolism pathway at several distinct events. For example, TDP-43 may influence transcription, splicing, miRNA production, and RNP formation, providing many avenues by which TDP-43 abnormalities may affect processing.

p190RhoGEF/RGNEF

Murine p190RhoGEF is a critical determinant of NF aggregate formation in the mouse (67,68). Normally, p190RhoGEF associates with NFL mRNA and imparts stability (67) but is sequestered to NFL protein subunits, removing it from the stabilizing RNP causing downregulation of NFL mRNA expression (68). Recently we have identified a human homologue to p190RhoGEF, called RGNEF, that interacts with human NFL mRNA only in ALS lysates and not in controls in *in vitro* assays (19).

Mutant SOD1

The first genetic linkage to ALS was made to mutations in the *SOD1* gene (69). While wild-type *SOD1* did not appear to interact with NFL mRNA, several mutant (mt)SOD1 forms interacted robustly and resulted in transcript destabilization (17). Destabilization of vascular endothelial growth factor (VEGF) and interleukin-8 mRNA by mtSOD1 has also been described (70,71) suggesting that this is a common action of this protein.

Alsin

Alsin is expressed as multiple splice variants, of which one form (ALS–LF) interacts with mtSOD1^{A4T}, mtSOD1^{G85R}, and mtSOD1^{G93A} (72). Knockout mice for alsin have defects in axonal transport (73).

CHMP2B

CHMP2B is a subunit of the endosomal sorting complexes required for transport (ESCRT). Mutations have been described in ALS and frontotemporal dementia (74,75), and may be related to faulty protein processing allowing the build-up of protein aggregates in cells (76). In *Drosophila* Huntington's disease models, decreased ESCRT levels cause a decrease in aggregate clearance (77,78). ESCRT proteins are involved in mRNA localization (79), miRNA production and localization, small RNA silencing processes (80,81), and autophagy (76).

Dynactin

Dynactin serves to link microtubules and cargos during dynein-mediated retrograde transport (82–84). Mutations have been associated with ALS (85,86) and appear to be localized to the N-terminal CAP-Gly region, which may disrupt dynein–dynactin complex association with microtubules, impair co-ordinated movement of the complex on microtubules (87,88), or prevent long-distance travel through drop-off of the complex from microtubules (88).

Peripherin

Peripherin has been described in neuronal inclusions in ALS (89). A splice variant of 61 kDa (Per61), in which retention of intron 4 results in a 32 amino acid insertion, is expressed abnormally in the mtSOD1 mouse model of ALS (90). In patients with ALS, a 28 kDa form of peripherin (Per28) is expressed through retention of introns 3 and 4, with intron 3 encoding a premature stop codon. When this variant is expressed in SW13 vimentin–/– cells or primary motor neurones, peripherin forms inclusions (91). Per28 was detected in human ALS spinal cord, co-localized with TDP-43 and peripherin (92). Taken together these data seem to point to abnormal splicing in ALS.

EAAT2

The astrocytic glutamate transporter EAAT2 is expressed as several splice variants, which may or may not be specific to ALS (93–96). Lauriat and McInnes determined that there was increased expression of a splice variant with a shortened 3′-UTR and EAAT2 variant b (EAAT2b) in the motor cortex in ALS (97). Shortening the 3′-UTR suggests that alterations in RBP recruitment may occur due to loss of normal *cis* elements. Another splice variant (HBGTII 5′ variant) bearing a longer 5′-UTR encoding an open reading frame was found to be upregulated in ALS. The longer 5′-UTR of this transcript may recruit ectopic RBPs and induce abnormal termination of translation through premature ribosome dissociation (97).

Progranulin

Progranulin mediates caspase cleavage of TDP-43 into 25 and 35 kDa forms detected in ALS and FTLD (98). Mutations in progranulin (including premature stop codons, frameshift mutations, deletions, exon–intron junction splice consensus site mutations) are thought to lead to haploinsufficiency through abnormal RNA processing (99–101).

Senataxin

Mutations in SETX have been described in a juvenile onset form of ALS (102). SETX encodes for a DNA/RNA helicase, a family of proteins required to unwind double-stranded DNA for repair or transcription and RNA (either RNA–RNA complexes or folded RNA) during both splicing and translation (103–105). Mutations in SETX have been postulated to result in dysfunction of helicase activity affecting DNA/RNA processing (102,106).

Angiogenin

Angiogenin interacts with the promoter region of ribosomal DNA sequences and modulates the transcription of ribosomal RNA (107). It is also a ribonucleolytic protein that can cleave transfer RNA and inhibit translation (108). Mutations in the protein have been described in both ALS and FTLD (109) and are thought to be associated with loss of function through either a dominant negative effect or through inhibition of angiogenesis (110,111). It is interesting to note that while mtSOD1 can destabilize VEGF mRNA, angiogenin is integral in modulating the transcription of VEGF mRNA (112).

14-3-3 proteins

14-3-3 proteins are ubiquitously expressed proteins that can interact with NFL mRNA (16). This family of proteins interacts with a multitude of other proteins, so it is probable that 14-3-3 proteins serve as scaffolding proteins in RNPs.

MicroRNA

Very little is known to date about the miRNA profile of ALS or FTLD. One study has determined that miR-206 is upregulated in ALS and miR-206–/– mice crossed to mtSOD1^{G93A} mice showed that miR-206 deficiency led to accelerated disease course, while miR-206 could aid in muscle reinnervation via the fibroblast growth factor signalling cascade (113).

Downstream effects

As can be seen by the complexity of the RNA metabolism pathways, the sheer number of events that could result in abnormal RNA processing, and the fact that many ALS linked proteins function in RNA metabolism, it follows that changes in these proteins could have profound effects on cellular functions. It will be important to determine the cargos and downstream targets affected by abnormal RNA processing in ALS to understand the disease mechanism. While RNA expression microarray approaches are well suited to these studies, the heterogeneity of disease tissues contributes to wide variation of RNA quality, quantity, and yields. Future studies will have to take into account that RBPs may interact with many mRNAs and small alterations in interactions may significantly affect cargos and downstream signalling pathways.

There are several mechanisms through which alterations in RNA metabolism may exert a physiological effect (Figure 22.4). First, sequestration of mRNA by abnormal, mutated, or overexpressed RBPs can either remove mRNA from the translationally competent pool or cause them to be overproduced through increased translation. Second, the absence of an RBP may allow for mRNA interaction with another RBP, which would not normally interact in the presence of the first protein. Third, the removal or mis-expression of proteins can exert specific effects on particular steps within the pathway, producing widespread downstream effects in a tissue-specific manner.

Spinal muscular atrophy is a prime example. The gene encoding SMN1 is deleted or mutated and causes a deficiency in normally functioning SMN1 protein (114). The SMN2 gene is alternatively spliced so that full length protein levels are insufficient (115), resulting in abnormalities in the SMN complex required for normal RNA splicing. In different tissues within the same individual, different patterns of splicing are seen.

In contrast, myotonic dystrophy is characterized by an expanded CUG repeat in the 3′ UTR of mRNA from the *DMPK* gene (116). These repeats abnormally sequester the muscleblind-like family of splicing regulators, which results in abnormal splicing of a large number of transcripts required for normal cellular functioning (117–119). Both outcomes lead to widespread splicing abnormalities and disease but in subtly different ways.

In ALS, alterations in RBPs may sequester mRNA preventing translation, or may leave mRNA open to alternative protein binding partners resulting in abnormal processing. It is also probable that mutations affect RNP complexes, through abnormal recruitment of proteins not normally found in the complex, or failure of recruitment of proteins, or failure to recruit proper cargo to the complex. Much more research is required to determine what downstream processes are affected; however, it seems clear that RNA metabolism is

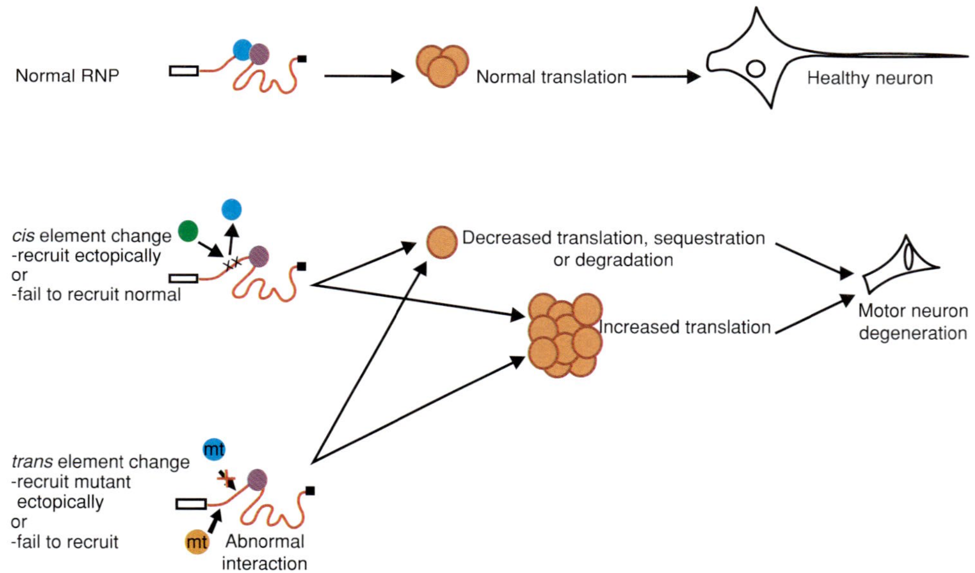

Fig. 22.4 Schematic depicting the several ways that alterations in either *cis* or *trans* elements may affect mRNA processing. With *cis* element changes proteins may be ectopically recruited, binding proteins that normally interact may not be recruited (or a combination of the two) resulting in abnormal protein production from the transcript. In *trans* element changes a mutated protein may ectopically interact with a region on the mRNA that is not a usual functioning *cis* element, or may not interact as it normally would, producing changes in mRNA metabolism leading to abnormal protein production. As many different changes may be elicited (as seen in Figure 22.3), the phenotype of the affected individual may vary drastically depending on where in the RNA pathway these changes occur; however, the outcome (cell death) may remain unchanged.

integrally intertwined with the disease process in ALS, and determining how to manipulate this system—either upstream or downstream of the RBPs—will be key to novel treatments for this disease.

Acknowledgements

Research supported by the ALS Society of Canada (Senior Investigator Bridge grant) and by the Canadian Institutes of Health Research. Many thanks to Dr C. Droppelmann for creative and fruitful discussions.

References

1. Arai T, Hasegawa M, Akiyama H, *et al.* (2006). TDP-43 is a component of ubiquitin-positive tau-negative inclusions in frontotemporal lobar degeneration and amyotrophic lateral sclerosis. *Biochem Biophys Res Commun*, **351**(3), 602–611.
2. Neumann M, Sampathu DM, Kwong LK, *et al.* (2006). Ubiquitinated TDP-43 in frontotemporal lobar degeneration and amyotrophic lateral sclerosis. *Science*, **314**(5796), 130–133.
3. Kwiatkowski TJ, Jr, Bosco DA, Leclerc AL, *et al.* (2009). Mutations in the FUS/TLS gene on chromosome 16 cause familial amyotrophic lateral sclerosis. *Science*, **323**(5918), 1205–1208.
4. Vance C, Rogelj B, Hortobagyi T, *et al.* (2009). Mutations in FUS, an RNA processing protein, cause familial amyotrophic lateral sclerosis type 6. *Science*, **323**(5918), 1208–1211.
5. Strong MJ. (2010). The evidence for altered RNA metabolism in amyotrophic lateral sclerosis (ALS). *J Neurol Sci*, **288**(1–2), 1–12.
6. Bergeron C, Beric-Maskarel K, Muntasser S, Weyer L, Somerville MJ, Percy ME. (1994). Neurofilament light and polyadenylated mRNA levels are decreased in amyotrophic lateral sclerosis motor neurons. *J Neuropathol Exp Neurol*, **53**(3), 221–230.
7. Wong NK, He BP, Strong MJ. (2000). Characterization of neuronal intermediate filament protein expression in cervical spinal motor neurons in sporadic amyotrophic lateral sclerosis (ALS). *J Neuropathol Exp Neurol*, **59**(11), 972–982.
8. Cote F, Collard JF, Julien JP. (1993). Progressive neuronopathy in transgenic mice expressing the human neurofilament heavy gene: a mouse model of amyotrophic lateral sclerosis. *Cell*, **73**, 35–46.
9. Xu Z, Cork LC, Griffin JW, Cleveland DW. (1993). Increased expression of neurofilament subunit NF-L produces morphological alterations that resemble the pathology of human motor neuron disease. *Cell*, **73**, 23–33.
10. Beaulieu JM, Jacomy H, Julien JP. (2000). Formation of intermediate filament protein aggregates with disparate effects in two transgenic mouse models lacking the neurofilament light subunit. *J Neurosci*, **20**(14), 5321–5328.
11. Sanelli T, Ge W, Leystra-Lantz C, Strong MJ. (2007). Calcium mediated excitotoxicity in neurofilament aggregate-bearing neurons *in vitro* is NMDA receptor dependant. *J Neurol Sci*, **256**(1–2), 39–51.
12. Sanelli T, Strong MJ. (2007). Loss of nitric oxide-mediated down-regulation of NMDA receptors in neurofilament aggregate-bearing motor neurons *in vitro*: implications for motor neuron disease. *Free Radic Biol Med*, **42**, 143–151.
13. Sanelli TR, Sopper MM, Strong MJ. (2004). Sequestration of nNOS in neurofilamentous aggregate bearing neurons *in vitro* leads to enhanced NMDA-mediated calcium influx. *Brain Res*, **1004**(1–2), 8–17.
14. Wen W, Sanelli T, Ge W, Strong W, Strong MJ. (2006). Activated microglial supernatant induced motor neuron cytotoxicity is associated with upregulation of the TNFR1 receptor. *Neurosci Res*, **55**, 87–95.

15. Barber SC, Mead RJ, Shaw PJ. (2006). Oxidative stress in ALS: a mechanism of neurodegeneration and a therapeutic target. *Biochim Biophys Acta*, **1762**(11–12), 1051–1067.
16. Ge WW, Volkening K, Leystra-Lantz C, Jaffe H, Strong MJ. (2007). 14-3-3 protein binds to the low molecular weight neurofilament (NFL) mRNA 3′ UTR. *Mol Cell Neurosci*, **34**, 80–87.
17. Ge WW, Wen W, Strong W, Leystra-Lantz C, Strong MJ. (2005). Mutant copper-zinc superoxide dismutase binds to and destabilizes human low molecular weight neurofilament mRNA. *J Biol Chem*, **280**, 118–124.
18. Strong MJ, Volkening K, Hammond R, *et al.* (2007). TDP43 is a human low molecular weight neurofilament (hNFL) mRNA-binding protein. *Mol Cell Neurosci*, **35**(2), 320–327.
19. Volkening K, Leystra-Lantz C, Strong MJ. (2010). Human low molecular weight neurofilament (NFL) mRNA interacts with a predicted p190RhoGEF homologue (RGNEF) in humans. *Amyotroph Lateral Scler*, **11**, 97–103.
20. Volkening K, Leystra-Lantz C, Yang W, Jaffee H, Strong MJ. (2009). Tar DNA binding protein of 43 kDa (TDP-43), 14-3-3 proteins and copper/zinc superoxide dismutase (SOD1) interact to modulate NFL mRNA stability. Implications for altered RNA processing in amyotrophic lateral sclerosis (ALS). *Brain Res*, **1305**, 168–182.
21. Perrone-Bizzozero N, Bolognani F. (2002). Role of HuD and other RNA-binding proteins in neural development and plasticity. *J Neurosci Res*, **68**(2), 121–126.
22. Bradrick SS, Gromeier M. (2009). Identification of gemin5 as a novel 7-methylguanosine cap-binding protein. *PLoS ONE*, **4**(9), e7030.
23. Joshi B, Cameron A, Jagus R. (2004). Characterization of mammalian eIF4E-family members. *Eur J Biochem*, **271**(11), 2189–2203.
24. Ford LP, Bagga PS, Wilusz J. (1997). The poly(A) tail inhibits the assembly of a 3′-to-5′ exonuclease in an *in vitro* RNA stability system. *Mol Cell Biol*, **17**, 398–406.
25. Pascale A, Amadio M, Scapagnini G, *et al.* (2005). Neuronal ELAV proteins enhance mRNA stability by a PKCalpha-dependent pathway. *Proc Natl Acad Sci USA*, **102**(34), 12065–12070.
26. Ratti A, Fallini C, Cova L, *et al.* (2006). A role for the ELAV RNA-binding proteins in neural stem cells: stabilization of Msi1 mRNA. *J Cell Sci*, **119**(Pt 7), 1442–1452.
27. Lai WS, Carballo E, Thorn JM, Kennington EA, Blackshear PJ. (2000). Interactions of CCCH zinc finger proteins with mRNA. Binding of tristetraprolin-related zinc finger proteins to Au-rich elements and destabilization of mRNA. *J Biol Chem*, **275**(23), 17827–17837.
28. Lai WS, Carballo E, Strum JR, Kennington EA, Phillips RS, Blackshear PJ. (1999). Evidence that tristetraprolin binds to AU-rich elements and promotes the deadenylation and destabilization of tumor necrosis factor alpha mRNA. *Mol Cell Biol*, **19**(6), 4311–4323.
29. Brewer G. (1991). An A + U-rich element RNA-binding factor regulates c-myc mRNA stability *in vitro*. *Mol Cell Biol*, **11**(5), 2460–2466.
30. Gherzi R, Lee KY, Briata P, *et al.* (2004). A KH domain RNA binding protein, KSRP, promotes ARE-directed mRNA turnover by recruiting the degradation machinery. *Mol Cell*, **14**(5), 571–583.
31. Kanai Y, Dohmae N, Hirokawa N. (2004). Kinesin transports RNA: isolation and characterization of an RNA-transporting granule. *Neuron*, **43**(4), 513–525.
32. Hirokawa N. (2006). mRNA transport in dendrites: RNA granules, motors, and tracks. *J Neurosci*, **26**(27), 7139–7142.
33. Kedersha N, Anderson P. (2007). Mammalian stress granules and processing bodies. *Methods Enzymol*, **431**, 61–81.
34. Zeitelhofer M, Macchi P, Dahm R. (2008). Perplexing bodies: the putative roles of P-bodies in neurons. *RNA Biol*, **5**(4), 244–248.
35. Houseley J, LaCava J, Tollervey D. (2006). RNA-quality control by the exosome. *Nat Rev Mol Cell Biol*, **7**(7), 529–539.

36. Parker R, Sheth U. (2007). P bodies and the control of mRNA translation and degradation. *Mol Cell*, **25**(5), 635–646.
37. Chen CY, Gherzi R, Ong SE, *et al.* (2001). AU binding proteins recruit the exosome to degrade ARE-containing mRNAs. *Cell*, **107**(4), 451–464.
38. Mukherjee D, Gao M, O'Connor JP, *et al.* (2002). The mammalian exosome mediates the efficient degradation of mRNAs that contain AU-rich elements. *EMBO J*, **21**(1–2), 165–174.
39. Stoecklin G, Mayo T, Anderson P. (2006). ARE-mRNA degradation requires the 5′-3′ decay pathway. *EMBO Rep*, **7**, 72–77.
40. Eystathioy T, Chan EK, Tenenbaum SA, Keene JD, Griffith K, Fritzler MJ. (2002). A phosphorylated cytoplasmic autoantigen, GW182, associates with a unique population of human mRNAs within novel cytoplasmic speckles. *Mol Biol Cell*, **13**(4), 1338–1351.
41. Anderson P, Kedersha N. (2006). RNA granules. *J Cell Biol*, **172**(6), 803–808.
42. Pillai RS. (2005). MicroRNA function: multiple mechanisms for a tiny RNA? *RNA*, **11**(12), 1753–1761.
43. Gregory RI, Yan KP, Amuthan G, *et al.* (2004). The Microprocessor complex mediates the genesis of microRNAs. *Nature*, **432**(7014), 235–240.
44. Liu X, Fortin K, Mourelatos Z. (2008). MicroRNAs: biogenesis and molecular functions. *Brain Pathol*, **18**, 113–121.
45. Jabri E. (2005). P-bodies take a RISC. *Nat Struct Mol Biol*, **12**(7), 564.
46. Rossi JJ. (2005). RNAi and the P-body connection. *Nat Cell Biol*, **7**(7), 643–644.
47. Nelson PT, Wang WX, Rajeev BW. (2008). MicroRNAs (miRNAs) in neurodegenerative diseases. *Brain Pathol* **18**, 130–138.
48. Orom UA, Nielsen FC, Lund AH. (2008). MicroRNA-10a binds the 5′UTR of ribosomal protein mRNAs and enhances their translation. *Mol Cell*, **30**(4), 460–471.
49. Walters RW, Bradrick SS, Gromeier M. (2010). Poly(A)-binding protein modulates mRNA susceptibility to cap-dependent miRNA-mediated repression. *RNA*, **16**, 239–250.
50. Elvira G, Wasiak S, Blandford V, *et al.* (2006). Characterization of an RNA granule from developing brain. *Mol Cell Proteomics*, **5**(4), 635–651.
51. Wang IF, Reddy NM, Shen CK. (2002). Higher order arrangement of the eukaryotic nuclear bodies. *Proc Natl Acad Sci USA*, **99**(21), 13583–13588.
52. Buratti E, Baralle FE. (2008). Multiple roles of TDP-43 in gene expression, splicing regulation, and human disease. *Front Biosci*, **13**, 867–878.
53. Buratti E, Brindisi A, Giombi M, Tisminetzky S, Ayala YM, Baralle FE. (2005). TDP-43 binds heterogeneous nuclear ribonucleoprotein A/B through its C-terminal tail: an important region for the inhibition of cystic fibrosis transmembrane conductance regulator exon 9 splicing. *J Biol Chem*, **280**(45), 37572–37584.
54. Buratti E, Baralle FE. (2001). Characterization and functional implications of the RNA binding properties of nuclear factor TDP-43, a novel splicing regulator of CFTR exon 9. *J Biol Chem*, **276**(39), 36337–36343.
55. Colombrita C, Zennaro E, Fallini C, *et al.* (2009). TDP-43 is recruited to stress granules in conditions of oxidative insult. *J Neurochem*, **111**(4), 1051–1061.
56. Freibaum BD, Chitta RK, High AA, Taylor JP. (2010). Global analysis of TDP-43 interacting proteins reveals strong association with RNA splicing and translation machinery. *J Proteome Res*, **9**(2), 1104–1120.
57. Moisse K, Mepham J, Volkening K, Welch I, Hill T, Strong MJ. (2009). Cytosolic TDP-43 expression following axotomy is associated with caspase 3 activation in NFL / mice: support for a role for TDP-43 in the physiological response to neuronal injury. *Brain Res*, **1296**, 176–186.
58. Wang IF, Wu LS, Chang HY, Shen CK. (2008). TDP-43, the signature protein of FTLD-U, is a neuronal activity-responsive factor. *J Neurochem*, **105**(3), 797–806.

59. Gitcho MA, Baloh RH, Chakraverty S, *et al.* (2008). TDP-43 A315T mutation in familial motor neuron disease. *Ann Neurol*, **63**(4), 535–538.
60. Rutherford NJ, Zhang YJ, Baker M, *et al.* (2008). Novel mutations in TARDBP (TDP-43) in patients with familial amyotrophic lateral sclerosis. *PLoS Genet*, **4**(9), e1000193.
61. Sreedharan J, Blair IP, Tripathi VB, *et al.* (2008). TDP-43 mutations in familial and sporadic amyotrophic lateral sclerosis. *Science*, **319**(5870), 1668–1672.
62. Van Deerlin VM, Leverenz JB, Bekris LM, *et al.* (2008). TARDBP mutations in amyotrophic lateral sclerosis with TDP-43 neuropathology: a genetic and histopathological analysis. *Lancet Neurol*, **7**(5), 409–416.
63. Winton MJ, Van Deerlin VM, Kwong LK, *et al.* (2008). A90V TDP-43 variant results in the aberrant localization of TDP-43 *in vitro*. *FEBS Lett*, **582**(15), 2252–2256.
64. Yokoseki A, Shiga A, Tan CF, *et al.* (2008). TDP-43 mutation in familial amyotrophic lateral sclerosis. *Ann Neurol*, **63**(4), 538–542.
65. Kabashi E, Lin L, Tradewell ML, *et al.* (2010). Gain and loss of function of ALS-related mutations of TARDBP (TDP-43) cause motor deficits *in vivo*. *Hum Mol Genet*, **19**(4), 671–683.
66. Iko Y, Kodama TS, Kasai N, *et al.* (2004). Domain architectures and characterization of an RNA-binding protein, TLS. *J Biol Chem*, **279**(43), 44834–44840.
67. Canete-Soler R, Wu J, Zhai J, Shamim M, Schlaepfer WW. (2001). p190RhoGEF Binds to a destabilizing element in the 3′ untranslated region of light neurofilament subunit mRNA and alters the stability of the transcript. *J Biol Chem*, **276**(34), 32046–32050.
68. Lin H, Zhai J, Canete-Soler R, Schlaepfer WW. (2004). 3′ untranslated region in a light neurofilament (NF-L) mRNA triggers aggregation of NF-L and mutant superoxide dismutase 1 proteins in neuronal cells. *J Neurosci*, **24**(11), 2716–2726.
69. Rosen DR, Siddique T, Patterson D, *et al.* (1993). Mutations in Cu/Zn superoxide dismutase gene are associated with familial amyotrophic lateral sclerosis. *Nature*, **362**(6415), 59–62.
70. Li B, Xu W, Luo C, Gozal D, Liu R. (2003). VEGF-induced activation of the PI3-K/Akt pathway reduces mutant SOD1-mediated motor neuron cell death. *Brain Res Mol Brain Res*, **111**(1–2), 155–164.
71. Lu L, Zheng L, Viera L, *et al.* (2007). Mutant Cu/Zn-superoxide dismutase associated with amyotrophic lateral sclerosis destabilizes vascular endothelial growth factor mRNA and downregulates its expression. *J Neurosci*, **27**(30), 7929–7938.
72. Kanekura K, Hashimoto Y, Niikura T, Aiso S, Matsuoka M, Nishimoto I. (2004). Alsin, the product of ALS2 gene, suppresses SOD1 mutant neurotoxicity through RhoGEF domain by interacting with SOD1 mutants. *J Biol Chem*, **279**(18), 19247–19256.
73. Gros-Louis F, Kriz J, Kabashi E, *et al.* (2008). Als2 mRNA splicing variants detected in KO mice rescue severe motor dysfunction phenotype in Als2 knock-down zebrafish. *Hum Mol Genet*, **17**(17), 2691–2702.
74. Parkinson N, Ince PG, Smith MO, *et al.* (2006). ALS phenotypes with mutations in CHMP2B (charged multivesicular body protein 2B). *Neurology*, **67**(6), 1074–1077.
75. Skibinski G, Parkinson NJ, Brown JM, *et al.* (2005). Mutations in the endosomal ESCRTIII-complex subunit CHMP2B in frontotemporal dementia. *Nat Genet*, **37**(8), 806–808.
76. Rusten TE, Simonsen A. (2008). ESCRT functions in autophagy and associated disease. *Cell Cycle*, **7**(9), 1166–1172.
77. Rusten TE, Filimonenko M, Rodahl LM, Stenmark H, Simonsen A. (2007). ESCRTing autophagic clearance of aggregating proteins. *Autophagy*, **4**(2), 233–236.
78. Filimonenko M, Stuffers S, Raiborg C, *et al.* (2007). Functional multivesicular bodies are required for autophagic clearance of protein aggregates associated with neurodegenerative disease. *J Cell Biol*, **179**(3), 485–500.

79. Irion U, St JD. (2007). Bicoid RNA localization requires specific binding of an endosomal sorting complex. *Nature*, **445**(7127), 554–558.
80. Lee YS, Pressman S, Andress AP, *et al.* (2009). Silencing by small RNAs is linked to endosomal trafficking. *Nat Cell Biol*, **11**(9), 1150–1156.
81. Gibbings DJ, Ciaudo C, Erhardt M, Voinnet O. (2009). Multivesicular bodies associate with components of miRNA effector complexes and modulate miRNA activity. *Nat Cell Biol*, **11**(9), 1143–1149.
82. Schroer TA. (2004). Dynactin. *Annu Rev Cell Dev Biol*, **20**, 759–779.
83. Hirokawa N, Takemura R. (2005). Molecular motors and mechanisms of directional transport in neurons. *Nat Rev Neurosci*, **6**(3), 201–214.
84. Shah JV, Flanagan LA, Janmey PA, Leterrier JF. (2000). Bidirectional translocation of neurofilaments along microtubules mediated in part by dynein/dynactin. *Mol Biol Cell*, **11**(10), 3495–3508.
85. Munch C, Rosenbohm A, Sperfeld AD, *et al.* (2005). Heterozygous R1101K mutation of the DCTN1 gene in a family with ALS and FTD. *Ann Neurol*, **58**(5), 777–780.
86. Munch C, Sedlmeier R, Meyer T, *et al.* (2004). Point mutations of the p150 subunit of dynactin (DCTN1) gene in ALS. *Neurology*, **63**(4), 724–726.
87. Culver-Hanlon TL, Lex SA, Stephens AD, Quintyne NJ, King SJ. (2006). A microtubule-binding domain in dynactin increases dynein processivity by skating along microtubules. *Nat Cell Biol*, **8**(3), 264–270.
88. Moore JK, Sept D, Cooper JA. (2009). Neurodegeneration mutations in dynactin impair dynein-dependent nuclear migration. *Proc Natl Acad Sci USA*, **106**(13), 5147–5152.
89. Migheli A, Pezzulo T, Attanasio A, Schiffer D. (1993). Peripherin immunoreactive structures in amyotrophic lateral sclerosis. *Lab Invest*, **68**(2), 185–191.
90. Robertson J, Doroudchi MM, Nguyen MD, *et al.* (2003). A neurotoxic peripherin splice variant in a mouse model of ALS. *J Cell Biol*, **160**(6), 939–949.
91. Xiao S, Tjostheim S, Sanelli T, *et al.* (2008). An aggregate-inducing peripherin isoform generated through intron retention is upregulated in amyotrophic lateral sclerosis and associated with disease pathology. *J Neurosci*, **28**(8), 1833–1840.
92. Sanelli T, Xiao S, Horne P, Bilbao J, Zinman L, Robertson J. (2007). Evidence that TDP-43 is not the major ubiquitinated target within the pathological inclusions of amyotrophic lateral sclerosis. *J Neuropathol Exp Neurol*, **66**(12), 1147–1153.
93. Flowers JM, Powell JF, Leigh PN, Andersen P, Shaw CE. (2001). Intron 7 retention and exon 9 skipping EAAT2 mRNA variants are not associated with amyotrophic lateral sclerosis. *Ann Neurol*, **49**(5), 643–649.
94. Honig LS, Chambliss DD, Bigio EH, Carroll SL, Elliott JL. (2000). Glutamate transporter EAAT2 splice variants occur not only in ALS, but also in AD and controls. *Neurology*, **55**(8), 1082–1088.
95. Lin CL, Bristol LA, Jin L, *et al.* (1998). Aberrant RNA processing in a neurodegenerative disease: the cause for absent EAAT2, a glutamate transporter, in amyotrophic lateral sclerosis. *Neuron*, **20**(3), 589–602.
96. Meyer T, Fromm A, Munch C, *et al.* (1999). The RNA of the glutamate transporter EAAT2 is variably spliced in amyotrophic lateral sclerosis and normal individuals. *J Neurol Sci*, **170**(1), 45–50.
97. Lauriat TL, McInnes LA. (2007). EAAT2 regulation and splicing: relevance to psychiatric and neurological disorders. *Mol Psychiatry*, **12**(12), 1065–1078.
98. Zhang YJ, Xu YF, Dickey CA, *et al.* (2007). Progranulin mediates caspase-dependent cleavage of TAR DNA binding protein-43. *J Neurosci*, **27**(39), 10530–10534.
99. Yu CE, Bird TD, Bekris LM, *et al.* (2010). The spectrum of mutations in progranulin: a collaborative study screening 545 cases of neurodegeneration. *Arch Neurol*, **67**(2), 161–170.

100. Baker M, Mackenzie IR, Pickering-Brown SM, *et al.* (2006). Mutations in progranulin cause tau-negative frontotemporal dementia linked to chromosome 17. *Nature*, **442**(7105), 916–919.
101. Cruts M, Gijselinck I, van der Zee J, *et al.* (2006). Null mutations in progranulin cause ubiquitin-positive frontotemporal dementia linked to chromosome 17q21. *Nature*, **442**(7105), 920–924.
102. Chen YZ, Bennett CL, Huynh HM, *et al.* (2004). DNA/RNA helicase gene mutations in a form of juvenile amyotrophic lateral sclerosis (ALS4). *Am J Hum Genet*, **74**(6), 1128–1135.
103. Cordin O, Banroques J, Tanner NK, Linder P. (2006). The DEAD-box protein family of RNA helicases. *Gene*, **367**, 17–37.
104. Linder P, Tanner NK, Banroques J. (2001). From RNA helicases to RNPases. *Trends Biochem Sci*, **26**(6), 339–341.
105. Tanner NK, Linder P. (2001). DExD/H box RNA helicases: from generic motors to specific dissociation functions. *Mol Cell*, **8**(2), 251–262.
106. Zhao ZH, Chen WZ, Wu ZY, *et al.* (2009). A novel mutation in the senataxin gene identified in a Chinese patient with sporadic amyotrophic lateral sclerosis. *Amyotroph Lateral Scler*, **10**(2), 118–122.
107. Tsuji T, Sun Y, Kishimoto K, *et al.* (2005). Angiogenin is translocated to the nucleus of HeLa cells and is involved in ribosomal RNA transcription and cell proliferation. *Cancer Res*, **65**(4), 1352–1360.
108. Yamasaki S, Ivanov P, Hu GF, Anderson P. (2009). Angiogenin cleaves tRNA and promotes stress-induced translational repression. *J Cell Biol*, **185**, 35–42.
109. Gellera C, Colombrita C, Ticozzi N, *et al.* (2008). Identification of new ANG gene mutations in a large cohort of Italian patients with amyotrophic lateral sclerosis. *Neurogenetics*, **9**, 33–40.
110. Wu D, Yu W, Kishikawa H, *et al.* (2007). Angiogenin loss-of-function mutations in amyotrophic lateral sclerosis. *Ann Neurol*, **62**(6), 609–617.
111. Greenway MJ, Andersen PM, Russ C, *et al.* (2006). ANG mutations segregate with familial and 'sporadic' amyotrophic lateral sclerosis. *Nat Genet*, **38**(4), 411–413.
112. Gao X, Xu Z. (2008). Mechanisms of action of angiogenin. *Acta Biochim Biophys Sin (Shanghai)*, **40**(7), 619–624.
113. Williams AH, Valdez G, Moresi V, *et al.* (2009). MicroRNA-206 delays ALS progression and promotes regeneration of neuromuscular synapses in mice. *Science*, **326**(5959), 1549–1554.
114. Lefebvre S, Burglen L, Reboullet S, *et al.* (1995). Identification and characterization of a spinal muscular atrophy-determining gene. *Cell*, **80**, 155–165.
115. Wirth B. (2000). An update of the mutation spectrum of the survival motor neuron gene (SMN1) in autosomal recessive spinal muscular atrophy (SMA). *Hum Mutat*, **15**(3), 228–237.
116. Brook JD, McCurrach ME, Harley HG, *et al.* (1992). Molecular basis of myotonic dystrophy: expansion of a trinucleotide (CTG) repeat at the 3′ end of a transcript encoding a protein kinase family member. *Cell*, **69**(2), 385.
117. Kuyumcu-Martinez NM, Cooper TA. (2006). Misregulation of alternative splicing causes pathogenesis in myotonic dystrophy. *Prog Mol Subcell Biol*, **44**, 133–159.
118. Leroy O, Wang J, Maurage CA, *et al.* (2006). Brain-specific change in alternative splicing of Tau exon 6 in myotonic dystrophy type 1. *Biochim Biophys Acta*, **1762**(4), 460–467.
119. Philips AV, Timchenko LT, Cooper TA. (1998). Disruption of splicing regulated by a CUG-binding protein in myotonic dystrophy. *Science*, **280**(5364), 737–741.

Chapter 23

Alterations in tau metabolism in amyotrophic lateral sclerosis with cognitive impairment

Michael J. Strong, Wencheng Yang, May Gohar, and Wendy L. Strong

As described throughout this text, the concept that amyotrophic lateral sclerosis (ALS) is a disorder solely of the motor system has been replaced by the understanding that it is often associated with one or more syndromes of frontotemporal dysfunction (1,2). Although these clinical manifestations can be attributed to a frontotemporal lobar degeneration (FTLD), not dissimilar in its features from that observed in a wide range of other frontotemporal dementias (FTD) (Figure 23.1), until recently the biological basis of the FTLD associated with ALS was unknown. To a large extent, this changed with the discovery that the transactive response DNA-binding protein of 43 kDa (TDP-43) is the core constituent of the ubiquitinated intraneuronal aggregates observed in the FTLDs with ubiquitin prominent pathology (FTLD-U), and that this property is shared with the ubiquitinated aggregates of ALS (3,4). As discussed by Cairns (Chapter 18), this has led to the current concept that ALS is best classified among the FTLDs in which TDP-43 deposition is the prominent pathology (FTLD/TDP) (5,6). The implication here is that the fundamental biological basis for the frontotemporal syndromes of ALS is thus a pathological transformation of TDP-43 metabolism. The controversy, however, is whether or not such pathological protein deposits of RNA binding protein simply reflect a more widespread alteration in RNA metabolism (7). As we will delineate in this chapter, there is another potential explanation for the pathogenesis of the frontotemporal syndromes of ALS, and more specifically that of ALS with cognitive impairment (ALSci), in that there is also substantive evidence that alterations in tau metabolism are present in ALSci.

As discussed by Cairns (Chapter 18), the neuropathological classification of the FTLDs can be largely dichotomized into those in which an impairment of the microtubule-associated protein tau (tau) is evident, and those in which it is not. For the latter, the neuropathological features can be further dichotomized into those in which alterations in TDP 43 metabolism are evident or those in which aggregates of the fused in sarcoma/translocated in liposcarcoma (FUS/TLS) are evident (5). A few undifferentiated cases remain.

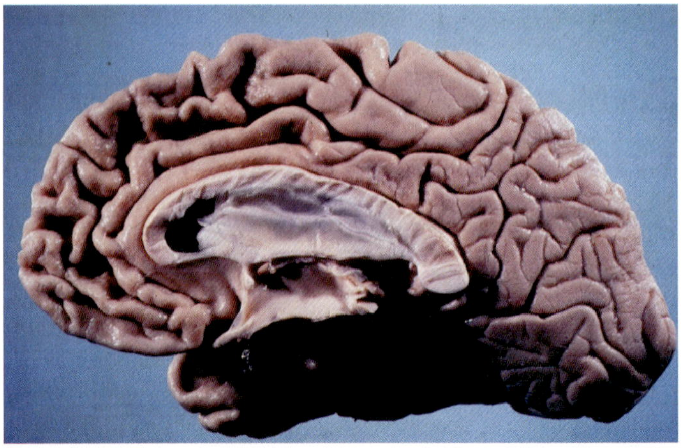

Fig. 23.1 Mesial surface of the brain of an individual with a frontotemporal syndrome and ALS. Note the prominent degree of atrophy of the mesial frontal lobe, including the anterior cingulate gyrus, while the more posterior aspects of the parietal and occipital lobes are spared. In this example, the precentral gyrus and supplementary motor cortex in which lower limb representation would be prominent also demonstrates very little atrophy compared with more anteriorly placed structures.

As discussed above, the frontotemporal syndromes of ALS are largely considered to be free of tau deposition, and thus classified as FTLD/TDP. However, this classification largely ignores a substantive literature with respect to alterations in tau metabolism in ALS. In this chapter, this literature along with more recent observations from our research on alterations in tau metabolism in ALS will be reviewed.

The tau proteins are cytoskeletal phosphoproteins of 40–60 kDa in which highly conserved C-terminal domains are responsible for tubulin binding mediated through a repeated element of 31 amino acids (8). Tau proteins promote both microtubule assembly and stabilization (9). Alternative splicing of the single chromosome 17 encoded tau gene yields six isoforms defined by the presence or absence of an exon 10-encoded multiphosphorylation repeat (3R versus 4R) and N-terminus insertions (0N, 1N, 2N). By determining whether the tau protein deposition reflects predominantly 3R, 4R, or both isoforms, whether the predominant form of tau being deposited is found within a guanidine soluble or insoluble fraction, and by matching this to the neuropathological findings, it is possible to create a molecular signature of the tauopathies (10). In addition to this, and specifically for Alzheimer's disease (AD), ultrastructural studies allow a further unique characterization in which the typical tau-containing neurofibrillary tangles (NFTs) of AD can be uniquely described as paired helical filaments in the insoluble tau isolate and a signature triplet insoluble hyperphosphorylated tau banding on Western blotting (11–14). Interestingly, and of relevance to our subsequent discussion of tau toxicity in ALS, the mechanism of toxicity in AD does not appear to be directly related to the formation of paired helical filaments, but rather to the ability of the non-fibrillized cytosolic hyperphosphorylated tau to sequester normal tau and lead to the disassembly of microtubules (15–19).

Historical evidence of alterations in tau metabolism in amyotrophic lateral sclerosis

The observation of tau deposition in ALS is not new. Forno and colleagues examined 10 patient with FTLD, including one patient with clinical evidence of motor neurone degeneration ante mortem and a further two with neuropathological evidence of such, and found tau and ubiquitin-immunoreactive glial inclusions negative for α-synuclein in non-motor cortical regions (20). In a family in which ALS and FTD coexisted, Martinaud and colleagues observed not only widespread tau deposition but that the dentate gyrus of the affected individuals was largely spared from the more typical ubiquitin-immunoreactive aggregates that were believed to be hallmarks of the non-motor pathology of ALS (21,22). In contrast, tau-immunoreactive aggregates were observed in the dentate gyrus, entorhinal cortex, and in the pyramidal layer of Ammon's horn. Astrocytic plaques and gliosis were not observed, while coiled bodies and neuropil threads were observed throughout the temporal white matter. As will be evident, this is very reminiscent of the pathology that we have subsequently observed in ALSci using novel polyclonal antibodies against tau.

In addition to these observations, widespread tau deposition was also readily observed in the western Pacific variants of ALS, including the Kii Peninsula of Japan. As described by Garruto (Chapter 1), the neuropathological hallmark of the hyperendemic focus of both ALS and parkinsonism in the western Pacific was the presence of NFTs morphologically identical to those observed in AD, including the presence of hyperphosphorylated tau (23–26). However, in contrast to AD, the NFT distribution was more widespread and included both cortical and subcortical structures. In addition, Lewy-like bodies containing α-synuclein, typical of Parkinson's disease, were observed in the amygdala (27,28). Similar features were observed among Japanese patients with the ALS/parkinsonian–dementia complex in the Kii peninsula (Muro disease) (29).

Alterations in tau metabolism in amyotrophic lateral sclerosis with cognitive impairment

It is of interest therefore that tau-immunoreactive neuronal and extraneuronal aggregates have been observed in ALSci (30) and in a number of cases of sporadic ALS (20,31–34). In addition, we have observed that tau isolated from ALSci harbours an unique threonine phosphorylation at residue 175 (phospho-^{175}Thr-tau) (35). As will be reviewed, these findings are in addition to the more traditional features of ALS that have been delineated by Highley and Ince (Chapter 19) and includes both non-neuronal tau aggregates such as astrocytic tau-immunoreactive aggregates and dystrophic neurites (30).

Although ALS is a disease of ageing, tau deposition in ALSci is not a function of ageing. In a quantitative and qualitative analysis of tau deposition across the age spectrum from birth to the ninth decade of life, we did not observe an age-dependent deposition of tau in the anterior cingulate gyrus (a region of specific interest to the phenomenology of ALS) and corresponding to the loss of neurones identified using H1-magnetic resonance imaging spectroscopy (36,37). In contrast, we did observe an age-dependent tau accumulation in the hippocampus, consistent with the earlier findings of Braak and Braak (38).

Having observed tau-immunoreactive neuronal and astrocytic aggregates in ALSci, as well as tau-immunoreactive dystrophic neurites, we then purified tau from both the cortical and subcortical frontal lobes of individuals with ALS or ALSci, and contrasted this to control (neurologically intact tau from the same region). In contrast to control cases in which very little if any tau could be observed in the insoluble tau fraction, all ALSci cases and a percentage of ALS cases without cognitive impairment, demonstrated tau within the insoluble fraction (35). Further, both 3R and 4R tau isoforms could be observed in the insoluble fraction in ALSci, while there was no evidence on Western blots of the typical triplet of paired helical filament in AD. In addition, tau isolated from patients with ALSci was resistant to dephosphorylation (35) and exhibited an enhanced rate of fibril formation compared with that observed from either neurologically intact control brain tissue or from ALS not associated with cognitive impairment (39). These findings suggested that post-translational modifications of tau had occurred. This hypothesis was validated when we then identified a novel phospho-epitope at threonine residue 175 (pThr^{175} tau) (35). The concept that tau was post-translationally modified in ALS was also supported by the finding of an increased expression of the protein kinase GSK3β, capable of phosphorylating tau, in tau aggregate bearing neurones (40).

To determine whether pThr^{175}tau is pathogenic, we subsequently constructed a pseudophosphorylated tau (Thr^{175}Asp-tau) that induces tau aggregate formation *in vitro* in both neuronal and non-neuronal cells (39). Although wild-type tau also formed fibrils, Thr^{175}Asp-tau fibrils formed significantly earlier than those observed in wild-type transfections and were associated with a greater extent of cell death. This occurred regardless of whether the construct harboured the 3R or 4R isoform. Inhibition of phosphorylation at Thr^{175} (Thr^{175}Ala-tau) inhibited fibril formation. We have subsequently demonstrated that inhibition of GSK3β activation using lithium chloride leads to inhibition of both tau fibril formation *in vitro* and cell death (Gohar *et al.*, current submission). This observation suggests it is not the aberrant phosphorylation at Thr^{175} giving rise to the fibril formation, but rather that this site is permissive to GSK3β activation, which then phosphorylates at a second site. Identifying this second site is the subject of current experiments.

While this is of considerable interest given the potential role of tau fibril formation in ALSci and specifically opens an avenue for consideration for pharmacotherapy of the frontotemporal syndromes, it still does not prove that tau pathology underlies these syndromes. To further examine this, we have developed a polyclonal antibody recognizing pThr^{175}tau (Yang *et al.*, current submission). Using this antibody and a panel of generic tau antibodies, we characterized tau deposition within ALS and ALSci, and compared this with control and Alzheimer's tau deposition (Figure 23.2). We observed a preferential deposition of tau within both neurones and glia in ALSci, not evident to the same extent in ALS. Intriguingly, we found that neuronal tau deposition was most prominent in the entorhinal cortex and amygdala, followed by the hippocampus and anterior cingulate gyrus.

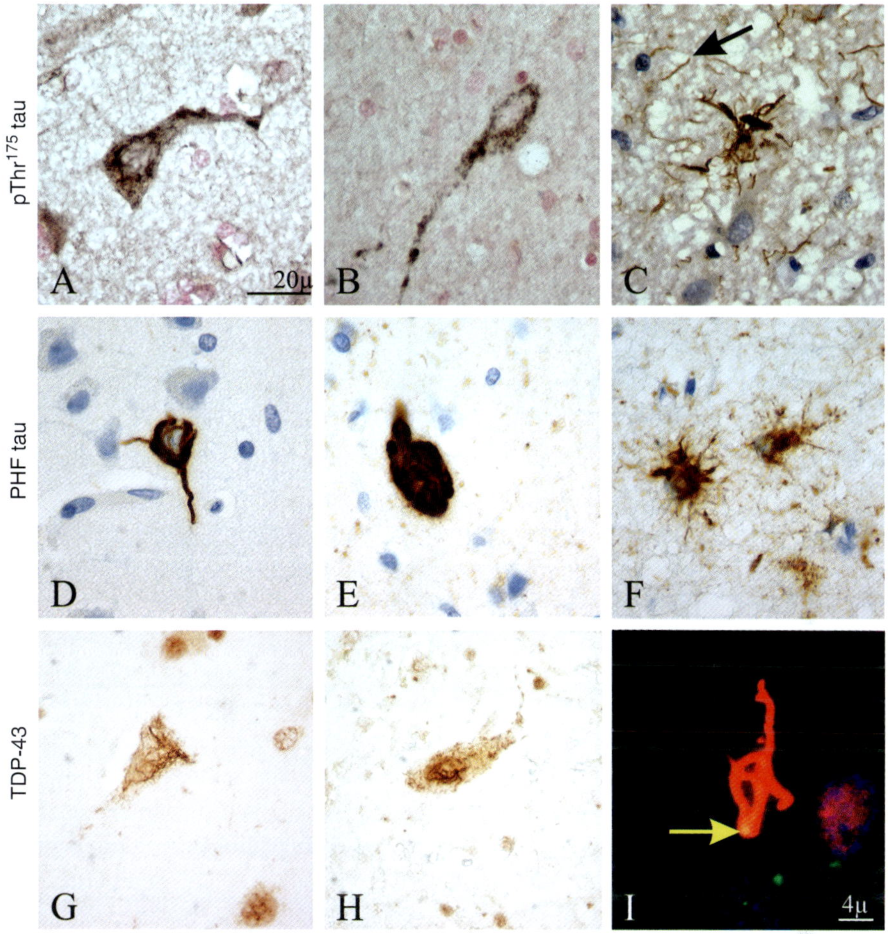

Fig. 23.2 Tau- and TDP-43-immunoreactive cortical pathology in ALSci. Antibodies recognizing pathological tau, including a novel polyclonal antibody against pThr175tau (A–C) and paired helical filament antibody (D,E) detect intraneuronal tau deposition within neurones of the superior frontal gyrus (A,D), anterior cingulate gyrus (B) and the entorhinal cortex (E). Prominent astrocytic tau immunoreactivity was also observed with both antibodies (C,F), as were dystrophic neurites (C, black arrow). TDP-43-immunoreactive intraneuronal skeins were observed in neurones of the superior frontal (G) and anterior cingulate (H) cortices. Using confocal microscopy, co-localization of TDP-43 and tau-immunoreactive skeins (I, yellow arrow) (TDP-43 red fluorochrome; tau green fluorochrome; co-localization as yellow).

Astrocytic tau deposition tended to follow a similar pattern. When we compared this with the pattern of TDP-43 deposition, we found no correlation between the presence or absence of cognitive impairment. Tau-immunoreactive neurones tended to demonstrate an upregulation of TDP-43 expression typical of that observed in response to neuronal injury (41) without the formation of pathological nuclear or cytosolic aggregates. Ubiquitin-immunoreactive neurones similarly followed the pattern of tau deposition.

Taken together, these features suggest that alterations in tau metabolism occur in ALS. They still do not, however, confirm that the abnormalities are pathogenic in and of themselves. In suggesting that this may be the case, however, transgenic mice expressing aberrantly phosphorylated tau develop tau aggregates and a neurobehavioural syndrome. It remains to be determined whether a similar syndrome will develop in $pThr^{175}$tau expressing transgenic mice.

Can the dichotomy of TDP-43 and tau deposition in amyotrophic lateral sclerosis with cognitive impairment be resolved?

In conclusion, there is substantive evidence that alterations in TDP-43 metabolism are associated with ALS and FTLD. This includes the presence of pathological intranuclear and intracytoplasmic aggregates that are not observed as a response to neuronal injury alone (41,42) (see also Buratti, Chapter 24). While there is thus justification in considering alterations in the metabolism of TDP-43 as being a significant component of ALS pathobiology, there are equally cogent reasons, as presented above, to also consider that tau metabolism is also fundamentally disturbed in ALSci.

The two findings are not mutually exclusive. Indeed, both tau pathology and pathological expression of TDP-43 has been well documented in AD (43,44). For the majority, TDP-43 appears to exist as either cytoplasmic or intranuclear inclusions distinct from the paired helical or straight filaments of tau. Only rare examples of incorporation of TDP-43 directly into the filamentous tau structures were observed. This set of observations might suggest that TDP-43 expression is upregulated in response to neuronal injury and that it is displaced by NFTs. Given that at least one of the primary pathologies of AD is a tauopathy (as discussed earlier), this suggests that the accumulation of TDP-43 is a secondary phenomenon. To date, none of the transgenic mouse models of AD have reported on the coexistence of tau pathology with TDP-43.

The failure of either rat or mouse transgenic models of either human wild-type or mutant TDP-43 to develop a tauopathy would support such a hypothesis. Instead, when expressed under the Thy-1 promoter, transgenic mice expressing wild-type TDP-43 develop a dose-dependent degeneration of spinal motor neurones and non-motor cortical and subcortical neurones consistent with the pattern of neurodegeneration in both FTLD and ALS (45). Although affected neurones developed ubiquitinated TDP-43 nuclear and cytoplasmic inclusions, none of the inclusions were immunoreactive for tau or α-synuclein. Mice overexpressing human TDP-43 driven by the Ca^{2}+/calmodulin-dependent kinase II (CaMKII) promoter develop a range of neuropathological features consistent with a FTLD, including impairments in learning and memory, motor dysfunction, and hippocampal atrophy (46). Although tau immunostaining was not commented upon is this report, the neuropathological features included an age-dependent development of TDP-43 and ubiquitin-immunoreactive neuronal cytoplasmic inclusions accompanied by the loss of nuclear TDP-43 immunoreactivity. Expression of the mutant TDP-43 (A315T mutation), driven by the prion promoter, gives rise to transgenic mice with ubiquitin-immunoreactive aggregates in spinal motor neurones and layer 5 pyramidal neurones of the frontal cortex (47). While the latter study failed to observe tau-immunoreactive aggregates, it is notable that no TDP-43 aggregates were observed either and the predominant phenotype was motor in nature. The conditional expression of mutant TDP-43 (M337V) in rats using the Tet-off system (as constitutive expression produces a lethal phenotype in founders) results in a robust motor neurone phenotype characterized by motor neurone degeneration with both astrocytic and microglial activation, but without evidence of brain involvement (48). Cortical pathology was only observed in the extreme late stages of the disease and was not characterized further. Taken together, these observations would suggest that the expression of mutant TDP-43 or of the human wild-type TDP-43 in either rats or mice is insufficient to induce tau pathology.

At this point, the experiment thus remains to be done in which transgenic mice expressing $pThr^{175}$tau are created and then the extent of TDP-43 pathology described. If such an experiment can confirm first that $pThr^{175}$tau is pathogenic *in vivo*, and secondly that this is accompanied by a heightened level of TDP-43 expression, then such a model will provide a valuable window into not only the development specific therapies for the frontotemporal syndromes of ALS, but also significantly advance our understanding of the disease process.

Acknowledgements

Research supported by the Michael Halls endowment for ALS research.

References

1. Strong MJ. (2008). The syndromes of frontotemporal dysfunction in amyotrophic lateral sclerosis. *Amyotroph Lateral Scler*, **9**, 323–338.
2. Strong MJ, Grace GM, Freedman M, *et al.* (2009). Consensus criteria for the diagnosis of frontotemporal cognitive and behavioural syndromes in amyotrophic lateral sclerosis. *Amyotroph Lateral Scler*, **10**, 131–146.
3. Neumann M, Sampathu DM, Kwong LK, *et al.* (2006). Ubiquitinated TDP-43 in frontotemporal lobar degeneration and amyotrophic lateral sclerosis. *Science*, **314**, 130–133.
4. Arai T, Hasegawa M, Akiyama H, *et al.* (2006). TDP-43 is a component of ubiquitin-positive tau-negative inclusions in frontotemporal lobar degeneration and amyotrophic lateral sclerosis. *Biochem Biophys Res Commun*, **351**, 602–611.
5. Mackenzie IR, Rademakers R, Neumann M. (2010). TDP-43 and FUS in amyotrophic lateral sclerosis and frontotemporal dementia. *Lancet Neurol*, **9**, 995–1007.
6. Mackenzie IR, Neumann M, Bigio EH, *et al.* (2010). Nomenclature and nosology for neuropathologic subtypes of frontotemporal lobar degeneration: an update. *Acta Neuropathol*, **119**, 1–4.
7. Strong MJ. (2010). The evidence for altered RNA metabolism in amyotrophic lateral sclerosis (ALS). *J Neurol Sci*, **288**, 1–12.
8. Himmler A, Dreschsel D, Kirschner MW, *et al.* (1989). Tau consists of a set of proteins with repeated C-terminal microtubule-binding domains and variable N-terminal domains. *Mol Cell Biol*, **9**, 1381–1388.
9. Weingarten MD, Lockwood AH, Hwo S-Y, *et al.* (1975). A protein factor essential for microtubule assembly. *Proc Natl Acad Sci USA*, **72**, 1858–1862.

10. Mott RT, Dickson DW, Trojanowski JQ, *et al.* (2005). Neuropathological, biochemical, and molecular characterization of the frontotemporal dementias. *J Neuropathol Exp Neurol*, **64**, 420–428.
11. Gong CX, Liu F, Grundke-Iqbal I, *et al.* (2005). Post-translational modifications of tau protein in Alzheimer's disease. *J Neural Trans*, **112**, 813–838.
12. Grundke-Iqbal I, Iqbal K, Tung Y-C, *et al.* (1986). Abnormal phosphorylation of the microtubule-associated protein (tau) in Alzheimer cytoskeletal pathology. *Proc Natl Acad Sci USA*, **83**, 4913–4917.
13. Grundke-Iqbal I, Iqbal K, Quinlan M, *et al.* (1986). Microtubule-associate protein tau. A component of Alzheimer paired helical filaments. *J Biol Chem*, **261**, 6084–6089.
14. Goedert M, Spillantini MG, Jakes R, *et al.* (1989). Multiple isoforms of human microtubule-associated protein tau: sequences and localization in neurofibrillary tangles of Alzheimer's disease. *Neuron*, **3**, 519–526.
15. del C.Alonso A, Li B, Grundke-Iqbal I, *et al.* (2006). Polymerization of hyperphosphorylated tau into filaments eliminates its inhibitory activity. *Proc Natl Acad Sci USA*, **103**, 8864–8869.
16. Köpke E, Tung Y-C, Shaikh S, *et al.* (1993). Microtubule-associated protein tau. Abnormal phosphorylation of a non-paired helical filament pool in Alzheimer disease. *J Biol Chem*, **268**, –24374.
17. del C.Alonso A, Zaidi T, Novak M, *et al.* (2001). Interaction of tau isoforms with Alzheimer's disease abnormally hyperphosphorylated tau and *in vitro* phosphorylation into the disease-like protein. *J Biol Chem*, **276**, 37967–37973.
18. del C.Alonso A, Zaidi T, Grundke-Iqbal I, *et al.* (1994). Role of abnormally phsophorylated tau in the breakdown of microtubules in Alzheimer disease. *Proc Natl Acad Sci USA*, **91**, 5562–5566.
19. Li B, Chohan MO, Grundke-Iqbal I, *et al.* (2007). Disruption of micrtubule network by Alzheimer abnormally hyperphosphorylated tau. *Acta Neuropathol*, **113**, 501–511.
20. Forno LS, Langston JW, Herrick MK, *et al.* (2002). Ubiquitin-positive neuronal and tau 2-positive glial inclusions in frontotemporal dementia of motor neuron type. *Acta Neuropathol*, **103**, 599–606.
21. Martinaud O, Laquerrière A, Guyant-Maréchal L, *et al.* (2005). Frontotemporal dementia, motor neuron disease and tauopathy: clinical and neuropathological study in a family. *Acta Neuropathol*, **110**, 84–92.
22. Wightman G, Anderson VER, Martin J, *et al.* (1992). Hippocampal and neocortical ubiquitin-immunoreactive inclusions in amyotrophic lateral sclerosis with dementia. *Neurosci Lett*, **139**, 269–274.
23. Malamud N, Hirano A, Kurland LT. (1961). Pathoanatomic changes in amyotrophic lateral sclerosis on Guam. *Arch Neurol*, **5**, 401–415.
24. Hirano A, Malamud N, Elizan TS, *et al.* (1966). Amyotrophic lateral sclerosis and Parkinsonism-dementia complex on Guam. Further pathologic studies. *Arch Neurol*, **15**, 35–51.
25. Hirano A, Arumugasamy N, Zimmerman HM. (1967). Amyotrophic lateral sclerosis. A comparison of Guam and classical cases. *Arch Neurol*, **16**, 357–363.
26. Hirano A, Dembitzer HM, Kurland LT, *et al.* (1968). The fine structure of some intraganglionic alterations: neurofibrillary tangles, granulovacuolar bodies, and 'rod-like' structures in Guam amyotrophic lateral sclerosis and parkinsonism-dementia complex. *J Neuropathol Exp Neurol*, **27**, 167–182.
27. Yamazaki M, Arai Y, Baba M, *et al.* (2000). Alpha-synuclein inclusions in amygdala in the brains of patients with the parkinsonism-dementia complex of Guam. *J Neuropathol Exp Neurol*, **59**, 585–591.
28. Forman MS, Schmidt ML, Kasturi S, *et al.* (2002). Tau and α-synuclein pathology in amygdala of Parkinsonsim-dementia complex patients of Guam. *Am J Pathol*, **160**, 1725–1731.

29. Kuzuhara S and Kokubo Y. (2005). Atypical parkinsonism of Japan: amyotrophic lateral sclerosis-parkinsonism-dementia complex of the Kii Peninsula of Japan (Muro Disease): an update. *Movement Disorders*, **S12**, S108–S113.
30. Yang W, Sopper MM, Leystra-Lantz C, *et al.* (2003). Microtubule-associated tau protein positive neuronal and glial inclusions in amyotrophic lateral sclerosis. *Neurology*, **61**, 1766–1773.
31. Itoh N, Ishiguro K, Arai H, *et al.* (2003). Biochemical and ultrastructural study of neurofibrillary tangles in amyotrophic lateral sclerosis/parkinsonism-dementia complex in the Kii peninsula of Japan. *J Neuropathol Exp Neurol*, **62**, 791–798.
32. Wakayama I, Kihira Y, Yoshida S, *et al.* (1993). Rare neuropil threads in amyotrophic lateral sclerosis and parkinsonism-dementia on Guam and in the Kii Peninsula of Japan. *Dementia*, **4**, 75–80.
33. Yokota O, Tsuchiya K, Oda T, *et al.* (2006). Amyotrophic lateral sclerosis with dementia: an autopsy case showing many Bunina bodies, tau-positive neuronal and astrocytic plaque-like pathologies, and pallido-nigral degeneration. *Acta Neuropathol*, **112**, 633–645.
34. Noda K, Katayama S, Watanabe C, *et al.* (1999). Gallyas- and tau-positive glial structures in motor neuron disease with dementia. *Clin Neuropathol*, **18**, 218–225.
35. Strong MJ, Yang W, Strong WL, *et al.* (2006). Tau protein hyperphosphorylation in sporadic ALS with cognitive impairment. *Neurology*, **66**, 1770–1771.
36. Yang W, Ang L-C, Strong MJ. (2005). Tau protein aggregation in the frontal and entorhinal cortices as a function of aging. *Dev Brain Res*, **156**, 127–138.
37. Strong MJ, Grace GM, Orange JB, *et al.* (1999). A prospective study of cognitive impairment in ALS. *Neurology*, **53**, 1665–1670.
38. Braak H and Braak E. (1991). Neuropathological staging of Alzheimer-related changes. *Acta Neuropathol*, **82**, 239–259.
39. Gohar M, Yang W, Strong WL, *et al.* (2009). Tau phosphorylation at ^{175}Thr leads to fibril formation. Implications for the tauopathy of amyotrophic lateral sclerosis. *J Neurochem*, **108**, 634–643.
40. Yang W, Leystra-Lantz C, Strong MJ. (2008). Upregulation of GSK3β expression in frontal and temporal cortex of ALS with cognitive impairment (ALSci). *Brain Res*, **1196**, 131–139.
41. Moisse K, Volkening K, Leystra-Lantz C, *et al.* (2009). Divergent patterns of cytosolic TDP-43 and neuronal progranulin expression following axotomy. *Brain Res*, **1249**, 202–211.
42. Moisse K, Mepham J, Volkening K, *et al.* (2009). Cytosolic TDP-43 expression following axotomy is associated with caspase 3 activation in NFL(-/-) mice: support for a role for TDP-43 in the physiological response to neuronal injury. *Brain Res*, **1296**, 176–186.
43. Wilson AC, Dugger BN, Dickson DW, *et al.* (2011). TDP-43 in aging and Alzheimer's disease - a review. *Int J Clin Exp Pathol*, **4**, 147–155.
44. Amador-Ortiz C, Lin W-L, Ahmed Z, *et al.* (2007). TDP-43 immunoreactivity in hippocampal sclerosis and Alzheimer's disease. *Ann Neurol*, **61**, 435–445.
45. Wils H, Kleinberger G, Janssens J, *et al.* (2010). TDP-43 transgenic mice develop spastic paralysis and neuronal inclusions characteristic of ALS and frontotemporal lobar degeneration. *Proc Natl Acad Sci USA*.
46. Tsai KJ, Yang CH, Fang YH, *et al.* (2010). Elevated expression of TDP-43 in the forebrain of mice is sufficient to cause neurological and pathological phenotypes mimicking FTLD-U. *J Exp Med*, **207**, 1661–1673.
47. Wegorzewska I, Bell S, Cairns NJ, *et al.* (2009). TDP-43 mutant transgenic mice develop features of ALS and frontotemporal lobar degeneration. *Proc Natl Acad Sci USA*, **106**, 18809–18814.
48. Zhou H, Huang C, Chen H, *et al.* (2010). Transgenic rat model of neurodegeneration caused by mutation in the TDP gene. *PLoS Genet*, **6**, e1000887.

Chapter 24

Transactive response DNA-binding protein of 43 kDa

Emanuele Buratti

The transactive response DNA-binding protein of 43 kDa

Transactive response DNA-binding protein of 43 kDa (TDP-43) is an ubiquitously expressed RNA-binding protein (RBP) belonging to the heterogeneous ribonucleoprotein (hnRNP) family and containing two RNA-recognition motif domains for target RNA binding and a glycine-rich C-terminal tail required for protein–protein interaction (the sequence of this protein and its functional regions are schematically depicted in Figure 24.1(A,B) (1). In normal conditions, TDP-43 is predominantly localized in the nucleus, but recent research has confirmed that this protein can also shuttle between this compartment and the cytoplasm (2,3), a property that may be important during axonal regeneration processes (4).

It has been long known that hnRNPs play crucial roles in many gene expression pathways such as DNA replication/repair, gene transcription, pre-mRNA splicing, mRNA export/retention, mRNA stability, and protein translation (5). From a pathological point of view, misregulation of their cellular roles has been known to play an important role in tumour development and progression (6). More recently, the role they play in RNA metabolism has extended their potential importance also with regards to neuropathological diseases. As many reviews have appeared on this subject, the reader is referred to them for a more general picture (7–9). Among these proteins, TDP-43 has emerged as a major neuropathological hallmark of amyotrophic lateral sclerosis (ALS) and a subgroup of the frontotemporal lobar degenerations (FTLD) (10). There are many still unresolved questions regarding the part played by this protein in disease, as will be later discussed in this chapter and extensively reviewed in several recent reports (11–13). Whatever the answers, however, it is essential to characterize as well as possible TDP-43 normal functions within cells.

Normal transactive response DNA-binding protein of 43 kDa functions in gene expression

In general, the functional role played by each hnRNP protein depends on individual characteristics (single-stranded or double-stranded RNA binding specificities, protein–protein interactions, etc.) that at their basic levels are mostly determined by

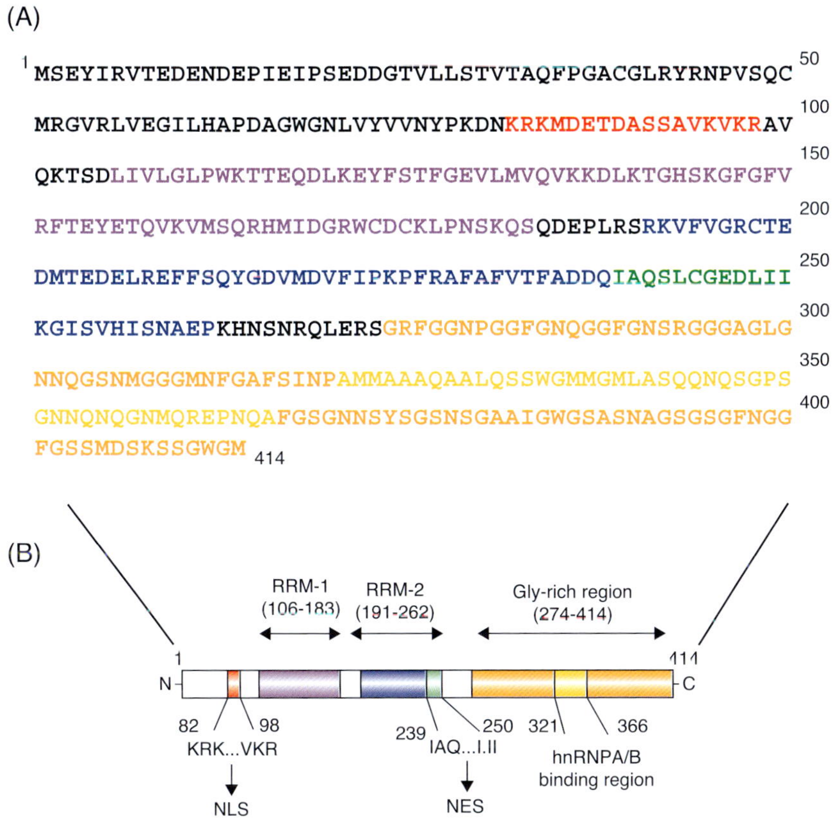

Fig. 24.1 The TDP-43 protein. (A) Shows the primary amino acid sequence of human TDP-43. Major features are highlighted. (B) Shows a schematic representation of TDP-43 protein structure reporting the major domain sequences highlighted in the sequence.

their structure. However, it should also be noted that hnRNPs are seldom 'fixed' in a single role within a particular cellular process and it is often observed that hnRNPs participate in different processes depending on a variety of additional influences provided by their cellular localization, relative abundance, binding context, and the interactions with themselves or other cellular components (6,14,15). TDP-43 is no exception to this rule and has had many diverse functional roles ascribed to it (Figure 24.2).

With regards to transcription, the role that TDP-43 plays in this process still remains pretty much undefined although originally, in fact, TDP-43 itself was identified as part of a research aimed at identifying novel HIV-1 inhibitors of transcription (16). However, aside from a promoter in the mouse *SP-10* gene where TDP-43 has been described to play a functional role as an insulator (17), no other examples have been uncovered of transcriptional regulation by this protein since its original discovery.

At the moment, the better characterized functional role of TDP-43 involves pre-mRNA splicing regulation. There are four systems in which TDP-43 has been described to play

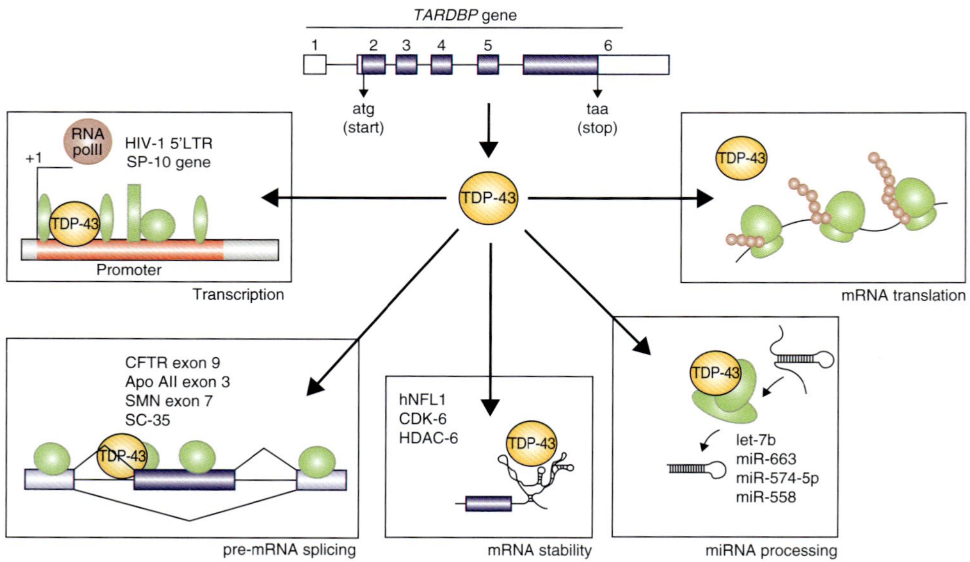

Fig. 24.2 Known functional roles of TDP-43. This figure shows the known functional roles of TDP-43. These include regulation of transcriptional processes, pre-mRNA splicing, mRNA stability, microRNA processing, and mRNA translation (although this property has only been validated *in vitro*).

an important role in deciding splicing outcomes. The first two have been extensively reviewed elsewhere (1) and involve the recognition of UG-repeated elements near the 3′ splice sites of exon 9 in the *CFTR* gene (18) and exon 3 in the *Apo AII* gene (19). In both these examples, TDP-43 has been described to act as negative splicing regulator. In this respect, it should be noted that TDP-43 splicing inhibition is dependent on its interaction with several other hnRNPs, such as A1/A2/B1/C, through its C-terminal tail (20). The C-terminal region responsible for the binding of these proteins to TDP-43 has been identified as the region spanning residues 321–366 (21). With regards to the other two splicing systems, it has been reported by Bose *et al.* that this protein plays a positive role in exon inclusion during the splicing regulation of *SMN1/2* exon 7 (22) and by Dreumont *et al.* that it helps in modulating the splicing-based, autoregulation mechanism of the SC35 splicing factor (23).

Besides splicing, TDP-43 has been found associated with both the human and mouse Drosha complexes (24,25), suggesting that this protein may also play a role in microRNA processing. In keeping with this hypothesis, depletion of TDP-43 has been recently shown to affect the cellular levels of two microRNAs, let-7b and miR-663, in a direct manner (26). Finally, and in addition to these well defined roles, TDP-43 functions have also been extended to the maintenance neurofilament stability (27,28), mRNA translation (29), and perhaps indirectly to protein geranylgeranylation (30).

Probably reflecting this great variety of functions, TDP-43 depletion from cells has been shown to affect major cellular properties such as cell-cycle regulation and the shape of the nuclear membrane (31). Moreover, Ayala *et al.* (31) have shown that several hundred factors significantly change their expression levels upon TDP-43 depletion in HeLa cells, most prominently the expression levels of the CDK6 transcript, a major controller of retinoblastoma protein (pRb) phosphorylation, and in the levels of other factors that are known to either directly interact with pRb (i.e. histone deacetylase 1, RBBP4, and CRI1) or act in response to pRb modulation (E2F8 and NAP1L1). A second microarray experiment in TDP-43 depleted HEK-293E cells (32), annexin 1 (ANXA1), and histone deacetylase 6 transcripts as major targets of TDP-43 depletion and several other targets such as chromogranin B, major vault protein, nicotinamide nucleotide adenylyltransferase 2, and secretogranin III. One interesting feature of these microarray experiments is represented by the observation that there is very little overlap with each other. Technical differences could be at the heart of many of these differences and, at this stage, it is still very difficult to separate real functional effects from potential artefactual ones. However, it is also possible that considerable heterogeneity may exist in different cell types and further work will hopefully better characterize this issue.

Pathological transactive response DNA-binding protein of 43 kDa

As previously mentioned, TDP-43 has emerged as the major neuropathological hallmark of ALS and a subgroup of the FTLD (10). It is noteworthy, however, that TDP-43 inclusions have also been described in Alzheimer's, Parkinson's, and Huntington diseases (33–35).

An unquestionable measure of its impact on neurodegeneration can be obtained by the fact that disease nomenclatures are being revised to better reflect these new clinical and pathological findings (36).

In the beginning, it was still an open question as to whether TDP-43 inclusions should have been considered as a simple pathological curiosity or whether they really played a role in disease origin and progression (37). This question was initially answered by several genetic findings in which TDP-43 mutations were identified in about 5% of familial ALS cases (38). The advent of animal models has further supported the potential role of TDP-43 in disease pathogenesis (discussed further below). What is clear is that in the patient's affected neurons, TDP-43 is abnormally mislocalized in the cytoplasm, ubiquitinated, hyperphosphorylated, and cleaved to generate C-terminal fragments (Figure 24.3A).

It is therefore likely that TDP-43 mislocalization coupled with post-translational modifications may play a pivotal role in neurodegeneration. These alterations might result in the loss of proper TDP-43 functions in the nucleus (loss-of-function effects) and/or, in the case of degradation, phosphorylation, and ubiquitination potentially toxic gain-of-function effects.

Transactive response DNA-binding protein of 43 kDa cleavage products, phosphorylation, and ubiquitination

Presently, five C-terminal degradation products of TDP-43 either by caspase or still unidentified proteases have been described and are schematically summarized in Figure 24.3(B) (39–41). It is currently believed that the presence of these fragments may produce pathological gain-of-function effects that contribute to neuronal loss. Studies in both a yeast disease model and human cell lines have supported this hypothesis (41–43). In addition to degradation, phosphorylation has been described to occur at specific amino acids, particularly S409/S410 (Figure 24.3C) (44). Phosphorylation at these two sites has been shown to be a consistent feature in all sporadic and familial ALS cases analysed so far (45). Although potentially very significant, at the moment there are very few data regarding the possible pathological effects of these aberrant phosphorylation events. Finally, also very little is known with regards to the effects of TDP-43 ubiquitination (10), although recent data have implicated this modification in affecting the clearance of this protein by autophagosomes (46). Hopefully, future experiments will address these issues in greater detail.

Transactive response DNA-binding protein of 43 kDa and stress granules

A very novel topic in TDP-43 research is represented by its potential involvement in stress granule formation. In conditions of oxidative stress, the regulation of gene expression at the post-transcriptional level causes an immediate block of the translation machinery with sequestration of the actively translating mRNAs in cytoplasmic foci, called stress granules. Stress granules are in dynamic equilibrium between polysomes and processing bodies (P-bodies) where translational arrest takes place and where TDP-43 has also been

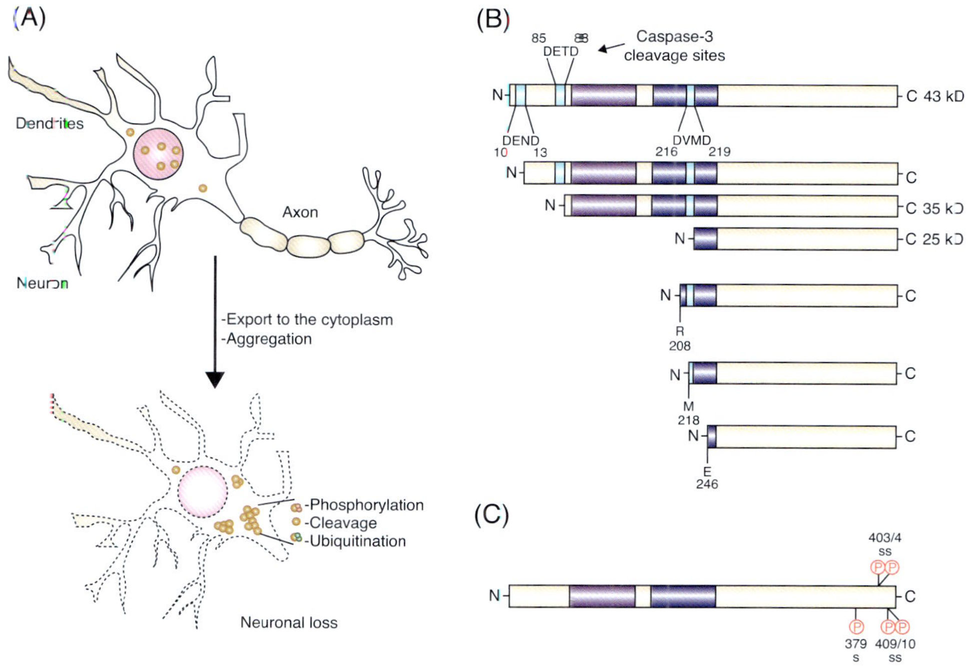

Fig. 24.3 Pathological TDP-43. (A) Shows that in normal conditions TDP-43 is continuously shuttling between the nucleus and the cytoplasm but is predominant in the nuclear compartment. In the disease state it is ubiquitinated, cleaved, phosphorylated, and exported to the cytoplasm to form insoluble aggregates. (B) Shows the known cleaved products of TDP-43 originating from caspase cleavage and by unknown proteases, which have been recently reported. (C) Shows the aberrant phosphorylation sites occurring following the aggregation of TDP-43 in the cytoplasm. These residues are never phosphorylated in normal tissues/conditions.

reported to colocalize (28). It has been shown using a motoneurone–hybridoma cell line (NSC34 cells) that different types of environmental insults are able to induce the assembly of TIAR- and HuR-positive stress granules, a subset of which also contains TDP-43 protein (47). The presence of TDP-43 in stress granules has been confirmed independently by parallel studies (28,48) and, in keeping with these conclusions, TDP-43 has been found to interact with several other stress granule protein components (48). More recently, stress granule formation has also been reported following overexpression of a 35 kDa isoform of TDP-43 that can be produced following the activation of in-frame alternative translational start sites downstream of the natural AUG (49). Overall, these data indicate that TDP-43 may play a role in the control of mRNA fate in the cytoplasmic compartment. For these reasons, beside direct cytotoxicity and loss-of-function effects, this pathway could be involved in the TDP-43 mediated pathogenesis.

Transactive response DNA-binding protein of 43 kDa mutations

Approximately 40 TDP-43 mutations associated with disease have been described to date, mostly in patients affected with familial and sporadic forms of ALS (reviewed in (38)), but also some in FTLD/motor neurone disease (MND) (50) and FTD cases without MND (51,52). These latter findings have been interpreted as suggesting that FTLD/TDPs (FTLD with TDP-43 pathology) and ALS represent two ends of a spectrum of diseases that might be better defined as TDP-43 proteinopathies. All mutations act in an apparently autosomal dominant pattern with regards to inheritance and, with only one exception (D169G), they are localized in the C-terminal end of the protein (Figure 24.4). This peculiarity highlights the importance of the C-terminal domain with regards to TDP-43 protein functions but, on the other hand, it may also indicate that the C-terminal domain might be the only domain of TDP-43 that can harbour mutations and still maintain TDP-43 essential functions in basic developmental processes. Based on the results of knockout animal models (see below), in fact, it is highly probable that mutations, which completely inactivate protein function, would probably be incompatible with life. In any case, many of the mutations identified so far have been analysed for their effect on toxicity in a variety of experimental systems (from cell lines to transgenic animal models) and the results are presented in Table 24.1. Taken together, the results of these experiments clearly demonstrate that some of these mutations are quite capable of accounting for at least part of the neurodegenerative effect mediated by TDP-43. It should also be remembered that the vast majority of patients do not carry a TDP-43 mutation and therefore their presence should not be considered essential for the origin or development of disease.

Transactive response DNA-binding protein of 43 kDa-based animal models

The development of several animal models has clearly shown the functional importance of TDP-43 in normal cellular functions. In this respect, it is worthy to note that the

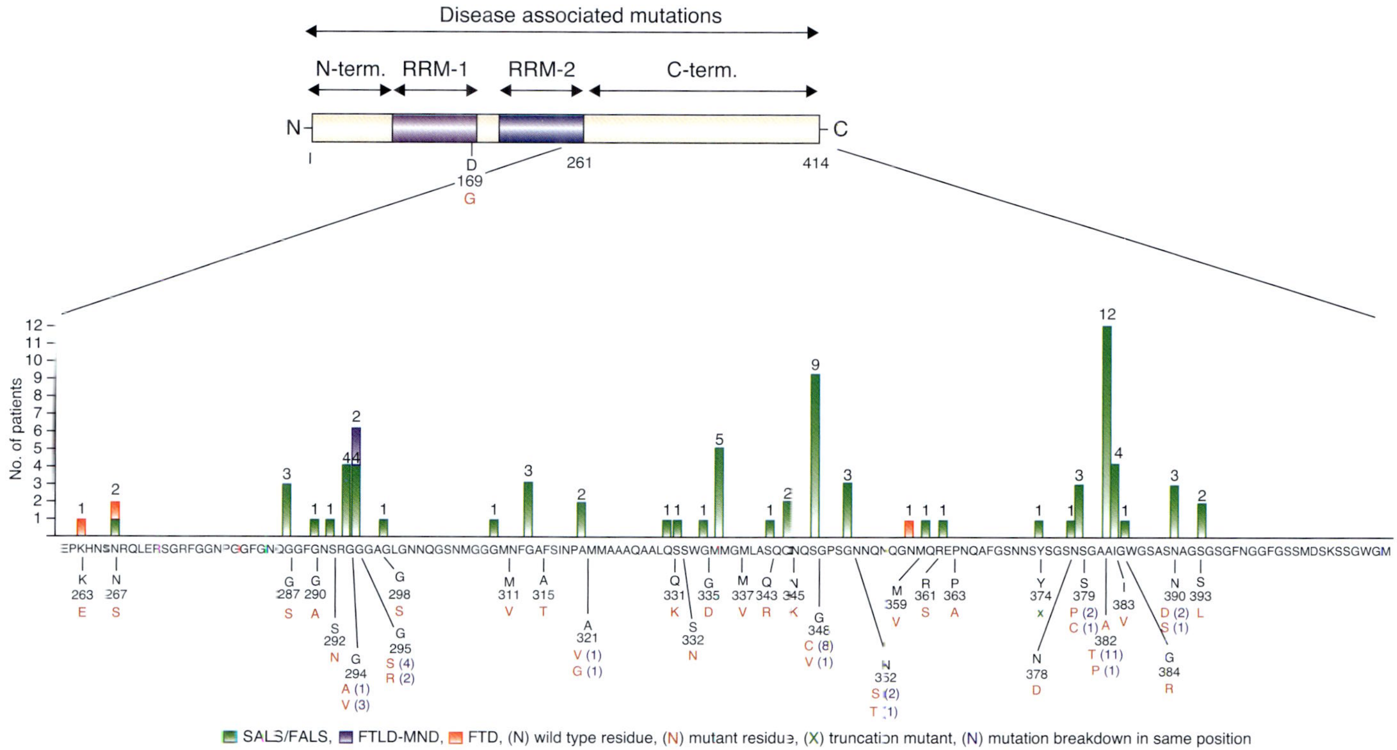

Fig. 24.4 TDP-43 mutations. Schematic diagram of the C-terminal tail of TDP-43 and of the missense/truncation mutations associated with disease (with the exception of D169G that is reported in the upper diagram) and associated with either familial/sporadic forms of ALS, FTLD/MND, and FTD without MND. The bar chart indicates the number or patients described that carry each of the identified mutation (in case of mutations found in different affected family members only one patient for family was computed).

Table 24.1 TARDBP mutations and their functional consequences

Mutation	Functional consequences of the mutation
p.D169G	Reduces binding to UBQLN factor. Promotes number of aggregates in SH-SY5Y cells.
p.K263E	ND
p.N267S	Reduced amounts of TDP-43 in patient lymphoblastoid cell line.
p.G287S	Increased CDK6 expression in fibroblasts.
p.G290A	ND
p.S292N	ND
p.G294V	ND
p.G294A	Promotes number of aggregates in SH-SY5Y cells.
p.G295S	ND
p.G295R	ND
p.G298S	ND
p.M311V	ND
p.A315T	Neurotoxic when injected in primary motor neurons and zebrafish embryos. Mice expressing the A315T protein develop a progressive and fatal neurodegenerative disease. This mutation is also toxic when expressed in rat primary cortical neurons. The proteomic pulldown profile of TDP-43 carrying this mutation is qualitatively indistinguishable from that of the wild-type protein.
p.A321V	Correlates with increased CDK6 expression in patient fibroblasts.
p.A321G	ND
p.Q331K	Causes neurotoxicity when injected in chicken embryos. When expressed in yeast, this mutation causes increased aggregation and toxicity *in vivo* with respect to wild-type TDP-43. When expressed in *Drosophila* model, this mutant protein displays less dendritic branching promotion activity than the human protein. Promotes number of aggregates in SH-SY5Y cells.
p.S332N	ND
p.G335D	ND
p.M311V	ND
p.M337V	Causes neurotoxicity when injected in chicken embryos. Displays increased degradation in lymphoblastoid cell line. Correlates with increased CDK6 expression in patient fibroblasts. When expressed in a rat animal model causes extensive neurodegeneration. In yeast, this mutation causes increased aggregation and toxicity *in vivo* with respect to wild-type TDP-43. When expressed in *Drosophila* model, the protein displays less dendritic branching promotion activity than the human protein. Promotes number of aggregates in SH-SY5Y cells. The proteomic pulldown profile of TDP-43 carrying this mutation is qualitatively indistinguishable from that of the wild-type protein.
p.Q343R	Probable increase in fragment production. When expressed in yeast, this mutation causes increased aggregation and toxicity *in vivo* with respect to wild-type TDP-43. Promotes number of aggregates in SH-SY5Y cells.
p.N345K	Increased degradation in lymphoblastoid cell line. When expressed in yeast, this mutation causes increased aggregation and toxicity *in vivo* with respect to wild-type TDP-43.

Table 24.1 (continued) TARDBP mutations and their functional consequences

Mutation	Functional consequences of the mutation
p.G348C	Increased degradation in lymphoblastoid cell line. Neurotoxic when injected in primary motor neurons and zebrafish embryos.
p.G348V	ND
p.N352S	ND
p.N352T	ND
p.M359V	ND
p.R361S	Increased degradation in lymphoblastoid cell line. When expressed in yeast, this mutation causes increased aggregation and toxicity *in vivo* with respect to wild-type TDP-43.
p.P363A	ND
p.Y374X	ND
p.N378D	ND
p.S379C	ND
p.S379P	ND
p.A382T	Neurotoxic when injected in primary motor neurons and zebrafish embryos. Increased degradation in patient fibroblasts.
p.A382P	ND
p.I383V	Increased degradation in lymphoblastoid cell line.
p.G384R	ND
p.N390D	Increased degradation in lymphoblastoid cell line. When expressed in yeast, this mutation causes increased aggregation and toxicity *in vivo* with respect to wild-type TDP-43. Promotes number of aggregates in SH-SY5Y cells.
p.N390S	Promotes number of aggregates in SH-SY5Y cells.
p.S393L	Increased degradation in patient fibroblasts.

ND, not determined.

removal of endogenous TDP-43 in *Drosophila* results in a paralytic phenotype (53), a result that has been recently confirmed in an independent fly cell line (54). Interestingly, disruption of TDP-43 expression severely impairs embryonic development in transgenic mice (55,56). Furthermore, expression of mutant forms of this protein in mice (57), rat (58), zebrafish (59), chicken (60), yeast (61), and neuronal cell lines (41,62) can reproduce neurodegenerative effects similar to those observed in human disease.

Conclusions

The emergence of TDP-43 as a novel player in neurodegeneration has provided beneficial effects at many levels. From a basic scientific point of view, the study of the importance of RNA metabolism in the control of neurodegeneration processes will probably become a very productive subject of research for many years to come. On the practical side, its identification will also move research closer to the clinic. In this respect, the main advance that we might expect in the near future is the use of 'new-entries' such as TDP-43 to devise new markers to monitor disease onset and progression. On a slightly longer time-scale, however, all this knowledge will possibly translate itself in the emergence of new pharmaceutical drugs that will specifically target these new proteins and the aberrant effects they mediate.

References

1. Buratti E, Baralle FE. (2008). Multiple roles of TDP-43 in gene expression, splicing regulation, and human disease. *Front Biosci*, **13**, 867–878.
2. Ayala YM, Zago P, D'Ambrogio A, *et al.* (2008). Structural determinants of the cellular localization and shuttling of TDP-43. *J Cell Sci*, **121**, 3778–3785.
3. Winton MJ, Igaz LM, Wong MM, Kwong LK, Trojanowski JQ, Lee VM. (2008). Disturbance of nuclear and cytoplasmic TAR DNA-binding protein (TDP-43). induces disease-like redistribution, sequestration, and aggregate formation. *J Biol Chem*, **283**, 13302–13309.
4. Moisse K, Mepham J, Volkening K, Welch I, Hill T, Strong MJ. (2009). Cytosolic TDP-43 expression following axotomy is associated with caspase 3 activation in NFL-/- mice: support for a role for TDP-43 in the physiological response to neuronal injury. *Brain Res*, **1296**, 176–186.
5. He Y, Smith R. (2009). Nuclear functions of heterogeneous nuclear ribonucleoproteins A/B. *Cell Mol Life Sci*, **66**, 1239–1256.
6. Carpenter B, MacKay C, Alnabulsi A, *et al.* (2006). The roles of heterogeneous nuclear ribonucleoproteins in tumour development and progression. *Biochim Biophys Acta*, **1765**, 85–100.
7. Strong MJ. (2010). The evidence for altered RNA metabolism in amyotrophic lateral sclerosis (ALS). *J Neurol Sci*, **288**, 1–12.
8. van Blitterswijk M, Landers JE. (2010). RNA processing pathways in amyotrophic lateral sclerosis. *Neurogenetics*, **11**(3), 275–290.
9. Anthony K, Gallo JM. (2010). Aberrant RNA processing events in neurological disorders. *Brain Res*, **1338**, 67–77.
10. Neumann M, Sampathu DM, Kwong LK, *et al.* (2006). Ubiquitinated TDP-43 in frontotemporal lobar degeneration and amyotrophic lateral sclerosis. *Science*, **314**, 130–133.
11. Chen-Plotkin AS, Lee VM, Trojanowski JQ. (2010). TAR DNA-binding protein 43 in neurodegenerative disease. *Nat Rev Neurol*, **6**, 211–220.
12. Buratti E, Baralle FE. (2009). The molecular links between TDP-43 dysfunction and neurodegeneration. *Adv Genet*, **66**, 1–34.
13. Gendron TF, Josephs KA, Petrucelli L. (2010). Review: transactive response DNA-binding protein 43 (TDP-43): mechanisms of neurodegeneration. *Neuropathol Appl Neurobiol*, **36**(2), 97–112.
14. Dreyfuss G, Kim VN, Kataoka N. (2002). Messenger-RNA-binding proteins and the messages they carry. *Nat Rev Mol Cell Biol*, **3**, 195–205.
15. Glisovic T, Bachorik JL, Yong J, Dreyfuss G. (2008). RNA-binding proteins and post-transcriptional gene regulation. *FEBS Lett*, **582**, 1977–86.
16. Ou SH, Wu F, Harrich D, Garcia-Martinez LF, Gaynor RB. (1995). Cloning and characterization of a novel cellular protein, TDP-43, that binds to human immunodeficiency virus type 1 TAR DNA sequence motifs. *J Virol*, **69**, 3584–96.
17. Abhyankar MM, Urekar C, Reddi PP. (2007). A novel CpG-free vertebrate insulator silences the testis-specific SP-10 gene in somatic tissues: role for TDP-43 in insulator function. *J Biol Chem*, **282**, 36143–36154.
18. Buratti E, Dork T, Zuccato E, Pagani F, Romano M, Baralle FE. (2001). Nuclear factor TDP-43 and SR proteins promote *in vitro* and *in vivo* CFTR exon 9 skipping. *EMBO J*, **20**, 1774–1784.

19. Mercado PA, Ayala YM, Romano M, Buratti E, Baralle FE. (2005). Depletion of TDP 43 overrides the need for exonic and intronic splicing enhancers in the human apoA-II gene. *Nucleic Acids Res*, **33**, 6000–6010.
20. Buratti E, Brindisi A, Giombi M, Tisminetzky S, Ayala YM, Baralle FE. (2005). TDP-43 binds heterogeneous nuclear ribonucleoprotein A/B through its C-terminal tail: an important region for the inhibition of cystic fibrosis transmembrane conductance regulator exon 9 splicing. *J Biol Chem*, **280**, 37572–37584.
21. D'Ambrogio A, Buratti E, Stuani C, *et al.* (2009). Functional mapping of the interaction between TDP-43 and hnRNP A2 *in vivo*. *Nucleic Acids Res*, **37**, 4116–4126.
22. Bose JK, Wang IF, Hung L, Tarn WY, Shen CK. (2008). TDP-43 Overexpression enhances exon 7 inclusion during the survival of motor neuron pre-mRNA splicing. *J Biol Chem*, **283**, 28852–28859.
23. Dreumont N, Hardy S, Behm-Ansmant I, *et al.* (2009). Antagonistic factors control the unproductive splicing of SC35 terminal intron. *Nucleic Acids Res*, **38**(4), 1353–1366.
24. Gregory RI, Yan KP, Amuthan G, *et al.* (2004). The Microprocessor complex mediates the genesis of microRNAs. *Nature*, **432**, 235–240.
25. Fukuda T, Yamagata K, Fujiyama S, *et al.* (2007). DEAD-box RNA helicase subunits of the Drosha complex are required for processing of rRNA and a subset of microRNAs. *Nat Cell Biol*, **9**, 604–611.
26. Buratti E, De Conti L, Stuani C, Romano M, Baralle M, Baralle FE. (2010). Nuclear factor TDP-43 can affect selected miRNA levels. *FEBS J*, **277**(10), 2268–81.
27. Strong MJ, Volkening K, Hammond R, *et al.* (2007). TDP43 is a human low molecular weight neurofilament (hNFL). mRNA-binding protein. *Mol Cell Neurosci*, **35**, 320–327.
28. Volkening K, Leystra-Lantz C, Yang W, Jaffee H, Strong MJ. (2009). Tar DNA binding protein of 43 kDa (TDP-43), 14–3-3 proteins and copper/zinc superoxide dismutase (SOD1). interact to modulate NFL mRNA stability. Implications for altered RNA processing in amyotrophic lateral sclerosis (ALS). *Brain Res*, **1305**, 168–182.
29. Wang IF, Wu LS, Chang HY, Shen CK. (2008). TDP-43, the signature protein of FTLD-U, is a neuronal activity-responsive factor. *J Neurochem*, **105**, 797–806.
30. Iguchi Y, Katsuno M, Niwa J, *et al.* (2009). TDP-43 depletion induces neuronal cell damage through dysregulation of Rho family GTPases. *J Biol Chem*, **284**, 22059–22066.
31. Ayala YM, Misteli T, Baralle FE. (2008). TDP-43 regulates retinoblastoma protein phosphorylation through the repression of cyclin-dependent kinase 6 expression. *Proc Natl Acad Sci USA*, **105**, 3785–3789.
32. Fiesel FC, Voigt A, Weber SS, *et al.* (2010). Knockdown of transactive response DNA-binding protein (TDP-43) downregulates histone deacetylase 6. *EMBO J*, **29**, 209–221.
33. Amador-Ortiz C, Lin WL, Ahmed Z, *et al.* (2007). TDP-43 immunoreactivity in hippocampal sclerosis and Alzheimer's disease. *Ann Neurol*, **61**, 435–445.
34. Nakashima-Yasuda H, Uryu K, Robinson J, *et al.* (2007). Co-morbidity of TDP-43 proteinopathy in Lewy body related diseases. *Acta Neuropathol*, **114**, 221–229.
35. Schwab C, Arai T, Hasegawa M, Yu S, McGeer PL. (2008). Colocalization of transactivation-responsive DNA-binding protein 43 and huntingtin in inclusions of Huntington disease. *J Neuropathol Exp Neurol*, **67**, 1159–1165.
36. Mackenzie IR, Neumann M, Bigio EH, *et al.* (2010). Nomenclature and nosology for neuropathologic subtypes of frontotemporal lobar degeneration: an update. *Acta Neuropathol*, **119**, 1–4.
37. Rothstein JD. (2007). TDP-43 in amyotrophic lateral sclerosis: pathophysiology or patho-babel? *Ann Neurol*, **61**, 382–384.
38. Pesiridis GS, Lee VM, Trojanowski JQ. (2009). Mutations in TDP-43 link glycine-rich domain functions to amyotrophic lateral sclerosis. *Hum Mol Genet*, **18**, R156–R162.
39. Zhang YJ, Xu YF, Dickey CA, *et al.* (2007). Progranulin mediates caspase-dependent cleavage of TAR DNA binding protein-43. *J Neurosci*, **27**, 10530–10534.

40. Igaz LM, Kwong LK, Chen-Plotkin A, *et al.* (2009). Expression Of TDP-43 C-terminal fragments *in vitro* recapitulates pathological features of TDP-43 proteinopathies. *J Biol Chem*, **284**, 8516–8524.
41. Nonaka T, Kametani F, Arai T, Akiyama H, Hasegawa M. (2009). Truncation and pathogenic mutations facilitate the formation of intracellular aggregates of TDP-43. *Hum Mol Genet*, **18**, 3353–3364.
42. Johnson BS, McCaffery JM, Lindquist S, Gitler AD. (2008). A yeast TDP-43 proteinopathy model: Exploring the molecular determinants of TDP-43 aggregation and cellular toxicity. *Proc Natl Acad Sci USA*, **105**, 6439–6444.
43. Zhang YJ, Xu YF, Cook C, *et al.* (2009). Aberrant cleavage of TDP-43 enhances aggregation and cellular toxicity. *Proc Natl Acad Sci USA*, **106**, 7607–7612.
44. Hasegawa M, Arai T, Nonaka T, *et al.* (2008). Phosphorylated TDP-43 in frontotemporal lobar degeneration and amyotrophic lateral sclerosis. *Ann Neurol*, **64**, 60–70.
45. Neumann M, Kwong LK, Lee EB, *et al.* (2009). Phosphorylation of S409/410 of TDP-43 is a consistent feature in all sporadic and familial forms of TDP-43 proteinopathies. *Acta Neuropathol*, **117**, 137–149.
46. Urushitani M, Sato T, Bamba H, Hisa Y, Tooyama I. (2010). Synergistic effect between proteasome and autophagosome in the clearance of polyubiquitinated TDP-43. *J Neurosci Res*, **88**, 784–797.
47. Colombrita C, Zennaro E, Fallini C, Weber M, Sommacal A, Buratti E, Silani V, Ratti A. (2009). TDP-43 is recruited to stress granules in conditions of oxidative insult. *J Neurochem*, **111**, 1051–1061.
48. Freibaum BD, Chitta RK, High AA, Taylor JP. (2010). Global analysis of TDP-43 interacting proteins reveals strong association with RNA splicing and translation machinery. *J Proteome Res*, **9**, 1104–1120.
49. Nishimoto Y, Ito D, Yagi T, Nihei Y, Tsunoda Y, Suzuki N. (2010). Characterization of alternative isoforms and inclusion body of the TAR DNA-binding protein-43. *J Biol Chem*, **285**, 608–619.
50. Benajiba L, Le Ber I, Camuzat A, *et al.* (2009). TARDBP mutations in motoneuron disease with frontotemporal lobar degeneration. *Ann Neurol*, **65**, 470–473.
51. Kovacs GG, Murrell JR, Horvath S, *et al.* (2009). TARDBP variation associated with frontotemporal dementia, supranuclear gaze palsy, and chorea. *Mov Disord*, **24**, 1843–1847.
52. Borroni B, Bonvicini C, Alberici A, *et al.* (2009). Mutation within TARDBP leads to frontotemporal dementia without motor neuron disease. *Hum Mutat*, **30**, E974–E983.
53. Feiguin F, Godena VK, Romano G, D'Ambrogio A, Klima R, Baralle FE. (2009). Depletion of TDP-43 affects Drosophila motoneurons terminal synapsis and locomotive behavior. *FEBS Lett*, **583**, 1586–1592.
54. Lu Y, Ferris J, Gao FB. (2009). Frontotemporal dementia and amyotrophic lateral sclerosis-associated disease protein TDP-43 promotes dendritic branching. *Mol Brain*, **2**, 30.
55. Sephton CF, Good SK, Atkin S, *et al.* (2010). TDP-43 Is a developmentally regulated protein essential for early embryonic development. *J Biol Chem*, **285**, 6826–6834.
56. Wu LS, Cheng WC, Hou SC, Yan YT, Jiang ST, Shen CK. (2010). TDP-43, a neuro-pathosignature factor, is essential for early mouse embryogenesis. *Genesis*, **48**, 56–62.
57. Wegorzewska I, Bell S, Cairns NJ, Miller TM, Baloh RH. (2009). TDP-43 mutant transgenic mice develop features of ALS and frontotemporal lobar degeneration. *Proc Natl Acad Sci USA*, **106**, 18809–18814.
58. Zhou H, Huang C, Chen H, *et al.* (2010). Transgenic rat model of neurodegeneration caused by mutation in the TDP gene. *PLoS Genet*, **6**, e1000887.
59. Kabashi E, Lin L, Tradewell ML, *et al.* (2010). Gain and loss of function of ALS-related mutations of TARDBP (TDP-43) cause motor deficits *in vivo*. *Hum Mol Genet*, **19**, 671–683.
60. Sreedharan J, Blair IP, Tripathi VB, *et al.* (2008). TDP-43 mutations in familial and sporadic amyotrophic lateral sclerosis. *Science*, **319**, 1668–1672.

61. Johnson BS, Snead D, Lee JJ, McCaffery JM, Shorter J, Gitler AD. (2009). TDP-43 is intrinsically aggregation-prone, and amyotrophic lateral sclerosis-linked mutations accelerate aggregation and increase toxicity. *J Biol Chem*, **284**, 20329–20339.

62. Barmada SJ, Skibinski G, Korb E, Rao EJ, Wu JY, Finkbeiner S. (2010). Cytoplasmic mislocalization of TDP-43 is toxic to neurons and enhanced by a mutation associated with familial amyotrophic lateral sclerosis. *J Neurosci*, **30**, 639–649.

Chapter 25

Progranulin

Jennifer Gass and Leonard Petrucelli

Progranulin (PGRN), a widely secreted growth factor, plays a role in the pathogenesis of multiple diseases, but new studies showing a link between a loss of PGRN and neurodegeneration have encouraged scientists searching for treatments. PGRN is involved in multiple biological functions, including cell growth and survival (1–3), embryogenesis (4,5), wound repair, and inflammation (1,6–9). Recent genetic evidence identified pathogenic mutations located within *GRN* as a major cause of frontotemporal lobar degeneration with ubiquitin-positive inclusions (FLTD-U) (10,11). These mutations, mostly non-sense, create a haploinsufficiency generating a loss of PGRN in these patients.

Currently, the role of PGRN in the central nervous system (CNS) remains relatively unknown; however, ongoing research in this area is furthering understanding. In humans, 6 kDa granulin repeats are derived from the precursor protein PGRN (1,12–14), which is also known as granulin–epithelin precursor (3), proepithelin (2), PC cell derived growth factor (15), and acrogranin (16).

While elevated levels of PGRN have been associated with various types of cancer (17–24), the loss of PGRN caused by mutations is linked to neurodegeneration. Determining how variations in the level of PGRN affect biological function is pertinent to potential treatment methods for FTLD-U and cancer. This chapter will highlight the functional and biochemical roles of PGRN, and how a decrease in PGRN neurotrophic support may lead to increased risk of cell death and neurodegenerative disease.

Progranulin structure and processing

PGRN is a 68.5 kDa glycoprotein composed of a secretory signal linked to seven-and-a-half tandem repeats of a 12-cysteine granulin motif, which are separated by interlinked spacer regions (Figure 25.1A) (25). The signal sequence allows PGRN to be secreted as an intact, full-length 88 kDa protein (8). The higher molecular weight of secreted PGRN is due to N-glycosylation at five potential sites (26).

Although the structure of full-length human PGRN is unknown, the granulins contain a distinct conformation consisting of four, stacked, β-hairpins that are joined by an axial rod of disulphide bridges (27,28). In the periphery, processing of the full-length PGRN into granulins occurs via proteolytic cleavage of the interlinked spacer regions by proteases. Currently, several proteases are known to cleave PGRN, including elastase (9), proteinase 3 (6), matrix metalloproteinase-14 (29), and ADAM metallopeptidase with thrombospondin

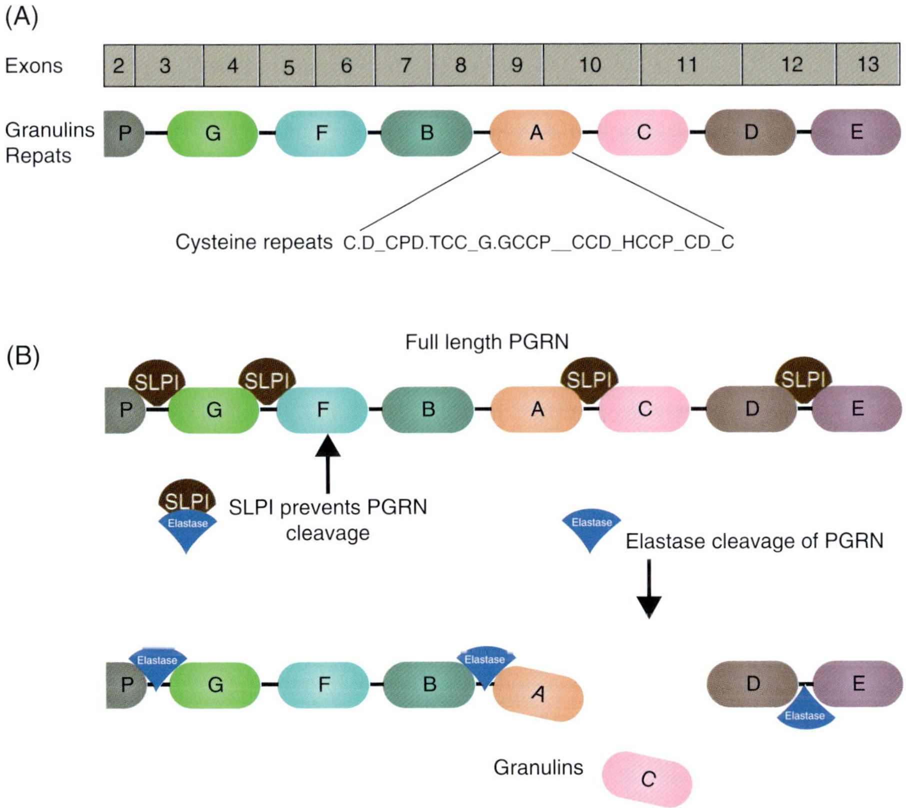

Fig. 25.1 PGRN structure and processing. (A) PGRN is made up of 593 amino acids with a predicted molecular weight of 68.5 kDa. However, due to heavy glycosylation it is secreted as an 88 kDa protein. PGRN is composed of 13 exons, 2–13 of which encode 7.5 granulin repeat peptides known as paragranulin and granulins (A–G). As shown, granulins are separated by interlinked spacer regions, and are composed of highly conserved cysteine repeats. (B) PGRN is cleaved at interlinker spacer regions by proteolytic enzymes, such as elastase, generating the granulin peptides. Secretory leucocyte protease inhibitor (SLPI) protects full-length PGRN by binding to both PGRN and elastase, therefore preventing cleavage into the 6 kDa granulins.

type 1 motif, 7 (30). The proteolytic processing of PGRN is also regulated by secretory leucocyte protease inhibitor (SLPI), a serine protease inhibitor secreted by neutrophils and macrophages (9). As depicted in Figure 25.1(B), SLPI prevents cleavage of PGRN by two distinct mechanisms (i.e. by directly binding to PGRN at cleavage sites and by binding to and inhibiting the protease elastase). Although it is unclear if this also occurs in the CNS, it is possible that elastase released from the microglia during injury will cleave PGRN, which can also be inhibited by SLPI released from astrocytes. Recently, it was also suggested that high-density lipoprotein HDL/apolipoprotein AI complex is able to suppress cleavage by binding to PGRN, but how or if this relates to the CNS has not been determined (31).

Progranulin function

Although PGRN expression occurs in a variety of body tissues, it is predominantly expressed in certain epithelial, immune, and neuronal cells in adult rats and mice (32). During embryogenesis, PGRN mRNA levels are highest at the blastocyst stage, indicating that PGRN is involved with early development (5). In addition, within the developing brain, PGRN has been shown to be widely expressed in the forebrain, retinal ganglia, olfactory bulbs, as well as the spinal cord. However, in the adult rodent brain, PGRN is mainly found in cerebellar Purkinje cells, pyramidal neurones of the cortex, and hippocampus, as well as in activated microglia, suggesting the function of PGRN is developmentally regulated (4,32). The findings may also indicate that a loss of PGRN expression could interfere with proper neurodevelopment.

It is believed that PGRN promotes neuronal cell survival due to its known function within the periphery and neurotrophic properties characteristic of other common growth factors. Although the functions of PGRN in the CNS are not completely understood, experiments in which PGRN is overexpressed in both cortical and motor neuronal cultures have shown increased cell viability (33,34). In addition, neurite outgrowth, which is increased by full-length PGRN, can be inhibited by application of recombinant SLPI, suggesting that SLPI inhibits full-length PGRN neurotrophic properties. An alternative explanation is that the presence of GRN is needed for proper outgrowth (33).

Recent identification of PGRN binding receptors will provide insight into the roles of PGRN in disease, in addition to therapeutics involved in regulating PGRN levels. Sortilin (Sort1), a Vsp10p-domain receptor, was the first receptor identified. This multifunctional receptor can act as a sorting receptor involved in protein transport typically between the Golgi apparatus and endosomes as well as a co-receptor in signal transduction. Carrasquillo *et al.* and Hu *et al.* both identified Sort1 independently and suggest that it is involved in endocytosis of PGRN and, therefore, regulating levels of PGRN (35,36). Additionally, identification of PGRN binding to tumor necrosis factor receptors (TNFR) suggests that PGRN acts as an antagonist for TNFα (37).

In the periphery, PGRN activates various growth factor signal transduction pathways involved in cell growth and survival, migration, and inflammation. For example, PGRN is able to phosphorylate p44/42 mitogen-activated protein kinase in the extracellular regulated kinase pathway, in addition to activating the phosphatidyl inositol-3 cascade by phosphorylating phosphatidyl inositol-3, protein kinase B/AKT, and $p70^{S6}$ (38–41). In wound repair, PGRN inhibits tumour necrosis factor-α induced signal transduction in neutrophils, thereby reducing inflammation (9). Thus, identification of signal transduction pathways influenced by PGRN within the CNS will be important for the development of future therapeutic approaches aimed at rescuing PGRN function in FTLD-U patients.

Progranulin mutations

The first mutations in *GRN* were discovered in 2006 after sequencing a 3.53 cM (6.19 Mb) linkage region containing 165 candidate genes (10,11). *GRN* was identified after thorough investigation of the 17q21 region, which is also home to microtubule associated protein tau (*MAPT*), the first gene identified to contain mutations causing FTLD (42). Patients with *MAPT* mutations are pathologically characterized by the accumulation of filamentous, hyperphosphorylated tau (43). Subsequent genetic analysis also identified other genes associated with FTLD, including *C9ORF72* and valosin-containing protein both located on chromosome 9 (44, 45, 46), and chromatin modifying protein 2B (*CHMP2B*) on chromosome 3 (47).

Multiple investigators have identified 69 different pathogenic mutations throughout *GRN*, as shown in Figure 25.2 (48). Non-sense, frameshift, and splice-site mutations promote premature termination of the coding sequence, which subsequently leads to degradation of the mutant RNA via non-sense-mediated decay (10,11,49). Kozak sequence mutations affect translation of PGRN, while other mutations cause full genomic deletions. A number of these mutations create a null allele that leads to haploinsufficiency of *GRN*. For example, an expression analysis of pathogenic mutation carriers revealed that reducing PGRN transcripts by 50% resulted in a 30–35% reduction in protein expression, with no detectable levels of the truncated PGRN products due to non-sense-mediated decay (10). An interesting exception is the missense mutation p.A9D, which due to its location within the hydrophobic core of the signal peptide, results in functional haploinsufficiency via loss of PGRN secretion (50).

While most pathogenic mutations result in a null allele of *GRN*, to date there are dozens of mutations of unknown pathogenicity (48). Thirty-four of these mutations are absent in controls, while 45 were discovered in controls suggesting that they are not pathogenic. These mutations are typically missense, silent, intronic, and regulatory variants, though it is unclear if these mutations lead to a loss of PGRN function similar to pathogenic null mutations. Lack of functional data on most of these mutations restricts our understanding of their possible contribution to disease; however, biochemical studies have determined that several missense mutations disrupt the normal function of PGRN. The missense mutations p.P248L and p.R432C display impaired secretion in comparison with wild-type PGRN when overexpressed *in vitro* (50). This decrease in secretion is likely due to improper transport through the secretory pathway leading to premature degradation of these PGRN mutants. *In silico* analysis of these mutations also suggests that they may severely disrupt the structure of PGRN leading to a haploinsufficiency (51). In addition, missense mutations of cysteine residues (p.C139R, p.C521Y) have been shown to impact PGRN production and possibly function. Cysteine residues mediate disulphide bond formation, and thus are extremely important to the secondary structure and stability of proteins. PGRN contains numerous cysteine repeat regions; consequently, mutations in cysteine residues could possibly lead to an altered secondary structure or instability of either PGRN or the resultant granulins. For example, functional analysis of p.C139R and p.C521Y PGRN mutants reveals improper protein mobility under non-reducing conditions, as well as abnormal cleavage (52). The loss of functional protein may result from variations in highly conserved cysteine residues that led to improper PGRN secondary structure.

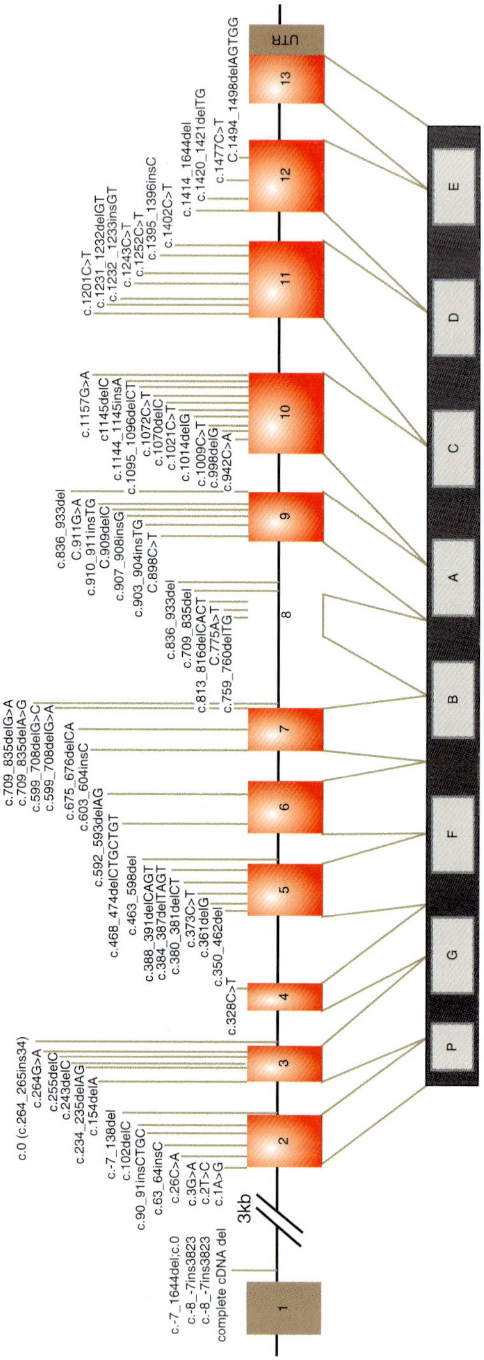

Fig. 25.2 Pathogenic *GRN* mutations associated with FTLD-U. At present, 69 pathogenic mutations have been discovered in patients with FTLD-U. These mutations range from complete protein deletions, non-sense, frameshift, splice-site, Kozak sequence, and signal peptide mutations. Pathogenic mutations have been shown to result in a haploinsufficiency caused by non-sense-mediated decay, which results in decreased PGRN expression. In the schematic diagram, clear lettered boxes within the full-length PGRN protein depict individual granulin repeats. Mutations are numbered relative to the largest PGRN transcript (GenBank accession number NM_002087.2).

In contrast to pathogenic null mutations, most missense, silent, and intronic variants do not result in a haploinsufficiency begging the question: Do *GRN* mutations possess another mechanism of pathogenicity other than the creation of a null allele? Without proper mutation segregation or *in vivo* functional data to help explain the mechanism of disease, it will be difficult to determine how or if these mutations are pathogenic. The possibility that these mutations may still influence the incidence of disease by acting as risk factors has not been excluded. In fact, the genetic variant (rs5848), which is located in the 3′-untranslated region of *GRN,* is believed to significantly increase the risk of FTLD-U (53,54). This region of *GRN* regulates expression through modulation of miRNA binding (53). T alleles at this site likely alter miRNA binding affinity for the human-specific miRNA miR-659. Study results show a decrease in PGRN protein levels, as well as a 3.2-fold increase in the risk of FTLD-U in patients with the TT genotype in comparison with patients expressing the control CC genotype (53). Attempts to replicate these data failed to show the same results, possibly due to differences in the patient populations that were studied (54,55). Despite the negative findings, it is likely this genetic variant influences the risk of disease given that patients with Alzheimer disease (AD) expressing the rs5848 variant exhibit decreased levels of PGRN (56), and the significant association between rs5848 variant and incidence of hippocampal sclerosis in patients with AD (57).

Several groups have reported decreased plasma levels of PGRN in mutation carriers when compared with patients without *GRN* mutations (58–60). In patients with null *GRN* mutations, PGRN reduction is about 75% with respect to non-mutation patients. Contrary to these results, PGRN mRNA levels are only reduced by 35–50% in patients with *GRN* mutations (10). This discrepancy in mRNA and plasma PGRN levels suggests abnormal metabolism of PGRN, though only full-length PGRN and not the cleaved granulins are detectable by this ELISA method. Perhaps under conditions of reduced PGRN expression, a greater percentage of full-length is converted into granulins, which could account for this difference (Figure 25.1B).

Disease susceptibility and pathology associated with progranulin mutations

The frequency of *GRN* mutations is estimated to be in the range of 1–11.7% of the total FTLD population, and 3.4–25.6% of familial cases (10,11,49,61–66). The high variability in frequencies is possibly due to the patient populations, as well as strong founder effects of the higher frequencies. In particular, large founder effects were caused by two different mutations IVS0+5G>C (11) and p.R493X. Mutation p.R493X was detected in 2% of the FTLD population studied and was suggested to arise from two founder haplotypes, one found in 27 families and the other in two families (67).

Disease onset from pathogenic mutations in *GRN* ranges from 48 to 83 years, with a mean age at onset about 59±7 years. Liability curve data demonstrate that 50% of *PGRN* mutation carriers are affected by the age of 60 years, while 90% are affected by 70 years of age, emphasizing the significant proportion of patients that remain unaffected until old age (49).

Disease duration in *GRN* mutation carriers is approximately 2.4 years shorter compared with *MAPT* mutation carriers, which is possibly due to a more rapid progression of the disease in these patients (68). The variable age at onset of disease in patients with *GRN* mutations may be indicative of the existence of other modifying factors—genetic or environmental—with a potential impact on disease progression and severity.

The brains of patients harbouring *GRN* mutations are characterized by severe atrophy in the frontal and temporal lobes, as well as atrophy of the parietal lobe (69). Often this atrophy is asymmetric. Brain volumes are also smaller, with a faster rate of whole brain atrophy compared with other patients with FTLD (70–73). *GRN* mutation carriers exhibit considerable heterogeneity among their symptoms. The behavioural variant of FTD (bvFTD) is the most common clinical phenotype reported in mutation carriers (49,64,74–77), but language dysfunction, such as primary progressive aphasia also accounts for a large percentage of patients with PGRN (11,72), as well as FTD with parkinsonism (75) and corticobasal syndrome (79–81).

PGRN is not detected within disease aggregates, unlike *MAPT* mutations that result in an accumulation of hyperphosphorylated tau. Shortly after the discovery of *GRN* mutations, transactive response DNA-binding protein of 43 kDa (TDP-43) was identified as the major protein associated with the ubiquitin-positive inclusions in FTLD-U and amyotrophic lateral sclerosis (ALS) (82). TDP-43 is normally a nuclear protein, but in disease is cleaved into 25 and 35 kDa fragments translocated to the cytoplasm (82,83) (see Buratti, Chapter 24, for a detailed discussion). Briefly, TDP-43 is involved in RNA binding, and additionally regulates a variety of cellular processes. Histological characterization of TDP-43 inclusions has revealed that patients with PGRN mutations present with a common FTLD/TDP subtype (see Cairns, Chapter 18, for a detailed discussion). This subtype is characterized by TDP-43-immunoreactive, neuronal cytoplasmic inclusions, short thin neurites in cortical

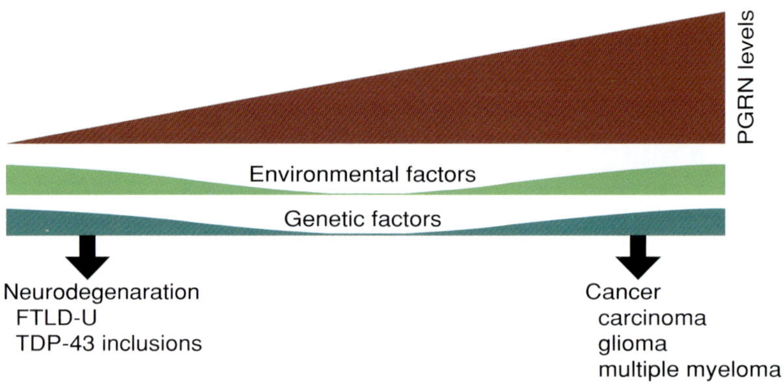

Fig. 25.3 Regulation of PGRN levels is important for successful ageing. PGRN upregulation is associated with several types of cancers. Conversely, mutations in PGRN result in decreased levels of PGRN, leading to neurodegeneration (FTLD-U) and the abnormal accumulation and cleavage of TDP-43. Although other unknown genetic and environmental factors also contribute to disease risk, determining how to restore PGRN levels, as well as how to maintain the proper level of expression, will be crucial to the development of future therapeutic approaches.

layer II, and lentiform neuronal intranuclear inclusions (70,84). The relationship between progranulin haploinsufficiency and TDP-43 pathology is currently unknown, though reduction in PGRN expression *in vitro* has been shown to induce caspase-dependent cleavage of TDP-43 into fragments similar to the 25 and 35 kDa species observed in humans (83). While caspase-mediated cleavage of TDP-43 has been replicated, it is still not confirmed if this is dependent on PGRN (85).

Progranulin, a risk factor for diseases other than frontotemporal lobar degeneration with ubiquitin

Although PGRN is a neurotrophin involved in the growth and survival of neurones, questions remain whether certain genetic variants of PGRN act as risk factors for multiple neurodegenerative diseases. PGRN haploinsufficiency is predominantly associated with FTLD-U; however, PGRN levels have been shown to be upregulated in AD, ALS, and Parkinson's disease (PD) (78,86,87). It is possible that in the above-mentioned neurodegenerative diseases, PGRN is upregulated by both activated microglia and neurones in response to CNS injury (88). While *GRN* null mutations have not been shown to be a major cause of AD, PD, or ALS, it is important to note in rare instances null mutations have been reported in clinically identified patients with AD and PD (78, 89). In addition, a number of *GRN* missense mutations have been reported in patients with AD and ALS (67,90). Some of these mutations were recently discovered in control samples (91), which argues against pathogenicity, but does not rule out the possibility these particular mutations modulate risk of disease. In conclusion, *GRN* mutations are not a major cause of AD, ALS, and PD, but it is possible that certain genetic variants of *GRN* serve as risk factors to other diseases.

Progranulin knockout animals

Investigators have generated and are beginning to characterize *GRN*-deficient mouse models to provide more information on the protein's function. Kayasuga and colleagues developed a PGRN-deficient mouse by disrupting the mouse *GRN* gene in mouse embryonic stem cells (92), resulting in a complete knockout (KO). Initial studies performed on these mice reveal enhanced aggressive behaviour, as well as a display of several features that correlate with FTLD (93). Ahmed and colleagues reported that *GRN*-deficient mice pathologically displayed characteristics of enhanced ageing, including the accumulation of aberrant ubiquitin-positive lipofuscin granules, which are formed by oxidative stress upon mitochondrial or lysosomal injury (94). Although these *GRN* KO mice do exhibit increased ubiquitin staining, they do not develop TDP-43 pathology characteristic of FTLD-U. However, aged *GRN* KO mice do develop focal neuronal loss associated with microgliosis and astrogliosis, which is a classic hallmark of neurodegeneration (94).

A conditional *GRN*-deficient mouse model has been generated by Yin and colleagues, who used Cre/loxP recombination to knockout PGRN in all tissues (7). These mice produce a hyperinflammatory response reportedly caused by decreases in anti-inflammatory cytokines and increases proinflammatory cytokines. This response appears to lead to microglial and astrocytic activation, which may account for the increase in cell death observed specifically in hippocampal neurones in this mouse model. Importantly, Yin and colleagues also report an increase in ubiquitin immunoreactivity, which colocalizes with phosphorylated TDP-43 (10). However, Ahmed and colleagues failed to detect TDP-43 pathology in their *GRN* KO model (94).

Additional work with *GRN*-deficient animals is needed to better characterize the role of PGRN in neuronal function and disease, in addition to evaluating a potential role for PGRN in the treatment or prevention of various neurodegenerative conditions. However, one of the most important questions that will need to be answered before active consideration of PGRN supplementation as a viable therapeutic option is whether it is possible to exploit the neuroprotective effects of PGRN, without the detrimental consequences of PGRN overexpression, in particular tumorigenesis.

Conclusions

Although the specific functions of PGRN have not been fully characterized, it is becoming apparent that the expression and function of PGRN is an important determinant of successful ageing. As we age, various genetic and environmental factors contribute to risk of disease, thereby also influencing disease onset and progression (Figure 25.3). Genetic mutations and alleles that confer risk of disease are widely studied modifiers of health. For example, as discussed within this chapter, reduction of PGRN levels in the brain as a result of mutations is a cause of FTLD-U, and may increase risk of other neurodegenerative diseases. The second factor, that of environmental insults, may be accrued throughout the life span of a neurone, though this component and its contribution to risk of disease is not well studied. Neurotrophic support is critical to the health of neurones, which are also likely to be comparatively sensitive to age-related accumulation of stress by virtue of their cell cycle senescence. Thus, a decrease in PGRN neurotrophic support may increase neuronal vulnerability to injury, inflammation, or other insults, leading to increased risk of cell death and disease. Such observations suggest that increasing PGRN levels, for example to patients at risk of FTLD-U, would be a potential therapeutic. Determining the balance of PGRN levels will be very important when developing therapeutics; doing so would mean understanding negative effects of elevated levels of PGRN that contribute to various types of cancer.

In working toward future therapeutics, several factors and relationships need to be considered. Further characterization of the specific functions of the various granulins, as well as how they impact/modulate signalling cascades within the CNS, will provide greater insight into the role of PGRN deficiency in neurodegeneration. Understanding why the loss of PGRN leads to degeneration specifically in the frontal and temporal lobes is crucial. Perhaps these regions of the brain are more vulnerable to insults, and the loss of trophic support exacerbates the effect. Alternatively, the neurotrophic functions performed by PGRN may be exclusive to PGRN in neurones affected in FTLD-U, and other neurotrophic factors may not be able to efficiently compensate for the deficiency. In either case, it is important to understand how *GRN* mutations and TDP-43 pathology are linked, as well as their respective roles in neurodegeneration. Answers to this question may broaden the understanding of pathogenesis in other neurodegenerative diseases.

References

1. Bateman A, Belcourt D, Bennett H, Lazure C, Solomon S. (1990). Granulins, a novel class of peptide from leukocytes. *Biochem Biophys Res Commun*, **173**(3), 1161–1168.
2. Plowman GD, Green JM, Neubauer MG, *et al.* (1992). The epithelin precursor encodes two proteins with opposing activities on epithelial cell growth. *J Biol Chem*, **267**(18), 13073–13078.
3. Xu SQ, Tang D, Chamberlain S, *et al.* (1998). The granulin/epithelin precursor abrogates the requirement for the insulin-like growth factor 1 receptor for growth *in vitro*. *J Biol Chem*, **273**(32), 20078–20083.
4. Daniel R, Daniels E, He Z, Bateman A. (2003). Progranulin (acrogranin/PC cell-derived growth factor/granulin-epithelin precursor) is expressed in the placenta, epidermis, microvasculature, and brain during murine development. *Dev Dyn*, **227**(4), 593–599.
5. Diaz-Cueto L, Stein P, Jacobs A, Schultz RM, Gerton GL. (2000). Modulation of mouse preimplantation embryo development by acrogranin (epithelin/granulin precursor). *Dev Biol*, **17**(2), 406–418.
6. Kessenbrock K, Frohlich L, Sixt M, *et al.* (2008). Proteinase 3 and neutrophil elastase enhance inflammation in mice by inactivating antiinflammatory progranulin. *J Clin Invest*, **118**(7), 2438–2447.
7. Yin F, Banerjee R, Thomas B, *et al.* (2010). Exaggerated inflammation, impaired host defense, and neuropathology in progranulin-deficient mice. *J Exp Med*, **207**, 117–128, S1–4.
8. He Z, Bateman A. (1999). Progranulin gene expression regulates epithelial cell growth and promotes tumor growth *in vivo*. *Cancer Res*, **59**(13), 3222–3229.
9. Zhu J, Nathan C, Jin W, *et al.* (2002). Conversion of proepithelin to epithelins: roles of SLPI and elastase in host defense and wound repair. *Cell*, **111**(6), 867–878.
10. Baker M, Mackenzie IR, Pickering-Brown SM, *et al.* (2006). Mutations in progranulin cause tau-negative frontotemporal dementia linked to chromosome 17. *Nature*, **442**(7105), 916–919.
11. Cruts M, Gijselinck I, van der Zee J, *et al.* (2006). Null mutations in progranulin cause ubiquitin-positive frontotemporal dementia linked to chromosome 17q21. *Nature*, **442**(7105), 920–924.
12. Bhandari V, Palfree RG, Bateman A. (1992). Isolation and sequence of the granulin precursor cDNA from human bone marrow reveals tandem cysteine-rich granulin domains. *Proc Natl Acad Sci USA*, **89**(5), 1715–1719.
13. Plowman GD, Whitney GS, Neubauer MG, *et al.* (1990). Molecular cloning and expression of an additional epidermal growth factor receptor-related gene. *Proc Natl Acad Sci USA*, **87**(13), 4905–4909.
14. Shoyab M, McDonald VL, Byles C, Todaro GJ, Plowman GD. (1990). Epithelins 1 and 2: isolation and characterization of two cysteine-rich growth-modulating proteins. *Proc Natl Acad Sci USA*, **87**(20), 7912–7916.
15. Zhou J, Gao G, Crabb JW, Serrero G. (1993). Purification of an autocrine growth factor homologous with mouse epithelin precursor from a highly tumorigenic cell line. *J Biol Chem*, **268**(15), 10863–10869.
16. Baba T, Hoff HB, 3rd, Nemoto H, *et al.* (1993). Acrogranin, an acrosomal cysteine-rich glycoprotein, is the precursor of the growth-modulating peptides, granulins, and epithelins, and is expressed in somatic as well as male germ cells. *Mol Reprod Dev*, **34**(3), 233–243.

17. Zhang H, Serrero G. (1998). Inhibition of tumorigenicity of the teratoma PC cell line by transfection with antisense cDNA for PC cell-derived growth factor (PCDGF, epithelin/granulin precursor). *Proc Natl Acad Sci USA*, **95**(24), 14202–14207.
18. Lu R, Serrero G. (1999). Stimulation of PC cell-derived growth factor (epithelin/granulin precursor) expression by estradiol in human breast cancer cells. *Biochem Biophys Res Commun*, **256**, 204–207.
19. Lu R, Serrero G. (2000). Inhibition of PC cell-derived growth factor (PCDGF, epithelin/granulin precursor) expression by antisense PCDGF cDNA transfection inhibits tumorigenicity of the human breast carcinoma cell line MDA-MB-468. *Proc Natl Acad Sci USA*, **97**(8), 3993–3998.
20. Liau LM, Lallone RL, Seitz RS, *et al.* (2000). Identification of a human glioma-associated growth factor gene, granulin, using differential immuno-absorption. *Cancer Res*, **60**(5), 1353–1360.
21. Markert JM, Fuller CM, Gillespie GY, *et al.* (2001). Differential gene expression profiling in human brain tumors. *Physiol Genomics*, **5**, 21–33.
22. Wang W, Hayashi J, Kim WE, Serrero G. (2003). PC cell-derived growth factor (granulin precursor) expression and action in human multiple myeloma. *Clin Cancer Res*, **9**(6), 2221–2228.
23. Jones MB, Michener CM, Blanchette JO, *et al.* (2003). The granulin-epithelin precursor/PC-cell-derived growth factor is a growth factor for epithelial ovarian cancer. *Clin Cancer Res*, **9**, 44–51.
24. Ong CH, Bateman A. (2003). Progranulin (granulin-epithelin precursor, PC-cell derived growth factor, acrogranin) in proliferation and tumorigenesis. *Histol Histopathol*, **18**(4), 1275–1288.
25. Bhandari V, Bateman A. (1992). Structure and chromosomal location of the human granulin gene. *Biochem Biophys Res Commun*, **188**, 57–63.
26. Songsrirote K, Li Z, Ashford D, Bateman A, Thomas-Oates J. (2010). Development and application of mass spectrometric methods for the analysis of progranulin N-glycosylation. *J Proteomics*, **73**(8), 1479–1490.
27. Hrabal R, Chen Z, James S, Bennett HP, Ni F. (1996). The hairpin stack fold, a novel protein architecture for a new family of protein growth factors. *Nat Struct Biol*, **3**(9), 747–752.
28. Tolkatchev D, Malik S, Vinogradova A, *et al.* (2008). Structure dissection of human progranulin identifies well-folded granulin/epithelin modules with unique functional activities. *Protein Sci*, **17**(4), 711–724.
29. Butler GS, Dean RA, Tam EM, Overall CM. (2008). Pharmacoproteomics of a metalloproteinase hydroxamate inhibitor in breast cancer cells: dynamics of membrane type 1 matrix metalloproteinase-mediated membrane protein shedding. *Mol Cell Biol*, **28**(15), 4896–4914.
30. Bai XH, Wang DW, Kong L, *et al.* (2009). ADAMTS-7, a direct target of PTHrP, adversely regulates endochondral bone growth by associating with and inactivating GEP growth factor. *Mol Cell Biol*, **29**(15), 4201–4219.
31. Okura H, Yamashita S, Ohama T, *et al.* (2010). HDL/apolipoprotein A-I binds to macrophage-derived progranulin and suppresses its conversion into proinflammatory granulins. *J Atheroscler Thromb*, **17**(6), 568–577.
32. Daniel R, He Z, Carmichael KP, Halper J, Bateman A. (2000). Cellular localization of gene expression for progranulin. *J Histochem Cytochem*, **48**(7), 999–1009.
33. Van Damme P, Van Hoecke A, Lambrechts D, *et al.* (2008). Progranulin functions as a neurotrophic factor to regulate neurite outgrowth and enhance neuronal survival. *J Cell Biol*, **181**, 37–41.
34. Ryan CL, Baranowski DC, Chitramuthu BP, *et al.* (2009). Progranulin is expressed within motor neurons and promotes neuronal cell survival. *BMC Neurosci*, **10**, 130.
35. Carrasquillo MM, Nicholson AM, Finch N, et al. (2010) Genome-wide screen identifies rs646776 near sortilin as a regulator of progranulin levels in human plasma. *Am J Hum Genet*, **87**(6) 890–897.

36. Hu F, Padukkavidana T, Vaegter CB, *et al.* (2010) Sortilin-mediated endocytosis determines levels of the frontotemporal dementia protein, progranulin. *Neuron*, **68**(4) 654–667.
37. Tang W, Lu Y, Tian QY, *et al.* (2011) The growth factor progranulin binds to TNF receptors and is therapeutic against inflammatory arthritis in mice. *Science*, **332**(6028) 478–484.
38. Monami G, Gonzalez EM, Hellman M, *et al.* (2006). Proepithelin promotes migration and invasion of 5637 bladder cancer cells through the activation of ERK1/2 and the formation of a paxillin/FAK/ERK complex. *Cancer Res*, **66**(14), 7103–7110.
39. Zanocco-Marani T, Bateman A, Romano G, Valentinis B, He ZH, Baserga R. (1999). Biological activities and signaling pathways of the granulin/epithelin precursor. *Cancer Res*, **59**(20), 5331–5340.
40. Kamrava M, Simpkins F, Alejandro E, Michener C, Meltzer E, Kohn EC. (2005). Lysophosphatidic acid and endothelin-induced proliferation of ovarian cancer cell lines is mitigated by neutralization of granulin-epithelin precursor (GEP), a prosurvival factor for ovarian cancer. *Oncogene*, **24**(47), 7084–7093.
41. He Z, Ismail A, Kriazhev L, Sadvakassova G, Bateman A. (2002). Progranulin (PC-cellderived growth factor/acrogranin) regulates invasion and cell survival. *Cancer Res*, **62**(19), 5590–5596.
42. Hutton M, Lendon CL, Rizzu P, *et al.* (1998). Association of missense and 5′-splice-site mutations in tau with the inherited dementia FTDP-17. *Nature*, **393**(6686), 702–705.
43. Spillantini MG, Bird TD, Ghetti B. (1998). Frontotemporal dementia and Parkinsonism linked to chromosome 17: a new group of tauopathies. *Brain Pathol*, **8**(2), 387–402.
44. Watts GD, Wymer J, Kovach MJ, *et al.* (2004). Inclusion body myopathy associated with Paget disease of bone and frontotemporal dementia is caused by mutant valosin-containing protein. *Nat Genet*, **36**(4), 377–381.
45. DeJesus-Hernandez M, Mackenzie IR, Bradely B, *et al.* (2011). Expanded GGGGCC hexanucleotide repeat in noncoding region of C9ORF72 causes chromosome 9p-linked FTD and ALS. *Neuron*, **72**(2), 245–256.
46. Renton AE, Majounie E, Waite A, *et al.* (2011). A hexanucleotide repeat expansion in C9ORF72 is the cause of chromosome 9p-21 linked ALS-FTD. *Neuron*, **72**(2), 257–268.
47. Skibinski G, Parkinson NJ, Brown JM, *et al.* (2005). Mutations in the endosomal ESCRTIII-complex subunit CHMP2B in frontotemporal dementia. *Nat Genet*, **37**(8), 806–808.
48. Alzheimer Disease & Frontotemporal Dementia Mutation Database. Available from: http://www.molgen.ua.ac.be/FTDMutations.
49. Gass J, Cannon A, Mackenzie IR, *et al.* (2006). Mutations in progranulin are a major cause of ubiquitin-positive frontotemporal lobar degeneration. *Hum Mol Genet*, **15**(20), 2988–3001.
50. Shankaran SS, Capell A, Hruscha AT, *et al.* (2008). Missense mutations in the progranulin gene linked to frontotemporal lobar degeneration with ubiquitin-immunoreactive inclusions reduce progranulin production and secretion. *J Biol Chem*, **283**(3), 1744–1753.
51. van der Zee J, Le Ber I, Maurer-Stroh S, *et al.* (2007). Mutations other than null mutations producing a pathogenic loss of progranulin in frontotemporal dementia. *Hum Mutat*, **28**(4), 416.
52. Wang J, Van Damme P, Cruchaga C, *et al.* (2010). Pathogenic cysteine mutations affect progranulin function and production of mature granulins. *J Neurochem*, **112**(5), 1305–1315.
53. Rademakers R, Eriksen JL, Baker M, *et al.* (2008). Common variation in the miR-659 binding-site of GRN is a major risk factor for TDP43positive frontotemporal dementia. *Hum Mol Genet*, **17**(23), 3631–3642.
54. Rollinson S, Rohrer JD, van der Zee J, *et al.* (2011). No association of PGRN 3′UTR rs5848 in frontotemporal lobar degeneration. *Neurobiol Aging*, **32**(4), 754–755.
55. Simon-Sanchez J, Seelaar H, Bochdanovits Z, Deeg DJ, van Swieten JC, Heutink P. (2009). Variation at GRN 3′-UTR rs5848 is not associated with a risk of frontotemporal lobar degeneration in Dutch population. *PLoS One*, **4**(10), e7494.

56. Fenoglio C, Galimberti D, Cortini F, *et al.* (2009). Rs5848 variant influences GRN mRNA levels in brain and peripheral mononuclear cells in patients with Alzheimer's disease. *J Alzheimers Dis*, **18**(3), 603–612.
57. Dickson DW, Baker M, Rademakers R. (2010). Common variant in GRN is a genetic risk factor for hippocampal sclerosis in the elderly. *Neurodegener Dis*, **7**(1–3), 170–174.
58. Ghidoni R, Benussi L, Glionna M, Franzoni M, Binetti G. (2008). Low plasma progranulin levels predict progranulin mutations in frontotemporal lobar degeneration. *Neurology*, **71**(16), 1235–1239.
59. Carecchio M, Fenoglio C, De Riz M, *et al.* (2009). Progranulin plasma levels as potential biomarker for the identification of GRN deletion carriers. A case with atypical onset as clinical amnestic Mild Cognitive Impairment converted to Alzheimer's disease. *J Neurol Sci*, **287**(1–2), 291–293.
60. Finch N, Baker M, Crook R, *et al.* (2009). Plasma progranulin levels predict progranulin mutation status in frontotemporal dementia patients and asymptomatic family members. *Brain*, **132**(Pt 3), 583–591.
61. Borroni B, Archetti S, Alberici A, *et al.* (2008). Progranulin genetic variations in frontotemporal lobar degeneration: evidence for low mutation frequency in an Italian clinical series. *Neurogenetics*, **9**(3), 197–205.
62. Bronner IF, Rizzu P, Seelaar H, *et al.* (2007). Progranulin mutations in Dutch familial frontotemporal lobar degeneration. *Eur J Hum Genet*, **15**(3), 369–374.
63. Bruni AC, Momeni P, Bernardi L, *et al.* (2007). Heterogeneity within a large kindred with frontotemporal dementia: a novel progranulin mutation. *Neurology*, **69**(2), 140–147.
64. Le Ber I, van der Zee J, Hannequin D, *et al.* (2007). Progranulin null mutations in both sporadic and familial frontotemporal dementia. *Hum Mutat*, **28**(9), 846–855.
65. Le Ber I, Camuzat A, Hannequin D, *et al.* (2008). Phenotype variability in progranulin mutation carriers: a clinical, neuropsychological, imaging and genetic study. *Brain*, **131**(Pt 3), 732–746.
66. Pickering-Brown SM, Rollinson S, Du Plessis D, *et al.* (2008). Frequency and clinical characteristics of progranulin mutation carriers in the Manchester frontotemporal lobar degeneration cohort: comparison with patients with MAPT and no known mutations. *Brain*, **131**(Pt 3), 721–731.
67. Schymick JC, Yang Y, Andersen PM, *et al.* (2007). Progranulin mutations and amyotrophic lateral sclerosis or amyotrophic lateral sclerosis-frontotemporal dementia phenotypes. *J Neurol Neurosurg Psychiatry*, **78**(7), 754–756.
68. Cruts M, Van Broeckhoven C. (2008). Loss of progranulin function in frontotemporal lobar degeneration. *Trends Genet*, **24**(4), 186–194.
69. Josephs KA, Ahmed Z, Katsuse O, *et al.* (2007). Neuropathologic features of frontotemporal lobar degeneration with ubiquitin-positive inclusions with progranulin gene (PGRN) mutations. *J Neuropathol Exp Neurol*, **66**(2), 142–151.
70. Mackenzie IR, Baker M, Pickering-Brown S, *et al.* (2006). The neuropathology of frontotemporal lobar degeneration caused by mutations in the progranulin gene. *Brain*, **129**(Pt 11), 3081–3090.
71. Mackenzie IR. (2007). The neuropathology and clinical phenotype of FTD with progranulin mutations. *Acta Neuropathol*, **114**, 49–54.
72. Rohrer JD, Warren JD, Barnes J, *et al.* (2008). Mapping the progression of progranulin-associated frontotemporal lobar degeneration. *Nat Clin Pract Neurol*, **4**(8), 455–460.
73. Rohrer JD, Ridgway GR, Modat M, *et al.* (2010). Distinct profiles of brain atrophy in frontotemporal lobar degeneration caused by progranulin and tau mutations. *Neuroimage*, **53**(3), 1070–1076.
74. Moreno F, Indakoetxea B, Barandiaran M, *et al.* (2009). 'Frontotemporoparietal' dementia: clinical phenotype associated with the c. 709lG>A PGRN mutation. *Neurology*, **73**(17), 1367–1374.
75. Tremolizzo L, Gelosa G, Galbussera A, *et al.* (2009). Higher than expected progranulin mutation rate in a case series of Italian FTLD patients. *Alzheimer Dis Assoc Disord*, **23**(3), 301.

76. Schlachetzki JC, Schmidtke K, Beckervordersandforth J, *et al.* (2009). Frequency of progranulin mutations in a German cohort of 79 frontotemporal dementia patients. *J Neurol*, **256**(12), 2043–2051.
77. Beck J, Rohrer JD, Campbell T, *et al.* (2008). A distinct clinical, neuropsychological and radiological phenotype is associated with progranulin gene mutations in a large UK series. *Brain*, **131**(Pt 3), 706–720.
78. Brouwers N, Nuytemans K, van der Zee J, *et al.* (2007). Alzheimer and Parkinson diagnoses in progranulin null mutation carriers in an extended founder family. *Arch Neurol*, **64**(10), 1436–1446.
79. Yu CE, Bird TD, Bekris LM, *et al.* (2010). The spectrum of mutations in progranulin: a collaborative study screening 545 cases of neurodegeneration. *Arch Neurol*, **67**(2), 161–170.
80. Benussi L, Ghidoni R, Pegoiani E, Moretti DV, Zanetti O, Binetti G. (2009). Progranulin Leu271LeufsX10 is one of the most common FTLD and CBS associated mutations worldwide. *Neurobiol Dis*, **33**(3), 379–385.
81. Masellis M, Momeni P, Meschino W, *et al.* (2006). Novel splicing mutation in the progranulin gene causing familial corticobasal syndrome. *Brain*, **129**(Pt 11), 3115–3123.
82. Neumann M, Sampathu DM, Kwong LK, *et al.* (2006). Ubiquitinated TDP-43 in frontotemporal lobar degeneration and amyotrophic lateral sclerosis. *Science*, **314**(5796), 130–133.
83. Zhang YJ, Xu YF, Dickey CA, *et al.* (2007). Progranulin mediates caspase-dependent cleavage of TAR DNA binding protein-43. *J Neurosci*, **27**(39), 10530–10534.
84. Sampathu DM, Neumann M, Kwong LK, *et al.* (2006). Pathological heterogeneity of frontotemporal lobar degeneration with ubiquitin-positive inclusions delineated by ubiquitin immunohistochemistry and novel monoclonal antibodies. *Am J Pathol*, **169**(4), 1343–1352.
85. Dormann D, Capell A, Carlson AM, *et al.* (2009). Proteolytic processing of TAR DNA binding protein-43 by caspases produces C-terminal fragments with disease defining properties independent of progranulin. *J Neurochem*, **110**(3), 1082–1094.
86. Irwin D, Lippa CF, Rosso A. (2009). Progranulin (PGRN) expression in ALS: an immunohistochemical study. *J Neurol Sci*, **276**(1–2), 9–13.
87. Pereson S, Wils H, Kleinberger G, *et al.* (2009). Progranulin expression correlates with dense-core amyloid plaque burden in Alzheimer disease mouse models. *J Pathol*, **219**(2), 173–181.
88. Naphade SB, Kigerl KA, Jakeman LB, Kostyk SK, Popovich PG, Kuret J. (2010). Progranulin expression is upregulated after spinal contusion in mice. *Acta Neuropathol*, **119**, 123–133.
89. Kelley BJ, Haidar W, Boeve BF, *et al.* (2010). Alzheimer disease-like phenotype associated with the c. 154delA mutation in progranulin. *Arch Neurol*, **67**(2), 171–177.
90. Brouwers N, Sleegers K, Engelborghs S, *et al.* (2008). Genetic variability in progranulin contributes to risk for clinically diagnosed Alzheimer disease. *Neurology*, **71**(9), 656–664.
91. Guerreiro RJ, Washecka N, Hardy J, Singleton A. (2010). A thorough assessment of benign genetic variability in GRN and MAPT. *Hum Mutat*, **31**(2), E1126–E1140.
92. Kayasuga Y, Chiba S, Suzuki M, *et al.* (2007). Alteration of behavioural phenotype in mice by targeted disruption of the progranulin gene. *Behav Brain Res*, **185**(2), 110–118.
93. Ghoshal N, Dearborn JT, Wozniak DF, *et al.* (2011) Core features of frontotemporal dementia recapitulated in progranulin knockout mice. *Neurobio Dis* doi:10.1016/j.nbd.2011.08.029
94. Ahmed Z, Sheng H, Xu YF, *et al.* (2010). Accelerated lipofuscinosis and ubiquitination in granulin knockout mice suggest a role for progranulin in successful aging. *Am J Pathol*, **177**, 311–324.

Index